THE DIETITIAN'S GUIDE TO VEGETARIAN DIETS

Issues and Applications

Mark Messina, PhD

Virginia Messina, MPH, RD
Nutrition Matters, Inc.
Port Townsend, Washington

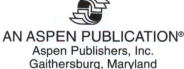

AN ASPEN PUBLICATION®
Aspen Publishers, Inc.
Gaithersburg, Maryland
1996

Library of Congress Cataloging-in-Publication Data

Messina, Mark.
The dietitian's guide to vegetarian diets : issues and
applications / Mark Messina, Virginia Messina.
p. cm.
Includes bibliographical references and index.
ISBN 0-8342-0635-8
1. Vegetarianism. 2. Diet. I. Messina, Virginia. II. Title.
[DNLM: 1. Vegetarianism. WB 430 M585d 1996]
RM236.M444 1996
613.2'62—dc20
DNLM/DLC
for Library of Congress
96-329
CIP

Aspen Publishers, Inc., is not affiliated with the
American Society of Parenteral and Enteral Nutrition

The authors have made every effort to ensure the accuracy of the information herein.
However, appropriate information sources should be consulted, especially for new or
unfamiliar drugs or procedures. It is the responsibility of every practitioner to evaluate
the appropriateness of a particular opinion in the context of actual clinical situations and
with due consideration to new developments. Authors, editors, and the publisher cannot
be held responsible for any typographical or other errors found in this book.

Editorial Resources: Ruth Bloom

Library of Congress Catalog Card Number: 96-329
ISBN: 0-8342-0635-8

Printed in the United States of America

1 2 3 4 5

Table of Contents

Preface

The Dietitian's Guide to Vegetarian Diets: Issues and Applications is designed to be used primarily by dietitians and other health care professionals as an aid in counseling vegetarian clients. It can also serve as a textbook for classroom study and as a resource for investigators who may benefit by having access to a comprehensive review of the vegetarian literature.

The book is divided into five parts. Part I provides an overview of the vegetarian population and the health status of this group. Chapter 1 discusses the demographics of vegetarians in the United States and describes the different types of vegetarian diets. The second chapter provides an overview of research on the health status of vegetarians, with particular attention to cancer, heart disease, diabetes, obesity, and hypertension.

Part II examines nutrient needs within the context of a vegetarian diet. Chapter 3 addresses issues specifically related to plant proteins and to meeting protein requirements on plant-based diets. Chapter 4 highlights the calcium intake of vegetarians and discusses calcium bioavailability from plant-based diets and dietary factors that are most likely to affect the calcium requirements of vegetarians. Chapters 5 and 6 include discussions of all essential vitamins and minerals with attention given to the bioavailability of these nutrients from plant foods, vegetarian intake, and the vitamin and mineral status of vegetarians. Special attention is paid to vitamin B_{12}, iron, and zinc. Chapter 7 describes food guides to meet nutrient needs of different groups of vegetarians.

Parts III and IV address the nutrient needs of specific groups of vegetarians. Chapters 8 through 12 discuss the adequacy of vegetarian diets and present meal planning guidelines for pregnant women, infants, children, adolescents and older people. Chapters 13 through 15 discuss research issues and practical applications to aid professionals working with vegetarian clients with cardiovascular disease, diabetes, or weight control problems and clients who are athletes. The last chapter in this section addresses practical issues of vegetarian food preparation.

The final part of the book includes a glossary of foods commonly consumed by vegetarians and eighteen appendixes that present in tabular form data on vegetarian and nonvegetarian micronutrient and macronutrient intakes, serum lipid levels, blood pressure, and anthropometry.

The continued growth of the vegetarian population means that most dietitians will be working with vegetarian clients. Questions related to vegetarianism are among those most frequently asked via The American Dietetic Association's nutrition hotline. It is our hope that by reviewing the current research on vegetarian diets and by translating this information into practical ideas for helping vegetarians to plan nutritious meals, we are able to help dietitians and other health care providers to better serve the needs of this important population group.

Acknowledgments

We are greatly indebted to a number of people who generously offered their time and effort in reviewing chapters and sections of this book. Thank you to Enette Larsen, MS, RD, University of Alabama; Dr. Peter Pellet, University of Massachusetts; Dr. Robert Heaney, Creighton University; Dr. Marilyn Abernathy, Framingham State University; and Dr. Milton Crane, Weimar Institute for reviewing chapters and providing us with valuable feedback and suggestions. We are especially indebted to Dr. Winston Craig, RD, Andrews University, who took time out of a busy schedule to review several chapters and who made himself available to discuss many questions and issues during manuscript preparation. And a special thank you to Dr. Reed Mangels, RD, whose expertise on vegetarian diets throughout the life cycle was invaluable and who provided much appreciated feedback on the section addressing vegetarian diets in pregnancy, infancy, and children.

A number of dietitians have been instrumental in educating consumers and health professionals on vegetarian nutrition issues. Their efforts have had a great impact on our own work and on this book. We offer warm thanks to Suzanne Havala, MS, RD, Mary Clifford, RD, and Cyndi Reeser, MPH, RD for all of their important work in this field.

Our editor at Aspen Publishers, Ruth Bloom, has earned our heartfelt thanks and admiration many times over for her hard work and her support throughout this project.

As always, we are thankful for the love, support, and encouragement of our families.

PART I

An Overview of Vegetarian Diet

CHAPTER 1

Demographics and Definitions

HISTORY OF VEGETARIANISM

The term *vegetarian* was not coined until the mid-1800s. The concept dates back to at least the sixth century BC, however, when the Greek philosopher Pythagoras, considered the father of vegetarianism, encouraged meatless eating among his followers as the diet that was most natural and healthful.[1] Other early philosophers, including Socrates, Plato, Horace, Ovid, and Virgil, all favored the idea of meatless diets.

It was many centuries before the Western world showed an interest in vegetarianism. The 19th century saw the birth of a true vegetarian movement that was largely Church related. In the year 1800, the Reverend William Cowherd, a minister of the Church of England, established the Bible Christians, a sect with Bible literalism at its foundation that embraced a vegetarian diet as the one prescribed by God in the book of Genesis.[2] Later Bible Christians traveled to Philadelphia and established a church there. Among the converts to the dietary philosophy of this group was Sylvester Graham, who toured the United States lecturing on the evils of meat, refined white bread, alcohol, coffee, extramarital sex, and tight pants. Although Graham was an advocate of meatless eating, his most important legacy was in encouraging the use of whole wheat flour, which came to be called graham flour. In the mid-1840s, Bible Christians in England established the Vegetarian Society of Great Britain, and the American church quickly followed suit by initiating the formation of the American Vegetarian Society.[2]

Another church group that had an extensive impact on the rise in vegetarianism in this country was the Seventh-day Adventist Church, founded by Ellen White in the 1840s. Mrs. White produced copious teachings on the relationship of physical health to religious life and encouraged church members to eat a vegetarian diet.[3] Today, approximately 50% of Seventh-day Adventists are vegetarians, and the church is active in health education, producing materials on nutrition and teaching classes on vegetarianism.

One church member was especially instrumental in establishing the popularity of vegetarianism in the late 19th and early 20th centuries. John Harvey Kellogg headed the Seventh-day Adventist-run Battle Creek Sanitarium in Battle Creek, Michigan, and was a protégé of Ellen White. Among Kellogg's greatest achievements were production of some of the first breakfast cereals—corn flakes and granola—to provide his patients with healthy breakfast options. He also invented nuttose, the first meat analog made from peanuts and flour, produced the first peanut butter, and was an early enthusiast of soymilk.[4]

Kellogg's sanitarium regimen, which he called biologic living and included a vegetarian diet, total abstinence from alcohol, caffeine, sugar, and strong spices, and emphasized exercise, hydrotherapy, fresh air, sunshine, good posture, simple dress, and good mental health, was popular with some of the most powerful personalities of the day. His sanitarium was visited by William Howard Taft, William Jennings Bryan, John D. Rockefeller, Alfred Dupont, J. C. Penney, Montgomery Ward, Thomas Edison, Henry Ford, George Bernard Shaw, and Admiral Richard Byrd.

As a result of the efforts of the diet reformers, interest in vegetarian diet was at a peak from the mid-19th century through the early part of the 20th century. Vegetarian sanitariums and eateries opened throughout the country. A popular vegetarian restaurant in New York City at the turn of the century was the Physical Culture and Strength Food Restaurant. Vegetarian organizations existed in Kansas City, St. Louis, Minneapolis, Boston, Pittsburgh, Chicago, Washington, DC, and many European countries.[5]

By the middle of the 20th century, however, with the discovery of vitamins and the production of government-sponsored food guides, meat-based diets were touted as the healthiest ways to eat. All food guides developed at the time encouraged generous consumption of both meat and dairy products. Nevertheless, the results of a 1943 Gallup poll showed that between 2.5 and 3.0 million Americans were vegetarians, representing 2% of the total population.[6] In 1944, the term *vegan* was coined for vegetarians who consumed no dairy or egg products, and the Vegan Society was formed in Great Britain in that year.[7]

Vegetarianism enjoyed a resurgence in popularity again in the 1960s and 1970s as a natural choice of the new health-conscious members of the counterculture. An important influence was macrobiotic teacher Michio Kushi. Even though vegetarianism was popular with young people, it had little mainstream appeal at that time.

Surprisingly, two influences that had little to do with health concerns served to popularize vegetarian diet among more diverse groups and led the way for a more mainstream view of meatless eating. The publication of Frances Moore Lappé's *Diet for a Small Planet* linked diet to global concerns and focused attention on the adverse effects of meat production on the planet.[8] Her book became an important influence on the way people viewed food choices. Second, the birth of the modern animal rights movement, heralded by the publication in 1975 of *Animal Liberation* by Peter Singer and the formation of the animal rights group People for the Ethical Treatment of Animals, focused new attention on the treatment of animals by the factory farming industry. Today, although most vegetarians identify health concerns as their primary reason for choosing a meatless diet, the environmental and ethical impacts of meat eating are probably largely responsible for the attention that has been directed toward vegetarian diets.

Over the past two decades, interest in vegetarian diets has remained strong. The number of vegetarians in the United States doubled between 1985 and 1992, when a Gallup poll revealed that 12 million American adults called themselves vegetarian.[9] It is likely that interest in vegetarian diet will continue, especially because diet-related problems such as heart disease and cancer continue to be pressing concerns today and because their link to diet is firmly established.

PROFILE OF VEGETARIANS

Early views among health professionals of the vegetarian population were usually unfavorable. In the early 1970s, those who reported on vegetarians often linked meatless diets with drug use (an observation that may have been accurate in some cases), and vegetarian communities were described as cults.[10–13] Food habits of vegetarians were not viewed positively. For example, the eating habits of young American vegetarians, which included avoidance of processed foods and extensive use of natural foods, were pronounced as bizarre in one 1971 article.[10] As recently as 1979, a study of simulated counseling sessions revealed that many dietitians encouraged meat consumption among their vegetarian clients.[14]

Today, the vegetarian population and its impact are decidedly different. Vegetarianism has become much more mainstream, and its proponents are somewhat older. Survey results indicate that the vegetarian population is slightly skewed toward the over-40 age group.[9] In addition, the three main reasons for choosing a vegetarian diet—improved health of vegetarians, environmental impact of diet, and inhumane practices of factory farming—are attracting increasing numbers of people from varied backgrounds to vegetarianism.

Dietitians who work with vegetarian clients should expect that this population will be somewhat diverse in outlook and background (Table 1–1). Some trends within the vegetarian population have been revealed in surveys, however. One study at the University of Texas showed that vegetarians are more knowledgeable about nutrition than meat eaters.[15] Another found that vegetarian subjects had read on average nearly six nutrition books compared with less than two nutrition books for nonvegetarians.[16] Not surprising, vegetarians also have a stronger internal locus of control regarding health issues. Vegetarians are more likely than meat eaters to disagree with the statement "Health is almost all a matter of luck." They are more likely to agree with the statement "How healthy you are mostly depends on how you look after yourself." Today's vegetarian is likely to have made a long-term commitment to this way of eating. A 1992 Gallup poll

Table 1–1 The U.S. Vegetarian Population

Characteristic	Vegetarians (%)	General Population (%)
Gender		
Female	68	52
Male	32	48
Education		
College graduate	30	25
High school graduate	45	56
No high school degree	21	18
Marital status		
Married	48	59
Single	24	22
Widowed	14	8
Divorced/separated	11	11
Have children under 18 years		
Yes	37	24
No	60	75
Income		
Under $35,000/year	56	55
Over $35,000/year	44	45
Occupation		
White collar	37	35
Not white collar	60	62
Age		
Under 40 years	42	49
Over 40 years	55	50

Source: Data from "The American Vegetarian: Coming of Age in the 90s—A Study of the Vegetarian Marketplace Conducted for *Vegetarian Times*" by Yankelovich, Skelly and White/Clancy, Shulman, Inc., 1992.

revealed that nearly half of all vegetarians had been eating this way for more than 10 years and that nearly one quarter had been vegetarian for more than 20 years.[9]

Vegetarian food preferences are of interest to anyone who works in a food- or medical-related capacity. Increasing interest in vegetarian foods is having a significant impact on food choices in the marketplace. A 1991 Gallup poll revealed that 20% of consumers who dine out were willing to eat only at restaurants that offer meatless options on the menu.[17] In the past decade, over 2,000 new soy-based meat and dairy alternatives have entered the market.[18] Although natural foods stores are found in many communities, most vegetarians shop at regular grocery stores.[9] Most school systems, particularly in urban areas, are likely to have vegetarian students in their cafeteria, and vegetarianism is growing in popularity on college campuses. According to the National Association of College and University Food Services, 15% of college students select a vegetarian meal in their dining hall daily.[19] Caterers, airlines, school food services, and hospitals need to be prepared to serve the vegetarian client.

TYPES OF VEGETARIAN DIETS

In working with vegetarian clients, it is of utmost importance to understand what a vegetarian diet is and to realize that several different styles of eating fall under this umbrella. At its broadest, a vegetarian diet is one that includes no meat, poultry, or fish. Beyond that, however, there are many variations on the vegetarian theme (Exhibits 1–1 and 1–2).

Lacto-Ovo Vegetarian Diets

Most vegetarians fall into this category. A lacto-ovo vegetarian diet includes dairy products and eggs but no animal flesh. Meat, poultry, and fish are avoided. A smaller subset of this group avoids eggs and are more accurately termed lacto-vegetarians. Likewise, some vegetarians may eat an ovo-vegetarian diet if they avoid dairy products but consume eggs.

When a lacto-ovo vegetarian eats a variety of whole foods, there is little concern about nutrient deficiencies. In the past, iron was often emphasized as a nutrient of concern in vegetarian plans. Vegetarian diets actually tend to be quite high in iron, however, and iron deficiency anemia does not appear to be any more common among vegetarians than among meat eaters.[20]

One cause for concern in lacto-ovo vegetarian diets can be overreliance on cheese, milk, and eggs. Particularly new vegetarians, those who are making the transition to this new pattern of eating and therefore may have lim-

Exhibit 1–1 Types of Vegetarian Diets

Types of Vegetarians	Foods Consumed	Foods Avoided	Comments
Lacto-ovo	Grains, legumes, vegetables, nuts, seeds, dairy, eggs	Meat, poultry, fish	Diet can be high in total fat if full-fat dairy products and eggs are used
Vegan	Grains, legumes, vegetables, fruits, nuts, seeds	Meat, poultry, fish, dairy, eggs; foods with small amounts of added animal products, such as casein or whey, are also generally avoided, as are foods that involve animal processing, such as white sugar, beer, and vinegar	Requires B_{12}-fortified foods or supplements; may also require vitamin D-fortified foods if sun exposure is inadequate
Macrobiotic	Grains, legumes, vegetables (nuts, seeds, fruits to a lesser extent); makes wide use of sea vegetables, soy products, and Asian condiments; seafood may be consumed	Meat, poultry, sometimes fish, dairy products, eggs, vegetables of nightshade family, tropical fruits, processed sweeteners	Guidelines for this diet may need to be adjusted to make it suitable for children Requires B_{12}-fortified foods or supplements; may also require vitamin D-fortified foods if sun exposure is inadequate
Fruitarian	Fruits, vegetables that are botanically fruits (tomatoes, eggplant, avocado, zucchini), nuts, seeds	Meat, fish, poultry, dairy foods, eggs, grains, legumes, most vegetables	Some modified versions of this pattern may allow grains and/or legumes; difficult to plan nutritionally adequate diets on strict fruitarian plans; not suitable for children

Exhibit 1–1 Continued

Types of Vegetarians	Foods Consumed	Foods Avoided	Comments
Raw foods	Vegetables, fruits, nuts, seeds, sprouted grains, sprouted beans, all consumed in the raw state; some adherents may use raw dairy products	Meat, fish, poultry, any cooked plant foods	Percentage of raw foods in the diet may actually vary among adherents from as little as 50% to 100%; completely raw foods diet not appropriate for children
Natural hygiene	Emphasis on raw vegetables and fruits; includes whole grains, legumes, nuts, sprouted grains, seeds, legumes	Varies; some regimens prohibit meat consumption, dairy, eggs	Emphasis on eating or avoiding certain combinations of foods

Exhibit 1–2 Sample Meal Plans for Different Types of Vegetarian Diets

Type of Diet	Breakfast	Lunch	Dinner	Snacks
Lacto-ovo	Cheerios with low-fat milk Whole wheat toast with fruit spread Sliced bananas Coffee	Veggie burger on hamburger roll with lettuce, tomato, ketchup Carrot sticks Apple juice Oatmeal cookies	Vegetable fajitas with zucchini, carrots, peppers, onions in soft corn tortillas Refried beans Tossed salad Fresh fruit cocktail	Nonfat yogurt mixed with fresh fruit Popcorn
Vegan	Scrambled tofu Rye bread toast with fruit spread Fresh fruit salad	Vegetable soup Whole wheat rolls Tossed salad with low-fat dressing Cantaloupe chunks	Pasta primavera with broccoli, carrots, pea pods Steamed kale French bread	Soymilk and fruit shake Rice cakes with almond butter

continues

Exhibit 1–2 Continued

Type of Diet	Breakfast	Lunch	Dinner	Snacks
Macrobiotic	Miso soup with tofu, daikon, carrots Oatmeal	Udon noodles seasoned with miso Steamed Brussels sprouts Peas and mushrooms	Miso soup with kombu and shiitake mushrooms Brown rice seasoned with umeboshi plum Steamed kale Baked winter squash	
Fruitarian*	Granola with raisins, almonds Sliced bananas Fresh pineapple and orange juice	Steamed eggplant and zucchini in tomato sauce Fruit salad with bananas, chopped figs, apples, chopped Brazil nuts Almond milk	Zucchini stuffed with sprouted wheat berries, raisins, walnuts with tahini dressing Apple slices spread with almond butter Sliced fresh papaya Fresh figs	
Raw foods	Granola with homemade almond milk Fresh fruit salad	Gazpacho soup Salad of fresh greens Almond-fig-oat bars (ground oats soaked in fruit juice, mixed with pureed figs and ground almonds, pressed into bars)	Salad of raw vegetables, sprouted lentils, and sprouted wheat berries, oil and lemon juice dressing, fresh herbs Freshly squeezed carrot juice Apple slices and celery spread with tahini	

*Modified, with limited amounts of grain.

ited skills in planning meals or may have concerns about protein intake, may base many meals on these animal products. Dairy products, particularly whole milk products and cheese, and eggs can contribute excessive saturated fat and cholesterol to meals and can displace the healthier fiber-rich plant foods in vegetarian menus. Counseling clients about the ease with which protein needs are met on vegetarian diets, helping them explore the use of nonfat dairy foods in their diet, and providing information about alternative sources of calcium can be ways to help them limit the use of fattier dairy foods and eggs.

Despite this concern, the health profile of lacto-ovo vegetarians is good. Nearly 98% of Seventh-day Adventist vegetarians, the most widely studied group of vegetarians in the United States, consume a lacto-ovo vegetarian diet. This population exhibits low rates of cancer, heart disease, obesity, diabetes, and hypertension compared with the general population.[21-25]

Vegan Diets

A much smaller number of vegetarians follow a vegan diet. Vegan diets are growing in popularity, however. Many ethical vegetarians in particular choose this pattern of eating, which avoids all animal products. Some vegans adopt this way of eating for health reasons as well. There is evidence that vegans have a lower risk of disease than lacto-ovo vegetarians.[26]

Vegans avoid meat, fish, poultry, dairy, and eggs. There are many other foods that may not be acceptable to many vegans, however. Foods that involve animal processing to any degree are often avoided. These may include honey, sugar, vinegar, wine, and beer. Vegan diets are likely to be lower in fat and higher in fiber than both nonvegetarian and lacto-ovo vegetarian diets.

Vegans will also differ in the degree to which they are willing to relax the confines of their diet. Some are likely to be careful label readers and will avoid foods with small amounts of added whey or casein or additives of nonspecific origin, such as monoglycerides or "natural flavorings." Many foods that are marketed directly to vegetarians are not acceptable to vegans. Veggie burgers may use egg whites as a binder, for example. Many soy cheeses contain the milk protein casein.

Although a strict vegan diet may appear complex, most vegans quickly identify the foods that are acceptable to them, make a usual habit of reading labels, and are able to plan healthy, satisfying meals within these guidelines. A dietitian who is counseling a vegan client needs to listen carefully to the client's own description of which foods are acceptable. Vegan meal plans make frequent use of ethnic cuisine, and many vegans are willing and eager to explore new foods and eating styles. As a result, an eating pattern that seems confining to some may actually be viewed as one with particularly expansive menu choices and culinary opportunities.

The nutrient of concern in vegan diets is vitamin B_{12}, which, for all practical purposes, is found only in foods of animal origin. Vitamin B_{12} deficiency is actually rare among vegans, for reasons discussed in Chapter 6.[27] A cautious approach to vitamin B_{12} nutrition is safest, however. All vegans need to identify a source of vitamin B12 in their diet. For vegans who do not use fortified foods, a supplement is the best choice, and dietitians should be able to identify locally available brands of B12 that are not derived from animal foods.

Vegan diets are often low in vitamin D. This is not a problem if vegans have adequate sun exposure, but this can be an unreliable means of maintaining normal vitamin D levels. Vegans can also obtain this vitamin from fortified foods. Many breakfast cereals are fortified, as are many brands of soymilk.

Because milk products are the most common source of calcium in the American diet, concern about the calcium content of vegan diets has been raised. Vegans typically consume less calcium than lacto-ovo vegetarians or omnivores, but there is evidence that they may need less of this nutrient (see Chapter 4). Vegans can meet the recommended dietary allowance for calcium, however, especially when fortified products such as calcium-fortified soymilks or orange juice are used.

Finally, zinc intake of vegans may be low, and zinc bioavailability is poorer in plant foods than in animal foods. Vegans need to give some attention to using zinc-rich foods in their menu planning.

Macrobiotic Diets

The general view of macrobiotics among health professionals has been a negative one. This stems from two concerns. First, it has been commonly believed that pure macrobiotics is a diet of rice only. The founder of macrobiotics, George Ohsawa, claims to have cured himself of disease by following such a diet. No modern macrobiotic teacher espouses an all-rice regimen, however; macrobiotic diets are actually quite varied. Second, observations of macrobiotic communities in the 1970s revealed serious nutrition deficiencies in infants and young children.[28,29] These were directly attributed to macrobiotic feeding practices that were not nutritionally adequate for children. Some of these practices are discussed in Chapters 9 and 10. For adults, however, a macrobiotic diet can be a safe and healthy approach to eating. With some modifications, described in Chapters 9 and 10, macrobiotics can also be an acceptable choice for children.

The macrobiotic philosophy is loosely linked to Buddhism and more strongly linked to the ancient Chinese principles of *yin* and *yang*. The foods that are central to macrobiotic cuisine reflect Asian influences. The diet makes extensive use of rice; sea vegetables; Asian condiments such as tamari, miso, and umeboshi plum; and root vegetables such as daikon and lotus root.

The macrobiotic life style focuses on principles of balance and harmony with nature and the universe. Foods consumed should be in season and locally produced if possible, so that climate and geography dictate the make-up of a macrobiotic diet to a large extent. People living in most of North America, Europe, Asia, parts of Latin America, and parts of Australia, however, all considered temperate zones, eat roughly the same diet.

Macrobiotic meals are based largely on grains, which make up between 50% and 60% of the diet. Vegetables, especially sea vegetables, play a central role in meals, and soups (especially miso soup) and beans are served in smaller amounts. Fruits, nuts, seeds, and breads are used in moderation and are not consumed every day. Foods that are avoided on a macrobiotic diet are vegetables of the nightshade family (potatoes, tomatoes, eggplant, and peppers), tropical fruits, and processed sweeteners. Some macrobiotics use limited amounts of fish.

Many people choose a macrobiotic diet because they believe that it is the healthiest way of eating. It has also been widely promoted as a diet with curative powers, particularly for diseases such as cancer. Although there is limited scientific support for this belief, there have been some observations that macrobiotic cancer patients live longer.[30,31]

Other Vegetarian Patterns

Although most vegetarians are likely to fall into the three categories described above, there are other vegetarian diets that bear mentioning because dietitians may occasionally encounter these eating patterns in their practices.

Fruitarian

As the name implies, fruitarian diets are based on fruits. The diet also includes nuts and seeds and will often make use of vegetables that are botanically fruits, such as squash, tomatoes, eggplant, peppers, and avocado. Planning fruitarian diets that meet nutrient needs is a challenge to the dietitian. Although fruits are high in many vitamins and minerals, they are devoid of protein and are generally low in some important nutrients, such as calcium. Followers of this diet can meet needs for both protein and calcium from the nuts and seeds used in meals, but the quantities that must be consumed would produce an excessively high fat intake. Those who follow a modified version of this pattern, which might include small amounts of grains, can meet nutrient needs more easily. This diet is generally not recommended and is never recommended for children.

Raw Foods Diet

Adherents to a raw foods diet believe that it most closely resembles the natural eating pattern of humans and that this diet preserves the integrity of food constituents, such as enzymes. Followers of this diet consume vegetables, fruits, nuts, seeds, and sprouted grains and beans, all in their raw state. The diet actually varies among adherents, who may consume anywhere from 50% to 100% of their foods as raw foods.

There is clearly some merit to consuming some raw foods in meals. Cooking can destroy significant amounts of nutrients in foods. Cooking also improves the digestibility of most foods, however, and destroys antinutritional factors. The premise for consuming a raw foods diet is not very well supported, but the diet can be safe if sprouted grains and beans are used. Diets that are 100% raw will take considerable planning to meet nutrient needs. Again, this diet is not recommended for children.

Natural Hygiene

A natural hygiene diet is a variation of a raw foods diet. It is based on vegetables, fruits, nuts, and sprouts (sprouted beans, grains, and seeds), eaten in their raw form for the most part. As natural hygiene has become more popular over the past several years, variations of this eating pattern have come into use. Many use cooked foods, and some use meat.

At the heart of this dietary philosophy are strict rules regarding food combining. Certain combinations of foods, such as starches and protein-rich foods, are avoided because it is believed that they cannot be efficiently digested at the same time. Fruits are nearly always consumed alone. The basic premises of natural hygiene, regarding the cleansing effects of certain foods and the importance of food combining, are largely unfounded. There are no particular health advantages of natural hygiene over other vegetarian meal patterns.

It is difficult to assess the nutritional adequacy of natural hygiene food plans because the diet varies so much among adherents. Where cooked grains and beans are used, a natural hygiene diet can be nutritionally adequate. The emphasis on raw foods would make the diet difficult to plan for children.

Semivegetarian or Nearly Vegetarian Diet

As interest in healthy vegetarian diets and optimal eating patterns grows, many people are limiting meat in their diet and calling themselves semivegetarians. The term *semivegetarian* can actually cover a wide range of eating practices. It includes individuals who may eat a variety of meat products but use them as condiments or consume them just a few times a week. It may include those who eat only certain animal products, such as fish or chicken, but eat them frequently. In counseling, it is important to ascertain the true extent of meat, fish, and poultry consumption because the nutrient composition of these diets can vary considerably from true vegetarian plans.

REFERENCES

1. Roe DA. History of promotion of vegetable cereal diets. *J Nutr.* 1986;116:1355–1363.

2. Spencer C. *The Heretics Feast.* London, England: Fourth Estate; 1993.

3. White EG. *Counsels on Diet and Foods: A Compilation from the Writings of Ellen G. White.* Hagerstown, Md: Review and Herald; 1938.

4. Shurtleff W, Aoyagi A. *History of Soybeans and Soyfoods.* Lafayette, Calif: Soyfoods Center (unpublished).

5. Unti B. *The Bible Christians and the Origins of Vegetarianism in North America.* Unpublished manuscript.

6. Hardinge MG, Crooks H. Non-flesh dietaries. *J Am Diet Assoc.* 1963;43:545–549.

7. Long A. The well nourished vegetarian. *New Sci.* 1981;89:330–333.

8. Lappe FM. *Diet for a Small Planet.* New York, NY: Ballantine; 1971.

9. *The American Vegetarian: Coming of Age in the 90s. A Study of the Vegetarian Marketplace Conducted for* Vegetarian Times *by Yankelovich, Skelly, and White/Clancy, Shulman, Inc.* 1992.

10. Dwyer JT, Mayer J. Vegetarianism in drug users. *Lancet.* 1971;2:1429–1430.

11. Dwyer JT, Mayer LDVH, Dowd K, Kandel RJ, Mayer J. The new vegetarians: The natural high? *J Am Diet Assoc.* 1971;65:529–535.

12. Dwyer JT, Mayer LDVH, Dowd K, Kandel RF, Mayer J. The new vegetarians. *J Am Diet Assoc.* 1973;62:503–509.

13. Erhard D. The new vegetarians. Part two: Zen macrobiotic movement and other cults based on vegetarianism. *Nutr Today.* 1974;9:20–27.

14. Strobe CM, Groll L. Professional knowledge and attitudes on vegetarianism: Implications for practice. *J Am Diet Assoc.* 1979;79:568–574.

15. Freeland-Graves JH, Greninger SA, Vickers J, Bradley CL, Young RK. Nutrition knowledge of vegetarians and nonvegetarians. *J Nutr Educ.* 1982;14:21–26.

16. Sims LS. Food-related value-orientations, attitudes, and beliefs of vegetarians and non-vegetarians. *Ecol Food Nutr.* 1978;7:23–25.

17. Interest in eating vegetarian foods at restaurants, June 1991. A Gallup Survey conducted for the National Restaurant Association. Washington, DC: National Restaurant Association; 1991.

18. Messina M, Messina V. Increasing use of soyfoods and their potential role in cancer prevention. *J Am Diet Assoc.* 1991;91:836–840.

19. Growing interest in vegetarianism among campus food services. *J Am Diet Assoc.* 1994;94:596.

20. Craig WJ. Iron status of vegetarians. *Am J Clin Nutr.* 1994;59(suppl):1233S–1237S.

21. Phillips RL. Role of life-style and dietary habits in risk of cancer among Seventh-Day Adventists. *Cancer Res.* 1975;35:3513–3522.

22. Phillips RL, Lemon FR, Beeson WL, Kuzma JW. Coronary heart disease mortality among Seventh-Day Adventists with differing dietary habits: A preliminary report. *Am J Clin Nutr.* 1978;31:S191–S198.

23. Phillips RL, Garfinkel L, Kuzma JW, Beeson WL, Lotz T, Brin B. Mortality among California Seventh-Day Adventists for selected cancer sites. *J Natl Cancer Inst.* 1980;65:1097–1107.

24. Mills PK, Beeson WL, Abbey DE, Fraser GE, Phillips RL. Dietary habits and past medical history as related to fatal pancreas cancer risk among Adventists. *Cancer.* 1988;61:2578–2585.

25. Snowdon DA. Animal product consumption and mortality because of all causes combined, coronary heart disease, stroke, diabetes, and cancer in Seventh-Day Adventists. *Am J Clin Nutr.* 1988;48:739–748.

26. Burr ML, Butland BK. Heart disease in British vegetarians. *Am J Clin Nutr.* 1988;48:830–832.

27. Ellis FR, Montegriffo VME. Veganism, clinical findings and investigations. *Eur J Clin Nutr.* 1979;23:249–255.

28. Dwyer JT, Palombo R, Thorne H, Valadian I, Reed RB. Preschoolers on alternate life-style diets. *J Am Diet Assoc.* 1978;72:264–270.

29. Dagnelie PC, van Staveren WA, Vergote FJVRA, et al. Nutritional status of infants aged 4 to 18 months on macrobiotic diets and matched omnivorous control infants: A population-based mixed longitudinal study. II. Growth and psychomotor development. *Eur J Clin Nutr.* 1989;43:325–338.

30. Carter JP, Saxe GP, Newbold V, Peres CE, Campeau RJ, Bernal-Green L. Hypothesis: Dietary management may improve survival from nutritionally linked cancers based on analysis of representative cases. *J Am Coll Nutr.* 1993;12:209–226.

31. Weisburger JH. Guest editorial: A new nutritional approach in cancer therapy in light of mechanistic understanding of cancer causation and development. *J Am Coll Nutr.* 1993;12:205–208.

CHAPTER 2

Health Consequences of Vegetarian Diets

Populations consuming vegetarian and semivegetarian diets have lower rates of the chronic diseases that typically plague Western countries, including some cancers, heart disease, and diabetes. Observations of vegetarians living in Western countries and of populations consuming plant-based diets in developing countries support this conclusion. Migration studies also support the overall health benefits of plant-based diets. The incidence of heart disease and many cancers increases when people from countries where plant-based diets are consumed relocate to countries with predominantly animal product–based diets. Similarly, when people in developing countries become more affluent and begin to add more animal products to their diet, rates of chronic disease increase.[1]

Many life style factors affect chronic disease risk; not surprising, determining the extent to which any given individual factor contributes to the better health of vegetarians is difficult. Nevertheless, the data strongly suggest that diet plays a major role. Identifying precisely which dietary factors are primarily responsible is also difficult, because so many dietary differences exist between vegetarians and nonvegetarians. It is therefore instructive to consider first some of these dietary differences within the context of what is known about the relationship between specific dietary components and disease risk (Table 2-1).

DIFFERENCES IN DIETARY COMPONENTS OF VEGETARIAN AND NONVEGETARIAN DIETS

Dietary Fat and Cholesterol

Differences in fat intake between vegetarians and nonvegetarians are not as striking as commonly thought. In the United States, fat intake ranges from

Table 2–1 Comparison of Vegetarian and Nonvegetarian Intakes of Protein, Fat, Carbohydrate, Cholesterol, and Fiber

Nutrient	Nonvegetarian	Lacto-Ovo Vegetarian	Vegan
Fat (% total calories)	34–38	30–36	28–33
Cholesterol (total grams)	300–500	150–300	0
Carbohydrate (% total calories)	<50	50–55	50–65
Dietary fiber (total grams)/day	10–12	20–35	25–50
Protein (% total calories)	14–18	12–14	10–12
Animal protein (% total protein)	60–70	40–60	0

about 34% to 38% of calories; in contrast, lacto-ovo vegetarians consume diets that are about 30% to 36% fat, and vegan diets are about 30% fat, although there is considerable variation among studies (see Appendix A). Thus even vegans consume diets that just barely conform to the rather conservative recommendations of the National Cancer Institute and the American Heart Association. Nevertheless, the relatively lower fat intake should provide some advantage to vegetarians, particularly because their diets are lower in saturated fat intake.

From studies involving direct comparisons (Appendix A), it is clear that omnivores consume considerably more saturated fat than vegetarians, but both lacto-ovo vegetarians and omnivores consume more saturated fat than polyunsaturated fat. In contrast, vegans consume more polyunsaturated fat than saturated fat. Cholesterol intake is also lower among vegetarians. Both these differences will certainly favorably affect heart disease risk. As shown in Appendix A, daily cholesterol intake among omnivores is generally between 300 and 500 mg. In lacto-ovo vegetarians, intake is typically between 150–300 mg, although there is a wide range among the studies. Strict vegan diets contain no cholesterol. Although dietary cholesterol affects blood cholesterol levels to a much lesser extent than saturated fat, cholesterol intake is directly linked to blood cholesterol levels in most individuals, especially at intakes ranging from 0 to 400 mg/day.[2]

Dietary Fiber and Carbohydrate Intake

Fiber intake differs markedly between vegetarians and nonvegetarians. Some national dietary surveys indicate that typical Americans consume as little as 10 to 12 g of fiber per day,[3] although many studies show higher intakes than this (see Appendix A). Vegetarians generally consume between 50% and 100% more fiber than nonvegetarians, and vegans consume more fiber than lacto-ovo vegetarians. Higher fiber intake is associated with a reduced risk of colon cancer and perhaps also breast cancer. The National Cancer Institute recommends that Americans consume between 20 and 35 g of fiber per day to reduce cancer risk. Fiber also appears to reduce heart disease risk, and soluble fiber lowers blood cholesterol levels. Not surprising, carbohydrate intake is also higher among vegetarians. Vegans consume roughly 50% to 65% of their calories in the form of carbohydrate, lacto-ovo vegetarians about 50% to 55%, and omnivores generally less than 50% (Appendix A).

Protein

Protein accounts for between 14% and 18% of calories in the diet of Western omnivores. Americans typically consume about twice the recommended dietary allowance (RDA; 0.8 g/kg body weight) for protein. Lacto-ovo vegetarians consume diets containing between 12% and 14% protein, and vegan diets are between 10% and 12% protein (Appendix A). Clearly, the type of protein consumed also differs. American omnivores derive about two thirds of their protein from animal foods; this has changed quite a bit from the turn of the century, when only half the protein was derived from animal sources.[4] In contrast to the omnivore diet, about 40% to 60% of the protein in lacto-ovo vegetarian diets is derived from animal products,[5-7] and vegans consume plant protein only. As discussed later, high-protein diets, particularly those high in animal protein, may increase risk for osteoporosis and kidney disease. Some evidence (although still speculative) suggests that high–animal protein diets also increase risk for some forms of cancer and heart disease.

Antioxidants

Antioxidants include nutrients, such as vitamins C and E, and nonnutrients, such as the carotenoids and flavonoids. Antioxidants may reduce risk of a wide array of diseases, including arthritis, cancer, and heart disease.[8] Vegetarians consume higher levels of the three primary vitamin antioxidants: β-carotene and vitamins C and E. In addition, because more plant foods are consumed, vegetarian diets are higher in phytochemicals (discussed later), which appear to be protective against chronic diseases such as cancer and heart disease; many of the phytochemicals are potent antioxidants.

CARDIOVASCULAR DISEASE

In 1925, British physician Sir John McNee described to his colleagues two cases of atherosclerosis, a "rare disease" that he had observed in the United

States.[9] Today, just 70 years later, cardiovascular disease kills more than 100 people each hour in this country.[10] About 40% of Americans die of cardiovascular disease, although mortality rates have come down quite significantly since the mid-1960s. There are a number of reasons for this decline; life style changes may have contributed, but the widespread use of cardiopulmonary resuscitation and improved medical procedures are also very important factors.

Blood cholesterol levels in Americans have dropped somewhat in recent years and now average about 205 mg/dL.[11] Nevertheless, about 20% of the population, approximately 37.2 million adult Americans, have blood cholesterol levels that place them at high risk for heart disease ($\geq$240 mg/dL).[10] The biologically normal or desirable level of blood cholesterol may be somewhere between 100 and 150 mg/dL.[12] Populations consuming plant-based diets often have levels within this range.

Mortality rates from heart disease differ markedly throughout the world; in fact, the death rate due to heart attack is 10 times higher in some countries than in others. For example, in Shanghai, China, just 1 of every 15 deaths is due to heart disease.[13] Although genetic factors affect heart disease risk, they are unlikely to account for a substantial portion of this worldwide variation. Even within countries, differences in mortality rates clearly suggest an environmental influence; for example, rural Chinese have only half the rate of heart disease of urban Chinese.[14]

Vegetarians and Heart Disease Risk

With the exception of only one study,[15] it is well established from studies in the United States,[16] Britain,[17-19] the Netherlands,[20] Norway,[21] Germany,[22] and Japan[23] that Seventh-day Adventists (approximately 50% of whom are vegetarians) and non–Seventh-day Adventist vegetarian men have approximately half the risk of death due to ischemic heart disease in comparison to the general population. Among Seventh-day Adventists, meat consumption is directly associated with fatal ischemic heart disease. Nonvegetarian Seventh-day Adventist men have a twofold to threefold increase in risk for coronary heart disease in comparison with vegetarian men. Risk among vegans is even lower than among lacto-ovo vegetarians.[16,24] Also, heart disease risk decreases among Seventh-day Adventists the longer they have been an Adventist.[24] Heart disease data for female vegetarians are less clear, although some research indicates rates are lower in women who eat no meat in comparison with omnivores.[25] However, recent results from the Adventist Health Study show that even after controlling for various risk factors, vegetarianism is associated with a greatly reduced risk for heart disease among men but not among women.[26]

Because smoking results in an approximately two- to threefold increase in cardiovascular disease risk, the lower rates of heart disease among vegetarians may be due, in part, to their avoidance of tobacco products (eg, less than 5% of Seventh-day Adventists smoke).[27] Even after controlling for smoking, however, heart disease rates are still much lower among vegetarians.[16,17,20,23] Hypertension also markedly increases heart disease risk by approximately the same factor as smoking. The lower incidence of hypertension among vegetarians, as discussed below, probably contributes to their reduced incidence of heart disease. Smokers who are hypertensive and hypercholesterolemic have 20 times the risk of heart disease of nonsmoking, normocholesterolemic, normotensive men.[28]

It is well established that diet influences blood cholesterol levels and that high blood cholesterol increases risk for heart disease (Figure 2–1). In 1991, the American Health Foundation in Valhalla, New York, concluded that a vegan diet could help both children and adults maintain low cholesterol levels.[29] The report found that, in comparison with omnivores, lacto-ovo

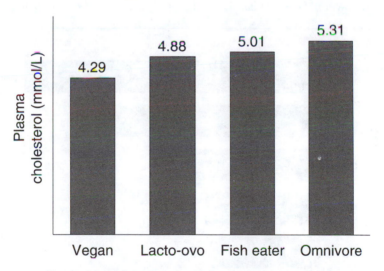

Figure 2–1 Effects of eating pattern on plasma cholesterol. Cholesterol values in vegans (N = 114), lacto-ovo vegetarians (N = 1,550), fish eaters (lacto-ovo vegetarians who ate fish, N = 415), and omnivores (N = 1,198). All groups included both men and women, but values were adjusted for age and gender. Average ages for each group ranged from 36 to 40 years. Cholesterol values for omnivores was significantly higher than for the other groups, values for fish eaters and lacto-ovo vegetarians were not significantly different from each other, but were higher than for vegans. *Source:* Data from Thorogood M, Carter R, Benfield L, et al. Plasma lipids and lipoprotein cholesterol concentrations in people with different diets in Britain. *Br Med J.* 1987;295:351–353.

vegetarians and vegans had blood cholesterol levels that were 14% and 35% lower, respectively. These findings were based on a review of only nine studies but are similar to findings from a larger group of studies presented in Appendix B. Former estimates have been that for every 1% decrease in blood cholesterol, heart disease risk decreases by about 2%. More recent estimates suggest, however, that as much as a 3% to 4% decrease in risk results from a 1% decrease in cholesterol levels[30] (Figure 2–2).

Although most studies did not, some studies reported lower high-density lipoprotein cholesterol (HDL-C) levels in vegetarians in comparison with omnivores (Appendix B). In a review of the relationship between diet and lipoproteins, Knuiman et al[31] concluded that replacing fat in the diet with carbohydrate lowers HDL-C levels. Ratios of total cholesterol (TC) to HDL-C are thought to be a better indicator of heart disease risk than TC levels alone, although TC:HDL-C ratios are quite similar across diverse populations with marked differences in coronary heart disease rates.[32,33] Populations with diets based largely on complex carbohydrates, however, generally have much less coronary artery disease than Western populations and have both lower TC and lower HDL-C levels. Low HDL-C levels may be a less important

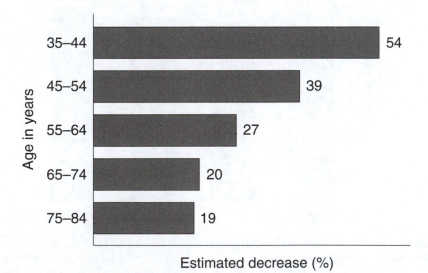

Estimated decrease (%)

Figure 2–2 Percentage reduction in heart disease risk in men according to age associated with a 10% decrease in blood cholesterol levels. The estimated decrease risk shown here for ischemic heart disease associated with a 0.6 mmol/L (about 10%) decrease in serum cholesterol is based upon the findings of 10 prospective studies that involved approximately 500,000 men and 18,000 ischemic heart disease events. *Source:* Data from reference 30.

factor in heart disease when TC levels are also low.[34] Clinical work indicates that low HDL-C alone does not necessarily result in accelerated atherosclerosis.[35] Nevertheless, a Japanese study found that although both coronary artery disease patients and patients without disease had similar and relatively low TC levels, patients with disease had significantly lower HDL-C.[36]

The role of very low-density lipoprotein cholesterol (VLDL-C, which carries mostly triglyceride) in coronary artery disease is controversial, but some data suggest that high triglyceride levels are a weak risk factor.[37] High triglyceride levels are often associated with low HDL-C levels, which would tend to increase risk further.[38] Consumption of high–complex carbohydrate diets is generally associated with higher levels of VLDL-C and lower HDL-C levels, although this may only be a transient phenomenon because long-term studies involving high-fiber, high-carbohydrate diets indicate that HDL-C values increase somewhat over time.[39] Some types of fiber have been shown to lower triglyceride without lowering HDL-C, and some studies have actually reported an increase in HDL-C in response to fiber.[40] Overall, studies indicate little if any difference in triglyceride levels between vegetarians and nonvegetarians (Appendix B).

Although vegetarians are leaner than omnivores and leanness results in lower TC, this is not the primary factor responsible for the lower cholesterol levels seen in vegetarians. In fact, Sacks et al[41] found that, even when vegetarian subjects were heavier than a similar group of omnivores, plasma lipoprotein levels were still markedly lower among the vegetarians.

As long ago as 1966, investigators observed that a vegan diet was effective in reducing angina in heart disease patients.[42] The lower heart disease rate and the lower blood cholesterol levels of vegetarians have prompted several investigators to examine the effects on blood cholesterol in subjects changing from a meat-based diet to a vegetarian diet. Not surprising, these studies have shown that adoption of a vegetarian diet lowers TC.[43–49] For example:

- Cooper et al[43] reported a 20 mg/dL (13%) decrease in TC in healthy normocholesterolemic subjects consuming a 20% fat, nearly vegan diet (the only animal product was skim milk). Weight did decrease on the vegetarian diet, although only slightly (1.6 lb in 3 weeks).
- Arntzenius and colleagues[49] found that, when omnivore heart disease patients adopted a vegetarian diet that was low in saturated fat and cholesterol and high in polyunsaturated fat, not only did serum cholesterol levels decrease by about 10% but the progression of atherosclerosis was slowed. In fact, 18 of 39 patients experienced no lesion growth.
- More recently, the potential benefits of a vegetarian diet on heart disease risk were demonstrated by Ornish et al.[48] This study involved a nearly vegan diet that was much lower in total fat (approximately 10%

of calories), saturated fat, and cholesterol than the American Heart Association's STEP 1 diet. It also included exercise, relaxation therapy, and other life style changes. TC decreased from 5.88 mmol/L to 4.45 mmol/L (25%). More important, this study demonstrated not only that plaque development could be halted through proper diet but that existing plaques could actually be reduced.

Other Factors Affecting Heart Disease Risk in Vegetarians

Protein

The higher polyunsaturated fat to saturated fat ratio of vegetarian diets compared to nonvegetarian diets primarily explains the decreased cholesterol level in habitual vegetarians and in omnivores adopting a vegetarian diet.[50,51] Nevertheless, there is some evidence, albeit weak, suggesting that meat protein, independent of dietary fat, may increase cholesterol levels. Subjects who consumed a 30% fat diet that included lean meat experienced only half the reduction in TC compared with subjects who consumed a lacto-ovo vegetarian diet and similar amounts of total fat, saturated fat, and cholesterol.[52] Other studies that have found animal products to be directly associated with an increase in blood cholesterol, however, have concluded that their hypercholesterolemic effects result from their fat and cholesterol content and not their protein content.[50,53,54]

Although the impact of dietary protein on blood cholesterol levels is controversial, Carroll[55] found that in animals fed diets containing similar amounts of fat, plant proteins are hypocholesterolemic in comparison with animal proteins. Also, a large amount of clinical work suggests that soy protein, in particular, is hypocholesterolemic.[56] However, the mechanism for this effect has not been established, nor is it clear whether it is the protein per se, or some component associated with soy protein that is hypocholesterolemic, such as the isoflavones that are abundant in soybeans.

Fiber

As noted previously, vegetarians consume between 50% and 100% more fiber than nonvegetarians, and soluble fiber has been shown to lower blood cholesterol levels. In a recent review by Glore et al,[57] 68 of 77 studies reported that soluble fiber decreased blood cholesterol by an average of about 10%. More impressive, however, are results from a prospective study in the U.S. involving more than 40,000 men showing that in comparison to men consuming ≈ 10 g of fiber/day, men consuming ≈ 30 g/day had approximately a 40% reduced risk of myocardial infarction.[58] This higher level of dietary fiber intake is similar to that consumed by vegetarians.

Antioxidants

The high antioxidant content of vegetarian diets may also influence heart disease among vegetarians. Many heart attacks occur in people with normal or only mildly elevated cholesterol. In fact, although smoking, high blood cholesterol, and high blood pressure are major risk factors for heart disease, these three risk factors may predict only about 30% of all cardiovascular events.[59] The oxidation of serum lipoproteins appears to be a critical factor in atherosclerosis. It is believed that only oxidized low-density lipoprotein (LDL) cholesterol (LDL-C) is taken up by macrophages that are found within the intima.[60] Also, only nonoxidized HDL-C is thought to remove cholesterol from deposits along the walls of the arteries.[61]

Recent work indicates that LDL-C oxidation is as important a risk factor for heart disease as elevated cholesterol. The primary antioxidant nutrient thought to protect LDL-C from oxidation is vitamin E; vitamin C may also have an important role by helping regenerate the reduced form of vitamin E.[62,63]

Vegetarians have higher blood levels of both vitamins E and C, and, not surprising, the ratio of vitamin E to cholesterol is higher among vegetarians in comparison with omnivores (see Chapter 6). Serum levels of β-carotene are also higher and a recent study found that higher serum levels of β-carotene were associated with a lower risk of acute myocardial infarction.[64] Additionally, *in vitro*, β-carotene has been shown to inhibit the oxidation of a lipoprotein(a), a modified form of LDL-C.[65] Lipoprotein(a) may also increase heart disease risk. Whether LDL-C in vegetarians is less prone to oxidation has yet to be demonstrated, but some findings are worthy of note:

- The consumption of a vegan diet (in combination with walking) was shown to reduce serum peroxide levels markedly, a possible indication of decreased system oxidation.[66]
- Vegans have been found to have lower concentrations of lipid peroxidation.[67]
- Vegetarians have been shown to have higher blood catalase activity and lower levels of conjugated dienes in comparison with omnivores, which could protect against both heart disease and cancer.[68]

In support of the importance of antioxidants is a recent study showing that, among 16 cohorts worldwide, flavonoid intake was associated with a reduced risk of cardiovascular disease.[69] Flavonoids are potent antioxidants and are widely distributed among fruits and vegetables and are also found in wine. In fact, the flavonoid content of red wine may be responsible for the French paradox, the relatively low rate of heart disease in France compared with other Western countries with similar intakes of saturated fat.[70] Vitamin E intake also has been proposed as a possible answer to the French paradox.[71] As indicated previously, many of the phytochemicals, the intake of which is higher among vegetarians, are potent antioxidants.

A considerable amount of data suggest that iron may increase heart disease risk because it can act as a prooxidant, thereby increasing LDL oxidation.[72] The lower iron stores seen in vegetarians (see Chapter 5) may be an additional factor in reducing heart disease risk. Also, Harvard researchers recently found that intake of heme iron, but not nonheme iron, was associated with a marked increase in heart disease risk[73] (Figure 2–3). The higher intake of antioxidants and the lower iron stores of vegetarians may work to inhibit LDL-C oxidation and to reduce heart disease risk.

Homocysteine

Considerable research indicates that increased serum levels of the amino acid homocysteine is an independent risk factor for vascular disease.[74] A recent

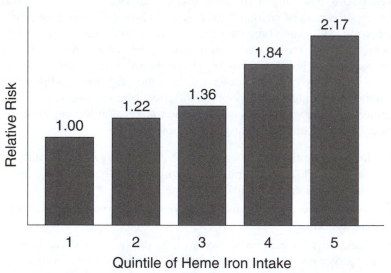

Figure 2–3 Association between heme iron intake and risk of myocardial infarction: Relative risk of myocardial infarction (fatal coronary heart disease and nonfatal myocardial infarction) for men not taking vitamin E supplements according to quintile of heme iron intake adjusted for energy intake. Average heme iron intake in quintile 5 was 2.1 mg/day. Data were based on 4 years of follow-up in 24,501 men (220 cases) aged 40 to 75 years with no previous history of cardiovascular disease. The relationship between heme iron intake and myocardial infarction was significant for trend ($P < 0.002$) using the Mantel extension test. Total iron intake was unrelated to risk, and in men taking vitamin E supplements, heme intake and myocardial infarction were unrelated. *Source:* Data from reference 73.

meta-analysis of 27 studies concluded that about 10% of coronary artery diseases was attributable to increased homocysteine and that a 5 μmol/L homocysteine increment elevates coronary artery disease by as much as cholesterol increases of 20 mg/dL. Low serum folate levels are associated with high homocysteine levels and folate administration can reduce serum homocysteine concentrations. It has been estimated that an additional 200 μg of folate can lower homocysteine levels by 4 μmol/L, and thereby reduce heart disease risk. Although no studies comparing homocysteine levels between vegetarians and nonvegetarians were identified, vegetarians consume considerably more folate than nonvegetarians (see Appendix J).

Factors Affecting Platelet Aggregation

A number of other factors unrelated to cholesterol are thought to affect heart disease risk. These include high fibrinogen levels,[75] and the tendency to form blood clots (platelet aggregation),[76,77] and the type and levels of various prostaglandins.[78] Many of these factors are affected by diet; for example, dietary fat, and saturated fat in particular, increase factor VII levels, which increases platelet aggregation.[79] In one study, when subjects were switched from a typical Danish diet (which is high in both total and saturated fat) to a low-fat, high-fiber diet, there was a marked increase in fibrinolytic activity, suggesting subjects were less likely to form blood clots.[79] Consistent with these findings, the consumption of dietary polyunsaturated fatty acids may reduce the tendency for platelets to form blood clots.[80] Conversely, saturated fat is thought to increase platelet aggregation.[81] Vegetarian diets may favorably affect these processes because they are lower in both total and saturated fat.

Ernst et al[82] found that vegetarians had reduced blood viscosity, although vegetarians in this study and in other studies[83–85] did not have lower fibrinogen levels. Similarly, in several studies no differences in platelet aggregation were noted between vegetarians and omnivores.[84–87] In a study of fibrositis/fibromyalgia patients placed on a vegetarian diet, however, fibrogen levels did decrease after 3 weeks.[88]

Specific Fatty Acids and Heart Disease

Plant foods do not contain arachidonic acid, whereas meat is rich in this fatty acid. Arachidonic acid leads to the synthesis of eicosanoids (hormones), such as the n-2 series prostacyclins and thromboxanes, that constrict the arteries and promote platelet aggregation, thereby increasing heart disease risk.[89] They are also proinflammatory, which is why fatty acids have been studied in relation to both heart disease and arthritis.[90]

Although vegetarians do not consume arachidonic acid, they do consume relatively more linoleic acid,[84,85,91] which is the precursor to arachidonic acid.

Also, the arachidonic acid intake of omnivores is relatively small, 100 to 1,000 mg/day.[84,92] Although some studies show that cells from vegetarians contain less arachidonic acid,[84,86,93] others show little or no difference[94] or even increased levels.[95] In one study, arachidonic acid levels were reduced significantly when omnivore subjects were placed on a vegan diet for 3 to 5 months after an initial 7- to 10-day fast, but levels returned to their initial values when subjects consumed a lacto vegetarian diet.[67] Conversely, when meat eaters were placed on a vegetarian diet, arachidonic acid levels increased.[87,96]

Vegetarian diets do not contain the long-chain polyunsaturated n-3 (omega 3) fatty acids, eicosapenaenoic acid (EPA) and docosahexaenoic acid (DHA) and the plasma cell concentration of the longer chain n-3 fatty acids has been found to be lower in vegetarians than in omnivores.[97] EPA and DHA, which are found predominately in certain types of fish, may have a role in reducing chronic diseases such as heart disease, via their conversion into the n-3 series prostacyclins and thromboxanes, which can favorably affect factors such as platelet aggregation. In contrast, and as noted above, vegetarian diets can be high in the essential fatty acid, linoleic acid, an n-6 fatty acid that can serve (via arachidonic acid) as a precursor to the n-2 series prostacyclins and thromboxanes. Also, linoleic acid competitively inhibits the conversion of the n-3 fatty acid, α-linolenic acid, which vegetarians do consume, into EPA and DHA, thereby decreasing the synthesis of the n-3 series prostacyclins and thromboxanes. The net effect (increased n-2 series and decreased n-3 series) may be an increased risk of heart disease. For this reason, there has been much discussion over the optimal dietary intake ratio of linoleic acid to α-linolenic acid. Estimates vary, but the World Health Organization recommends that this ratio should between 5:1 and 10:1.[98]

Although there are few rich plant sources of α-linolenic acid (Table 2–2), the biological requirement for α-linolenic acid is small (≈0.5% of calories)[99] and the limited data indicate that vegetarian intake is sufficient to meet these biological requirements (Appendix F). It is also clear from these data, however, that in some cases, the linoleic acid to α-linolenic acid ratio may be too high. Ratios can be improved by substituting carbohydrate or monounsaturated fats for linoleic acid and by increasing intake of α-linolenic acid. Good sources of α-linolenic acid include soybeans, soy products, and especially linseed oil and flax seed (Table 2–2). Although α-linolenic acid comprises a substantial portion of the total fat content of many vegetables, because of their overall low total fat content, vegetables are only modest sources.

Finally, although *trans* fatty acids have been studied for more than a decade, there has been renewed interest in these fatty acids, in part because of a study by Willet et al, which found that the consumption of margarine, which is high in *trans* fatty acids, was associated with a marked increase in coronary heart disease risk among women.[100] *Trans* fatty acids are found in both the vegetable

Table 2–2 Total Fat, Total Polyunsaturated Fat, and α-Linolenic Acid Content (g/100 g edible portion) of Selected Foods

Food	Total Fat	Polyunsaturated (PUFA)	α-Linolenic Acid	PUFA:α-Linolenic Acid
Nuts and Seeds				
Butternuts (dried)	57.0	42.7	8.7	4.9
Walnuts, English/Persian	61.0	39.1	6.8	5.8
Legumes				
Beans, common	1.5	0.9	0.6	1.5
Soybeans, dry	21.3	12.3	1.6	7.7
Vegetables				
Leeks, freeze-dried, raw	2.1	1.2	0.7	1.7
Soybeans, green, raw	6.8	3.8	3.2	1.2
Kale, raw	0.7	0.3	0.2	1.5
Broccoli, raw	0.4	0.2	0.1	2.0
Cauliflower, raw	0.2	trace	0.1	1.0
Fats and Oils				
Soybean oil	100	57.9	6.8	8.5
Soybean oil, partially hydrogenated	100	27.6	2.6	10.6
Walnut oil	100	63.3	10.4	6.1
Wheat germ oil	100	61.7	6.9	8.9
Rapeseed oil (Canola)	100	33.3	11.1	3.0
Linseed oil	100	66.0	53.3	1.2
Margarine, hard, soybean	100	20.9	1.5	13.9

Source: United States Department of Agriculture. Human Nutrition Service, HNIS/PT. 103. Provisional table on the content of omega-3 fatty acids and other fat components in selected foods.

and animal kingdom but are also formed as a result of the partial hydrogenation of vegetable oils, the principle one being elaidic acid which is the *trans* form of oleic acid.

Few data are available on the intake of *trans* fatty acids by vegetarians. Draper et al reported that the daily intake of *trans* fatty acids by British male and female lacto-ovo vegetarians was 5.4 and 3.4 g respectively, and for vegan male and females, it was 2.7 and 2.8 g.[101] In comparison, British male and female nonvegetarians reportedly consume 5.5 and 3.9 g of *trans* fatty acids per day, respectively.[101] In a Swedish study involving small numbers of subjects, nonvegetarian, lacto-vegetarian and vegan diets reportedly contained 2.0%, 1.3% and 0.5% of their calories as *trans* fatty acids (only *trans*-octadecenoic acids were determined).[102] Finally, the level of *trans* (18:n-9) fatty acids in the subcutaneous fat of lacto-ovo vegetarians was reported by Crane et al[103] to be about one-third lower than that of nonvegetarians. In contrast, no *trans* fatty acids were detected in the subcutaneous fat of vegans on a strict diet containing no refined foods.

Summary

Exhibit 2–1 summarizes the factors in vegetarian diets that may reduce heart disease risk.

HYPERTENSION

There are striking differences in blood pressure among populations worldwide. In industrialized societies, blood pressure typically increases with advancing age, and the prevalence of hypertension is high. Migrant studies demonstrate an environmental influence on blood pressure in that blood pressure rises in children and adults after they move from indigenous cultures to areas having a diet and life style more characteristic of economically developed societies. Also, in some agrarian societies, sizable age-related blood pressure changes do not occur in most adults, and the prevalence of hypertension among the elderly remains low.[104]

In the United States, more than 60 million adults and children have or are being treated for high blood pressure ($\geq$140/90 mmHg); more than half of all women over 55, and more than two thirds of all women 65 and older, have hypertension.[10] More than 30,000 Americans die each year of complications related to hypertension; it is a major risk factor for heart disease.[10]

An interest in the possible blood pressure–lowering effect of a vegetarian diet dates back to 1917 when Hamman[105] concluded that meat was harmful for patients with hypertension. Subsequently, in 1926 Donaldson[106] reported that blood pressures of vegetarian college students increased significantly

Exhibit 2–1 Factors among Vegetarians That Reduce or Are Hypothesized To Reduce Risk for Heart Disease

- Reduced saturated fat intake
- Reduced cholesterol intake
- Higher fiber intake
- Higher antioxidant intake
- Lower heme iron intake and lower iron stores
- Lower incidence of obesity
- Lower blood pressure
- Lower intake of animal protein
- Decreased tendency to form blood clots
- Reduced blood viscosity
- Higher folate intake

within 2 weeks of adding meat to their diet. Four years later, Saile[107] reported that German vegetarian monks had lower blood pressures at all ages than monks who ate meat. About that same time, Heun[108] observed a mean decline in systolic blood pressure of 60 mm and a decrease in diastolic blood pressure of 28 mm in 14 severely hypertensive patients who were treated with a fruit and vegetable diet. These observations are consistent with studies showing that vegetarian Buddhist monks did not experience the rise in blood pressure with age seen in omnivore controls matched for age, sex, and body mass index (BMI) and that the duration of vegetarianism was inversely related to blood pressure.[109,110]

Appendix C lists studies in which blood pressure in vegetarians was compared with that in omnivores (see also Figure 2–4). In many of these studies vegetarians had both lower systolic and diastolic blood pressure. Although differences between vegetarians and omnivores were generally between 5 and 10 mm Hg, this degree of difference may have a significant impact on

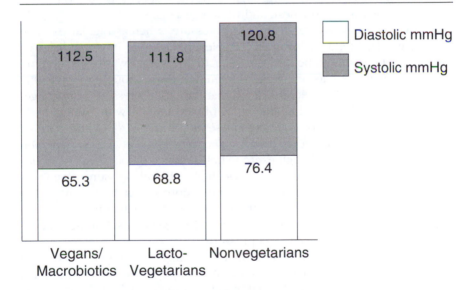

Figure 2–4 Differences in blood pressure between vegetarians and meat eaters. There were 226 vegans (macrobiotics), 63 lacto vegetarians, and 458 nonvegetarians. The vegans and lacto vegetarians had adhered to their dietary patterns for approximately 2 and 3 years, respectively. The systolic and diastolic blood pressures of both groups of vegetarians were significantly lower than those of the omnivores (*P* < 0.001), and the diastolic pressure of vegans was significantly lower than that of the lacto vegetarians (*P* < 0.02). Significant differences between vegetarians and nonvegetarians existed after controlling for body weight. *Source:* Data from Sacks FM, Kass EH. Low blood pressure in vegetarians: effets of specific foods and nutrients. *Am J Clin Nutr.* 1988;48:795–800.

morbidity or mortality. In 55- to 59-year-old men, a reduction in systolic blood pressure of only 5 mm Hg has been estimated to result in a 7% reduction in major coronary events.[111] Similarly, a reduction in blood pressure of only 4 mm Hg was found to cause a marked reduction in mortality from all causes in the Hypertension Detection and Follow-Up Program.[112] Also, differences in blood pressure between vegetarians and nonvegetarians were likely minimized because of the selection criteria for study subjects.

Not only is average blood pressure lower in vegetarians, but the extent of actual hypertension appears to be lower as well. For example, Ophir et al[113] reported that 42% of the nonvegetarians studied had hypertension (140/90) compared with only 13% of the vegetarians. The prevalence of blood pressure over 160/95 was 13 times higher in the nonvegetarians (26% versus 2%).[113] In another study, 37% of the nonvegetarians but only 14% of the vegetarians had a history of physician-diagnosed hypertension.[114] Similarly, the prevalence of hypertension requiring current medication use was 44% and 22% among African American and white nonvegetarian subjects, respectively, but only 18% and 7% among African American and white vegetarians.[115]

Obesity is positively related to blood pressure, whereas regular exercise and weight loss tend to lower it.[116,117] Nevertheless, in most studies that found blood pressure to be lower in vegetarians, weight was controlled for, and in two where it was not, weight differences were thought to have little if any impact.[118,119] Ophir et al[113] found that the blood pressure of nonvegetarians is appreciably higher than that of vegetarians with similar body weights. Only when subjects were obese (ie, above 20% of the average weight) were no differences in blood pressure between vegetarians and nonvegetarians seen. Although exercise helps reduce blood pressure, Rouse et al[120] found that Mormon women had higher blood pressures than Seventh-day Adventist women, even though the Mormons exercised more. For men, there were no differences in the frequency of activity among Mormon omnivores, Adventist omnivores, and Adventist vegetarians, but the vegetarians had the lowest systolic blood pressure.

Rouse et al[43] were the first to evaluate the effects of a vegetarian diet on blood pressure in a controlled setting. After controlling for age, obesity, heart rate, weight change, and initial blood pressure, they found that systolic and diastolic blood pressures decreased by 5 to 6 mm Hg and 2 to 3 mm Hg, respectively, when normotensive omnivore subjects were placed on a lacto-ovo vegetarian diet. In a later study involving a similar design, mean systolic and diastolic blood pressures decreased 6.8 and 2.7 mm Hg on a lacto-ovo vegetarian diet.[121] Other studies have also reported hypotensive effects of a vegetarian diet in normotensive subjects,[122] mildly hypertensive subjects,[123] and hypertensive subjects.[45]

Several studies have tried to determine the dietary component of vegetarian diets that is responsible for their hypotensive effect, but the absence of neither meat[124,125] nor milk protein[126] appears to be responsible. Controlled studies involving relatively specific nutrient changes while holding energy intake constant suggest that the effects are not due independently to the ratio of polyunsaturated to saturated fat or cholesterol,[127–129] fiber,[130] or protein.[124] Also, changes in potassium, magnesium, and calcium appear to be too small to account for the observed blood pressure differences.[43] Although blood pressure in agrarian societies with primarily vegetarian diets and low sodium intakes is lower than in industrialized nations, the sodium intake of vegetarians in industrialized countries is similar to that of omnivores (see Appendix G). Thus sodium intake does not appear to be the explanation for blood pressure differences between omnivores and vegetarians.

The lower glycemic index of vegetarian diets has been suggested as one possible explanation for lower blood pressure in vegetarians.[131] The lower blood pressure of vegetarians may be partly effected through a blood glucose-insulin sympathoadrenal mechanism, as postulated by Landsberg and Young.[132] They suggested that the lower blood pressures of vegetarians may be related to the slower delivery of glucose to the blood as a result of an increased consumption of complex carbohydrates and a decreased sucrose intake. Sacks and Kass[133] suggested that modest intake of animal products may be a marker for a large intake of other potentially beneficial nutrients from vegetable products that collectively have a hypotensive effect. It is almost certain that it is the combination of nutrient changes incurred when changing to a vegetarian diet that elicits the blood pressure-lowering response.[134,135]

CANCER

Cancer is this nation's second leading cause of death, but sometime early next century cancer is expected to surpass heart disease as the number 1 killer. One of every three Americans born today will develop some form of cancer. There are, however, striking dissimilarities in cancer rates among countries. In fact, individual cancer rates vary as much as 100-fold among populations, according to the *Surgeon General's Report on Nutrition and Health*.[136] Although genetic differences among populations may contribute to international variations in cancer rates, the evidence that these differences are largely life style–related is persuasive and is based on migration studies, intracountry variations, and trends within countries. Some estimates suggest that as much as 50% to 90% of the cancer in this country could be eliminated if Americans adopted the life style and diet of low-risk countries.[137]

According to the National Cancer Institute, diet is related to one third of all cancer deaths. Since the 1970s, comparisons among countries have repeatedly found that the consumption of high-fat, animal-based diets is associated with higher rates of a wide range of cancers, particularly breast, colon, and prostate cancer. The National Cancer Institute has issued a set of dietary guidelines for reducing cancer risk. These call for Americans to reduce their fat intake and to increase their intake of fiber, fruits, and vegetables. Vegetarian diets come much closer to meeting these guidelines than typical omnivore diets.

There are many biologic mechanisms by which a vegetarian diet may affect cancer risk; for example, some work suggests that vegetarians have higher levels of natural killer cells, which may make the immune system more effective in destroying developing tumors.[138] Low-fat diets have been shown to stimulate the activities of natural killer cells.[139]

Cancer Rates in Vegetarians

That vegetarians have an overall lower cancer rate than the general population is beyond dispute. What is not clear is the extent to which diet is responsible for this difference. Vegetarians are generally more health conscious, smoke less, drink less alcohol, are often more highly educated, and are leaner than the general population. Consequently, differences in cancer rates between vegetarians and nonvegetarians are probably the result of a multitude of factors.

Much of our understanding about vegetarian cancer rates comes from studies involving Seventh-day Adventists. Approximately half the Adventists in the cancer age range (>40 years) are adult converts to the church, with the remaining half either being born into an Adventist home or joining the church before the age of 20.[140] About 50% of Seventh-day Adventist church members are vegetarians, and approximately 98% of these are lacto-ovo vegetarians. Consequently, this means that there is little information about the cancer rates of vegans.

Initial reports that Seventh-day Adventists have lower overall cancer mortality rates, and specifically lower rates for cancers of the lung, esophagus, bladder, stomach, colon-rectum, pancreas, breast, cervix, and ovary, as well as leukemia, were not adjusted for socioeconomic status.[141,142] This is important because the church members tend to be of above-average socioeconomic status, and people of higher socioeconomic status in the United States are generally at a lower cancer risk.

In a study involving more than 22,000 California Seventh-day Adventists and 112,000 white California non–Seventh-day Adventists adjusted for socioeconomic status, lower mortality rates were found only for colorectal cancers (both sexes), lung cancer (both sexes), and other smoking-related cancers (men only).[140] Breast cancer mortality rates were slightly lower, but not significantly so. Given the church's proscription against smoking, the lower lung cancer rate and the lower rate of other smoking-related cancers are expected. Even so, Phillips et al[143] found that lung cancer mortality was lower among Adventists in California not only in comparison with the general population but also in comparison with nonsmoking, non-Adventist Californians, although meat per se did not appear to contribute to this decreased incidence.[144]

Seventh-day Adventist women, on average, have children at a later age, a factor that appears to increase breast cancer risk and may obscure any protective effects of diet. Conversely, any decrease in breast cancer mortality, should it exist, may be due to the better survival rates among Adventists resulting from earlier breast cancer diagnosis among these women in comparison with the general population.[145]

A recent British study involving more than 6,000 individuals found the cancer mortality rate among vegetarians for all cancers combined to be only half that of the general population.[146] When vegetarians were compared with an omnivore population that was similar in life style habits, the cancer mortality rate was still 40% lower, indicating that diet is an important factor. The decreased mortality rate held true even after correction for smoking, BMI, and socioeconomic status.

Lower overall cancer mortality rates have also been observed in another British study[147] and in German,[148] Japanese Adventist,[149] Japanese non-Adventist,[150] and Swedish[151] vegetarians. Among the Japanese Adventists, overall cancer mortality was reduced in men and women, but not significantly so in women. The only cancer found to be reduced significantly when analyzed individually, however, was cancer of the respiratory system.[149] In the Swedish vegetarian study of 9,000 subjects, relative risk of all cancers was decreased, in particular the cancer rates for digestive organs, pancreas, and liver.[151]

A prospective study of more than 122,000 Japanese non–Seventh-day Adventists found that those subjects who abstained from smoking, alcohol, and meat and who ate green and yellow vegetables had the lowest mortality rates for all causes, including cancer.[149] In a similar group who ate meat, higher rates were seen for cancer of the esophagus, lung, and pancreas (breast cancer was not evaluated). When people stopped eating meat, risk of stomach cancer risk decreased. It was also found that the combined effect of eating green and yellow vegetables and abstaining from meat decreased colon cancer risk (Figure 2–5).

In the study of German vegetarians cited above, vegetarians were more highly educated than the general population, and results were not controlled for socioeconomic status. Longer duration of vegetarianism (20 years or more) was associated with a marked (relative risk, 0.44, both sexes combined) decrease in overall cancer risk, however. Surprisingly, semivegetarians (those who consumed fish and meat occasionally) had a lower relative risk of cancer than strict vegetarians.[148]

Similar results were reported by Kinlen et al,[147] who found a lower proportion of deaths due to respiratory diseases and lung cancer, as well as a lower proportion of deaths due to colorectal cancer, among members of the

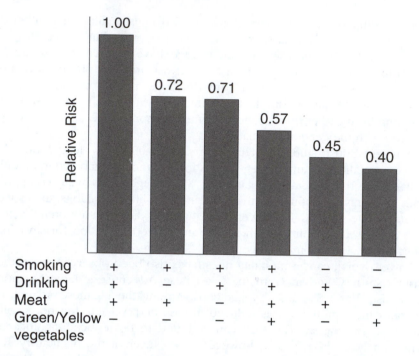

Figure 2–5 Effects of individual life style habits on risk of dying of cancer in Japanese men. The standardized morality rates shown here are based on 16 years of follow-up results from a prospective cohort study involving 122,261 men. Dietary intake data were gathered during home visits by public health nurses and midwives using standardized forms. Not drinking alcohol ($P < 0.05$), not eating meat ($P < 0.01$), and consuming green and yellow vegetables ($P < 0.01$) were independently associated with a statistically significantly decreased risk of cancer. Those factors plus not smoking were significant at $P < 0.001$. *Source:* Data from reference 149.

Vegetarian Society in Great Britain in comparison with the general population of England and Wales. No differences were seen in breast cancer rates, and rates for stomach cancer were actually higher among the vegetarians. When only long-term vegetarians were considered, however (ie, those who had been vegetarians for at least 15 years), only the increased deaths due to stomach cancer and the decreased risk of lung cancer remained significant. Stomach cancer is the most common cancer worldwide and occurs most frequently among populations consuming more plant-based diets. This relationship is thought to stem from the use of salted and pickled foods, however. Recent theories about stomach cancer suggest that it is due in part to the presence of the bacterium *Helicobacter pylori*. It is unlikely that vegetarianism per se increases risk, since as noted above, when Japanese subjects stopped eating meat, the risk of stomach cancer risk decreased.[149]

Vegetarians and Breast Cancer

There is relatively little evidence that Western vegetarians have less breast cancer than Western nonvegetarians. Worldwide, however, populations that consume plant-based diets have much less breast cancer than those with more Western-type diets. For example, death rates due to breast cancer in the United States are about five times greater than in China, four times greater than in Japan, and three times greater than in Mexico.[152] Interestingly, among the rural Chinese the consumption of animal foods just 1½ to 3 times per week is associated with an increase in breast cancer in comparison with women consuming animal products less than once a week (Figure 2–6).[153]

There is also evidence that vegetarian diets or nearly vegetarian diets produce hormonal changes that seem to protect against breast cancer. High blood estrogen levels increase breast cancer risk, and differences in life-long exposure to estrogen have been suggested as the partial or complete explanation for the variation in breast cancer mortality among countries.[154] Several

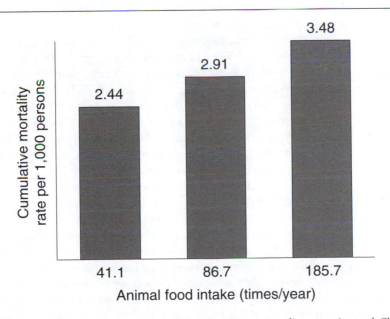

Figure 2–6 Animal product intake and breast cancer mortality rates in rural China. Data were derived from 64 rural counties in China. Breast cancer morality rates were obtained during a 1973–1975 nationwide survey in China. Animal foods included meat, fish, and eggs. Adjustments for the percentage of the population employed in industry, used as an indicator for standard of living, did not substantially alter the association between breast cancer mortality and animal food intake. By multiple regression analysis, animals foods were significantly related to breast cancer mortality ($P = 0.03$). *Source:* Data from reference 153.

studies have reported that vegetarians have lower blood levels of estrogen,[155-157] perhaps because dietary fat and fiber intakes are associated with increases and decreases, respectively, in estrogen levels.[158-160]

Several lines of evidence suggest that high-fat diets increase breast cancer risk. For example, Howe et al,[161] in an analysis of 12 case-control studies, concluded that dietary fat was significantly and positively associated with breast cancer, but this view has been challenged in recent years. Most important, a recent pooled analysis of prospective studies involving over 300,000 women and nearly 5,000 cases found that fat intake, even when comparing women consuming as little 20% of their calories in the form of fat with women consuming more than 40% fat diets, was unrelated to breast cancer risk.[162] It has been pointed out, however, that Western studies failing to show a relationship between fat intake and breast cancer risk have included relatively few individuals with low fat intakes. Nevertheless, international comparisons among countries do not suggest that there is any threshold effect of fat on breast cancer mortality rates, so that even moderate reductions in fat intake might be expected to produce lower breast cancer rates if fat is a factor in these rates.

The role of fiber in relation to breast cancer risk also is not clear. As noted previously, fiber may decrease breast cancer risk, possibly by binding estrogen as it undergoes enterohepatic circulation.[163] Consistent with this are results from an Australian study showing that women with high fiber intakes (at least 28 g of fiber daily) had less than half the risk of breast cancer compared with women with much lower fiber intakes.[164] In contrast, a study of 89,000 nurses failed to find any protective effect of fiber intake on breast cancer risk.[165] In this study, however, women with fiber intakes as low as 22 g/day were placed in the high-fiber intake group.

Pike et al[154] has estimated that later menses and earlier menopause may explain as much as 80% of the difference in breast cancer mortality rates between Japan and the United States. Other investigators have also concluded that later age at onset of menses reduces risk for breast cancer.[166] Vegetarians begin menstruation at a later age than omnivores.[167,168] Also, in Asian countries, where diets are more plant based, women have longer menstrual cycles; that is, there is a longer length of time between periods of ovulation. Longer menstrual cycles are also linked to lower risk of breast cancer. Both these factors, longer menstrual cycles and later onset of menstruation, mean that women are exposed to less estrogen over their lifetimes.

Some evidence indicates that dietary fat shortens menstrual cycle length whereas fiber increases it.[159,169,170] Emerging evidence, although still speculative, suggests that phytoestrogens (plant estrogens) can influence hormonal status. Many foods, particularly soyfoods, contain components with estrogenic activity.[171] One recent study found that premenopausal women who were fed soy experienced an increase in menstrual cycle length by an average of about 2.5 days.[172] Genistein, one of the phytoestrogens in soybeans, has been shown to inhibit the growth of a wide range of cancer cells in vitro; therefore, soyfoods could contribute to the lower breast cancer rate in some Asian countries.[173]

Vegetarians and Colon Cancer

Diet appears to be more strongly linked to colon cancer than to any other type of cancer. Several studies indicate that vegetarians experience lower colon cancer rates than omnivores. American Seventh-day Adventists have an approximately 40% decreased risk of colorectal cancer, and researchers suspect that this is due to diet and/or some other life style factor common to Adventists.[174] Lower colon cancer mortality rates have also been observed among Adventists residing in the Netherlands[20] and Denmark,[175] although not in Holland[176] or Japan.[149]

Several dietary factors may contribute to the lower colon cancer rates among vegetarians. Diet affects several biologic mechanisms that may influence colon cancer risk. The higher fiber intake of vegetarians is thought to play a significant role. In fact, it has been estimated that the risk of colon cancer in the United States could be reduced by 31% if fiber intake was increased by an average of just 13 g/day[177] (Figure 2–7). This would still represent a fiber intake below that of most vegetarians.

The environment of the colon differs significantly in vegetarians compared with nonvegetarians in ways that could favorably affect colon cancer risk:

- Colon cell proliferation is reduced in vegetarians.[178]
- Vegetarians have a lower concentration of potentially carcinogenic bile acids.[179–182] Vegans have lower bile acid levels than lacto-ovo vegetarians.[180,183] Dietary fat increases, whereas dietary fiber decreases, bile acid levels.[184]
- Some evidence suggests that vegetarians have fewer intestinal bacteria that convert the primary bile acids into the more carcinogenic secondary bile acids.[185–189]
- Colon pH is lower in vegetarians, which would tend to decrease the activity of enzymes responsible for converting primary bile acids into secondary bile acids.[190–191]
- Vegetarians have larger and heavier feces and experience more frequent elimination,[192–194] which may limit contact between potential carcinogens and the lining of the colon.[195] Fecal weight, which is related to fiber intake, is inversely related to the incidence of colon cancer among countries.[196]
- Vegetarians have lower levels of enzymes that hydrolyze conjugated xenobiotics, thereby enhancing the elimination of potential colon car-

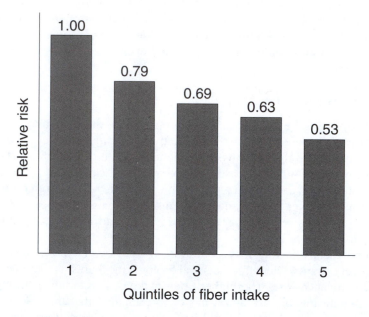

Figure 2–7 Relationship between fiber intake and risk of colon and rectal cancer. Data are based on 13 studies involving 5,225 cases and 10,349 controls. The inverse trend between fiber intake and colorectal cancer risk was statistically significant ($P < 0.001$). If causality is assumed, these data suggest that increasing fiber intake by approximately 13 g/day could reduce risk of colorectal cancer by approximately 31% in the United States. Dietary fiber intake in the highest quintile was approximately 31 g/day. *Source:* Data from reference 177.

cinogens.[155,179] Most studies indicate that vegetarians have lower levels of fecal mutagens.[197–200]

Other Cancers

Seventh-day Adventists have less lung cancer than non-Adventists. One reason undoubtedly is the church's proscription against smoking, although Adventists have even less lung cancer than nonsmoking non-Adventists.[143] Lung cancer risk among Adventists, however, appears to be similar whether or not they are vegetarian.[142]

Nevertheless, in a Japanese study of more than 122,000 people, meat intake increased lung cancer risk in people who smoked,[23] and in a large case-control study of nonsmoking women, saturated fat intake increased lung cancer risk by a factor of 6.[201] One protective factor for vegetarians may be their higher dietary intake of β-carotene, which is thought to protect against lung cancer,[202,203] although a recent trial found that β-carotene supplementation did not decrease lung cancer risk in long-term smokers.[204]

Prostate cancer is typically highest in Western countries, a finding that may be related to fat intake as well as to other dietary factors. Interestingly, in Japan the incidence of histologic prostate cancer is similar to that in the United States, but the Japanese incidence of clinical prostate cancer is much lower. Apparently, the growth of prostate tumors is slower, and/or the onset of tumors is later, in Japanese men.[205] Diet may be one factor for this. Some studies have found that high-fiber intake decreases, whereas high-fat intake increases, risk of prostate cancer.[205–207] Animal fat in particular may raise risk.[208] There is also some evidence, although the data are inconsistent, that vegetarian diet may affect hormone levels in a way that lowers prostate cancer risk.[209–212] A recent study found that low-fat diets slow the growth of tumors established from human prostatic adenocarcinoma cells in an animal model.[213] And, in male mice, soybeans added to the typical laboratory diet delayed the onset of prostatic dysplasia, an effect possibly resulting from the antiestrogenic effect of soy.[214] Finally, carotenoids such as lycopene may decrease prostate cancer risk (see section on phytochemicals).

Animal Products and Cancer

An important issue related to diet and cancer is whether animal products specifically increase cancer risk. International studies show that meat- and dairy-based diets are associated with an increased incidence of breast, colon, prostate, renal, and endometrial cancer.[215] Other types of studies have produced similar findings.[216,217] High intakes of animal products are associated with diets that are lower in plant products overall, however, and specifically lower in fiber, complex carbohydrates, and phytochemicals, and higher in fat.

The conclusion from a comprehensive review by Phillips et al[218] published in 1983 was that there was insufficient evidence definitively indicating that meat itself increases cancer risk. Similar conclusions were reached by Klurfeld[219] and Kritchevsky.[220] Studies of members of the Mormon church support this conclusion. Mormons, who do eat meat but do not smoke or drink, have colon cancer rates similar to those of Seventh-day Adventists.[221] Similarly, in a study of 25,000 Adventists, intake of meat, cheese, or milk did not specifically increase cancer risk.[174,222] Nevertheless, several important studies have found that animal product intake is specifically associated with an increase in cancer risk, particularly colon cancer:[223]

- In one large study of Seventh-day Adventists, although there was no relationship between animal product consumption and breast cancer, both meat and egg consumption raised risk for ovarian cancer. The combined effect of eating meat, eggs, milk, and cheese increased cancer risk by a factor of 3.5.[224]

- Adventists who consumed meat, fish, or poultry three times or more per week were 2.5 times more likely to develop bladder cancer than those who consumed it fewer than three times per week.[225]
- A Harvard study of 88,000 nurses found that meat intake, especially red meat, raised the risk for colon cancer.[226]
- In the Health Professional Follow-Up Study, researchers looked at the meat intake of 50,000 male health professionals. Those who ate red meat (beef, pork, and lamb) more than four times per week had more than a threefold increase in risk of colon cancer compared with those who ate meat less than once per month.[227]

Although the data on the relationship between animal food intake and cancer are conflicting, much attention has been directed toward the role of meat in producing heterocyclic amines (HCAs). HCAs are potent mutagens that are formed when meat is cooked at high temperatures, especially when it has been grilled.[228] Most research has emphasized the relationship between HCAs and colon cancer. In experimental models, however, HCAs have been shown to increase risk for a wide array of cancers, including cancer of the liver, lung, breast, and small and large intestines.[229] Higher temperatures increase HCA formation, whereas microwaving foods produces only small amounts of mutagens. HCAs are also present in pan scrapings and fat drippings.[230]

A case-control study found that total meat intake, frequent consumption of brown gravy, and a preference for a heavily grilled meat surface each independently increased the risk of colorectal cancer.[231] There does not appear to be a clear association between the temperature at which meat is prepared and cancer risk, however.[232,233]

Finally, although speculative, some data suggest that dietary cholesterol, by increasing the level of cholesterol in the large intestinal lumen, increases colon cancer risk. Cholesterol can undergo extensive oxidation in foods.[234,235]

DIABETES

There are striking variations in the prevalence of diabetes throughout the world. In some populations it is rare or almost nonexistent,[236] whereas in others as much as 50% of the population is thought to be diabetic.[237] Although some groups are genetically susceptible to this disease (eg, Native Americans), it is clear that life style and diet affect the risk for diabetes. Within a given ethnic population, most often the incidence of diabetes among rural dwellers is lower than among urban dwellers (Figure 2–8),[238] a difference that exists even after controlling for weight.[239] Similarly, migration studies show that Westernization of the diet and life style, as is seen in

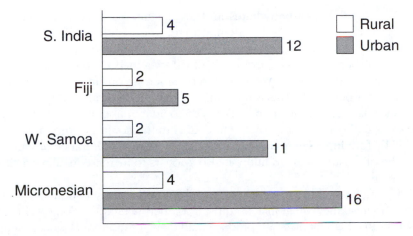

Figure 2–8 Percentage prevalence of diabetes mellitus, rural versus urban populations. Values are for men only aged 30 to 64 years age adjusted for the world population, although similar differences exist for women. Diabetes prevalence is based upon the World Health Organization criteria for glucose intolerance. *Source:* Data from reference 238.

Japanese who move to Hawaii and California and in Yemenites who migrated to Israel, is associated with an increased incidence of diabetes.[240]

In the United States, at least 13 million people, or 5% of the population, are diabetic, although it remains undiagnosed in probably half these people. In fact, as much one third of the world's diabetics reportedly live in this country.[241] Most of the US diabetics have non–insulin-dependent diabetes mellitus (NIDDM), and most are overweight. Obesity is the single most important risk factor for NIDDM,[240] and weight loss in overweight diabetics is the most effective treatment. Abdominal and upper body fat appears to be particularly important; in fact, a high waist-to-hip ratio, which is a relative measure of upper body fat, has been shown to be a risk factor for NIDDM independent of BMI, which measures only relative weight, not body fat distribution.[242,243]

International comparisons generally show that the prevalence of diabetes correlates positively with serum cholesterol levels and with intake of fat, animal fat, protein, animal protein, and sugar and correlates negatively with intakes of carbohydrates and vegetable fat.[244,245] The impact of diet on diabetes was evident during both world wars when food shortages were associated with as much as a 50% decline in diabetes-related mortality.[246]

In 1979, the American Diabetes Association revised its dietary recommendations to suggest that diabetics move away from the typical high-fat, high-protein diet that previously had been recommended to one that is high in fiber and complex carbohydrates and low in fat. Forty years before that switch, however, Himsworth[247] demonstrated the beneficial effects of high carbohydrate intake on glucose tolerance. Recommended carbohydrate intake for diabetics increased from 20% of calories in 1920 to 60% in 1986.[241]

The American Diabetes Association recommends consuming 20 to 35 g of dietary fiber per day.[248] This is much higher than the typical omnivore intake but is similar to the vegetarian intake of 25 to 50 g of fiber per day. Although the overall effect is minor, soluble fiber aids in the control of blood glucose levels by forming a gel in the intestine and delaying the entrance of glucose into the bloodstream; in addition, it also appears to increase insulin sensitivity directly.[249–251]

Reduced fat intake, particularly saturated fat, is especially important for diabetics because they are at increased risk for atherosclerosis.[252] Some evidence suggests that high-fat diets can produce mild diabetes (abnormal glucose tolerance) in lean, healthy men.[253,254] High fiber intake may protect against increased triglycerides in diabetics.[255,256] Diets high in monounsaturated fat (ie, Mediterranean diet) also seem to have benefits for diabetics[257] and may be particularly helpful for individuals who experience elevated triglycerides in response to high carbohydrate intakes.

There is some evidence that vegetarians are less likely to develop diabetes. Rates of diabetes among Seventh-day Adventists are less than half (47% for men, 45% for women) those of the general population. Within the Adventist population, vegetarians have lower rates of diabetes than nonvegetarians. In a large prospective study involving more than 25,000 Adventists, the prevalence of diagnosed diabetes at the outset, after adjusting for age and weight, was 1.9 and 1.4 times higher in nonvegetarian men and women, respectively, than in vegetarian men and women.[258] During the 21-year follow-up of individuals without a history of diabetes, the age-adjusted risk of diabetes appearing on a death certificate for nonvegetarians compared with vegetarians was 2.2 for men and 1.4 for women. After adjusting for weight, however, this risk remained high in nonvegetarian men (1.8) but was no longer elevated in women (1.1).

As indicated above, the protective effects of vegetarian diet against diabetes appear to be more evident in men than women. In men, meat consumption was directly associated with an increased risk of diabetes. Relative risks for men consuming meat 1 to 2 days per week, 3 to 5 days per week, and 6 days or more per week were 1.3, 1.5, and 2.4, respectively, compared with vegetarian men.[258] Among women, only those consuming meat six times or more per week were at an increased risk relative to vegetarian women. In this study, nonvegetarian men and women were 1.9 and 1.6 times as likely to be overweight compared with vegetarian men and women.

Meat consumption has been shown to be positively related to blood glucose levels, and saturated fat intake may increase insulin secretion and possibly lead to insulin insensitivity.[118,259] Diets based on whole grains, beans, vegetables, and fruits with isocaloric reductions of meat and total fat significantly reduce insulin requirements for most diabetic patients.[260] Research indicates that high complex carbohydrate, high-fiber diets increase peripheral insulin sensitivity in both young and old individuals and in normal and diabetic subjects.[251,260] The data do not permit one to conclude that meat per se raises the risk of diabetes, however, although vegetarian diets have been shown to be effective in treating diabetes (see Chapter 14).[261,262]

OBESITY

More than one of every four adult Americans are significantly overweight.[263] The prevalence of obesity (generally defined as 20% or more overweight) reaches 50% in some minority populations, particularly Native American, African American, and Hispanic women.[264] Obesity is much more common in American women below the poverty line, whereas in men it is more common above the poverty line.[265]

At any given time, approximately 25% of men and 50% of women diet to lose weight.[266] In 1989, Americans spent over $30 billion trying to lose weight, but with little success.[267] Unfortunately, although short-term success is common, one third to two thirds of the weight is regained within 1 year, and almost all is regained within 5 years.[265] The health care costs to this country of the morbidity related to obesity were estimated to be $39 billion in 1986.[268]

Distribution of weight is an important determinant of obesity-associated morbidity. Distribution in the abdominal area is often referred to as the apple form, whereas peripheral distribution in the femoral area (hips and buttocks) is called the pear shape. It is the apple shape that represents a health risk for overall mortality, heart disease, cancer, diabetes, and hypertension.[269-272]

Both genetics and life style affect weight. BMI differs among countries and among individual ethnic groups residing in different locations. Vegetarians tend to be leaner than nonvegetarians. For example, in a study involving 25,000 Seventh-day Adventists, nonvegetarian men and women were 1.9 and 1.6 times more likely to be overweight than vegetarians.[258] There are many inconsistencies within the literature, however.

Research on the BMI and body fat content of vegetarians compared with nonvegetarians is summarized in Appendixes D and E. Collectively, these studies indicate that vegetarians are either similar to nonvegetarians or have lower BMIs and/or less body fat. Differences between vegetarians and nonvegetarians were likely minimized, however, because of the selection criteria for study subjects (ie, obese people were often ineligible). Overall, male vegetarians compared more favorably with male nonvegetarians than female vegetarians did with female nonvegetarians. Although there are many factors that may contribute to the lower BMI/body fat of vegetarians, differences in the levels of physical activity do not appear to be one because several studies indicated little if any difference between the two groups in this regard.[106,120,273–276]

Several studies have looked at vegan body weight. Freeland-Graves et al[277] reported that the average weight of vegans was 12 to 14 lb less than that of lacto-ovo vegetarians, lacto vegetarians, and nonvegetarians. Hardinge and Stare[278] found that male and female vegans weighed about 20 lb less than their lacto-ovo vegetarian and omnivorous controls. Finally, Sanders et al[98] reported that vegans were lighter than omnivores; on average, vegans weighed 91% and omnivores 102% of the standard weight for height. Also, triceps skinfold measurements were much lower in vegans.

The relationship between diet and obesity is poorly understood. Some data suggest that eating less calorically dense diets is advantageous for weight control.[279–283] This suggests that vegetarian diets, which are somewhat lower in fat and much higher in fiber, are likely to be associated with fewer weight problems. The extent to which dietary carbohydrate is actually converted into fat *in vivo* has also been questioned.[283] A low conversion rate would favor vegetarian diets because of their high carbohydrate content. Furthermore, vegetarians may have a higher metabolic rate than nonvegetarians. In a study of young vegetarians (mid-20s, 10 lacto-ovo vegetarians and 7 vegans), resting metabolic rate (RMR) was 11% higher in vegetarians than in nonvegetarians. This was at least partly due to a higher level of plasma norepinephrine, which could result from the higher carbohydrate and lower fat intake of vegetarians.[284]

Previous studies found a trend toward a higher RMR in male[285] but not female[286] vegetarians. Also, based on differences in urinary amino acid excretion, Hubbard et al[287] speculated that vegans had higher amino acid metabolic activity. Vegetarian diet per se, however, may be no more effective in producing weight loss than other dietary patterns that emphasize low fat and high carbohydrate intake.[288–290]

KIDNEY DISEASE

Although not all studies are in agreement, some research indicates that high dietary protein may exacerbate existing kidney disease or increase the risk for disease in susceptible individuals. Protein increases the glomerular filtration rate (GFR) in healthy individuals.[291] In healthy people (those who do not have kidney disease), factors that increase the GFR may negatively affect kidney health, especially in those who are susceptible to kidney disease or in the elderly because kidney function decline is seen in aging. In 1982, Brenner et al[292] first hypothesized that glomerular capillary hypertension, which is associated with increased GFR, results from an unrestricted intake of protein-rich foods and can lead to the progressive decrease of renal function seen in aging.

Some recent studies support this hypothesis of Brenner et al.[292] For example, in a group of 2,500 older subjects who reported experiencing previous kidney problems, consuming an additional 15 g of protein was associated with a 25% increase in overall mortality during the 14-year follow-up period.[293] Because of their lower protein content, vegetarian diets may reduce risk for developing kidney disease. The GFR of healthy vegetarians is lower than that of healthy nonvegetarians (based on creatinine clearance), and, not unexpected, vegans have an even lower GFR than lacto-ovo vegetarians.[294]

Recent findings indicate that the type of protein consumed may also affect kidney function. GFR was shown to be 16% higher in healthy subjects after eating a meal containing animal protein in comparison with a meal containing soy protein.[295] Similarly, challenging the kidneys of healthy subjects with a high dose of meat protein adversely affected a variety of kidney function parameters in comparison with a challenge with soy protein.[296] Kontessis et al found that in normotensive, nonproteinuric subjects with IDDM, consuming a diet in which all of the protein was derived from plant foods resulted in more favorable effects on renal function than consuming a diet in which 70% of protein was derived from animal products. Beneficial effects may have been due to differences in plasma concentrations of amino acids and insulin-like growth factor I.[297]

Although protein has the undesirable effect of raising GFR in healthy people, its effect in kidney disease is to slow GFR, a sign of declining kidney function. Results from a study of diabetic nephrotic patients indicated that protein consumption at levels similar to those seen in the general US population led to progressive decline in GFR. Those patients whose protein intake was close to the RDA had a more stable GFR.[298] Because vegetarian protein intake is typically much closer to the RDA than omnivore intake, vegetarian diets may have a role in the management of kidney disease. The consumption of a vegetarian diet that included soy protein was shown to reduce urinary protein excretion in nephrotic patients, a sign of improved kidney function.[299] The protective effect of protein restriction is most apparent in diabetic nephropathy[300] and advanced renal disease.[301] A recent study supports the possible benefits of vegetarian diet for kidney function in diabetic subjects (Figure 2–9).[297]

Because the pathology of kidney disease is now thought to be similar to that of atherosclerosis, reducing high serum cholesterol levels and inhibiting cholesterol oxidation is thought to be important for reducing risk of developing kidney disease and for preventing the deterioration of kidney function in patients with existing kidney disease.[302] Consequently, vegetarian diet may offer additional protection against kidney disease because choles-

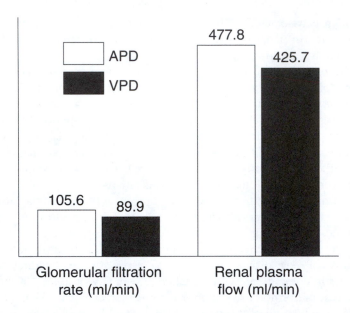

Figure 2–9 Effects of vegetarian diet on kidney function in diabetic subjects. Kidney function was studied in nine normotensive, nonproteinuric individuals with noninsulin dependent diabetes mellitus fed in random order for 4 weeks either an animal protein diet (APD) (protein intake 1.1 g/kg/day) or a vegetable protein diet (VPD) (0.95 g/kg/day) with similar caloric densities. Differences in glomerular filtration rate and renal plasma flow between the two dietary periods were significantly significant (P < 0.05, Wilcoxon's signed-rank test). *Source:* Data from reference 297.

terol levels are lower in vegetarians and because their intake of antioxidants is higher than that of omnivores, as discussed previously. The combination of reduced intakes of saturated fat, protein, and animal protein and higher intake of antioxidants suggests that vegetarian diets may be useful in both prevention and treatment of kidney disease.

RENAL STONES

Renal stones affect about 12% of Americans and are much more common in men than women.[303] Renal stones may be 10 times more common today than they were at the beginning of this century[304] and are thought to be a public health problem primarily in affluent countries.[305] About 80% of all renal stones are comprised of calcium oxalate, sometimes with a nucleus of calcium phosphate. Oxalate is present in foods and is also synthesized endogenously. Contrary to a long-held belief, consuming diets high in calcium does not appear to increase risk for renal stones; rather, calcium seems to reduce the risk.[306] The reason may be that calcium binds oxalates in foods and in the intestines, making less oxalate available for renal stone formation.

As discussed in Chapter 4, protein in general, and animal protein in particular, may promote urinary calcium excretion.[307] This may explain why people who have recurrent bouts of kidney stones tend to eat diets high in animal protein.[308–311] One recent prospective study involving 45,000 men found a 30% increased risk of renal stone formation associated with above-average protein intakes.[306] Not surprising, vegetarians may have a lower incidence of renal stone formation. A survey of approximately 2,500 British vegetarians, 73% of whom were lacto-ovo vegetarians, found that the prevalence of urinary stone formation was roughly half that of the general population.[312] Brockis et al[308] found that increased intake of animal protein was associated with an increase in the urinary output of compounds that raised risk of renal stone formation by 250%. Based on such evidence, Robertson et al[310] suggested advocating a more vegetarian diet as a means of reducing the risk of stone recurrence. Meat protein in particular appears to cause an imbalance between promoters and inhibitors of urinary crystallization by at least five mechanisms.[313]

Although most kidney stones are comprised primarily of calcium oxalate, they may also be formed of uric acid. Uric acid is derived primarily from the metabolism of purines, which are highly concentrated in meat, although some plant foods (eg, lentils) are also high. Breslau et al[314] found that, when subjects switched from a vegetarian diet in which most of the protein came from soy and some cheese, to a mixed diet containing both animal and plant protein, to one in which protein came predominantly from animal sources, dietary purine intake increased from 1 to 2 to 72 mg/day, respectively. Others have found that a diet rich in animal protein causes a doubling of urinary excretion of urate.[315] Citrate, an organic acid that is abundant in plant foods, interferes with kidney stone formation.[316] Urinary pH also influences stone formation. Animal proteins tend to decrease urinary pH,[317] and a low pH is thought to increase risk of forming both types of kidney stones. For these reasons, vegetarian diets may offer additional protection against renal stone formation.

GALLSTONES

Gallstones are the major cause of gallbladder disease in the United States, affecting approximately 10% of the population; they are as much as 3 times more common in women as in men. Cholesterol is one of the main components of gallstones.

In Japan, the incidence of gallstones increased by a factor of 5 between 1950 and 1975.[318] During this time the intake of animal protein and fat increased by 129% and 190%, respectively. In contrast, rural Africans, who consume a largely vegan diet, rarely if ever develop gallstones.[319] Similarly, vegetarians are much less likely to develop gallstones than meat eaters.

In a study of more than 800 women between the ages of 40 and 69 years, Pixley et al[320] found that only 12% of the vegetarians but 25% of the nonvegetarians had gallstones. Many factors have long been thought to be risk factors for gallstones, but of these only obesity, gender, and aging have been confirmed.[321] Even after controlling for these factors, however, vegetarians were still only half as likely to develop gallstones as meat eaters.[320]

Why vegetarians have a reduced risk is not known for certain. Some studies have found that higher intakes of calories, saturated fat, and simple sugars increase risk, whereas moderate alcohol consumption and fiber decrease risk.[322] Legume intake[323] and the intake of plant foods containing lecithin may also help prevent gallstones.[324] An additional advantage for vegetarians may be their leanness because obesity increases risk for gallstones. Although speculative, vegetable protein, in particular soy protein, may also have some advantages for reducing the risk of developing gallstones.[325]

DIVERTICULAR DISEASE

Diverticular disease has been referred to as a deficiency disease of Western civilization, referring to the lack of fiber in Western diets.[326] It is characterized by pouching and inflammation of the wall of the bowel. This defect is common in Western industrialized nations and is estimated to occur in 30% to 40% of people aged 50 and over in the United States. Symptomatic diverticular disease results in 200,000 hospitalizations in this country annually.[327] As recently as 1916, however, the disease was not prevalent enough to merit a mention in medical textbooks. Research indicates that diverticulitis is less common in vegetarians.[328]

In a study conducted in 1979, both male and female vegetarians aged 45 to 59 years and older were only 50% as likely to have diverticulitis as nonvegetarians.[328] The effects of vegetarian diets on diverticular disease are probably due to their increased fiber content, especially the insoluble cereal fibers, such as wheat bran. Bran has been shown to be useful in the treatment of diverticular disease,[329] although a recent study suggests that fiber from fruits and vegetables is also important.[330] In that study, vegetarians consumed 41.5 g of fiber per day, whereas meat eaters consumed only 21.4 g/day. Fiber increases fecal bulk and presumably decreases colon pressure, so that the products of digestion are more easily propelled through the colon.[331] Stool weights of vegetarians were shown to be two to three times those of omnivores and of individuals with diverticular disease in one study.[332]

Other factors common to Western diets may also play a role in promoting diverticulitis. A recent study involving more than 47,000 US health professionals found that high-fat diets increased risk of diverticulitis independent of fiber intake.[322] Men on a high-fat, low-fiber diet were more than twice as likely to develop the disease. Even more striking, men on a high–red meat, low-fiber diet were more than three times as likely to develop diverticulitis, suggesting that meat per se may increase risk. These findings support a previous observation that red meat intake may promote growth of bacteria that produce a toxic metabolite or a spasmogen that weakens the wall of the colon and favors the formation of diverticula.[333]

OTHER CONDITIONS

Vegetarians may be less likely to suffer from a number of other conditions, although the evidence is not nearly as strong as for those diseases discussed above.

Arthritis

Arthritis is a general term for inflammation of the joints. Rheumatoid arthritis is the most common form of arthritis, and it can result in irreversible damage to joints. It is thought to be an autoimmune disease. More than 40 million Americans suffer from arthritis. A few studies have suggested some relief from a vegan diet that includes substantial amounts of raw foods.[334–337] In one study, patients began with a 7- to 10-day fast followed by a gluten-free, vegan diet for 3 to 5 months and then a lacto-ovo vegetarian diet for 6 months.[337] There was significant reduction in pain and stiffness among the patients. Unfortunately, the studies on diet and arthritis suffer from a number of design weaknesses, so that it is not possible to draw any firm conclusions about the effects of vegetarianism on this disease.[338,339]

Gout

The formation of crystals in the joints results in an inflammatory disease known as gout. These crystals contain uric acid, a breakdown product of purines. Only about 15% of the urate formed each day comes from dietary sources. The majority comes from the normal turnover of nucleic acids. Alcohol appears to be the main dietary component associated with gout, but a diet restricted in purines can also be of some help. High-purine foods include fish, liver, and kidneys. All meats are moderately high in purines, as are some legumes. There may be some advantage to gout patients of consuming a predominantly grain-based diet.

Multiple Sclerosis

Multiple sclerosis is a degenerative disease of the central nervous system that affects more than 200,000 Americans. The signs and symptoms of multiple sclerosis include numbness, impaired vision, tremor, and lack of coordination. There are no studies on vegetarian diet and multiple sclerosis, but saturated fat may have an impact. Patients who consumed less than 20 g of saturated fat per day had many fewer symptoms than those who ate more than 20 g of saturated fat per day.[340] Another study found that progression of the disease was slowed in people who ate a diet higher in polyunsaturated fat but low in total fat.[341]

Dementia

Dementia is a major economic and public health problem. As much as 50% of the over-65 population may have mild forms of this condition, with 5% suffering from severe dementia.[342] The US economic burden attributable to senile dementia is estimated to be approximately $20 billion for the care of these persons. One preliminary report indicated that vegetarian diet may offer some benefits because, among Seventh-day Adventists, those who ate meat were found to be more than twice as likely to develop dementia.[343] If they had been eating meat for many years, they were more than three times as likely to show symptoms. One theory is that free radicals might be involved in the onset of dementia.[344] Because vegetarian diets are higher in the antioxidants that protect against free radical damage, this might also contribute to a reduced risk of senile dementia among vegetarians.

Constipation and Hemorrhoids

A specific definition of constipation is likely to vary from person to person, but technically constipation is characterized by hard stools and elimination fewer than three times per week. Constipation affects approximately 4.5 million Americans. The consumption of adequate liquids and fiber is the best approach to avoiding constipation. Insoluble fiber, such as that found in wheat bran, is especially helpful.[345] When people become constipated, they strain to pass stools. This can result in hemorrhoids, which are clusters of enlarged veins near the rectum. Because vegetarians consume 50% to 100% more fiber as meat eaters, they are less likely to suffer from either constipation or hemorrhoids.

Tooth Decay

Vegetarians may have better dental health than meat eaters, although the data are inconsistent. Several studies of Seventh-day Adventist children and non-Adventist vegetarians have shown that they have fewer dental cavities, although the reasons for this are not clear.[346,347]

Duodenal Ulcers

Ulcers of the duodenum are about 10 times more common than gastric ulcers, and they affect about 10% of the US population. Ulcer formation occurs when breaks in the mucosal barrier expose the underlying tissue to the corrosive action of acid and pepsin. The bacterium *Helicobacter pylori* is present in the majority of patients with ulcers,[348] but diet may be a contributing factor.[349] A recent prospective study of close to 50,000 male health professionals found that fiber intake, particularly fiber from legumes, fruits, and vegetables, was inversely associated with risk of duodenal ulcer (0.55 relative risk for men in the highest versus lowest quintiles of fiber intake).[350] Animal work also suggests that the consumption of flavonoids, phenolic phytochemicals present in fruits and vegetables, may help prevent the development of ulcers.[351]

THE DAIRY CONNECTION

More than 95% of vegetarians use dairy products. Thus comparisons of vegetarians with omnivores often focus on the health benefits of avoiding meat and are less likely to examine the impact of dairy foods on health and disease. Although much of the information is still speculative, some health risks have been associated with consumption of cow's milk.

Diabetes

Early consumption of cow's milk, as regular cow's milk or in infant formulas based on cow's milk, may increase risk for insulin-dependent diabetes mellitus in genetically susceptible infants. These infants may produce antibodies to milk protein that destroy pancreatic β cells, which are responsible for insulin production.[352,353] According to the Work Group on cow's milk protein and diabetes mellitus, "The avoidance of cow's milk protein for the first several months of life may reduce the later development of IDDM or delay its onset in susceptible individuals."[354] Although most work has focused on infants and young children, a recent study of children up to 14 years of age found that the consumption of cow's milk throughout childhood was associated with a twofold increased risk of diabetes.[355]

Ovarian Cancer

Some studies have found an association between dairy products and ovarian cancer,[356–358] although other studies do not support this relationship.[359,360] The biologically proposed explanation for this association involves the toxic effect of galactose-1-phosphate (from the galactose contained in lactose) on ovarian cells. Although galactose in the body undergoes metabolism, some individuals may have low levels of galactose-1-phosphate uridyltransferase, which would result in higher levels of galactose-1-phosphate.

Colic

Sensitivity to milk proteins can cause colic, a digestive problem in infants that causes great discomfort. Even breastfed infants can suffer from this problem when the nursing mother is using dairy products. Removing milk from the mother's diet has been shown to reduce symptoms of colic in breastfed infants.[361] Also, although very speculative, milk protein intolerance has been suggested as one possible link to sudden infant death syndrome.[362]

Contaminants

Microorganisms such as *salmonella* and *listeria monocytogenes* that can cause illness have been isolated from milk and other dairy products. In some cases, the bacteria contaminate the milk after pasteurization.[363] Soft cheeses are especially vulnerable to contamination,[364] and the Centers for Disease Control and Prevention recommend that pregnant women, older people, and those with weakened immune systems in particular should avoid these cheeses.[365]

Milk (Lactose) Intolerance

Many people are unable to digest the milk sugar lactose. Drinking milk can cause cramping, diarrhea, and nausea in these people. The incidence of lactose intolerance among children is relatively low, however. (Lactose intolerance is discussed in Chapter 4.)

Milk and Anemia

In children, overreliance on milk can lead to iron-deficiency anemia. This is because milk, which is extremely low in iron, may displace iron-rich foods in the diet if milk consumption is excessive. In young infants, protein from cow's milk can cause intestinal bleeding, which can lead to anemia.[366] Also, the calcium in milk markedly inhibits iron absorption.[367]

Milk and Vitamin D Toxicity

Federal regulations specify that 10 µg of vitamin D should be added to each quart of milk. Because large volumes of milk are fortified at one time, however, improper mixing of vitamin D may occur, resulting in some portions containing excessive amounts of vitamin D. In fact, in one incident of vitamin D toxicity, milk samples were found to contain 500 times the amount of vitamin D permitted by the government (see Chapter 6).

Heart Disease

The consumption of whole milk and dairy products is associated with an increased risk of ischemic heart disease in international comparisons. There is actually a much stronger correlation, however, between heart disease and dairy products excluding fat than between dairy fat and heart disease.[368,369] The proposed biologic explanation for this relationship is the high lactose content of milk. One cup of milk contains about 11 g of lactose.[370]

It has been suggested that the galactose component of lactose can participate in the Maillard reaction, the reaction that occurs between sugars and individual amino acids and can be observed, for example, when milk is heated at high temperatures. According to this hypothesis, galactose can attach to proteins that line the arterial walls, and this in turn may cause lipoproteins and cholesterol to become attached as well. Consistent with this hypothesis are two observations: First, galactose forms this reaction more readily than glucose,[371] and second, in animals lactose but not glucose increases atherosclerosis.[372] Nevertheless, the connection between galactose or lactose and heart disease is highly speculative.

Cataracts

The association between cataracts and dairy foods is speculative, but galactose has been referred to as a cataractogenic sugar.[373] As long ago as 1935, it was shown conclusively that diets high in galactose or lactose produced cataracts in rats.[374] More recent studies have confirmed these findings.[375] Although rats are much more sensitive to galactose, in humans galactose can cause cataracts.[376] In cases of classic galactosemia, ingestion of milk for just 4 to 8 weeks leads to the development of cataracts.[377] In India, where cataracts are the cause of 39% of all blindness, studies of subjects with cataracts and no other clinical abnormalities revealed that 7 of 15 such subjects had an impaired tolerance to galactose.[378] Galactose can be converted into the alcohol galactitol, which disrupts the structure of the lens;[379] galactitol has been found in the cataracts of galactosemic subjects at postmortem examination.[380,381]

Classic galactosemia occurs only rarely, perhaps in as few as 1 or 2 of every 100,000 infants, and is due to genetic deficiencies of two different enzymes involved in the metabolism of galactose. As many as 1 out of every 1,000 people have low levels of these enzymes[382] (which would be undiagnosed), however, and several researchers have proposed that lactose intake increases risk of developing cataracts in these individuals.[383,384] Consistent with this hypothesis are clinical findings from a recent study showing that drinking large amounts of milk was a risk factor for developing senile cataracts in people with a decreased ability to metabolize galactose,[385] but overall the evidence is inconclusive.[386]

Finally, dietary antioxidants, including carotenoids and vitamin C (both of which are consumed in much greater amounts by vegetarians than by omnivores), have been inversely associated with risk of cataracts, presumably because they reduce the accumulation of oxidized and denatured proteins in the eye.[387]

Milk and Bovine Somatotropin

Bovine somatotropin (BST) use can increase milk yield by 15% to 20% and can improve production efficiency (a measure of the amount of milk produced relative to the amount of feed consumed) by approximately 10%.[388] On November 5, 1993, the Food and Drug Administration approved the use of BST; that same day, in a press release, the American Dietetic Association declared that "the evidence is clear that BST does not change the composition of milk, and consumers should have complete confidence in the milk supply."[389] Nevertheless, there is considerable consumer concern about the use of BST.

Although a thorough discussion of this complex issue is beyond the scope of this book, two concerns about BST bear mentioning. First, some reports suggest that BST increases the incidence of mastitis, which is an infection of the mammary glands. Increased infection results in increased antibiotic use. The Government Accounting Office, in a report on BST, referred to this as a new category of indirect human food safety risks.[390] Second, BST works largely by stimulating the production of insulin-like growth factor type I (IGF-I), and some have argued that IGF-I would have biologic activity in humans and possibly could result in adverse effects.[391]

PHYTOCHEMICALS

The Golden Age of Nutrition refers to the exciting period of nutrition history that spanned the first half of this century, when the vitamins in foods were isolated and linked to deficiency diseases. Before that, scientists were well aware that acute diseases were associated with the lack of certain foods, as was evidenced by the famous British Navy experiments linking citrus fruit consumption to the prevention of scurvy. As early as the 16th century, Chinese sailors grew leafy green vegetables aboard ships to prevent scurvy.

The actual discovery of the vitamins allowed physicians to utilize these compounds in extensive public health endeavors to cure or prevent disease in impoverished areas through simple and inexpensive administration of vitamin preparations. By 1950, all the essential nutrients known today had been discovered, and the search for new dietary compounds of relevance had largely ended. In fact, in the 1940s Oxford University decided not to establish a nutrition department because it was believed that researchers essentially already knew all that was to be known about nutrition.[392]

Although the search for new vitamins and nutrients came to a halt, scientists from disciplines outside nutrition, such as plant biochemists and pharmacognosists, were well aware that foods contain many other substances that have potent biologic activity. It has been only within the past 5 to 10 years or so, however, that the nutrition community has begun to appreciate this. Now, the physiologic effects of these nonnutritive, biologically active dietary components, often called phytochemicals, is one of the most active areas of research in the field of nutrition.

Phytochemicals do not fit the classic definition of a nutrient. That is, their absence in the diet is not linked to acute deficiency disease, and they provide no calories. Increasingly, however, the phytochemicals are being viewed collectively as contributing to optimal health. The recognition of the importance of phytochemicals has opened an exciting new area of nutrition research because there are literally thousands of phytochemicals in foods. In fact, this new era of nutrition can be viewed as the Second Golden Age of Nutrition. The phytochemicals are, in a sense, the vitamins and minerals of the 21st century.

Phytochemicals are plant secondary metabolites, and because they are found only in plant foods, vegetarian diets are phytochemical rich. For example, soybeans contain chemicals called isoflavones; one isoflavone in particular, called genistein, has been found to inhibit the growth of a wide range of cancer cells *in vitro*.[393] Cruciferous vegetables (cabbage, turnips, broccoli, and the like) contain several chemical classes of compounds, such as indoles and isothiocyanates, that have also demonstrated anticancer potential.[394]

The sulfur compounds in garlic and onions, the lignans in flax seed, saponins in legumes, and the phenolic acids and flavonoids widely present in plant foods have all shown potential to decrease risk for several diseases, most notably heart disease and cancer. Plant pigments include over 600 different types of carotenoids, many of which have anticancer activity. In fact, the anticancer activity often attributed to β-carotene may, in fact, be the result of the combined effect of other dietary carotenoids. For example, lycopene, the primary carotenoid in tomatoes, is as potent an antioxidant as β-carotene[395] and was recently shown to decrease prostate cancer risk.[396] The biologic activities of the thousands of phytochemicals differ, but many phytochemicals are potent antioxidants, can influence xenobiotic metabolism, and the metabolism of endogenous hormones, and influence signal transduction. Also, a wide range of plant components have demonstrated estrogenic/antiestrogenic activity.[397]

When one considers that approximately 25% of the active ingredients of prescribed medicines in North America and England come from plants, it is apparent that plants are chemical factories. The National Cancer Institute screens hundreds of plant substances each year in an attempt to identify anticancer agents, and throughout much of the world plants represent the primary form of health care. Because all plants contain phytochemicals, and because vegetarians, particularly vegans, consume more plant foods than omnivores, the higher intake of phytochemicals may represent a previously unrecognized health advantage to vegetarian eating. Steinmetz and Potter, authors of a comprehensive review on phytochemicals, note that "Vegetables and fruits contain the anticarcinogenic cocktail to which we are adapted. We abandon it at our peril."[394(p438)] To this, it seems prudent to add the reminder that grains, legumes, nuts and seeds also contain phytochemicals and that a diet that makes liberal use of all types of plant foods will provide a wide array of phytochemicals and likely potential health benefits as a result.

CONCLUSION

Vegetarians have lower rates of cancer (particularly colon and lung cancer), heart disease, hypertension, diabetes, gallstones, kidney disease, and colon disease. The extent to which vegetarian diet plays a role in the better health of vegetarians is not easy to determine, but the evidence indicates that it is an important contributing factor in many instances (Exhibit 2–3).

Exhibit 2–3 The Vegetarian Health Advantage

Vegetarians have lower rates of:

- cancer
- heart disease
- diabetes
- obesity
- hypertension
- gallstones
- kidney stones

continues

Protective factors in vegetarian diets:

- Vegetarians eat less total fat and less saturated fat. High-fat and/or high–saturated fat diets are linked to an increased risk for diabetes, heart disease, obesity, and possibly cancer. American omnivores eat a diet that is 34% to 38% fat, lacto-ovo vegetarians eat a 30% to 36% fat diet, and vegans eat a diet that is about 30% fat.
- Vegetarians eat less cholesterol. Dietary cholesterol raises risk for heart disease and possibly for cancer. American omnivores consume about 400 mg of cholesterol per day, lacto-ovo vegetarians consume diets containing about 150 to 300 mg of cholesterol, and vegan diets exclude foods containing cholesterol.
- Vegetarians eat more fiber. Dietary fiber lowers risk for cancer and heart disease, helps control blood glucose levels, and possibly reduces risk for diabetes. Typical Americans eat only about 12 g of fiber each day. Vegetarians eat about 50% to 100% more fiber than nonvegetarians.
- Vegetarians consume more antioxidants. Antioxidants may reduce risk for cancer, heart disease, and possibly arthritis and cataracts. Dietary antioxidants include vitamin E, vitamin C, and carotenoids as well as the many phytochemicals in plants. Vegetarian diets are typically about 50%, 100%, and higher in vitamins C and E and are phytochemical rich.
- Vegetarians consume adequate protein but less total protein and less animal protein. Omnivores consume a diet that is 14% to 18% protein, lacto-ovo vegetarians consume diets comprising 12% to 14% protein, and vegan diets are only 10% to 12% protein. Excess protein, especially animal protein, may be linked to higher risk for osteoporosis, kidney stone formation, and kidney disease. Animal protein may raise blood cholesterol levels.

Vegetarian diets differ in many ways from omnivore diets. They are lower in fat (particularly saturated fat), protein, and animal protein and are higher in fiber, complex carbohydrates, antioxidants, and phytochemicals. All these factors may contribute to the health-promoting effects of vegetarian diets. Animal product intake per se may also directly increase risk of some chronic diseases. It is clear that vegetarian eating patterns adhere more closely to guidelines for optimal diet and are similar to the diets of populations with reduced chronic disease risk.

REFERENCES

1. World Health Organization Study Group on Diet, Nutrition and Prevention of Noncommunicable Diseases. Diet, nutrition and the prevention of chronic diseases. *Nutr Rev.* 1991;49:291–301.
2. Hopkins PN. Effects of dietary cholesterol on serum cholesterol: A meta-analysis and review. *Am J Clin Nutr.* 1992;55:1060–1070.
3. Lanza E, Jones DY, Block G, Kessler L. Dietary fiber intake in the US population. *Am J Clin Nutr.* 1987;46:790–797.

4. Committee on Diet and Health, Food and Nutrition Board, Commission on Life Sciences, National Research Council. *Diet and Health. Implications for Reducing Chronic Disease Risk.* Washington, DC: National Academy Press; 1989.

5. Nieman DC, Sherman SK, Underwood BC, et al. Hematological, anthropometric, and metabolic comparisons between vegetarian and nonvegetarian elderly women. *Int J Sports Med.* 1989;10:243–250.

6. Nieman DC, Underwood BC, Sherman KM, et al. Dietary status of Seventh-Day Adventist vegetarian and nonvegetarian elderly women. *J Am Diet Assoc.* 1989;89:1763–1769.

7. Shickle D, Lewis PA, Charny M, Farrow S. Differences in health, knowledge and attitudes between vegetarians and meat eaters in a random population sample. *J R Soc Med.* 1989;82:18–20.

8. Cross CE. Oxygen radicals and human disease. *Ann Intern Med.* 1987;107:526–545.

9. Burkitt DP, Walker ARP, Painter NS. Dietary fiber and disease. *JAMA.* 1974;229:1068–1074.

10. American Heart Association. *Heart and Stroke Facts: 1995 Statistical Supplement.* Dallas, Tex: American Heart Association National Center; 1994.

11. National Cholesterol Education Program, National Heart, Lung and Blood Institute, National Institutes of Health. Declining serum total cholesterol levels among US adults. The National Health and Nutrition Examination Surveys. *JAMA.* 1993;269:3002–3008.

12. Brown MS, Goldstein JL. A receptor-mediated pathway for cholesterol homeostasis. *Science.* 1986;232:34–47.

13. Chen A, Peto R, Collins R, MacMahon S, Lu J, Li W. Serum cholesterol concentration and coronary heart disease in population with low cholesterol concentrations. *Br Med J.* 1991;303:276–282.

14. Ministry of Public Health. *Health Statistics Information in China 1949–1988.* Ministry of Public Health, People's Republic of China; 1990.

15. Kinlen LJ, Hermon C, Smith PG. A proportionate study of cancer mortality among members of a vegetarian society. *Br J Cancer.* 1983;48:355–361.

16. Phillips RL, Lemon FR, Beeson L, Kuzma JW. Coronary heart disease mortality among Seventh-Day Adventists with differing dietary habits: A preliminary report. *Am J Clin Nutr.* 1978;31:S191–S198.

17. Burr ML, Sweetnam PM. Vegetarianism, dietary fiber, and mortality. *Am J Clin Nutr.* 1982;36:873–877.

18. Burr ML, Butland BK. Heart disease in British vegetarians. *Am J Clin Nutr.* 1988;48:830–832.

19. Thorogood M, Mann J, Appleby, McPherson K. Risk of death from cancer and ischaemic heart disease in meat and non-meat eaters. *Br Med J.* 1994;308:1667–1671.

20. Berkel J, de Waard F. Mortality pattern and life expectancy of Seventh-Day Adventists in the Netherlands. *Int J Epidemiol.* 1983;12:455–459.

21. Waaler HT, Hjort PF. Low mortality among Norwegian Seventh-Day Adventists 1960–1977. A message on lifestyle and health? *Tidsskr Nor Laegeforen.* 1981;101:623–627.

22. Chang-Claude J, Frentzel-Beyne R, Eilber U. Mortality pattern of German vegetarians after 11 years of follow-up. *Epidemiology.* 1992;3:395–401.

23. Hirayama T. Mortality in Japanese with life-styles similar to Seventh-Day Adventists: Strategy for risk reduction by life-style modification. *Natl Cancer Inst Monogr.* 1985;69:143–153.

24. Snowdon DA, Phillips RL, Fraser GE. Meat consumption and fatal ischemic heart disease. *Prev Med.* 1984;13:490–500.

25. Fraser GE. Determinants of ischemic heart disease in Seventh-day Adventists: A review. *Am J Clin Nutr.* 1988;48:833–836.

26. Fraser GE, Linsted KD, Beeson WL. Effect of risk factor values on lifetime risk at first coronary event. *Am J Epid*. 1995;142:746–758.

27. Phillips RL, Kuzma JW, Beeson WL, Lotz T. Influence of selection versus lifestyle on risk of fatal cancer and cardiovascular disease among Seventh-Day Adventists. *Am J Epidemiol*. 1980;112:296–314.

28. Neaton JD, Wentworth D. Serum cholesterol, blood pressure, cigarette smoking, and death from coronary heart disease. *Arch Intern Med*. 1992;152:56–64.

29. Resnicow K, Barone J, Engle A, et al. Diet and serum lipids in vegan vegetarians: A model for risk reduction. *J Am Diet Assoc*. 1991;91:447–453.

30. Law MR, Wald NJ, Wu T, Hacksaw A, Bailey A. Systematic underestimation of association between serum cholesterol concentration and ischaemic heart disease in observational studies: Data from the BUPA study. *Br Med J*. 1994;308:363–366.

31. Knuiman JT, West CE, Katan MB, Hautvast JGAT. Total cholesterol and high density lipoprotein cholesterol levels in populations differing in fat and carbohydrate intake. *Arteriosclerosis*. 1987;7:612–619.

32. Knuiman JT, Hermus RJJ, Hautvast JGAJ. Serum total and high density lipoprotein (HDL) cholesterol concentrations in rural and urban boys from 16 countries. *Atherosclerosis*. 1980;36:529–537.

33. Connor WE, Cerqueira MT, Connor RW, Wallace RB, Malinow MR, Casdorph HR. The plasma lipids, lipoproteins and diet of the Tarahumara Indians of Mexico. *Am J Clin Nutr*. 1978;31:1131–1142.

34. Masarei JRL, Rouse IL, Lynch WJ, Robertson K, Vandongen R, Beilin LJ. Vegetarian diets, lipids and cardiovascular risk. *Aust NZ J Med*. 1984;14:400–404.

35. Rader DJ, Ikewaki K, Duverger N, Feurstein I, Zech L, Connor W, Brewer HB Jr. Very low high-density lipoproteins without coronary atherosclerosis. *Lancet*. 1993;342:1455–1458.

36. Kukita H, Imamura Y, Hamada M, Joh T, Kokubu T. Plasma lipids and lipoproteins in Japanese male patients with coronary artery disease and in their relatives. *Atherosclerosis*. 1982;42:21–29.

37. NIH Consensus Development Panel on Triglyceride, High-Density Lipoprotein, and Coronary Artery Disease. Triglyceride, high-density lipoprotein, and coronary heart disease. *JAMA*. 1993;269:505–510.

38. Sprecher DL, Feigelson HS, Laskarzewski PM. The low HDL cholesterol/high triglyceride trait. *Arterioscler Thromb*. 1993;13:495–504.

39. Anderson JW, Story L, Sieling B, Chen W-JL. Hypocholesterolemic effects of high-fibre diets rich in water-soluble fibres. *J Can Diet Assoc*. 1984;45:140–149.

40. Mackay S, Ball MJ. Do beans and oat bran add to the effectiveness of a low-fat diet? *Eur J Clin Nutr*. 1992;46:641–648.

41. Sacks FM, Castelli WP, Donner A, Kass EH. Plasma lipids and lipoproteins in vegetarians and controls. *N Engl J Med*. 1975;292:1148–1151.

42. Ellis FR, Sander TAB. Angina and vegan diet. *Am Heart J*. 1977;93:803–807.

43. Cooper RS, Goldberg RB, Trevisan M, et al. The selective lipid-lowering effect of a vegetarianism on low density lipoproteins in a cross-over experiment. *Atherosclerosis*. 1982;44:293–305.

44. Rouse IL, Armstrong BK, Beilin LJ, Vandongen R. Blood-pressure-lowering effect of a vegetarian diet: Controlled trial in normotensive subjects. *Lancet*. 1983;i:5–9.

45. Masarei JRL, Rouse JL, Lynch WJ, Robertson K, Vandongen R, Beilin LJ. Effects of a lacto-ovo vegetarian diet on serum concentrations of cholesterol, triglyceride, HDL-C, HDL₂-C, HDL₃-C, apoprotein-B and Lp(a). *Am J Clin Nutr*. 1984;40:468–479.

46. Lindahl O, Lindwall L, Spangberg A, Stenram A, Ockerman PA. A vegan regimen with reduced medication in the treatment of hypertension. *Br J Nutr.* 1984;52:11–20.

47. Fernades J, Dijkhuis-Stoffelsma R, Groot PHE, Grose WFA, Ambagtsheer JJ. The effect of a virtually cholesterol-free, high-linoleic-acid vegetarian diet on serum lipoproteins of children with familial hypercholesterolemia type (type II-A). *Acta Paediatr Scand.* 1981;70:677–682.

48. Ornish D, Brown SE, Scherwitz LW, et al. Can lifestyle changes reverse coronary heart disease? *Lancet.* 1990;336:129–133.

49. Arntzenius AC, Kromhout D, Barth JD, et al. Diet, lipoproteins, and the progression of coronary atherosclerosis. *N Engl J Med.* 1985;312:805–811.

50. Sacks FM, Handysides GH, Marais GE, Rosner B, Kass EH. Effects of a low-fat diet on plasma lipoprotein levels. *Arch Intern Med.* 1986;146:1573–1577.

51. Roshanai F, Sanders TAB. Assessment of fatty acid intakes in vegans and omnivores. *Hum Nutr Appl Nutr.* 1984;38a:345–354.

52. Kestin M, Rouse JL, Correll RA, Nestel PJ. Cardiovascular disease risk factors in free-living men: Comparison of two prudent diets, one based on lactoovovegetarianism and the other allowing lean meat. *Am J Clin Nutr.* 1989;50:280–287.

53. Sacks FM, Donner A, Castelli WP, et al. Effect of ingestion of meat on plasma cholesterol of vegetarians. *JAMA.* 1981;246:640–644.

54. Sacks FM, Ornish D, Rosner B, McLanahan S, Castelli WP, Kass EH. Plasma lipoprotein levels in vegetarians. The effect of ingestion of fats from dairy products. *JAMA.* 1985;254:1337–1341.

55. Carroll KK. Dietary protein in relation to plasma cholesterol levels and atherosclerosis. *Nutr Rev.* 1978;36:1–5.

56. Anderson JW, Johnstone BM, Cook-Newell ME. Meta-analysis of the effects of soy protein intake on serum lipids. *N Engl J Med.* 1995;333:276–282.

57. Glore SR, Van Treeck DV, Knehans AW, Guild M. Soluble fiber and serum lipids: A literature review. *J Am Diet Assoc.* 1994;94:425–436.

58. Rimm EB, Ascherio A, Giovannucci E, et al. Vegetable, fruit, and cereal fiber intake and risk of coronary heart disease among men. *JAMA.* 1996;275:447–451.

59. Heller RF, Chinn S, Tunstall-Pedoe HD, Rose G. How well can we predict coronary heart disease? *Br Med J.* 1984;288:1409–1411.

60. Steinberg D, Witztum JL. Lipoproteins and atherogenesis. *J Am Diet Assoc.* 1990;264:3047–3052.

61 Nagano U, Arai H, Kita T. High density lipoprotein loses its effect to simulate efflux of cholesterol from foam cells after oxidative modification. *Proc Natl Acad Sci USA.* 1991;88:6457–6461.

62. Jackson RL, Ku G, Thomas CE. Antioxidants: A biological defense mechanism for the prevention of atherosclerosis. *Med Res Rev.* 1993;13:161–182.

63. Retsky KL, Freeman MW, Frei B. Ascorbic acid oxidation product(s) protect human low density lipoprotein against atherogenic modification. *J Biol Chem.* 1993;268:1304–1309.

64. Kardinaal AFM, Aro A, Kark JD, et al. Association between β-carotene and acute myocardial infarction depends on polyunsaturated fatty acid status. *Arterioster Thromb Vasc Biol.* 1995;15:726–732.

65. Naruszewica M, Selinger E, Davignon J. Oxidative modification of lipoprotein(a) and the effect of β-carotene. *Metabolism.* 1992;41:1215–1224.

66. Hostmark AT, Lystad E, Vellar OD, Hovi K, Berg JE. Reduced plasma fibrinogen, serum peroxides, lipids, and apolipoproteins after a 3-week vegetarian diet. *Plant Foods Hum Nutr.* 1993;43:55–61.

67. Haugen MA, Kjeldsen-Kragh J, Bjerve KS, Hostmark AT, Forre O. Changes in plasma phospholipid fatty acids and their relationship to disease activity in rheumatoid arthritis patients treated with a vegetarian diet. *Br J Nutr.* 1994;72:555–566.

68. Krajcovicová M, Simoncic R, Bederová A, Ondreicka R, Klvanová J. Selected parameters of lipid metabolism in young vegetarians. *Ann Nutr Metab.* 1994;38:331–335.

69. Hertog MGL, Kromhout D, Aravants C, et al. Flavonoid intake and long-term risk of coronary heart disease and cancer in the Seven Countries Study. *Arch Intern Med.* 1995;155:381–386.

70. Fuhrman B, Lavy A, Aviram M. Consumption of red wine with meals reduces the susceptibility of human plasma and low-density lipoprotein to lipid peroxidation. *Am J Clin Nutr.* 1995;61:549–554.

71. Bellizzi MC, Franklin MF, Duthie GG, James WPT. Vitamin E and coronary heart disease: The European paradox. *Eur J Clin Nutr.* 1994;48:822–831.

72. Beard JL. Are we at risk for heart disease because of normal iron status? *Nutr Rev.* 1993;51:112–115.

73. Ascherio A, Willet WC, Rimm EB, Giovannucci EL, Stampler MJ. Dietary iron intake and risk of coronary disease among men. *Circulation.* 1994;89:969–974.

74. Boushey CJ, Beresford SAA, Omenn GS, Motulsky A. A quantitative assessment of plasma homocysteine as a risk factor for vascular disease. *JAMA.* 1995;274:1049–1057.

75. Mehta J, Mehta P. Role of blood platelets and prostaglandins in coronary artery disease. *Am J Cardiol.* 1981;48:366–373.

76. Weksler BB, Nachman RL. Platelets and atherosclerosis. *Am J Med.* 1981;71:331–333.

77. Kinsella JE, Lokesh B, Stone RA. Dietary *n*-3 polyunsaturated fatty acids and amelioration of cardiovascular disease: Possible mechanisms. *Am J Clin Nutr.* 1990;52:1–28.

78. Mitropoulos KA, Miller GJ, Martin JC, Reeves BEA, Cooper J. Dietary fat induces changes in factor VII coagulant activity through effects on plasma free stearic acid concentration. *Arterioscler Thromb.* 1994;14:214–222.

79. Marckmann P, Sandstrom B, Jespersen J. Favorable long-term effect of a low-fat/high-fiber diet on human blood coagulation and fibrinolysis. *Arterioscler Thromb.* 1993;13:505–511.

80. Renaud S, Godsey F, Dumont E, et al. Influence of long-term diet modification on platelet function and composition in Moselle farmers. *Am J Clin Nutr.* 1986;43:136–150.

81. Renaud S, de Lorgeril M. Dietary lipids and their relation to ischaemic heart disease: From epidemiology to prevention. *J Intern Med.* 1989;225:39–46.

82. Ernst E, Pietsch L, Matrai A, Eisenberg J. Blood rheology in vegetarians. *Br J Nutr.* 1986;56:555–560.

83. Haines AP, Chakrabarti R, Fisher D, Meade TW, North WRS, Stirling Y. Haemostatic variables in vegetarians and nonvegetarians. *Thromb Res.* 1980;19:139–148.

84. Sanders TAB, Roshanai F. Platelet phospholipid fatty acid composition and function in vegans compared with age- and sex-matched omnivore controls. *Eur J Clin Nutr.* 1992;46:823–831.

85. Pan W-H, Chin C-J, Sheu C-T, Lee M-H. Homostatic factors and blood lipids in young Buddhist vegetarians and omnivores. *Am J Clin Nutr.* 1993;58:354–359.

86. Fisher M, Levine PH, Weiner B, et al. The effect of vegetarian diets on plasma lipid and platelet levels. *Arch Intern Med.* 1986;146:1193–1197.

87. Chetty N, Bradlow BA. The effects of a vegetarian diet on platelet function and fatty acids. *Thromb Res.* 1983;30:619–624.

88. Barsotti G, Morelli E, Cupisti A, Bertoncini P, Giovannetti S. A special, supplemented "vegan" diet for nephrotic patients. *Am J Nephrol.* 1991;11:380–385.

89. Kinsella JE, Lokesh B, Stone RA. Dietary *n-3* polyunsaturated fatty acids and amelioration of cardiovascular disease: Possible mechanisms. *Am J Clin Nutr.* 1990;52:1–28.

90. Willet WC, Stampfer MJ, Manson JE, et al. Intake of trans fatty acids and risk of coronary heart disease among women. *Lancet.* 1993;341:581–585.

91. Hardinge MG, Crooks H, Stare FJ. Nutritional studies of vegetarians. *Am J Clin Nutr.* 1962;10:516–524.

92. Garg A, Bonanome A, Grundy SM, Zhang ZJ, Uriger RH. Comparison of a high carbohydrate diet with a high monounsaturated fat diet in patients with non-insulin-dependent diabetes mellitus. *N Engl J Med.* 1988;319:829–834.

93. Phinney SD, Odin RS, Johnson SB, Holman RT. Reduced arachidonate in serum phospholipids and cholesteryl esters associated with vegetarian diets in humans. *Am J Clin Nutr.* 1990;51:385–392.

94. Melchert HU, Limsthayourat N, Mihajlovic H, Eichberg J, Thefeld W, Rottka H. Fatty acid patterns in triglycerides, diglycerides, free fatty acids, cholesteryl esters, and phosphatidylcholine in serum from vegetarians and non-vegetarians. *Atherosclerosis.* 1987;65:159–166.

95. Sanders TAB, Ellis FR, Dickerson DJWT. Studies of vegans: The fatty acid composition of plasma choline phosphoglycerides, erythrocytes, adipose tissue, and breast milk, and some indicators of susceptibility to ischemic heart disease in vegans and omnivore controls. *Am J Clin Nutr.* 1978;31:805–813.

96. Sinclair AJ, O'Dea K, Dunstan G, Ireland PD, Niall M. Effects on plasma lipids and fatty acid composition of very low fat diets enriched with kangaroo meat. *Lipids.* 1987;22:523–529.

97. Dickerson JWT, Sanders TAB, Ellis FR. The effects of a vegetarian and vegan diet on plasma and erythrocyte lipids. *Qual Plant—Pl Fds Hum Nutr.* 1979;xxxix:85–94.

98. WHO and FAO Joint Consultation: Fats and Oils in Human Nutrition. *Nutr Rev.* 1994;202–205.

99. Bjerve KS, Mostad IL, Thoresen L. Alpha-linolenic acid deficiency in patients on long-term gastric-tube feeding: estimation of linolenic acid and long-chain unsaturated n-3 fatty acid requirement in man. *Am J Clin Nutr.* 1987;45:66–77.

100. Willet WC, Stampfer MJ, Manson JE, et al. Intake of *trans* fatty acids and risk of coronary heart disease among women. *Lancet.* 1993;341:581–585.

101. Draper A, Lewis J, Malhotra N, Wheeler E. The energy and nutrient intakes of different types of vegetarian: A case for supplements. *Br J Nutr.* 1993;69:3–19.

102. Åkesson B, Johansson B-M, Sevenson M, Öckerman P-A. Content of *trans*-octadecenoic acid in vegetarian and normal diets in Sweden, analyzed by the duplicate portion technique. *Am J Clin Nutr.* 1981;34:2517–2520.

103. Crane MG, Zielinski R, Aloia R. Cis and trans fats in omnivorous, lacto-ovo-vegetarians, and vegans. *Am J Clin Nutr.* 1988;48:920 (abstr P2).

104. King H, Collins A, Ling L, et al. Blood pressure in Papua New Guinea: A survey of two highland villages in the Asaro Valley. *J Epidemiol Community Health.* 1985;39:215–219.

105. Hamman L. Hypertension. Its clinical aspects. *Med Clin North Am.* 1917;1:155–176.

106. Donaldson AN. The relation of protein foods to hypertension. *Calif West Med.* 1926;24:328–331.

107. Saile F. Uber den Einfluss der vegetarischen Ernahrung auf den Blutdruck. *Med Klin.* 1930;26:929–931.

108. Heun E. Vegetarian fruit juices in therapy in obesity and hypertension. *Forsch Ther.* 1936;12:403–411.

109. Ko YC. Blood pressure in Buddhist vegetarians. *Nutr Rep Int.* 1983;28:1375–1383.

110. Melby CL, Goldflies DG, Toohey ML. Blood pressure differences in older black and white long-term vegetarians and nonvegetarians. *J Am Coll Nutr.* 1993;12:262–269.

111. Wilkins JR, Calabrese EJ. Health implications of a 5 mm Hg increase in blood pressure. In Calabrese EJ, Tuthill RW, Condie L, eds. *Inorganics in Drinking Water and Cardiovascular Disease.* Princeton, NJ: Princeton Scientific; 1985:85–100.

112. Hypertension Detection and Follow-Up Program Cooperative Group. Five-year findings of the Hypertension Detection and Follow-Up Program I. Reduction in mortality of persons with high blood pressure, including mild hypertension. *JAMA.* 1979;242:2562–2571.

113. Ophir O, Peer G, Giland J, Blum M, Aviram A. Low blood pressure in vegetarians: The possible role of potassium. *Am J Clin Nutr.* 1983;37:755–762.

114. Melby CL, Hyner GC, Zoog B. Blood pressure in vegetarians and non-vegetarians: A cross-sectional analysis. *Nutr Res.* 1985;5:1077–1082.

115. Melby CL, Goldflies DG, Hyner GC, Lyle RM. Relation between vegetarian/nonvegetarian diets and blood pressure in black and white adults. *Am J Public Health.* 1989;79:1283–1288.

116. Wadsworth MEJ, Cripps HA, Midwinter RE, Colley JRT. Blood pressure in a national birth cohort age 36 related to social and familial factors, smoking and body mass. *Br Med J.* 1985;291:534–536.

117. Nelson L, Jennings GL, Esler MD, Korner PL. Effect of changing levels of physical activity on blood pressure and haemodynamics in essential hypertension. *Lancet.* 1986;2:473–476.

118. Gear JS, Mann JI, Thorogood M, Carter R, Jelfs R. Biochemical and haematological variables in vegetarians. *Br Med J.* 1980;280:1414–1415.

119. Anholm AC. The relationship of a vegetarian diet to blood pressure. *Prev Med.* 1978;7:35. Abstract.

120. Rouse IL, Armstrong BK, Beilin LJ. The relationship of blood pressure to diet and lifestyle in two religious populations. *J Hypertens.* 1983;1:65–71.

121. Margetts BM, Beilin LJ, Vandongen R, Armstrong BK. Vegetarian diet in mild hypertension: A randomized controlled trial. *Br Med J.* 1986;293:1468–1471.

122. Sciarrone SEG, Strahan MT, Beilin LJ, Burke V, Rogers P, Rouse IL. Biochemical and neurohormonal responses to the introduction of a lacto-ovovegetarian diet. *J Hypertens.* 1993;11:849–860.

123. Rouse IL, Beilin LJ, Mahoney DP, et al. Nutrient intake, blood pressure, serum and urinary prostaglandins and serum thromboxane B_2 in a controlled trial with a lacto-ovo-vegetarian diet. *J Hypertens.* 1986;4:241–250.

124. Prescott SL, Jenner DA, Beilin LJ, Margetts BM, Vandongen R. A randomized controlled trial of the effect of blood pressure on dietary non-meat protein versus meat protein in normotensive omnivores. *Clin Sci.* 1989;74:665–672.

125. Prescott SL, Jenner DA, Beilin LJ, Margetts BM, Vandongen R. Controlled study of the effects of dietary protein on blood pressure in normotensive humans. *Clin Exp Pharmacol Physiol.* 1987;14:159–162.

126. Brussaard JH, Van Raaij JM, Stasse-Wolthuis M, Katan MB, Haurvast JG. Blood pressure and diet in normotensive volunteers: Absence of an effect of dietary fiber, protein or fat. *Am J Clin Nutr.* 1981;34:2023–2029.

127. Margetts BM, Beilin IJ, Armstrong BK, Vandongen R, Croft KD. Dietary fat intake and blood pressure: A double blind controlled trial of changing polyunsatured fat to saturated fat ratio. *J Hypertens.* 1984;2(suppl 3):201–203.

128. Margetts BM, Beilin LJ, Armstrong BK, et al. Blood pressure and dietary polyunsaturated and saturated fats: A controlled trial. *Clin Sci.* 1985;69:165–175.

129. Sacks FM, Rouse IL, Stampfer MJ, Bishop LM, Lenherr CF, Walther RF. Effect of dietary fats and carbohydrates on blood pressure of mildly hypertensive patients. *Hypertension.* 1987;10:452–460.

130. Margetts BM, Beilin LJ, Vandongen R, Armstrong BK. A randomized controlled trial of the effect of dietary fibre on blood pressure. *Clin Sci.* 1987;72:343–350.

131. Sciarrone EG, Strahan MT, Beilin LJ, Burke V, Rogers P, Rouse LJ. Ambulatory blood pressure and heart rate responses to vegetarian meals. *J Hypertens.* 1993;11:227–285.

132. Landsberg L, Young JB. The role of the sympathetic nervous system and catecholamines in the regulation of energy metabolism. *Am J Clin Nutr.* 1983;38:1018–1024.

133. Sacks FM, Kass EH. Low blood pressure in vegetarians: Effects of specific foods and nutrients. *Am J Clin Nutr.* 1988;48:795–800.

134. Beilin LJ. State of the art lecture. Diet and hypertension: Critical concepts and controversies. *J Hypertens.* 1987;5(suppl):S447–S457.

135. Beilin LJ, Burke V. Vegetarian diet components, protein and blood pressure: Which nutrients are important? *Clin Exp Pharmacol Physiol.* 1995;22:195–198.

136. US Department of Health and Human Services. *The Surgeon General's Report on Nutrition and Health.* Washington, DC: Department of Health and Human Services, Public Health Service; 1988.

137. Muir C, Waterhouse J, Mack T, Powell J, Whelan S. *Cancer Incidence in Five Continents.* Lyons, France: International Agency for Research on Cancer; 1987;5. IARC scientific publication 88.

139. Malter M, Schriever G, Eilber U. Natural killer cells, vitamins, and other blood components of vegetarian and omnivorous men. *Nutr Cancer.* 1989;12:271–278.

138. Barone J, Herbert JR, Reddy MM. Dietary fat and natural-killer-cell activity. *Am J Clin Nutr.* 1989;50:861–867.

140. Phillips RL, Garfinkel L, Kuzma JW, Beeson WL, Lotz T, Brin B. Mortality among California Seventh-Day Adventists for selected cancer sites. *J Natl Cancer Inst.* 1980;65:1097–1107.

141. Lemon FR, Walden RT, Woods RW. Cancer of the lung and mouth in Seventh-Day Adventists. A preliminary report on a population study. *Cancer.* 1964;17:486–497.

142. Phillips RL. Role of lifestyle and dietary habits in risk of cancer among Seventh-Day Adventists. *Cancer Res.* 1975;35:3513–3522.

143. Phillips RL, Kuzma JW, Beeson WL, et. al. Influence of selection versus lifestyle on risk of fatal cancer and cardiovascular disease among Seventh-Day Adventists. *Am J Epidemiol.* 1980;112:296–314.

144. Fraser GE, Beeson WL, Phillips RL. Diet and lung cancer in California Seventh-Day Adventists. *Am J Epidemiol.* 1991;133:683–693.

145. Zollinger TW, Phillips RL, Kuzma JW. Breast cancer survival rates among Seventh-Day Adventists and non-Seventh-Day Adventists. *Am J Epidemiol.* 1984;119:503–509.

146. Thorogood M, Mann J, Appleby P, McPherson K. Risk of death from cancer and ischaemic heart disease in meat and non-meat eaters. *Br Med J.* 1994;308:1667–1671.

147. Kinlen LJ, Hermon C, Smith PG. A proportionate study of cancer mortality among members of a vegetarian society. *Br J Cancer*. 1983;48:355–361.

148. Chang-Claude J, Frentzel-Beyme R. Dietary and lifestyle determinants of mortality among German vegetarians. *Int J Epidemiol*. 1993;22:228–236.

149. Kuratsune M, Ikeda M, Hayashi T. Epidemiologic studies on possible health effects of intake of pyrolyzates of foods, with reference to mortality among Japanese Seventh-day Adventists. *Environ Health Perspect*. 99.

150. Hirayama T. Mortality in Japanese with life-styles similar to Seventh-Day Adventists: Strategy for risk reduction by life-style modification. *Natl Cancer Inst Monogr*. 1985;69:143–153.

151. Halling H, Carstensen J. Cancer incidence among a group of Swedish vegetarians. *Cancer Detect Prev*. 1984;7:425. Abstract.

152. American Cancer Society. *Cancer Facts and Figures—1994*. Atlanta, Ga: American Cancer Society; 1994.

153. Guo W-D, Chow W-H, Zheng W, Li J-Y, Blot WJ. Diet, serum markers and breast cancer mortality in China. *Jpn J Cancer Res*. 1994;85:572–577.

154. Pike MC, Spicer DV, Dahmoush L, Press MF. Estrogens, progestogens, normal breast cell proliferation, and breast cancer risk. *Epidemiol Rev*. 1993;15:17–35.

155. Goldin BR, Adlercreutz H, Gorbach SL, et. al. Estrogen excretion patterns and plasma levels in vegetarian and omnivorous women. *N Engl J Med*. 1982;307:1542–1547.

156. Adlercreutz H, Fotsis T, Bannwart C, Hamalainen E, Bloigu S, Otlus A. Urinary estrogen profile determination in young Finnish vegetarian and omnivorous women. *J Steroid Biochem*. 1986;24:289–296.

157. Barbosa JC, Shultz TD, Filley SJ, Nieman DC. The relationship among adiposity, diet, and hormone concentrations in vegetarian and nonvegetarian postmenopausal women. *Am J Clin Nutr*. 1990;51:798–803.

158. Prentice RL, Thompson D, Clifford C, Gorbach S, Goldin B, Byar D. Dietary fat reduction and plasma estradiol concentration in healthy postmenopausal women. *J Natl Cancer Inst*. 1990;82:129–134.

159. Goldin BR, Woods MN, Spiegelman DL, et al. The effect of dietary fat and fiber on serum estrogen concentrations in premenopausal women under controlled dietary conditions. *Cancer*. 1994;74:1125–1131.

160. Rose DP, Goldman M, Connolly JM, Strong LE. High-fiber diet reduces serum estrogen concentrations in premenopausal women. *Am J Clin Nutr*. 1991;54:520–525.

161. Howe GR, Hirohata T, Hislop G, et al. Dietary factors and risk of breast cancer: Combined analysis of 12 case-control studies. *J Natl Cancer Inst*. 1990;82:561–569.

162. Hunter DJ, Spiegelman D, Adami H-O, et al. Cohort studies of fat intake and risk of breast cancer—A pooled analysis. *N Engl J Med*. 1996;334:356–61.

163. Shultz TD, Howie BJ. In vitro binding of steroid hormones by natural and purified fibers. *Nutr Cancer*. 1986;8:141–147.

164. Baghurst PA, Rohan TE. High-fiber diets and reduced risk of breast cancer. *Int J Cancer*. 1994;56:173–176.

165. Willett WC, Hunter DJ, Stampfer MJ, et al. Dietary fat and fiber in relation to risk of breast cancer. *JAMA*. 1992;268:2037–2044.

166. De Waard F, Trichopoulos D. A unifying concept of the etiology of breast cancer. *Int J Cancer*. 1988;41:666–669.

167. Sanchez A, Kissinger DG, Phillips RL. A hypothesis on the etiological role of diet on age of menarche. *Med Hypotheses*. 1981;7:1339–1345.

168. Kissinger DG, Sanchez A. The association of dietary factors with the age of menarche. *Nutr Res*. 1987;7:471–479.

169. Jones DY, Judd JT, Taylor PR, Campbell WS, Nair PP. Influence of dietary fat on menstrual cycle and menses length. *Clin Nutr.* 1987;41C:341–345.

170. Reichman ME, Judd JT, Taylor PR, Nair PP, Jones DY, Campbell WS. Effect of dietary fat on length of the follicular phase of the menstrual cycle in a controlled diet setting. *J Clin Endocrinol Metab.* 1992;74:1171–1175.

171. Price KR, Fenwick GR. Naturally occurring oestrogens in foods-A review. *Food Addit Contam.* 1985;2:73–106.

172. Cassidy A, Bingham S, Setchell KDR. Biological effects of a diet of soy protein rich in isoflavones on the menstrual cycle of premenopausal women. *Am J Clin Nutr.* 1994;60:333–340.

173. Messina MJ, Persky V, Setchell KDR, Barnes S. Soy intake and cancer risk: A review of the in vitro and in vivo data. *Nutr Cancer.* 1994;21:113–121.

174. Phillips RL, Snowdon DA. Association of meat and coffee use with cancers of the large bowel, breast, and prostate among Seventh-Day Adventists: Preliminary results. *Cancer Res.* 1983;43(suppl):2403s–2408s.

175. Jensen OM. Cancer risk among Danish male Seventh-Day Adventists and other temperance society members. *J Natl Cancer Inst.* 1983;70:1011–1014.

176. Fonnebo V, Helseth A. Cancer incidence in Norwegian Seventh-Day Adventists 1961–1986. *Cancer.* 1991;68:666–671.

177. Howe GR, Benito E, Castelleto R, et al. Dietary intake of fiber and decreased risk of cancers of the colon and rectum: Evidence from the combined analysis of 13 case-control studies. *J Natl Cancer Inst.* 1992;84:1887–1896.

178. Lipkin M, Uehara K, Winawer S, et al. Seventh-Day Adventist vegetarians have a quiescent proliferative activity in colonic mucosa. *Cancer Lett.* 1985;26:139–144.

179. Reddy BS, Wynder EL. Large-bowel carcinogenesis: Fecal constituents of populations with diverse incidence rates of colon cancer. *J Natl Cancer Inst.* 1973;50:1437–1442.

180. Nair PP, Turjman N, Goodman GT, Guidry C, Calkins BM. Diet, nutrition intake, and metabolism in populations at high and low risk for colon cancer. *Am J Clin Nutr.* 1984;40:931–936.

181. Turjman N, Goodman GT, Jaeger B, Nair P. Diet, nutrition intake and metabolism in populations at high and low risk for colon cancer. *Am J Clin Nutr.* 1984;40:937–941.

182. Korpela JT, Adlercreutz H, Turunen MJ. Fecal free and conjugated bile acids and neutral sterols in vegetarians, omnivores, and patients with colorectal cancer. *Scand J Gastroenterol.* 1988;23:277–283.

183. van Faassen A, Bol J, van Dokkum W, Pikaar NA, Ockhuizen T, Hermus RJJ. Bile acids, neutral steroids, and bacteria in feces as affected by a mixed, a lacto-ovovegetarian, and a vegan diet. *Am J Clin Nutr.* 1987;46:962–967.

184. Cummings JH, Wiggins HS, Jenkins DJA, et al. Influence of diets high and low in animal fat on bowel habit, gastrointestinal transit time, fecal microflora, bile acid and fat excretion. *J Clin Invest.* 1978;61:953–963.

185. Aries VG, Crowther JS, Drasar BS, Hill MJ, Ellis FR. The effect of a strict vegetarian diet on the faecal flora and faecal steroid concentration. *J Pathol.* 1972;103:54–56.

186. Hill MJ, Aries VG. Faecal steroid composition and its relationship to cancer of the large bowel. *J Pathol.* 1971;104:129–139.

187. Finegold SM, Sutter VL, Sugihara PT, Elder HA, Lehmann SM, Phillips RL. Fecal microflora in Seventh Day Adventist populations and control subjects. *Am J Clin Nutr.* 1977;30:1781–1792.

188. Finegold SM, Attebery HR, Sutter VL. Effect of diet on human fecal flora: Comparison of Japanese and American diets. *Am J Clin Nutr.* 1974;27:1456–1469.

189. Finegold SM, Flora DJ, Attebery HR, Sutter VL. Fecal bacteriology of colonic polyp patients and control patients. *Cancer Res.* 1975;35:3407–3417.

190. Thornton JR. High colonic pH promotes colorectal cancer. *Lancet.* 1981;8229:1081–1082.

191. van Dokkum W, de Boer BCJ, van Faassen A, Pikaar NA, Hermus RJJ. Diet, faecal pH and colorectal cancer. *Br J Cancer.* 1983;48:109–110.

192. van Faassen A, Hazen MJ, van den Brandt PA, van den Bogaard AE, Hermus RJJ, Janknegt RA. Bile acids and pH values in total feces and in fecal water from habitually omnivorous and vegetarian subjects. *Am J Clin Nutr.* 1993;58:917–922.

193. Davies GJ, Crowder M, Reid B, Dickerson JWT. Bowel function measurements of individuals with different eating patterns. *Gut.* 1986;27:164–169.

194. Burkitt DP, Walker ARP, Painter NS. Effect of dietary fibre on stools and transit times, and its role in the causation of disease. *Lancet.* 1972;2:1408–1411.

195. Glober GA, Kamiyama S, Nomura A, Shimada A, Abba BC. Bowel transit times and stool weight in populations with different colon-cancer risks. *Lancet.* 1977;2:110–111.

196. Cummings JH, Bingham SA, Heaton KW, Eastwood MA. Fecal weight, colon cancer risk, and dietary intake of nonstarch polysaccharides (dietary fiber). *Gastroenterology.* 1992;103:1783–1789.

197. Reddy BS, Sharma C, Wynder E. Fecal factors which modify the formation of fecal comutagens in high- and low-risk population for colon cancer. *Cancer Lett.* 1980;10:123–132.

198. Reddy BS, Sharma C, Darby L, Laakso K, Wynder EL. Metabolic epidemiology of large bowel cancer. Fecal mutagens in high- and low-risk population for colon cancer. *Mutat Res.* 1980;72:511–522.

199. Kuhnlein U, Bergstrom D, Kuhnlein H. Mutagens in feces from vegetarians and nonvegetarians. *Mutat Res.* 1981;85:1–12.

200. Nader CJ, Potter JD, Weller RA. Diet and DNA-modifying activity in human fecal extracts. *Nutr Rep Int.* 1981;23:113–117.

201. Alavanja MCR, Brown CC, Swanson C, Brownson RC. Saturated fat intake and lung cancer risk among nonsmoking women in Missouri. *J Natl Cancer Inst.* 1993;85:1906–1916.

202. Colditz GZ, Stampfer MJ, Willett WC. Diet and lung cancer: A review of the epidemiologic evidence in humans. *Arch Intern Med.* 1987;14:157–160.

203. Zeigler RG, Mason TJ, Stemhagen A, et al. Carotenoid intakes, vegetables, and the risk of lung cancer among white men in New Jersey. *Am J Epidemiol* 1986;123:1080–1091.

204. The α-Tocopherol, β-Carotene Cancer Prevention Study Group. The effect of vitamin E and β-carotene on the incidence of lung cancer and other cancers in male smokers. *N Engl J Med.* 1994;330:1029–1035.

205. Nomura AMY, Kolonel LN. Prostate cancer: A current perspective. *Am J Epidemiol.* 1991;13:200–227.

206. Slattery ML, Schumacher MC, West DW, Robinson LM, French TK. Food-consumption trends between adolescent and adult years and subsequent risk of prostate cancer. *Am J Clin Nutr.* 1990;52:752–757.

207. Snowdon DA, Phillips RL, Choi W. Diet, obesity, and risk of fatal prostate cancer. *Am J Epidemiol.* 1984;120:244–250.

208. Rose DP, Boyar AP, Wynder EL. International comparisons of mortality rates for cancer of the breast, ovary, prostate, and colon, and per capita food consumption. *Cancer.* 1986;58:2363–2371.

209. Hill PB, Wynder EL. Effect of a vegetarian diet and dexamethasone on plasma prolactin, testosterone and dehydroepiandrosterone in men and women. *Cancer Lett.* 1979;7:273–282.

210. Howie BJ, Schultz TD. Dietary and hormonal interelationships among vegetarian Seventh-Day Adventists and nonvegetarian men. *Am J Clin Nutr.* 1985;42:127–134.

211. Ross JK, Pusateri DJ, Schultz TD. Dietary and hormonal evaluation of men at different risks for prostate cancer: Fiber intake, excretion, and composition, with in vitro evidence for an association between steroids, hormones and specific fiber components. *Am J Clin Nutr.* 1990;51:365–370.

212. Pusateri DJ, Roth WT, Ross JK, Shultz TD. Dietary and hormonal evaluation of men at different risks for prostate cancer: Plasma and fecal hormone-nutrient interrelationships. *Am J Clin Nutr.* 1990;51:371–377.

213. Wang Y, Corr JG, Thaler HT, et al. Decreased growth of established human prostate LNCaP tumors in nude mice fed a low-fat diet. *J Natl Cancer Inst.* 1995;87:1456–1462.

214. Mäkelä SI, Pylkkänen LH, Santti RSS, Adlercreutz H. Dietary soybean may be antiestrogenic in male mice. *J Nutr.* 1995;125:437–445.

215. Armstrong B, Doll R. Environmental factors and cancer incidence and mortality in different countries, with special reference to dietary practice. *Int J Cancer.* 1975;15:617–631.

216. Kolonel LN. Fat and colon cancer: How firm is the evidence? *Am J Clin Nutr.* 1987;45:336–341.

217. Lubin JH, Wax Y, Modan B. Role of fat, animal protein, and dietary fiber in breast cancer etiology: A case-control study. *J Natl Cancer Inst.* 1986;77:605–611.

218. Phillips RL, Snowdon DA, Brin BN. Cancer in vegetarians. In: Wynder EL, Leville GA, Weisburger JH, Livingston GE, eds. *Environmental Aspects of Cancer. The Role of Macro and Micro Components of Foods.* Westport, Conn: Food and Nutrition Press; 1983:53–72.

219. Klurfeld DM. Human nutrition and health. Implications of meat with more muscle and less fat. In: Hafs HD, Zimbelman RG, eds. *Low-Fat Meats.* Orlando, Fla: Academic Press;1994.

220. Pearson AM, Dutson TB. Meat and health. *Adv in Meat Research.* 1990;6:89–103.

221. Lyon JL, Sorenson AW. Colon cancer in a low-risk population. *Am J Clin Nutr.* 1978;31(suppl):227–230.

222. Phillips RL, Snowdon DA. Dietary relationships with fatal colorectal cancer among Seventh-Day Adventists. *J Natl Cancer Inst.* 1985;74:307–317.

223. Gerhardsson de Verdier M, Hagman U, Peter RK, Steineck G, Overvik E. Meat, cooking methods and colorectal cancer: A case-referent study in Stockholm. *Int J Cancer.* 1991;49:1–6.

224. Snowdon DA. Animal product consumption and mortality because of all causes combined, coronary heart disease, stroke, diabetes, and cancer in Seventh-Day Adventists. *Am J Clin Nutr.* 1988;48:739–748.

225. Mills PK, Beeson WL, Phillips RL, Fraser GE. Bladder cancer in a low risk population: Results from the Adventist Health Study. *Am J Epidemiol.* 1991;133:230–239.

226. Willet WC, Stamper MJ, Colditz GA, Rosner BA, Speizer FE. Relation of meat, fat, and fiber intake to the risk of colon cancer in a prospective study among women. *N Engl J Med.* 1990;323:1664–1672.

227. Giovannucci E, Rimm EB, Colditz GA, et al. A prospective study of dietary fat and risk of prostate cancer. *J Natl Cancer Inst.* 1993;85:1571–1579.

228. Hatch FT, Knize MG, Moore DH II, Felton JS. Quantitative correlation of mutagenic and carcinogenic potencies for heterocyclic amines from cooked foods and additional aromatic amines. *Mutat Res.* 1992;271:269–287.

229. Wakabayashi K, Nagao M, Esumi H, Sugimura T. Food-derived mutagens and carcinogens. *Cancer Res.* 1992;52(suppl):2092s–2098s.

230. Gross GA, Turesky RJ, Fay LB, Stillwell WG, Skipper PL, Tannenbaum SR. Heterocyclic aromatic amine formation in grilled bacon, beef and fish in grill scrapings. *Carcinogenesis.* 1993;14:2313–2318.

231. Gerhardsson de Verdier M, Hagman U, Peter RK, Steineck G, Overvik E. Meat, cooking methods and colorectal cancer: A case-referent study in Stockholm. *Int J Cancer.* 1991;49:1–6.

232. Lyon JL, Mahoney AW. Fried foods and risk of colon cancer. *Am J Epidemiol.* 1988;128:1000–1006.

233. Young TB, Wolf DA. Case-control study of proximal and distal colon cancer and diet in Wisconsin. *Int J Cancer.* 1988;42:167–175.

234. Kendall CW, Koo M, Sokoloff E, Rao AV. Effect of dietary oxidized cholesterol on azoxymethane-induced colonic preneoplasia in mice. *Cancer Lett.* 1992;66:241–248.

235. van de Bovenkamp P, Kosmeijer-Schuil TG, Katan MB. Quantification of oxysterols in Dutch foods: Egg products and mixed diets. *Lipids.* 1988;23:1079–1085.

236. Hazlett BE. Historical perspective: The discovery of insulin. In: Davidson JK, ed. *Clinical Diabetes Mellitus, a Problem Oriented Approach.* 2nd ed. New York, NY: Thieme Medical; 1991:2–10.

237. Knowler WC, Pettitt DJ, Bennett PH, Williams RC. Diabetes mellitus in the Pima Indians: Genetic and evolutionary considerations. *Am J Physiol.* 1983;62:107–114.

238. King H, Rewers M. Diabetes in adults is now a Third World problem. *Bull World Health Org.* 1991;69:643–648.

239. Zimmet P. The global epidemiology of diabetes mellitus. *Tohoku J Exp Med.* 1983;141(suppl):41–54.

240. West KN. *Epidemiology of Diabetes and Its Vascular Lesions.* New York, NY: Elsevier/North-Holland; 1978.

241. Nutrition recommendations and principles for people with diabetes mellitus. *Diabetes Care.* 1994;17:519–522.

242. Björntorp P. Abdominal obesity and the development of non-insulin-dependent diabetes mellitus. *Diabetes Metab Rev.* 1988;4:615–622.

243. Dowse GK, Zimmet PZ, Gareeboo H, et al. Abdominal obesity and physical inactivity are risk factors for NIDDM and impaired glucose tolerance in Indian, Creole, and Chinese Mauritians. *Diabetes Care.* 1991;14:271–282.

244. West KM, Kalbfleisch JM. Influence of nutritional factors on prevalence of diabetes. *Diabetes.* 1971;20:99–108.

245. West KM, Kalbfleisch JM. Glucose tolerance, nutrition, and diabetes in Uruguay, Venezuela, Malaya, and East Pakistan. *Diabetes.* 1966;15:9–18.

246. Himsworth HP. Diet in the etiology of human diabetes. *Proc R Soc Med.* 1949;42:9–12.

247. Himsworth HP. The dietetic factor determining the glucose tolerance and sensitivity to insulin in healthy men. *Clin Sci.* 1935;2:67–94.

248. American Diabetes Association. Principles of nutrition and dietary recommendations for individuals with diabetes mellitus. *Diabetes Care.* 1994;17:519–522.

249. Munoz JM. Fiber and diabetes. *Diabetes Care.* 1994;7:297–300.

250. Pedersen O, Hjollund E, Lindskov HO, Helms P, Sorensen NG, Ditzel J. Increased insulin receptor binding to monocytes from insulin-dependent diabetic patients after a low-fat, high-starch, high-fiber diet. *Diabetes Care.* 1982;5:284–291.

251. Hjollund E, Pedersen O, Richelsen B, Beck-Nielsen H, Sorensen NS. Increased insulin binding to adipocytes and monocytes and increased insulin sensitivity of glucose transport and metabolism in adipocytes from non-insulin dependent diabetics after a low-fat/high-starch/high-fiber diet. *Metabolism.* 1983;32:1067–1075.

252. Pyörala K, Loast M, Uusitupa N. Diabetes and atheroclerosis: An epidemiologic view. *Diabetes Metab Rev.* 1987;3:463–524.

253. Anderson JW, Herman RH, Zakin D, et al. Effect of high glucose and high sucrose diets on glucose tolerance of normal men. *Am J Clin Nutr.* 1973;26:600–607.

254. Hales CN, Randall PJ. Effects of low-carbohydrate diet and diabetes mellitus on plasma concentration of glucose, non-esterified fatty acids, and insulin during oral glucose-tolerance tests. *Lancet.* 1963;1:790–794.

255. Riccardi G, Rivellese AA. Effects of dietary fiber and carbohydrate on glucose and lipoprotein metabolism in diabetic patients. *Diabetes Care.* 1991;14:1115–1125.

256. Rivellese AA, Auletta P, Marotta G, et al. Long term metabolic effects of two dietary methods of treating hyperlipidemia. *Br Med J.* 1994;308:227–231.

257. Garg A, Bantle JP, Henry RR, et al. Effects of varying carbohydrate content of diet in patients with non-insulin-dependent diabetes mellitus. *JAMA.* 1994;271:1421–1428.

258. Snowdon DA, Phillips RL. Does a vegetarian diet reduce the occurrence of diabetes? *Am J Public Health.* 1985;75:507–512.

259. Collier G, O'Dea K. The effect of coingestion of fat on the glucose, insulin, and gastric inhibitory polypeptide responses to carbohydrate and protein. *Am J Clin Nutr.* 1983;37:941–944.

260. Anderson JW, Zeigler JA, Deakins DA, et al. Metabolic effects of high-carbohydrate, high-fiber diets for insulin-dependent diabetic individuals. *Am J Clin Nutr.* 1991;54:936–943.

261. Barnard RJ, Massey MR, Cherny S, et al. Longterm use of high-complex-carbohydrate high-fiber diet and exercise in the treatment of NIDDM patients. *Diabetes Care.* 1983;6:268–273.

262. Barnard RJ, Lattimore L, Holly RG, Cherny S, Pritkin N. Response of non-insulin-dependent diabetic patients to an intensive program of diet and exercise. *Diabetes Care.* 1982;5:370–374.

263. Sichieri R, Everhart JE, Hubbard VS. Relative weight classifications in the assessment of underweight and overweight in the United States. *Int J Obes.* 1992;16:303–312.

264. Williamson DF, Kahn HS, Remington PL, Anda RF. The 10-year incidence of overweight and major weight gain in US adults. *Arch Intern Med.* 1990;150:665–672.

265. NIH Technology Assessment Conference Panel. Methods for voluntary weight loss and control. *Ann Intern Med.* 1992;116:942–949.

266. Levy AS, Heaton AW. Weight control practices of US adults trying to lose weight. *Ann Intern Med.* 1993;119:661–666.

267. Steiger JD. Testimony before the Subcommittee on Regulation, Business Opportunities and Energy of the House Committee on Small Business, March 26, 1990.

268. Colditz GA. Economic costs of obesity. *Am J Clin Nutr.* 1992;55:503S–507S.

269. Kaye SA, Folsom AR, Sprafka JM, Prineas RJ, Wallace RB. Increased incidence of diabetes mellitus in relation to abdominal adiposity in older women. *J Clin Epidemiol.* 1991;44:329–334.

270. Bjorntorp P. The associations between obesity, adipose tissue distribution and disease. *Acta Med Scand.* 1988;723(suppl):121–134.

271. Folsom AR, Kaye SA, Sellers TA, et al. Body fat distribution and 5-year risk of death in older women. *JAMA.* 1993;269:483–487.

272. Van Noord PAH, Seidell JC, Tonkelaar ID, Halewijn EAB-V, Ouwehand IJ. The relationship between fat distribution and some chronic diseases in 11,825 women participating in the DOM-project. *Int J Epidemiol.* 1990;19:564–570.

273. McKenzie J. Profile on vegans. *Plant Foods Hum Nutr.* 1971;2:79–88.

274. Armstrong B, Van Merwyk AJ, Coates H. Blood pressure in Seventh-Day Adventist vegetarians. *Am J Epidemiol.* 1977;105:444–449.

275. Slattery ML, Jacobs DR, Hilner JE Jr, et al. Meat consumption and its association with other diet and health factors in young adults: The CARDIA study. *Am J Clin Nutr.* 1991;54: 930–935.

276. Janelle KC, Barr SI. Nutrient intakes and eating behavior scores of vegetarian and nonvegetarian women. *J Am Diet Assoc.* 1995;95:180–189.

277. Freeland-Graves JH, Bodzy PW, Eppright MA. Zinc status of vegetarians. *J Am Diet Assoc.* 1980;77:655–661.

278. Hardinge MG, Stare FJ. Nutritional studies of vegetarians. *J Clin Nutr.* 1954;2:73–82.

279. Pi-Sunyer F. Effect of the composition of the diet on energy intake. *Nutr Rev.* 1990;48: 94–105.

280. Prewitt TE, Schmeisser D, Bowen PE, et al. Changes in body weight, body composition, and energy intake of women fed high- and low-fat diets. *Am J Clin Nutr.* 1991;54:304–310.

281. Romieu I, Willet WC, Stampfer MJ, et al. Energy intake and other determinants of relative weight. *Am J Clin Nutr.* 1988;47:406–412.

282. Dreon DM, Frey-Hewitt B, Ellsworth N, Williams PT, Terry RB, Wood PD. Dietary fat:carbohydrate ratio and obesity in middle-aged men. *Am J Clin Nutr.* 1988;47:995–1000.

283. Flatt JP. McCollum Award Lecture, 1995. Diet, lifestyle, and weight maintenance. *Am J Clin Nutr.* 1995;62:820–836.

284. Toth MJ, Poehlman ET. Sympathetic nervous system activity and resting metabolic rate in vegetarians. *Metabolism.* 1994;43:621–625.

285. Poehlman ET, Arciero PJ, Melby CS, et al. Resting metabolic rate and postprandial thermogenesis in vegetarians and nonvegetarians. *Am J Clin Nutr.* 1988;48:209–213.

286. Oberlin P, Melby CL, Poehlman ET. Resting energy expenditures in young vegetarian and nonvegetarian women. *Nutr Res.* 1990;10:39–49.

287. Hubbard R, Haddad E, Berk L, Peters W, Tan S. Urinary amino acid level differences between adult human omnivores and vegans. *FASEB J.* 1994;8(suppl):A464. Abstract.

288. Hakala P, Karvetti R-L. Weight reduction on lactovegetarian and mixed diets. *Eur J Clin Nutr.* 1988;43:421–430.

289. Caswell K, Linet OJ, Metzler C, Vantassel M. Effect of lacto-ovo-vegetarian diet on compliance and success of weight reduction program. *Am J Diet Assoc.* 1991;87:1718. Abstract.

290. Lindroos A-K, Hallgren P, Sullivan M, Jagerburg O, Sjostrom L. Comparisons between a vegetarian and a non-vegetarian weight reducing regime on weight reduction and cardiovascular risk factors in obese women. Presented at the First European Congress on Obesity; June 5–6, 1988; Stockholm, Sweden.

291. Bosch JP, Saccaggi A, Lauer A, Ronco C, Belldonne M, Glabman S. Renal functional reserve in humans. Effect of protein intake on glomerular filtration rate. *Am J Med.* 1983;75:943–950.

292. Brenner BM, Meyer TW, Hostetter TH. Dietary protein intake and the progressive nature of kidney disease: The role of hemodynamically medicated glomerular injury in the pathogenesis of progressive glomerular sclerosis in aging, renal ablation, and intrinsic renal disease. *N Engl J Med.* 1982;307:652–659.

293. Dwyer JT, Madans JH, Tumbull B, et al. Diet, indicators of kidney disease, and later mortality among older persons in the NHANES I epidemiologic follow-up study. *Am J Public Health.* 1994;84:1299–1303.

294. Wiseman MJ, Hunt R, Goodwin A, Gross JL, Keen H, Viberti GC. Dietary composition and renal function in healthy subjects. *Nephron.* 1987;46:37–42.

295. Kontessis P, Jones S, Dodds R, et al. Renal, metabolic and hormonal responses to ingestion of animal and vegetable proteins. *Kidney Int.* 1990;38:136–144.

296. Dhaene M, Sabot J-P, Philippart Y, Doutrelepont J-M, Vanherweghem J-L. Effects of acute protein loads of different sources on glomerular filtration rate. *Kidney Int.* 1987;32(suppl 22):S25–S28.

297. Kontessis PS, Bossinakou I, Sarika L, et al. Renal, metabolic, and hormonal responses to proteins of different origin in normotensive, nonproteinuric type I diabetic patients. *Diabetes Care.* 1995;18:1233–1240.

298. Raal FJ, Kalk WJ, Lawson M, et al. Effect of moderate dietary protein restriction on the progression of overt diabetic nephropathy: A 6-mo prospective study. *Am J Clin Nutr.* 1994;60:579–585.

299. D'Amico G, Gentile MG, Manna G, et al. Effect of vegetarian soy diet on hyperlipidemia in nephrotic syndrome. *Lancet.* 1992;339:1131–1134.

300. Zeller K, Whittaker E, Sullivan L, Raskin P, Jacobson HR. Effect of restricting dietary protein on the progression of renal failure in patients with insulin dependent diabetes. *N Engl J Med.* 1991;324:78–84.

301. Ihle BU, Becker GJ, Whitworth JA, Kincaid-Smith PS. Effect of protein restriction on the rate of progression of renal insufficiency. *N Engl J Med.* 1989;321:1773–1777.

302. Gröne EF, Walli AK, Gröne H-J, Miller B, Seidel D. The role of lipids in nephrosclerosis and glomerulosclerosis. *Atherosclerosis.* 1994;107:1–13.

303. Johnson CM, Wilson DM, O'Fallon WM, Malek RS, Kurland LT. Renal stone epidemiology: A 25-year study in Rochester, Minnesota. *Kidney Int.* 1979;16:624–631.

304. Danileson BG. Renal stones—Current viewpoints on etiology and management. *Scand J Urol Nephrol.* 1985;19:1–5.

305. Goldfarb S. Diet and nephrolithiasis. *Annu Rev Med.* 1994;45:235–241.

306. Curhan GC, Willet WC, Rimm EB, Stampfer MJ. A prospective study of dietary calcium and other nutrients and the risk of symptomatic kidney stones. *N Engl J Med.* 1993;328:833–838.

307. Kerstetter JE, Allen LH. Dietary protein increases urinary calcium. *J Nutr.* 1990;120:134–136.

308. Brockis JG, Levitt AJ, Cruthers SM. The effects of vegetable and animal protein diets on calcium, urate and oxalate excretion. *Br J Urol.* 1982;54:590–593.

309. Martini LA, Heilberg IP, Cuppari L, et al. Dietary habits of calcium stone formers. *Braz J Med Biol Res.* 1993;26:805–812.

310. Robertson WG, Peacock M, Heyburn PJ, et al. Should recurrent calcium oxalate stone formers become vegetarians? *Br J Urol.* 1979;51:427–431.

311. Jibani MM, Bloodworth LL, Foden E, Griffiths KD, Galpin OP. Predominantly vegetarian diet in patients with incipient and early clinical diabetic nephropathy: Effects on albumin excretion rate and nutritional status. *Diabetic Med.* 1991;8:949–953.

312. Robertson WG, Peacock M, Marshall DH. Prevalence of urinary stone disease in vegetarians. *Eur Urol.* 1982;8:334–339.

313. Jaeger PH. Prevention of recurrent calcium stones: Diet versus drugs. *Miner Electrolyte Metab.* 1994;20:410–415.

314. Breslau NA, Brinkley L, Hill KD, Pak CYC. Relationship of animal protein-rich diet to kidney stone formation and calcium metabolism. *J Clin Endocrinol Metab.* 1988;66:140–146.

315. Fellstrom B, Danielson BG, Karlstrom B, Lithell H, Ljunghall S, Vessy B. The influence of a high dietary intake of purine-rich animal protein on urinary urate excretion and super-saturation in renal stone disease. *Clin Sci.* 1983;64:399–405.

316. Nikkila M, Koivula T, Jokela H. Urinary citrate excretion in patients with urolithiasis and normal subjects. *Eur Urol.* 1989;16:382–385.

317. Dwyer J, Foulkes E, Evans M, Ausman L. Acid/alkaline ash diets: Time for assessment and change. *J Am Diet Assoc.* 1985;85:841–845.

318. Kameda H, Ishihara F, Shibata K, Tsukie E. Clinical and nutritional study on gallstone disease in Japan. *Jpn J Med.* 1984;23:109–113.

319. Burkitt DP, Tunstall M. Gallstones: Geographical and chronological features. *J Trop Med Hyg.* 1975;78:140–144.

320. Pixley F, Wilson D, McPherson K, Mann J. Effect of vegetarianism on development of gall stones in women. *Br Med J.* 1985;291:11–12.

321. Bennion LJ, Grundy SM. Risk factors for the development of cholelithiasis in man. *N Engl J Med.* 1978;299:1161–1167.

322. Smith DA, Gee MI. A dietary survey to determine the relationship between diet and cholelithiasis. *Am J Clin Nutr.* 1979;32:1519–1526.

323. Thijs C, Knipschild P. Legume intake and gallstone risk: Results from a case-control study. *Int J Epidemiol.* 1990;19:660–663.

324. Tompkins RK, Burke LG, Zollinger RM, Cornwell DG. Relationship of biliary phospholipid and cholesterol concentrations to the occurrence and dissolution of human gallstones. *Ann Surg.* 1970;172:936–945.

325. Ozben T. Biliary lipid composition and gallstone formation in rabbits fed on soy protein, cholesterol, casein and modified casein. *Biochem J.* 1989;263:293–296.

326. Painter NS, Burkitt DP. Diverticular disease of the colon: A deficiency disease of Western civilization. *Br Med J.* 1971;2:450–454.

327. Thompson WG, Patel DG. Clinical picture of diverticular disease of the colon. *Clin Gastroenterol.* 1986;15:903–916.

328. Gear JSS, Fursdon P, Nolan DJ, et al. Symptomless diverticular disease and intake of dietary fibre. *Lancet.* 1979;1:511–514.

329. Painter NS, Almeida AZ, Colebourne KW. Unprocessed bran in treatment of diverticular disease of the colon. *Br Med J.* 1972;2:137–140.

330. Aldoori WH, Giovannucci EL, Rimm EB, Wing AL, Trichopoulos DV, Willet WC. A prospective study of diet and the risk of symptomatic diverticular disease in men. *Am J Clin Nutr.* 1994;60:757–764.

331. Manousos O, Day NE, Tzonou A, et al. Diet and other factors in the aetiology of diverticulitis: An epidemiologic study in Greece. *Gut.* 1985;26:544–549.

332. Segal I, Solomon A, Hunt JA. Emergence of diverticular disease in the urban South African Black. *Gastroenterology.* 1977;72:215–219.

333. Heaton KW. Diet and diverticulosis: New leads. *Gut.* 1986;26:541–543.

334. Hamberg VJ, Lindahl O, Lindwall L, Ockerman PA. Fasting and vegetarian diet in the treatment of rheumatoid arthritis—A controlled study. *Rheuma.* 1982;4:9–14.

335. Lithell H, Bruce A, Gustafsson IB, et al. A fasting and vegetarian diet treatment trial on chronic inflammatory disorders. *Acta Dermatol Venereol.* 1983;63:397–403.

336. Skoldstam L. Fasting and vegan diet in rheumatoid arthritis. *Scand J Rheumatology.* 1986;15:219–223.

337. Kjeldsen-Kragh J, Haugen M, Borchgrevink CF, et al. Controlled trial of fasting and one-year vegetarian diet in rheumatoid arthritis. *Lancet.* 1991;338:899–902.

338. Abuzakouk M, O'Farrelly C. Diet, fasting, and rheumatoid arthritis. *Lancet.* 1992;339:68.

339. Panavi GS. Diet, fasting, and rheumatoid arthritis. *Lancet.* 1992;339:69.

340. Swank RL, Dugan BB. Effect of low saturated fat diet in early and late cases of multiple sclerosis. *Lancet.* 1990;336:37–39.

341. Fitzgerald G, Harbige LS, Forti A, Crawford MA. The effect of nutritional counseling on diet and plasma FFA status in multiple sclerosis patients over 3 years. *Appl Nutr.* 1987;41A:297–310.

342. Evans DA, Funkenstein HH, Albert MS, et al. Prevalence of Alzheimer's disease in a community population of older persons. Higher than previously thought. *JAMA.* 1989;262:2551–2556.

343. Glem P, Beeson WL, Fraser GE. The incidence of dementia and intake of animal products: Preliminary findings from the Adventist Health Study. *Neuroepidemiology.* 1993;12:28–36.

344. Harman D. Free radical theory of aging: A hypothesis on pathogenesis of senile dementia of the Alzheimer's type. *Age.* 1993;16:23–30.

345. Odes HS, Lazovski H, Stern I, Madar Z. Double-blind trial of a high dietary fiber, mixed grain cereal in patients with chronic constipation and hyperlipidemia. *Nutr Res.* 1993;13:979–985.

346. Glass RL, Hayden J. Dental caries in Seventh-Day Adventist children. *J Dent Child.* 1966;33:22–23.

347. Harris R. Biology of children of Hopewood House. *J Dent Res.* 1963;42:1387–1398.

348. Tovey FL, Yiu YC, Husband EM, Baker L, Jayaraj AP. *Helicobacter pylori* and peptic ulcer recurrence. *Gut.* 1992;34:1293.

349. Tovey FI. Diet and duodenal ulcer. *J Gastroenterol Hepatol.* 1994;9:177–185.

350. Aldoori WH, Giovannucci EL, Stampfer MJ, Rimm EB, Wing AL, Willet WC. A prospective study of diet and the risk of duodenal ulcer in men. *Am J Clin Nutr.* 1995;61:897. Abstract.

351. Izzo AA, Di Carlo G, Mascolo N, Capasso F, Autore G. Antiulcer effect of flavonoids. Role of endogenous PAF. *Phytother Res.* 1994;8:179–181.

352. Dahl-Jørgensen K, Joner G, Hanssen KF. Relationship between cow's milk consumption and incidence of IDDM in childhood. *Diabetes Care.* 1991;14:1081–1083.

353. Gerstein HC. Cow's milk exposure and type I diabetes mellitus. *Diabetes Care.* 1993;17:13–19.

354. Work Group on Cow's Milk Protein and Diabetes Mellitus, Drash AL, Kramer MS, Swanson J, Udall JN Jr. Infant feeding practices and their possible relationship to the etiology of diabetes mellitus. *Pediatrics.* 1994;94:752–754.

355. Fava D, Leslie RDG, Pozzilli P. Relationship between dairy product consumption and incidence of IDDM in childhood in Italy. *Diabetes Care.* 1994;17:1488–1490.

356. Cramer DW, Willet WC, Bell DA, et al. Galactose consumption and metabolism in relation to the risk of ovarian cancer. *Lancet.* 1989;2:66–71.

357. Cramer DW, Harlow BL. Commentary: Re: "A case-control study of milk drinking and ovarian cancer risk." *Am J Epidemiol.* 1991;134:454–456.

358. Harlow BL, Cramer DW, Geller J, Willett WC, Bell DA, Welch WR. The influence of lactose consumption on the association of oral contraceptive use and ovarian cancer risk. *Am J Epidemiol.* 1991;134:445–453.

359. Mettlin CJ, Piver MS. A case-control study of milk-drinking and ovarian cancer risk. *Am J Epidemiol.* 1990;132:871–876.

360. Herrinton LJ, Weiss NS, Beresford SAA, et al. Lactose and galactose intake and metabolism in relation to the risk of epithelial ovarian cancer. *Am J Epidemiol.* 1995;141:407–416.

361. Lake AM, Whitington PF, Hamilton SR. Dietary protein-induced colitis in breast-fed infants. *J Pediatr.* 1982;101:906–910.

362. Coombs RRA, Holgate ST. Allergy and cot death: With special focus on allergic sensitivity to cow's milk and anaphylaxis. *Clin Exp Allergy.* 1990;20:359–366.

363. Ryan CA, Nickels MK, Hargrett-Bean NT, et al. Massive outbreak of antimicrobial-resistant salmonellosis traced to pasteurized milk. *JAMA.* 1987;258:3269–3274.

364. Tham WA, Danielsson-Tham MM-L. *Listeria monocytogenes* isolated from soft cheese. *Vet Med.* 1988;122:539–540.

365. CDC traces listeriosis to soft cheeses. *Nation's Health.* May–June 1992: 18.

366. Fomon SJ, Ziegler EF, Nelson SE, Edwards BB. Cow milk feeding in infancy: Gastrointestinal blood loss and iron nutritional status. *J Pediatr.* 1981;98:540–545.

367. Hallberg L, Rossander-Hultén, Brune M, Gleerup A. Calcium and iron absorption: Mechanism of action and nutritional importance. *Eur J Clin Nutr.* 1991;46:317–327.

368. Segall JJ. Dietary lactose as a possible risk factor for ischaemic heart disease: Review of epidemiology. *Intern J Cardiol.* 1994;46:197–207.

369. Segall JJ. Is milk a coronary health hazard? *Br J Prev Soc Med.* 1977;31:81–85.

370. Paul AA, Southgate DAT. *The Composition of Foods.* 4th ed. London, England: NMSO; 1978.

371. Bunn HF. Reaction of monosaccharides with proteins: Possible evolutionary significance. *Science.* 1981;213:22–24.

372. Kritchevsky D, Davidson LM, Kim HK, et al. Influence of type of carbohydrate on atherosclerosis in baboons fed semi-purified diets plus 0.1% cholesterol. *Am J Clin Nutr.* 1890;33:1869–1887.

373. Bunce GE. Nutrition and cataract. *Nutr Rev.* 1979;37:337–343.

374. Mitchell HS, Dodge WM. Cataract in rats fed high lactose rations. *J Nutr.* 1935;9:37–49.

375. Keiding S, Mellengaard L. Dose dependence of galactose cataract in the rat. *Acta Ophthalmol.* 1972;50:174–182.

376. Harding VJ, Grant GA, Glaister D. Metabolism of galactose; behavior of rat towards moderate amounts of galactose. *Biochem J.* 1934;28:257–263.

377. Rennert OM. Disorders of galactose metabolism. *Ann Clin Lab Sci.* 1977;7:443–448.

378. Bhat KS, Gopolan C. Human cataract and galactose metabolism. *Nutr Metab.* 1974;17:1–8.

379. Van Heyningen R. Formation of polyols by the lens of the rat with "sugar" cataract. *Nature* (London). 1959;184:194–195.

380. Quan-Ma R, Wells HJ, Wells WW, Sherman FE, Egan TJ. Galactitol in the tissues of a galactosemic child. *Am J Dis Child.* 1966;112:477–478.

381. Gitzelman R, Curtius HC, Schneller I. Galactitol and galactose-1-phosphate in the lens of a galactosemic infant. *Exp Eye Res.* 1967;6:1–3.

382. Skalka HW, Prchal JT. Presenile cataract formation and decreased activity of galactosemic enzymes. *Arch Ophthalmol.* 1967;98:269–273.

383. Montelone JA, Beutler E, Montelone PL, Uz CL, Casey EC. Cataracts, galactosuria, and galactosemia due to galactokinase deficiency in a child: Studies of a kindred. *Am J Med.* 1971;50:403–407.

384. Beutler E, Krill A, Comings D, Trinidad F. Galactokinase deficiency: An important cause of familial cataracts in children and young adults. *J Lab Clin Med*. 1970;76:1006.

385. Jacques PF, Phillips J, Hartz SC, Chylack LT Jr. Lactose intake, galactose metabolism and senile-cataract. *Nutr Res*. 1990;10:225–265.

386. Couet C, Jan P, Debry G. Lactose and cataract in humans: A review. *J Am Coll Nutr*. 1991;10:79–86.

387. Hankinson SE, Stampfer MJ, Seddon JM, et al. Nutrient intake and cataract extraction in women: A prospective study. *Br Med J*. 1992;305:335–339.

388. Chalupa W, Galligan DT. Nutrition implications of somatotropin for lactation. *J Dairy Sci*. 1989;72:2510–2524.

389. The American Dietetic Association supports Food and Drug Administration's approval of BST. Chicago, Ill: American Dietetic Association; 1993.

390. General Accounting Office. *FDA's Review of Recombinant Bovine Growth Hormone*. Washington, DC: General Accounting Office.

391. Epstein SS. Potential public health hazards of biosynthetic milk hormones. *Int J Health Sci*. 1990;20:73–84.

392. Lloyd B. Nourishing a nation. In: Gale M, Lloyd B, eds. *Sinclair: The Founders of Modern Nutrition*. Berkshire, England: McHarrison Society; 19xx:xx–xx.

393. Messina MJ, Persky V, Setchell KDR, Barnes S. Soy intake and cancer risk: A review of the in vitro and in vivo data. *Nutr Cancer*. 1994;21:113–131.

394. Steinmetz KA, Potter JD. Vegetables, fruit, and cancer. II. Mechanisms. *Cancer Causes Control*. 1991;2:427–442.

395. Di Mascio P, Kaiser S, Sies H. Lycopene as the most efficient biological carotenoid singlet oxygen quencher. *Arch Biochem Biophys*. 1989;274:532–538.

396. Giovannucci E, Ascherio A, Rimm EB, et al. Intake of carotenoids and retinol in relation to risk of prostate cancer. *J Natl Cancer Inst*. 1995;87:1767–1776.

397. Price KR, Fenwick GR. Naturally occurring estrogens in foods—A review. *Food Addit Contam*. 1985;2:73–106.

PART II

Vegetarian Nutrition

CHAPTER 3

Protein

A HISTORICAL PERSPECTIVE ON PROTEIN

Protein plays numerous and varied roles in the body. Half of our water-free body weight is protein, and about half of this is found in muscle tissue. Protein functions as hormones, enzymes, blood components (eg, albumin), and antibodies and is part of every cell membrane.

Historically, dietary protein has been most closely associated with animal foods. Throughout the world, however, populations have thrived on largely plant-based diets. Nevertheless, biases against the value of plant proteins prevail. For 25 years after the Second World War, much of the emphasis in the nutrition community was on eliminating the "world protein gap." The work of the Nutrition Division of the Food and Agriculture Organization (FAO) during this period was based on the assumption that deficiency of protein in the diet is the most serious and widespread problem in the world.[1] By 1975, however, it was clear that the world protein gap was a myth and that what really existed was a food and calorie gap. Throughout the world, protein deficiency is nearly always linked to calorie deficiency; that is, it is the result of inadequate calorie intake, not consumption of poor-quality proteins.[2]

There are two reasons why such an unwarranted emphasis was placed on protein during this period. First, early estimates of protein needs of infants were greatly exaggerated. Between 1948 and 1974, these estimates decreased by about two thirds, from more than 3 g/kg body weight to a little over 1 g/kg body weight.[1] Second, there was a marked underappreciation of the value of plant proteins and their ability to meet protein needs. Unfortunately, this emphasis on protein in general, and on animal protein in particular, influenced views on protein nutriture not just in developing countries but in developed countries as well. This has contributed to unsupported concerns still being raised today over the ability of vegetarian diets to provide adequate protein.

Ironically, a best-selling book of the early 1970s that purported to dispel myths about protein actually served to reinforce concerns about the quality of plant proteins.[3] Frances Moore Lappé's *Diet for a Small Planet* focused on the principle of protein complementarity, that is, the principle that the protein quality of a meal could be enhanced by combining proteins with different amino acid patterns. Unfortunately, this book created the impression that protein complementarity was an arduous task requiring careful planning and consideration. In a later edition, Lappé corrected this impression. "In combating the myth that meat is the only way to get high-quality protein, I reinforced another myth. I gave the impression that in order to get enough protein without meat, considerable care was needed in choosing foods. Actually, it is much easier than I thought."[4(p162)] Nevertheless, the notion that plant foods need to be precisely and specifically combined at each meal to support adequate protein nutrition had taken firm hold in the minds of American consumers and professionals, and it still persists among many today.

An overemphasis on dietary protein has roots that predate modern understanding of protein nutrition by a century. When scientists first discovered protein in the late 19th century, they assigned it a name based on the Greek word *proteios*, which means "primary" or "in the first place."[5] Throughout the 1800s it was believed that the source of energy for all muscular movement was produced by the oxidation of protein. The customary diets of heavy laborers and athletes were found to be high in protein, and this was accepted by nutritionists as a physical necessity. Even as late as 1939, nutritionist J. S. McLester, in his book *Nutrition and Diet in Health and Disease,* credited the consumption of large amounts of animal protein (far in excess of the current recommended dietary allowance [RDA]) for the accomplishments of Western civilization.[6]

Animal food remains a symbol of prestige and status throughout the world. In developing countries, where traditional diets generally contain little meat and dairy foods, as the standard of living rises, so does consumption of these foods. This occurs despite warnings by the World Health Organization (WHO) that this trend will undoubtedly lead to the same chronic disease patterns that plague the West.[7]

PROTEIN REQUIREMENTS

On a by weight basis, protein is about 16% nitrogen. This permits protein requirements to be estimated by conducting nitrogen balance studies because nitrogen is relatively easy to quantify. Protein needs are estimated by comparing the amount of nitrogen lost in the urine, feces, and sweat with the amount of nitrogen (protein) consumed, thus giving the amount retained and therefore the amount of protein required. Protein requirements and allowances have been debated throughout most of this century; in fact, it may be that the requirements for protein have received more scrutiny than those for any other nutrient. Disagreements have arisen for several reasons, including the following:

- Subtle signs of protein inadequacy are difficult to detect.
- Humans appear to be able to adapt relatively easily to different intakes of protein.
- Energy intake greatly influences protein requirements.
- Nitrogen balance studies are error prone.

Recently, however, newer methodologies that involve assessing amino acid oxidation have helped resolve some of these issues.

According to the most recent version of the RDAs, the adult dietary requirement for protein is 0.8 g/kg body weight.[8] This figure includes a considerable safety margin. There is a 25% increase to account for individual variation, so that the RDA for protein is sufficient to meet the needs of 97.5% of the healthy population. In addition, the RDA was rounded up from 0.75 g/kg to 0.8 g/kg to simplify calculations. Numerous nitrogen balance studies conducted over the past few decades, however, have concluded that the biologic requirement for protein is less than the current RDA value. As long ago as 1920, even diets with protein sources derived almost entirely from plant foods, such as wheat, oats, and corn, were shown to be sufficient to maintain nitrogen balance when consumed at a level of 0.5 g of protein per kilogram body weight.[9] In fact, there are published reports of subjects living on protein intakes approximating about half the RDA.[10] WHO recommends that 0.6 g/kg body weight is adequate to meet protein needs of most adults, although this figure does not allow for individual variability. Nevertheless, even when the generous RDA figures are used, it is clear that protein needs represent only a small percentage of the total caloric intake.

According to the National Research Council, the recommended energy intake for a 79-kg man (174 lb) aged 25 to 50 years is 2,900 kcal/day. This individual would require only 63.2 g of protein per day (0.8 g/kg × 79 kg), which represents less than 9% of total caloric intake (63.2 g/day × 4 cal/g = 252.8 cal/day; 252.8 cal/day ÷ 2,900 cal/day × 100 = 8.7%). On this basis alone, it is clear that vegetarians should have no problem meeting protein requirements because most plant foods, even those considered relatively low in protein, contain at least this much protein on a percentage of calories basis (Table 3-1).

Recent surveys indicate that between 14% and 18% of the calories in typical US diets are derived from protein, far in excess of the RDA.[11–13] Studies of vegetarians report that between 12% and 14% and between 10% and 12% of the calories of lacto-ovo vegetarians and vegans, respectively, are derived from protein (see Appendix A). Thus it appears that the total protein intake of vegetarians is well above dietary requirements.

Of course, the biologic requirement is not for protein per se but for amino acids and nitrogen. Of the 20 amino acids used for protein synthesis, 9 are considered indispensable or essential. The quality of a protein influences dietary protein requirements; consumption of low-quality proteins can increase overall protein requirements. The RDA for protein assumes a mixture of both animal and vegetable proteins. Because vegans derive all their protein from plant foods, the current RDA is not necessarily applicable to this group.

VEGETARIAN DIETS AND PROTEIN DIGESTIBILITY

Protein quality is determined by two factors: protein digestibility and amino acid content. In Western diets, digestibility is generally of lesser importance than amino acid pattern because most proteins are digested and

Table 3–1 Protein Content (% of kcal) of Selected Plant Foods

Food/Serving Size	Protein (%)	Protein (g) per Serving
Brown rice (1 cup)	8.5	4.9
White rice (1 cup)	7.4	4.1
Barley, pearled (1 cup)	9.4	16.4
Garbanzo beans (1 cup)	21.6	14.5
Lentils (1 cup)	31.0	17.9
Lima beans (1 cup)	27.1	14.7
Tofu, raw (½ cup)	42.5	10.0
Soymilk (1 cup)	33.4	6.6
Peanuts, dried (1 oz)	18.1	7.3
Broccoli, raw (½ cup)	43.3	1.3
Carrots, raw (1 medium)	9.0	0.7
Green beans, boiled (1 cup)	21.8	1.2
Bread, whole wheat (1 slice)	15.7	2.4
Bagel (1)	14.7	6.0
Apple, raw, with skin (1 medium)	1.5	0.3
Banana, raw (1 medium)	4.6	1.2

Source: Data from *Bowes & Church's Food Value of Portions Commonly Used,* 16th ed., by J. Pennington, Lippincott-Raven, © 1994.

absorbed fairly well. In North America, protein derived from plant-based diets, consisting largely of whole grains, beans, and vegetables, is about 85% digestible, whereas the protein from mixed diets based on refined grains and meat products, typical of most omnivores, is about 95% digestible.[14] The digestibility of selected diets and foods is shown in Table 3–2. In some countries, such as India, overall protein digestibility is relatively low (about 75%) because fewer refined plant products are consumed. Note that the digestibility of dried beans, which are an excellent plant source of protein, is relatively low (also about 75%).

Differences in digestibility may arise as a result of inherent differences in the way the amino acids in a protein are linked together, or they may be due to nonprotein factors, such as fiber or polyphenolic compounds (eg, tannins, which are plentiful in tea). In addition, a variety of processing conditions, such as heat, oxidation, and the addition of organic solvents and acids, can all adversely affect digestion. Table 3–2 shows that ready-to-eat wheat and rice cereals are digested less well than unprocessed wheat and rice. Vegetarian diets in particular may be high in components that tend to decrease protein digestibility, such as fiber.[15]

Table 3–2 Digestibility of Different Diets and Individual Foods

Type of Diet/Food	Digestibility (%)
Diet	
North American, typical mixed diet	94
North American, lacto vegetarian	88
North American, lacto-ovo vegetarian	93
Brazil (rice, beans, meat, eggs, vegetables)	78
Guatemala (black beans, corn tortillas, rice, wheat rolls, cheese, eggs, vegetables)	77
India (rice, red gram dahl, milk powder, vegetables)	75
Food	
Oats, ready-to-eat cereals	72
Dried beans (various types)	75
Rice, ready-to-eat cereals	75
Wheat, ready-to-eat cereals	77
Soybeans	78
Soybean flour	86
Wheat, whole	87
Rice, polished	89
Bread, whole wheat	92
Meat, poultry, fish, eggs, milk	95
Bread, white wheat	97

Source: Data from Sarwar G. Digestibility of protein and bioavailability of amino acids in foods. *Wld Rev Nutr Diet.* 1987;54:26–70.

There is one additional consideration: individual amino acids may not be as available or digestible as the total protein in a food.[16] For example, 90% of the total protein in wheat is digestible, but only 80% of the lysine is.[17] Consequently, the overall digestibility of a protein may be an overestimate of the actual digestibility of the individual amino acids.

Based on the assumption that 95% of the protein in mixed omnivore diets is digestible compared with 85% in vegetarian diets, it appears that vegetarians, primarily vegans, would need to consume between 10% and 15% more protein than omnivores, or about 0.9 g of protein per kilogram body weight. Little if any adjustment is needed for lacto-ovo vegetarians, who derive about one-half of their protein from animal products. Protein digestibility is just one factor affecting protein quality, however, and as indicated previously, in Western diets the amino acid pattern of a protein is likely to play a larger role in determining protein quality.

ASSESSING PROTEIN QUALITY

A variety of methods have been used to evaluate protein quality. Until recently, the protein efficiency ratio (PER) was the official US procedure for evaluating protein quality and was used for regulations regarding food labeling and for the protein RDA. The PER estimates protein requirements by measuring the growth of laboratory animals, most often rats, in response to a given amount of protein. Rats grow at a much faster rate than infants, however, and therefore they have a much higher protein requirement. Equally important, rats have different requirements for individual amino acids than humans.[18] For certain amino acids, such as methionine, the rat requirement is a full 50% higher.[19] The value of legume protein and soy protein, in particular, has been underestimated by the use of the PER because the limiting amino acid in beans is methionine.

In recognition of the inadequacy of the PER and the expense and time required to conduct these tests, a number of health agencies, including the FAO/WHO[20] and the Food and Drug Administration,[21] have adopted the protein digestibility corrected amino acid score (PDCAAS) as an official assay for evaluating protein quality. The PDCAAS, which may have some flaws,[22,23] is the amino acid score using amino acid requirements for 2- to 5-year-old children with a correction factor for digestibility:

$$\text{PDCAAS} = \frac{\text{Amino acid content (mg/g protein) in food protein} \times \text{digestibility}}{\text{Amino acid content in 1985 FAO/WHO/United Nations University pattern for children ages 2 to 5 years}}$$

PDCAASs for various proteins are shown in Table 3–3.

Table 3–3 Protein Digestibility Corrected Amino Acid Scores (PDCAAS) for Selected Plant and Animal Foods

Food	PDCAAS
Casein	1.00
Egg white	1.00
Beef	1.00
Soy protein concentrate	0.99
Pea flour	0.69
Kidney beans (canned)	0.68
Pinto beans (canned)	0.57
Rolled oats	0.57
Whole wheat	0.40
Lentils (canned)	0.51
Wheat gluten	0.25
Whole wheat flour plus pea flour (50:50)	0.82
Whole wheat flour plus soy protein (50:50)	0.72

Source: Data from Protein Quality Evaluation, Report of the Joint FAO/WHO Expert, Food, and Agricultural Organization of the United Nations, Rome, Italy; 1990 and Sarwar G, McDonough FE. Evaluation of Protein Digestibility—Corrected Amino Acid Score Method for Assessing Protein Quality of Foods. *Journal of Association of Official Analytical Chemistry,* 73:347-356, 1990.

PLANT PROTEINS AND NITROGEN BALANCE

Plant proteins tend to be limiting in one or more amino acids. Cereals are low in lysine and threonine, whereas legumes are low in the sulfur amino acids methionine and cysteine. Proteins are typically considered complete if they supply all the essential amino acids necessary to meet biologic requirements when consumed at the recommended level of total protein intake. Basic nutrition texts generally refer to animal proteins as complete and to plant proteins as incomplete. This terminology not only is of little practical relevance but is also misleading, however.

With the exception of gelatin, all proteins contain all the amino acids. Meeting biologic requirements for amino acids in the case of a low-quality protein simply means that more of that particular protein must be consumed. How much more will depend on the amino acid content of the protein in question. For example, Young and colleagues[24] found that, to maintain nitrogen balance in 16 young men, twice as much wheat protein as beef protein (96 versus 178 mg of nitrogen per kilogram body weight) was required. Similarly, about 35% more rice protein than egg protein was required to achieve nitrogen balance in young men (0.65 versus 0.87 g/kg).[25] Because of the high quality of soybean protein, similar amounts of protein were required to maintain subjects in nitrogen balance when derived from soy compared with cow's milk[26] or beef.[27]

Differences in the amount of plant versus animal protein required to achieve nitrogen balance are not trivial, but they do not justify the inferior category to which plant proteins are commonly relegated. The quality of many plant proteins is reasonably good, and protein requirements can easily be met without using animal foods, especially when mixed plant proteins are used.

The ability of plant protein to meet protein needs when fed as the sole source of protein was demonstrated in the Michigan State University Bread Study. University students aged 19 to 27 years were fed diets for 50 days that provided 70 g of protein per day, 90% to 95% of which was derived from wheat flour, with the remaining protein coming from fruits and vegetables.[28] Results indicated that, on average, subjects were in nitrogen balance. Several other studies,[29-32] although not all,[33] have also found that wheat protein can meet protein needs. This helps to explain the lack of protein deficiency (although marasmus still occurs) in the Middle East, where at one time bread provided 70% to 95% of the calories in the diet.[34-37] Similarly, studies have also found that when rice contributes a large percentage of the calories in the diet, as it does in many Asian countries (as much as 75%),[38,39] nitrogen balance is maintained.[39,40]

There is one point worth noting about the Michigan State University Bread Study. The length of this study was considerably longer than is typical for nitrogen balance studies. This is important because short-term studies fail to allow for adaptation to low-protein diets. In fact, subjects in the Michigan State Bread Study were in negative nitrogen balance during the first 2 weeks but gradually entered into nitrogen balance. A fairly immediate physiologic response to conserve body protein when challenged with a low protein intake is to reduce the rate at which individual amino acids are catabolized.[41] In rats, for example, the catabolism of lysine is decreased by as much as 50% in response to a lysine-deficient diet.[42] The ability to reuse the nitrogen from the catabolism of amino acids is also enhanced when protein is in short supply.[43] This flexibility allows the body to adapt to different levels of protein intake. It is well known that in malnourished children protein catabolism and synthesis are slowed.[44]

Several other nitrogen balance studies involving single plant proteins other than wheat, such as those using potato protein[45,46] and corn protein,[47] have also found that subjects were able to achieve nitrogen balance. However, even though these subjects were in nitrogen balance, the amounts of essential amino acids in the diets did not appear to meet newly established estimates of amino acid requirements, which are based in part on the oxidation of individual amino acids.[48-50] In spite of our ability to adapt to low-protein diets, there is some concern that chronic low protein intakes may result in subtle adverse effects. That is, the level of protein and individual amino acids in these diets may be sufficient for one to survive but not necessarily to thrive.[50] Balance studies may not provide the best estimate of individual amino acid and total protein requirements for optimal health. Nevertheless, these studies lend credence to observations that plant proteins support protein needs. Furthermore, because vegetarians actually consume a variety of plant protein foods, requirements can be met with ease on diets that contain no animal products. The benefit of protein complementarity is one factor that enhances protein quality of foods.

PROTEIN COMPLEMENTARITY

Historically, recommendations to vegetarians included instructions to combine complementary proteins at each meal to ensure adequate protein intake. More recently, the American Dietetic Association, in its position paper on vegetarian diets, noted "Plant sources of protein alone can provide adequate amounts of the essential and nonessential amino acids, assuming that dietary protein sources from plants are reasonably varied and that caloric intake is sufficient to meet energy needs. . . . Conscious combining of these foods within a given meal as the complementary protein dictum suggests is unnecessary."[51(p1317)] Experts in protein nutrition largely concur with this, although recommendations for children may be less flexible.[41,48]

These more flexible guidelines take into consideration the contribution of the pool of indispensable amino acids that is maintained by the body.[52,53] This reserve provides free amino acids that can be used to complement dietary proteins. This pool comes from as many as three sources:

1. enzymes secreted into the intestine to digest proteins
2. intestinal cells sloughed off into the intestine
3. a pool of free amino acids, particularly lysine, in the intracellular spaces of the skeletal musculature.

These three sources may be quite significant. In fact, the amount of endogenous protein present in the gut may be much greater than the amount of protein we ingest.[54] Also, it has been estimated that after a protein-rich meal as much as 60% of the adult daily requirement for lysine may be deposited in the intracellular spaces of the skeletal musculature within 3 hours.[48,55] Consequently, if one were to consume at one sitting a meal composed primarily of beans, which are high in lysine, there would be plenty of stored lysine to be used for protein synthesis if a meal comprising primarily grains was consumed later in the day. As a result, complementary plant proteins can still combine to produce proteins of a higher quality even when they are not consumed at the same time.

Animal studies first demonstrating the benefits of protein complementarity were conducted some 50 years ago.[56,57] From these studies and others,[58] it has been shown that feeding complementary proteins between 10 hours and 1 day apart does not promote growth in comparison with feeding these proteins simultaneously. Complementary effects were observed, however, when rats were fed complementary proteins (rice and mung beans) approximately 5 hours apart.[59] In humans, though, it is still unclear as to how far apart proteins can be eaten to derive the benefits of complementary amino acid patterns. In children, the effects of adding beans to a corn diet were somewhat less when the supplement was given at intervals of more than 6 hours.[48]

Additional research is required to address definitively the effects of timing on the benefits of protein complementarity in humans. It is somewhat surprising, given the amount of research involving vegetarian issues, that studies to resolve this issue have not been conducted. Perhaps this is because the answer may be of little practical significance for two reasons. First, populations consuming largely plant-based diets tend to eat complementary proteins as part of their normal eating pattern. Some examples include rice and soybean products in Asian countries, chick peas and tahini (sesame butter) in Middle Eastern countries, and pinto beans and corn tortillas in Latin American countries. Second, although combining proteins can reduce the amount of dietary protein required to meet biologic requirements,[60–62] adults can meet essential amino acid requirements by eating a variety of foods, even if those foods do not complement one another. Table 3–4 illustrates the estimated amounts of rice and beans needed to meet essential amino acid requirements for adults without considering the benefits of protein complementarity. In reality, of course, the proteins in these foods will complement each other and will combine with the body's amino acid pool so that protein needs are met even more easily.

Protein combining may be of significance for infants and young children, however. Infants and young children have higher protein needs (infants, 1.2 to 1.5 g/kg; adults, 0.8 g/kg), although their energy requirements are also higher on a body weight basis. Some work suggests that their requirement for essential amino acids is also much higher,[8,63,64] although there is some dispute about this. Additionally, many plant foods are high in bulk, so that consuming enough of these foods to meet protein and calorie needs may be somewhat more difficult. The consumption of refined foods may help circumvent this problem. Also, children do eat more frequently than adults, so that some complementary effects are likely to occur even without conscious effort toward combining proteins at each meal.

Table 3–4 Estimated Amounts of Rice and Lentils Needed To Meet Biologic Requirements for Essential Amino Acids without the Benefits of Protein Complementarity*

Food	Rice	Lentils
Protein content (% calories)	8	28
Protein (g) per cup	5.5	18
Lysine content (mg/g protein)	31	64
Sulfur amino acid content (mg/g protein)	37	25
Score[†] (limiting amino acid = lysine)	62	
Score[†] (limiting amino acid = sulfur amino acid)		86
Usable lysine (mg) per cup	170	714
	$(5.5\ g \times 31\ mg/g)$	$(18\ g \times 64\ mg/g)$
		$\times 0.62$
Usable sulfur amino acid (mg) per cup	175	450
	$(5.5\ g \times 37\ mg/g)$	$(18\ g \times 25)$
	$\times 0.86$	

*According to the RDAs, when the recommended level of protein intake is consumed (0.75 g/kg), lysine and sulfur amino acid (SAA) requirements are 58 and 25 mg per gram of protein, respectively. Thus a 70-kg person requires 3,045 mg of lysine [(70 kg x 0.75 g/kg) x 58 mg/g = 3,045 mg] and 1,313 mg of SAA [(70 kg x 0.75 g/kg) x 25 mg/g = 1313 mg]. Therefore, without considering protein complementarity, the consumption of 6 cups of rice (1,020 mg) and 3 cups of beans (2,142 mg) will provide 3,162 mg of lysine and 2,400 mg of SAA (1,050 mg from rice and 1,350 mg from beans), thereby meeting biologic requirements for essential amino acids. These calculations, however, do not consider digestibility. If one assumes that these foods are only 85% digestible, then an additional cup of beans would be required. Of course, in reality a vegetarian diet would include many other sources of protein; for example, one slice of bread contains 2 g of protein. Also, there will almost certainly be some reduction in the amount of protein required as a result of complementarity.

†Amino acid score refers to the percentage adequacy for the amino acid in greatest deficit.

CONCLUSION

Other than allowances for the lower digestibility of plant proteins, there appears to be little reason to think that protein intake should be markedly increased on vegetarian diets. A reasonable adjustment to the current RDA value, allowing for the lower digestibility and perhaps the somewhat poorer amino acid pattern of plant proteins, would be about 25%, or 1.0 g of protein per kilogram body weight. This value is consistent with nitrogen balance studies involving plant-based diets.[65–67] Based on this recommendation, vegetarians need to consume diets that are approximately 10% protein on a caloric basis. Both lacto-ovo vegetarians and vegans consume diets that contain at least this amount (Appendix A). Of course, the "vegetarian RDA" assumes an adequate caloric intake, as does the standard RDA. Energy intake positively influences nitrogen retention; for example, the consumption of excess calories (700 to 1,000 excess calories per day) reduces the amount of protein required to achieve nitrogen balance by approximately 30% and 50% for animal and plant proteins, respectively.[25]

The notion that strictly plant-based diets can adequately meet protein is not new. In 1946, based on a series of nitrogen balance studies, Hegsted concluded "it is most unlikely that protein deficiency will develop in apparently healthy adults on a diet in which cereals and vegetables supply adequate calories."[68(p282)] As many Americans shift toward semivegetarian or completely vegetarian diets and even vegan diets, meeting protein needs is likely to be a concern voiced by increasing numbers of clients. Dietitians can assure these clients that such concerns are unnecessary. In fact, the opposite would appear to be the case. Consuming protein via plant foods will almost certainly result in lower fat, saturated fat, and cholesterol intakes and a higher fiber and complex carbohydrate intake. As discussed in Chapter 2, diets composed primarily of plant foods are likely to reduce risk of several chronic diseases.

Protein should be an issue of little concern to vegetarians. Protein needs are easily met when the diet includes a variety of plant foods and calorie intake is adequate. The protein intake of vegetarians, even with slightly elevated needs, is adequate. As noted in Table 3–1, with the exception of fruits many plant foods are high in protein when expressed on a caloric basis. In fact, because of the high fat content of animal foods, many plant foods are actually higher in protein than animal products, such as regular ground beef (32% of calories) and whole milk (21% of calories).

New vegetarians often express concern about this nutrient, however. A nutritional analysis of their food record can often help assure them that protein needs are being adequately met. Many vegetarians will need to be updated on the newer information about protein combining.

The following points can help in counseling vegetarians on meeting protein needs:

- All plant proteins are complete in that they provide all the essential amino acids needed for health. Classifying proteins as incomplete or complete is misleading.
- Eating combinations of plant foods helps improve the overall quality of the proteins in those foods. Old ideas about eating certain combinations of foods at each meal are outdated, however.
- Protein combining means eating a variety of protein-rich foods throughout the day (eg, several servings every day of grains, beans, vegetables, and possibly nuts or seeds). The proteins in these foods combine with one another and with a pool of endogenous amino acids in the body to provide adequate, high-quality protein.

- Consuming adequate calories is important for meeting protein needs. When caloric intake is inadequate, protein needs increase.
- Almost without exception, people, including vegetarians, consume more protein than required. There is no advantage to eating excess protein.

REFERENCES

1. Carpenter KJ. The history of enthusiasm for protein. *J Nutr.* 1986;116:1364–1370.
2. Sukahatme PV. Size and nature of the protein gap. *Nutr Rev.* 1970;28:223–226.
3. Lappé FM. *Diet for a Small Planet.* New York, NY: Ballantine; 1971.
4. Lappé FM. *Diet for a Small Planet.* New York, NY: Ballantine; 1982.
5. Chenault AA. *Nutrition and Health.* New York, NY: Holt, Rinehart & Winston; 1983.
6. McLester JS. *Nutrition and Diet in Health and Disease.* Philadelphia, Pa: Saunders; 1939.
7. World Health Organization (WHO). *Diet, Nutrition, and the Prevention of Chronic Diseases* (Technical Report Series 797). Geneva, Switzerland: WHO; 1990.
8. National Research Council. *Recommended Dietary Allowances.* 10th ed. Washington, DC: National Academy Press; 1989.
9. Sherman HC. Protein requirement of maintenance in man and the nutritive efficiency of bread protein. *J Biol Chem.* 1920;41:97–109.
10. Strieck FR. Metabolic studies in a man who lived for years on a minimum protein diet. *Ann Intern Med.* 1937;11:643–650.
11. US Department of Agriculture. *Nationwide Food Consumption Survey 1977–1978. Food Intakes: Individuals in 48 States. Year 1977–1978* (report 1–1). Hyattsville, Md: Consumer Nutrition Division, Human Nutrition Information Service, Department of Agriculture; 1983.
12. US Department of Agriculture. *Nationwide Food Consumption Survey. Continuing Survey of Food Intakes by Individuals. Men 19–50 Years, 1 Day, 1985* (report 85–3). Hyattsville, Md: Nutrition Monitoring Division, Human Nutrition Information Service, Department of Agriculture; 1986.
13. US Department of Agriculture. *Nationwide Food Consumption Survey. Continuing Survey of Food Intakes by Individuals. Women 19–50 Years and Their Children 1–5 Years, 4 Days, 1985* (report 85–4). Hyattsville, Md: Nutrition Monitoring Division, Human Nutrition Information Service, Department of Agriculture; 1987.
14. Joint Food and Agricultural Organization/World Health Organization/United Nations University Expert Consultation. (World Health Organization Technical Report Series 724.) Geneva, Switzerland: World Health Organization; 1985.
15. Acosta PB. Availability of essential amino acids and nitrogen in vegan diets. *Am J Clin Nutr.* 1988;48:868–874.
16. Sarwar G, Peace RW. Comparisons between true digestibility of total nitrogen and limiting amino acids in vegetable proteins fed to rats. *J Nutr.* 1986;116:1172–1184.
17. Eggum BO. Digestibility of plant proteins: Animal studies. In: Finley JW, Hopkins DT, eds. *Digestibility and Amino Acid Availability of Cereals and Oilseeds.* St Paul, Minn: American Association of Cereal Chemists; 1985:275–283.

18. Steinke FH. Measuring protein quality of foods. In: Wilcke HL, Hopkins DT, Waggle DH, eds. *Soy Protein and Human Nutrition*. New York, NY: Academic Press; 1979.

19. Sarwar G, Peace RW, Botting HG. Corrected relative net protein ratio (CRNPR) method based on differences in rat and human requirements for sulfur amino acids. *J Am Oil Chem Soc*. 1985;68:689–693.

20. Food and Agricultural Organization (FAO). *Protein Quality Evaluation*. Rome, Italy: FAO; 1990.

21. 21 CFR, Part 101, et al. Part III. Food Labeling, 1991.

22. Sarwar G, Peace RW. The protein quality of some enteral products is inferior to that of casein as assessed by rat growth methods and digestibility—Corrected amino acids scores. *J Nutr*. 1994;124:2223–2232.

23. Sarwar G, Peace RW. Protein quality of enteral nutritionals: A response to Young. *J Nutr*. 1995;125:1365–1366.

24. Young VR, Fajardo L, Murray E, Rand WM, Scrimshaw NS. Protein requirements of man: Comparative nitrogen balance response within the submaintenance-to-maintenance range of intakes of wheat and beef proteins. *J Nutr*. 1975;105:534–542.

25. Inque G, Fujita Y, Nhyama Y. Studies on protein requirements of young men fed egg protein and rice protein with excess and maintenance energy intakes. *J Nutr*. 1973;103:1673–1687.

26. Scrimshaw NS, Wayler AH, Murray E, Steinke FH, Rand WM, Young VR. Nitrogen balance response in young men given one of two isolated soy proteins or milk proteins. *J Nutr*. 1983;113:2492–2497.

27. Wayler A, Queiroz E, Scrimshaw NS, Steinke FH, Rand WM, Young VR. Nitrogen balance studies in young men to assess the protein quality of an isolated soy protein in relation to meat proteins. *J Nutr*. 1983;113:2485–2491.

28. Bolourchi S, Friedman CM, Mickelsen O. Wheat flour as a source of protein for adult human subjects. *Am J Clin Nutr*. 1968;21:827–835.

29. Edwards CH, Booker LK, Rumph CH, Wright WG, Ganapathy SN. Utilization of wheat by adult man: Nitrogen metabolism, plasma amino acids and lipids. *Am J Clin Nutr*. 1971;24:181–193.

30. Hegsted DM, Trulson MF, Stare FJ. Role of wheat and wheat products in human nutrition. *Physiol Rev*. 1954;34:221–258.

31. Begum A, Radhakrishnan N, Pereira SM. Effect of amino acid composition of cereal bread diets on growth of preschool children. *Am J Clin Nutr*. 1970;23:1175–1183.

32. Widdowson EM, McCance RA. *Studies on the Nutritive Value of Bread and on the Effect of Variation in the Extraction Rate of Flour on Growth of Undernourished Children* (Special Report Series 287). London, England: Medical Research Council; 1954.

33. Fujita Y, Yamamoto T, Rikimaru T, Inoue J. Effect of low protein diets on free amino acids in plasma of young men: Effect of wheat gluten diet. *J Nutr Sci Vitaminol*. 1979;25:427–439.

34. Browe JH, Butts JS, Youmans P, et al. A nutrition survey of the armed forces of Iran. *Am J Clin Nutr*. 1961;9:478–514.

35. Pelshenke PF. Bread as a daily food. *Cereal Sci Today*. 1961;7:325.

36. Sen Gupta PN, et al. *Household Food Consumption and Nutrition Surveys No 1–11*. Tehran, Iran: Food and Nutrition Institute; 1962–1967.

37. Sarry LI. Protein foods in Middle Eastern Diets. In: *Meeting Protein Needs of Infants and Children*. Washington, DC: National Research Council; 1961.

38. Food and Agricultural Organization (FAO). *Rice: Grain of Life, World Food Problems.* Rome, Italy; FAO; 1966.

39. Lee C, Howe JM, Carlson K, Clark HE. Nitrogen retention of young men fed rice with or without supplementary chicken. *Am J Clin Nutr.* 1971;24:318–323.

40. Clark HE, Howe JM, Lee CH-J. Nitrogen retention of adult human subjects fed a high protein rice. *Am J Clin Nutr.* 1971;24:324–328.

41. Young VR, Pellet PL. Protein intake and requirements with reference to diet and health. *Am J Clin Nutr.* 1987;45:1323–1343.

42. Yamashita K, Ashida K. Lysine metabolism in rats fed lysine-free diet. *J Nutr.* 1969;99:267–273.

43. Langran M, Moran BJ, Murphy JL, Jackson AA. Adaptation to a diet low in protein: Effect of complex carbohydrate upon urea kinetics in normal man. *Clin Sci.* 1992;82:191–198.

44. Young VR, Scrimshaw NS. Human protein and amino acid metabolism and requirements in relation to protein quality. In: Bodwell CE, ed. *Evaluation of Proteins for Humans.* Westport, Conn: AVI; 1977:11–54.

45. Markakis P. The nutritive quality of potato protein. In: Friedman M, ed. *Protein Nutritional Quality of Foods and Feeds.* New York, NY: Dekker; 1975:471–487.

46. Kon SK, Kleen A. The value of whole potato protein in human nutrition. *Biochem J.* 1928;22:258.

47. Clark HE, Allen PE, Meyers SM, Tuckett SE, Yamamura Y. Nitrogen balances of adults consuming *Opaque*-2 maize protein. *Am J Clin Nutr.* 1967;20:825–833.

48. Young VR, Pellet PL. Plant proteins in relation to human protein and amino acid nutrition. *Am J Clin Nutr.* 1994;59(suppl):1203–1212.

49. Young VR, Bier DM, Pellet PL. A theoretical basis for increasing current estimates of the amino acid requirements in adult man, with experimental support. *Am J Clin Nutr.* 1989;50:80–92.

50. Young VR, Marchini JS. Mechanisms and nutritional significance of metabolic responses to altered intakes of protein and amino acids, with reference to nutritional adaptation in humans. *Am J Clin Nutr.* 1990;51:270–289.

51. Havala S, Dwyer J. Position of the American Dietetic Association: Vegetarian diets. *J Am Diet Assoc.* 1993;93:1317–1319.

52. Nasset ES. Amino acid homeostasis in the gut lumen and its nutritional significance. *World Rev Nutr Diet.* 1972;14:134–153.

53. Nassett ES. Role of the digestive tract in the utilization of protein and amino acids. *JAMA.* 1957;164:172–177.

54. Nassett ES, Ju JS. Mixture of endogenous and exogenous protein in the alimentary tract. *J Nutr.* 1961;74:461–465.

55. Bergstrom J, Furst P, Vinnars E. Effect of a test meal, without and with protein, on muscle and plasma free amino acids. *Clin Sci.* 1990;79:331–337.

56. Geiger E. The role of the time factor in feeding supplementary proteins. *J Nutr.* 1948;36:813–819.

57. Henry KM, Kon SK. The supplementary relationships between the proteins of dairy products and those of bread and potato as affected by the method of feeding. With a note on the value of soya bean protein. *J Dairy Res.* 1946;14:330–339.

58. Mills EB, Canolty NL. Role of the time factor in protein complementation. *Nutr Rep Int.* 1984;30:311–322.

59. Sanchez A, Hernado I, Shavlik GW, Register UD, Hubbard RW, Burke KI. Complementation of proteins from one meal to the next. *Nutr Res.* 1987;7:629–635.

60. Chick H. Nutritive value of a vegetable protein and its enhancement by admixture. *Br J Nutr.* 1951;5:261–265.

61. Bressani R, Elias LG, Gomez Brenes RA. Improvement of protein quality by amino acid and protein supplementation. In: Bigwood EJ, ed. *Protein and Amino Acid Functions.* Oxford, England: Pergamon; 1972; 2:475–540.

62. Bricker M, Mitchell HH, Kinsman GM. The protein requirements of adult human subjects in terms of the protein contained in individual foods and food combinations. *J Nutr.* 1945;30:269–283.

63. Food and Agricultural Organization/World Health Organization/United Nations University. *Energy and Protein Requirements* (Technical Report Series 724). Geneva, Switzerland: World Health Organization; 1985.

64. Food and Agricultural Organization/World Health Organization. *Energy and Protein Requirements* (Technical Report Series 522). Geneva, Switzerland: World Health Organization; 1973.

65. Agarwal DK, Agarwal KN, Shankar R, Bhatia BD, Mishra KP, Tripathi BN. Determination of protein requirements of vegetarian diet in healthy female volunteers. *Indian J Med Res.* 1984;79:60–67.

66. Yañez E, Uauy R, Zacarías I, Barrera G. Long-term validation of 1 g of protein per kilogram body weight from a predominantly vegetable mixed diet to meet the requirements of young adult males. *J Nutr.* 1986;116:865–872.

67. Patwardhan VN, Mukundan R, Rama Sastri BV. Studies in protein metabolism. The influence of dietary protein on the urinary nitrogen excretion. *Indian J Med Res.* 1949;37:327–346.

68. Hegsted DM, Tsongas AG, Abbott DB, Stare FJ. Protein requirements of adults. *J Lab Clin Med.* 1946;31:261–284.

CHAPTER 4

Calcium

There is much debate over the dietary requirement for calcium for both the general population and vegetarians. Many factors, including overall diet, affect calcium needs. Consequently, vegetarians, particularly vegans, may have different calcium needs than omnivores. The complexity of bone health and the multitude of factors that affect it, however, make it difficult to establish the precise calcium needs of vegetarians.

OSTEOPOROSIS

Osteoporosis is a wideworld problem of immense magnitude; in 1990, there were 1.66 million hip fractures worldwide, two thirds of which were in women.[1] Osteoporosis is particularly problematic in industrialized countries. The United States, for example, has one of the highest rates of hip fracture in the world, and between 15 and 20 million Americans have osteoporosis.[2] About 50,000 Americans die each year of complications related to osteoporosis.[3] Women are at especially high risk; one of every five American women over the age of 65 has one or more fractured bones.[4]

The rate of hip fracture increases dramatically with age. Because differences in peak bone mass are an important determinant of later risk of developing osteoporosis, this condition is often considered a pediatric disease with a geriatric outcome. The relatively smaller peak bone mass of women compared with men places them at higher risk of fracture later in life.

Developing and maintaining optimal bone health represent the interplay between bone mineralization and resorption, a complex process that is affected by a wide array of factors. Bones are extremely dynamic and constantly remodeling; as much as 15% of the total bone mass turns over annually,[5] and about 700 mg of calcium exits and enters the bones every day.[6]

This active remodeling process gives bone the ability to repair any damage caused by the daily stresses to which it is exposed. It has been estimated that adequate nutrition can reduce the impact of osteoporosis by as much as 50% or more.[7]

Until the end of the third decade of life or so, bone physiology favors bone acquisition and bone mass. Between the ages of 35 and 45, peak bone mass is generally maintained, whereas beyond this age resorption dominates, and bone mass gradually decreases. After the age of 45, humans lose as much as 0.5% of their total bone mass every year.[8] For women, this process increases dramatically after menopause as a result of the decrease in circulating estrogen levels. Women can lose bone mass at an annual rate of between 2% and 5% in the 10 years starting just before and after menopause.[9]

The adult human body contains between 1,000 and 1,500 g of calcium, approximately 99% of which is found in bones and teeth. Most of the remaining 1% is found in the soft tissue with smaller amounts in the bloodstream. Adequate calcium is critical for optimal bone health; this is particularly true during the years when bones are forming so that peak bone density is maximized. Although bone mineral density and bone mass are not the only factors determining risk of fracture, they are the predominant ones.[10–12]

Many people, particularly girls and women, do not meet the recommended dietary allowance (RDA) for calcium. Women in the 19- to 50-year age group and teenage girls consume roughly two thirds[13] and less than two thirds[14] of the RDA for calcium, respectively. Yet a National Institutes of Health consensus development conference panel recently recommended increasing the RDA for children aged 1 to 10 years from 800 mg to 1,200 mg and for those aged 11 to 24 years and postmenopausal women who are not on estrogen replacement therapy to 1,500 mg.[15]

Adoption of these guidelines by the National Research Council would mean that, to meet the RDA, many Americans would need to rely on calcium-fortified foods or calcium supplements. There has been expressed concern about the use of calcium supplements because large amounts of calcium can interfere with iron absorption. This problem can be resolved by consuming calcium supplements separately from iron-containing foods or iron pills. Also, recent data suggest the inhibitory effect of calcium on iron absorption may be primarily an acute effect.

CALCIUM AND OSTEOPOROSIS

Although calcium is crucial to bone health, the relationship of calcium intake to bone mass and osteoporosis is not as straightforward as one might expect. In fact, internationally calcium intake appears not to be the predominant factor in determining bone status. There is actually an inverse relationship between the incidence of hip fracture and calcium intake worldwide[16] (Figure 4–1). It is more meaningful, however, to look within cultures, since so many differences that affect bone health exist among cultures. Uncertainty over the relative importance of calcium for optimal bone health are clearly reflected in the different recommendations for calcium intake among countries (Table 4–1).

There is also some disagreement over the extent to which prospective and case-control studies support the beneficial effect of high calcium intakes on bone health (bone mass). Some researchers have pointed out, however, that high calcium intakes show no benefit only in those studies in which calcium intake was not controlled or in which subjects were early menopausal women.[17] What is clear is that there are many important factors that can affect calcium balance, and thus bone health besides calcium intake. This may be especially relevant for vegans since they consume less calcium than nonvegetarians. Life style differences, including diet, may compensate totally or partially for the lower calcium intake of vegans.

CALCIUM ABSORPTION AND THE RDA

The RDA for calcium is based on two assumptions.[18] One is that the average person typically loses between 200 and 250 mg of calcium in feces,

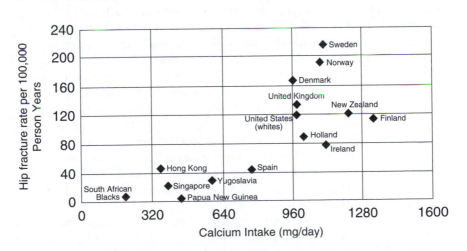

Figure 4–1 Relationship between calcium intake and hip fracture rate among countries. The fracture rate is per 100,000 person years for women over age 50 years adjusted to 1987 U.S. female population. *Sources:* Data from reference 16. In some cases fracture data from more than one survey were indicated; in those cases, data from only the most recent survey were used. Calcium intakes are based on FAO data.

Table 4–1 Calcium Recommendations

	Calcium RDA (mg)					
Population	United States	Canada	United Kingdom	Japan	Korea	World Health Organization
Children	800	550–700	600	400	500–700	450
Adolescents	1200	1000–1100	700	900	800	650
Adults	800	700–800	500	600	600	450
Pregnant women	1200	1200	1200	1000	1000	1100

urine, and perspiration each day. The second is that the average person absorbs between 30% and 40% of the calcium in the diet. If an adult consumes 800 mg of calcium, then he or she can expect to absorb between 240 and 320 mg of calcium, enough to replace the amount lost.

Both the need for calcium at a particular time and the amount of calcium in the diet will affect how much calcium is absorbed. For example, if calcium intake is high—greater than 800 mg/day—only about 15% will be absorbed.[19] Bear in mind, though, that the decrease in absorption efficiency with increasing intakes is a gradual one, such that higher intakes still result in greater absolute calcium absorption. When calcium needs are high, absorption rates go up. For example, young infants have a high calcium need as a result of new bone growth and can absorb as much as 75% of the calcium in their diet.[18] There is also considerable individual variation, however. That is, even individuals with similar calcium needs and intakes can differ markedly in the amount of calcium they absorb.[20]

Calcium absorption is a complicated process. Calcium in food is usually linked to other substances and must be released. It was formerly thought that because many elderly people do not produce adequate amounts of gastric acid, calcium absorption may be impaired.[21,22] This seems to be relevant only in the case of low-solubility calcium supplements, however, such as calcium carbonate.[23] When calcium is ingested with a meal, the lack of gastric acid does not inhibit calcium absorption.[24,25] The elderly have lower levels of vitamin D and/or fewer vitamin D receptors, however, which may account for their poorer calcium absorption.[25]

Serum calcium concentrations are tightly regulated and are maintained at about 100 mg/L (2.5 mmol/L), primarily through the action of parathyroid hormone. When serum calcium begins to decline, vitamin D is hydroxylated in the liver and kidney, producing the active form of vitamin D, 1,25-dihydroxyvitamin D, which aids in calcium absorption. Vitamin D is important for calcium absorption, although primarily at low calcium intakes, but it also acts directly to stimulate calcium uptake by the bones.[26] Perhaps for these reasons, higher intakes of vitamin D have been shown to be related to improved bone health.[27-29] The role of vitamin D on bone health is discussed in more detail in Chapter 6. Calcitonin, which is produced by the thyroid gland, is also involved in regulating serum calcium.

Most individuals appear to require between 400 and 800 mg of calcium per day; for example, in one study differences in bone health were noted only between those women consuming less than 405 mg and more than 777 mg of calcium per day.[30] Because of individual variations in nutrient needs, however, some individuals may need as much as or more than 1,500 mg of calcium per day.[31]

Because the percentage of calcium absorbed increases in response to low calcium intakes, damage due to low calcium intakes is mitigated to some extent. Although it may take as long as 2 months for absorption rates to increase in response to low calcium intakes,[32] it only takes 1 day for the body to decrease the amount of calcium excreted in the urine.[33] It has been suggested that it may take as long as 2 years for the bones themselves to adjust fully to a lower calcium intake by slowing the rate at which calcium exits and enters the bones,[34] but recent research suggests that this process may occur within a matter of weeks.[35] What is not clear, however, is whether low calcium intakes over prolonged periods of time result in any subtle adverse effects on bone health.

CALCIUM EXCRETION

Certainly, the ability to partially adapt to low calcium intakes provides at least a partial explanation for why hip fracture rates are not increased, and are even lower, in countries where calcium consumption is relatively low compared with the United States. It may be that variations in calcium excretion play an even bigger role, however.

The kidneys filter about 8,000 mg of calcium per day, and although some loss of calcium is normal, about 98% is reabsorbed.[36] With such large amounts of calcium filtered, it is clear that any factor that causes the kidneys to excrete even slightly more calcium can have a detrimental effect on bone health. In fact, research based on data from more than 500 women shows that urinary calcium loss accounts for more than 50% of the variation in calcium balance among individuals (see Figure 4-2).[37] Urinary loss was three times as important in affecting calcium balance as calcium intake. Excessive calcium loss is particularly important because the relative efficiency of calcium absorption decreases as calcium intake increases. Consequently, to compensate for a urinary loss of 50 mg of calcium, it may be necessary to consume an additional 250 to 350 mg of calcium (assuming an absorption

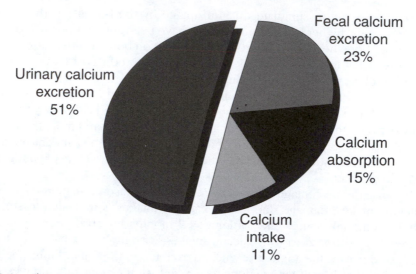

Figure 4–2 Relative impact of factors on the variation in calcium balance among middle-aged women. These data are based on balance/kinetic studies in over 500 healthy, middle-aged women. *Source:* Data from Heaney RP. Cofactors influencing the calcium requirement—Other nutrients. Presented at the NIH Consensus Development Conference on Optimal Calcium Intake. June 6–8, 1994. Bethesda, Maryland.

---

rate of 15% to 20%). Two factors that markedly increase calcium excretion are protein and sodium; both these factors are relevant to the bone status of vegans.

Protein and Calcium Balance

Worldwide, there is a positive correlation between animal protein intake and the incidence of hip fracture[16] (Figure 4–3). In 1968, Wachman and Bernstein[38] first proposed that high animal protein intake could lead to osteoporosis. As long ago as 1920, a diet containing large amounts of meat was found to increase urinary calcium greatly.[39] Vegans consume less protein than either lacto-ovo vegetarians or omnivores. Only about 10% to 12% of calories in vegan diets are derived from protein versus about 12% to 14% for lacto-ovo vegetarians and 14% to 18% for omnivores.

The effect of protein on calcium excretion is quite marked. In one study, for example, when subjects were fed 142 g of protein they were in negative calcium balance despite consuming 1,400 mg of calcium per day, but they were in positive calcium balance when consuming only 500 mg of calcium and 48 g of protein.[40] Similarly, when young men consumed roughly 600 mg

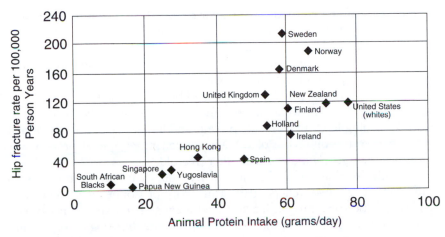

Figure 4–3 Relationship between animal protein intake and hip fracture rate among counrties. The fracture rate is per 100,000 person years for women over age 50 years adjusted to 1987 U.S. female population. *Sources:* Data are from reference 16. In some cases fracture data from more than one survey were indicated; in those cases, data from only the most recent survey were used. Animal protein intakes are based on FAO data.

of calcium on a low-protein diet they were in positive calcium balance, but when they ate a similar diet containing meat the same amount of calcium did not support calcium balance.[41] It has been estimated that excessive protein intake could account for the 1.0% to 1.5% loss in bone mass per year that is typically seen in postmenopausal women.[42]

The hypercalciuric effect of protein is generally attributed to the sulfur amino acids methionine and cysteine, which are metabolized to sulfate and hydrogen, resulting in an acid ash. The effect of the sulfur amino acids on calcium excretion has been demonstrated experimentally; methionine supplementation results in a lowering of urinary pH and an increase in urinary calcium excretion.[43] In contrast, when the diet is supplemented with the sulfur amino acid taurine, which is not metabolized to sulfate and hydrogen, there is no increase in calcium loss.[44] Consistent with these observations, chemically induced acidosis caused healthy adults to excrete three times as much calcium in one study.[45] The skeletal system is involved in the buffering system and in the process calcium is leached from bone and excreted in the urine. Protein also directly causes an increase in glomeruler filtration rate, which also increases calcium excretion to some extent.[40]

Some research indicates that the sulfur amino acids account for only part of the hypercalciuric effect of animal foods, such as meat, and that other organic acids in animal foods also play a role.[46] More recent research suggests, however, that the sulfur amino acids are primarily responsible for the increased acid production and calcium excretion.[47]

Diets that contain meat are more acid producing than vegetarian diets, and lacto-ovo vegetarian diets are more acid producing than vegan diets.[48] A recent study found that acid levels increased by a factor of about 5 on a diet containing meat and eggs compared with a lacto vegetarian diet (no meat or eggs) containing low but adequate protein and a diet containing about half the protein of the omnivore diet.[43] When even more animal protein was consumed, acid levels increased another fivefold.[43]

Generally, increasing protein intake by 100% causes calcium loss to double as well.[49] Researchers at the University of Connecticut found that increasing a person's protein intake by 50 g caused an extra 60 mg of calcium to be excreted.[50] Over the course of a lifetime, this degree of calcium loss may significantly increase bone loss and the risk of osteoporosis because bones contain only between 1,000 and 1,500 g of calcium.[51] In Western populations, a protein intake higher than 75 g/day is likely to produce excessive calcium loss.[51] On average, for every gram of protein consumed, calcium loss increases by about 1 mg.

Vegetarian diets are lower in total protein than omnivore diets. The protein content of these diets differs as well. Animal proteins are relatively high in sulfur amino acids, whereas legume proteins are relatively low; consequently, diets in which beans provide a substantial portion of the protein will result in less calcium being excreted. In one study, when subjects consumed diets with similar amounts of calcium and total protein, they excreted 150 mg of calcium in their urine per day when protein was derived from animal products and only 103 mg when protein was derived entirely from soy.[52] Because some vegetarians are likely to consume legumes as a substitute for meat, their intake of sulfur amino acids will be relatively less. Although the relative sulfur amino acid content of grains is similar to that of most animal foods, as indicated previously some research suggests that plant foods in general are less likely to cause urinary calcium excretion.[53–55]

The phosphorus that normally accompanies high protein animal foods mitigates the effects of protein on urinary calcium loss. According to Spencer et al,[56] experiments using isolated proteins such as casein, which is devoid of phosphorus, do not accurately reflect dietary conditions. Even though the phosphorus in animal products mitigates the hypercalciuric effect of animal products, according to Heaney it increases fecal calcium loss such that the net effects of animal protein on calcium balance are still negative.[57,58] The preponderance of evidence suggests excess dietary protein increases calcium excretion, although not all studies are in agreement.[59–61]

The ratio of calcium to protein in a diet may be the best predictor of bone health and may be more important than total calcium intake.[62] Eating less total protein probably reduces calcium requirements and promotes bone health. Using the RDA values for both calcium (in milligrams) and protein (in grams), for an adult woman weighing 137 lb (50 kg) the ideal ratio is 16:1.[18] In contrast, the ratio of calcium to protein in the diet of the average adult woman in this country is only 9:1 according to one national survey.[63] This is because protein intake generally exceeds the RDA, whereas calcium intake is typically less than the RDA. Meat is high in protein and generally contains little calcium; therefore, meat-based diets produce an undesirable ratio. Conversely, milk and dairy products have a calcium to protein ratio of about 36:1, which is quite good.

Not surprising, in studies directly comparing dietary intake, calcium-to-protein ratios of lacto-ovo vegetarian diets are equal to or higher than those of omnivores because the former contain dairy foods but no animal flesh (with the exception of eggs). Findings vary, but the ratio is about 15:1 to 17:1 versus 10:1 to 12:1 for omnivores (see Table 4–2 and Appendix G). As noted previously, vegans consume less calcium, but also less protein, than nonvegetarians; their ratio is about 9:1 to 12:1. Consequently, their ratio is much better than expected given their lower calcium intake, although it is not as high as for omnivores.

Table 4–2 Protein, Calcium, Phosphorus, and Sodium Intakes of Vegetarians and Nonvegetarians—Summary of Data Presented in Appendix G.

Group/ Gender	% Protein	Calcium (mg)	Calcium (mg): Protein (g)	Phosphorus (mg)	Calcium: Phosphorus	Sodium (mg)
LOV F	12–14	900–1,000	15–17	1,200–1,300	0.70–0.80	2,000–2,500
NV-F	14–18	800–900	11–12	1,100–1,200	0.65–0.75	2,000–2,500
LOV-M	12–13	1,100–1,300	15–17	1,600–2,000	0.75–0.80	3,000–3,800
NV-M	14–17	1,100–1,200	10–12	1,500–2,000	0.55–0.65	3,000–3,600
VEG-F	10–12	400–600	9–11	900–1,200	0.50–0.65	1,800–2,400
VEG-M	10–12	600–700	9–12	1,300	0.58	2,800

Abbreviations: LOV, lacto-ovo vegetarian; VEG, vegan; NV, nonvegetarian.

Protein values represent the percentage of calories derived from protein. For vegan men, phosphorus and sodium values are derived from only one study. Data should be viewed only as an approximation of values in Appendix F. Ranges presented do not actually represent the ranges reported in Appendix G, but were chosen as a means of reflecting both the range and the average value for each category. Table does not include data for studies that combined genders and/or vegetarian groups.

Data from reference 1 in Appendix G were not included in the values shown for VEGs because they were inconsistent with the remaining data, which were limited.

Sodium and Calcium Balance

High sodium intakes may markedly increase risk of osteoporosis.[64] Sodium intakes vary considerably among populations. In one worldwide survey, sodium intake varied by as much as a factor of 1,000 among different geographic regions.[65] In the United States sodium intake is quite high, about 5 to 10 times more than the estimated biologic requirement of 500 mg/day.[14] High sodium intakes increase calcium excretion by inhibiting proximal renal tubular calcium reabsorption. For every gram or so of sodium ingested, urinary calcium loss increases by between 20 and 40 mg.[7] In fact, based on findings from a recent 2-year longitudinal study of bone density in 124 postmenopausal women, it was estimated that when urinary sodium excretion is reduced by 50% from 3,450 mg/d to 1,725 mg/d the effect on bone density is equivalent to an increase in dietary calcium intake of 891 mg.[66] Similarly, in a study of younger women (aged 8 to 13 years), urinary sodium excretion was found to be the biggest determinant of urinary calcium excretion.[67]

Not only do protein and sodium individually increase urinary calcium loss, but a recent animal study found that there was a marked synergistic effect between the two factors such that a high-sodium, high-protein diet increased calcium excretion by a factor of 3 compared with a low-sodium, low-protein diet.[68] Additive effects of protein and sodium on calcium excretion have been observed in human subjects.[69] Estimates are that a young woman consuming a low-protein, low-sodium diet may require only 450 mg of calcium to maintain calcium balance, whereas that same woman consuming a high-protein, high-sodium diet may need as much as 2,000 mg of calcium per day.[37,70] Estimates are that a single fast-food hamburger, because of its high protein and sodium content, can cause a negative calcium balance of about 22 mg.[71]

The extent to which the hypercalciuric effects of sodium are pertinent to differences in calcium requirements between vegetarians and omnivores is not clear because dietary intake data are somewhat limited. Also, it is very difficult to accurately quantify sodium intake. Some data suggest that only about 10% of the sodium consumed comes naturally from the food we eat. Fifteen percent comes from salt added during cooking and at the table, and fully 75% comes from salt added during processing and manufacturing.[72,73] Although many agrarian societies, whose diets are primarily vegetarian, consume less sodium than the typical industrialized society,[74,75] the sodium intake of lacto-ovo vegetarians appears to be similar to or only slightly lower than that of omnivores. There are only limited data on vegans, although their sodium intake does appear to be somewhat lower than that of nonvegetarians (see Table 4–2 and Appendix G).

BONE HEALTH OF VEGETARIANS

Some research,[76–78] but not all,[79–82] suggests that lacto-ovo vegetarians have greater bone density than meat eaters. In women aged 50 to 87, lacto-ovo vegetarians were found to lose about 50% to 60% less bone mass in comparison with omnivores,[78,83] although a recent study did not confirm these findings.[81] This difference is not seen in older men or in younger age groups, however.[78,79] Although the evidence that lacto-ovo vegetarians have stronger bones than meat eaters appears equivocal, it is clear that their bones are at least as strong.

There is little information about the bone health of vegans. One study, which involved only 11 women, found that bone density was lower in elderly vegans (age 60 to 90) in comparison with nonvegan vegetarians.[82] Subjects were classified as vegans if they had followed this diet for as little as 2 years, however. Thus the relevance of these findings to life-long vegans is certainly questionable. The bone density of semivegan rural Chinese who consumed few or no dairy products was somewhat lower than rural Chinese who consumed dairy and had calcium intakes similar to those of the vegans.[83] No information was provided about the dietary sources of calcium in the vegan diets, however, so that calcium bioavailability is unknown. Also, calcium intakes were only between 300 and 400 mg/day, much less than the calcium intake of vegans in industrialized countries.[83]

As noted previously, comparisons among countries have shown that the consumption of diets relatively low in calcium is not associated with higher hip fracture rates. Nevertheless, the bone mineral density of these populations (eg, the Chinese and Japanese) is similar to or lower than that of Western populations with relatively higher calcium intakes.[84,85] Because there are no studies on the bone density of life-long vegans, it is not possible to draw definitive conclusions about the adequacy of calcium intake among Western vegans. This is especially true because so many life style factors affect calcium balance and bone health (Table 4–3).

Because their calcium intake is low relative to both lacto-ovo vegetarians and omnivores, vegans certainly will absorb more of the calcium they ingest. In fact, one study found that vegetarians are generally more efficient at absorbing calcium than omnivores.[86] It is not known, however, whether this improved absorption compensates fully for a low calcium intake or to what extent the lower protein, and perhaps somewhat lower sodium, intake of vegans reduce their calcium requirements. Consequently, it is prudent to recommend that vegans strive to meet the current RDA for calcium, particularly because some research indicates that calcium intake above the RDA is beneficial.

Table 4–3 Life Style Factors That Affect Bone Health

Factors That May Increase Calcium Needs or Risk for Osteoporosis	Factors That May Decrease Calcium Needs or Enhance Bone Health	Factors That May Increase or Decrease Osteoporosis Risk
Protein	Estrogen	Genetics/heredity
Phytates	Heavier weight	Lactation
Advanced age	Boron	
Smoking	Potassium	
Oxalates	Vitamin D	
Caffeine	Exercise	
Diabetes	Male gender	
Fiber	Lactose	
Sodium		
Alcohol		
Childbearing		
Premature menopause		

MEETING THE CALCIUM RDA ON PLANT-BASED DIETS

Dietary recommendations in Western countries tend to be biased toward the inclusion of dairy products in the diet, so that these foods are commonly and erroneously believed to be dietary essentials. Most American consumers adhere to those recommendations to some extent. In the United States, dairy products directly and indirectly provide about 75% of the calcium in the diet.[87] In other parts of the world, dairy foods may play limited roles in the diet or be absent altogether. This is due in part to availability and custom but also to the high incidence of lactose intolerance in most non–northern European populations (Figures 4–4 and 4–5).

Estimates are that about two thirds of the world's adult population has difficulty digesting milk.[88,89] In fact, nutritional anthropologists suggest that until 10,000 years ago or so all human adults were lactose intolerant.[88,89] The ability to digest milk well into adulthood is probably the result of a genetic mutation among northern European populations. In the rest of the world, including Asia, North and South America, Africa, and along the Mediterranean, populations continued to develop normally; that is, they continued to lose their ability to digest milk as they matured. Thus historically milk has played a limited role in the diet of humans. Insufficient lactase, the enzyme needed to digest lactose, is the normal condition for most adult humans[88,89] (Figure 4–5). To some extent, however, the prevalence of lactase insufficiency is exaggerated because most adults are able to tolerate small amounts of dairy foods even in populations where lactase insufficiency rates are high.[90] Also, a recent study found that among individuals who described

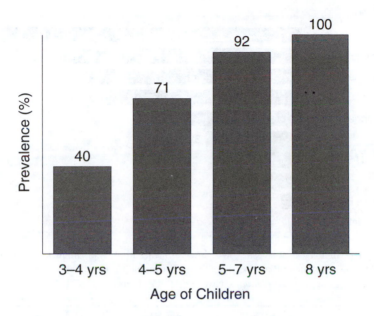

Figure 4–4 Percentage of Pima Indian children unable to digest lactose at various ages. *Source:* Data from Johnson JD, Simoons FJ, Hurwitz R, et al. Lactose malabsorption among the Pima Indians in Arizona. *Gastroenterol.* 1977;73:1299–1304.

themselves as lactose intolerant, most did not experience symptoms in response to 1 cup of milk when measured objectively.[91]

PLANT SOURCES OF CALCIUM

Although populations that consume dairy products have higher intakes of calcium than those that do not, many plant foods are rich sources of calcium. In fact, Eaton and Nelson[92] have estimated that plants provided most of the calcium in our ancestral diets and that we evolved in a calcium-rich environment. Average calcium intakes may have been as high as 3,000 mg/day on diets that included no dairy foods.[92] Although wild plants are generally much higher in calcium than cultivated ones, commonly consumed plants such as broccoli and kale are high in calcium.

There are some misconceptions about the bioavailability of calcium from plant sources. Although the calcium in some high-oxalate vegetables—most notably spinach, Swiss chard, beet greens, and rhubarb—is largely unavailable, this situation represents the exception rather than the norm. The absorption efficiency of calcium from a meal is fairly constant, between 25%

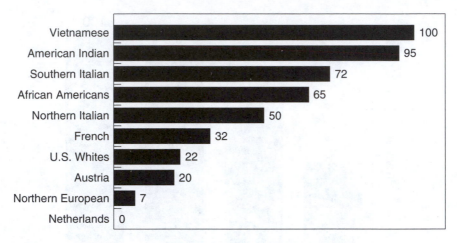

Figure 4–5 Incidence of lactose intolerance among different populations. *Source:* Data from Flatz G. Genetics of lactose digestion in humans. In: Harris H and Hirschhorn K, eds. *Advances in Human Genetics.* New York, NY: Plenum; 1987:1–77.

and 35%, regardless of the food source of the calcium, except for the high-oxalate foods.[93] Table 4–4 illustrates that calcium absorption from plants is generally quite good. On average, only about 20% of the calcium from legumes but as much as 50% of the calcium from green leafy vegetables is absorbed.

In addition, calcium is well distributed in the food supply, although many foods contain relatively small amounts of this nutrient. Foods that are fortified with calcium, including some breakfast cereals, orange juice, and soymilks, are also increasingly available. Some baked goods contain the preservative calcium propionate, which can contribute to calcium intake as well.

There has been some concern that vegans cannot meet calcium needs without consuming unusually large quantities of vegetables such as kale. No one food needs to be emphasized in the diet to meet calcium requirements, however. Consuming a variety of foods, including normal servings of some that are relatively rich in this nutrient, makes it reasonably easy to meet calcium needs on plant diets.

Many dietary factors in addition to oxalate affect calcium bioavailability. Two that are of importance for vegetarians are fiber and phytate, although in typical American diets these compounds are thought not to affect calcium absorption very much.[18] Vegetarians, however, typically consume 50% to 100% more fiber (see Appendix A) and two to three times the amount of phytate as nonvegetarians.[94–96] However, of substances tested thus far, only wheat bran has antiabsorber effects (i.e., it decreases calcium absorption

Table 4–4 Availability of Calcium from Cow's Milk and Selected Plant Foods

Food Source*	Calcium Content (mg)	Fractional Absorption (%)**	Estimated Absorbable Calcium (mg)/Serving
Broccoli	35	52.6	18.4
Brussel sprouts	19	63.8	12.1
Chinese cabbage	79	53.8	42.5
Green cabbage	25	64.9	16.2
Kale	47	58.8	27.6
Milk (one cup)	300	32.1	96.3
Mustard greens	64	57.8	37.0
Pinto beans	44.7	17.0	7.6
Sesame seeds (1 oz)	37	20.8	7.7
Turnip greens	99	51.6	51.1
Tofu, calcium set	258	31.0	80.0

*Serving size equals ½ cup unless otherwise indicated.
**Absorption rates were adjusted for load (absolute amount of calcium).
Source: Data from Weaver CM, Plawecki KL. Dietary calcium: Adequacy of a vegetarian diet. *Am J Clin Nutr.* 1994;59:(suppl):1238–1241.

from milk when eaten together).[97] In foods, components such as oxalate and phytate are already bound to calcium and so they are unlikely to interfere with calcium absorption from other foods.[98]

There is disagreement over the extent to which high-fiber diets may impair calcium absorption. Initial observations about the detrimental effects of fiber (whole wheat bread) on calcium balance were made more than 50 years ago.[99] Some investigators, however, have concluded that fiber does not have a significant effect,[100–102] whereas others have concluded that it does.[35,103–105] In one study, fiber supplementation markedly decreased calcium absorption and reduced calcium balance in young men, although, apparently in response to the lower bioavailability, bone turnover was slowed, suggesting that subjects were adapting to the lower calcium bioavailability.[35] Similarly, although the calcium content of a high-fiber, plant-based rural Mexican diet was higher than that of an urban Mexican diet, both calcium absorption and calcium balance were poorer on the rural diet.[106] Total fiber may be less important than the amount of insoluble fiber in the diet, which is more likely to bind calcium.[107] For example, the calcium from kale is well absorbed, although this is a high-fiber food.[108] Fiber may impair calcium absorption, but the effect when the entire diet is considered is probably minor.

Many high-fiber foods are also high in phytate. Phytate may adversely affect calcium absorption more than fiber.[109] When grain products are leavened with yeast, which hydrolyzes the bond between phytate and calcium, the calcium is better absorbed.[110] Studies also reveal, however, that even the calcium in unleavened bread products is better absorbed than the calcium from milk, although bread is relatively low in calcium.[111] Also, foods that are naturally high in phytate and fiber tend to have higher mineral contents than refined food, so that the overall amount of available calcium may be greater in the unprocessed foods. Finally, the oxalate, fiber, and phytate content of a food does not always dictate calcium bioavailability. For example, the calcium in soybeans is well absorbed despite the fact that this food is high in all three of these components.[112]

Osteoporosis is frequently less common in countries where most calcium is derived from high-fiber, high-phytate plant foods. Although many other factors—including genetics, physical activity, childbearing practices, and overall diet—affect the rates of osteoporosis around the world, these observations support the notion that diets based on plant foods can support adequate bone health. Past biases against plants as a source of calcium need to be reevaluated in light of more recent findings.

OTHER FACTORS THAT AFFECT BONE HEALTH/FRACTURE RATE

A number of other factors, in addition to those already discussed, appear to have significant effects on bone health and/or fracture rate.

Genetics

Blacks have denser bones than whites and excrete less calcium than whites independent of calcium load.[112] Also, the bone density of parents influences that of their offspring.[113,114] Recent research indicates that up to 75% of the difference in bone mass/density due to genetics is the result of a change in a single gene.[115]

Height

A recent study involving 50,000 male health professionals in the United States found that men 6 ft and taller were twice as likely to experience a hip fracture than men 5 ft 9 in or shorter.[116] Somewhat related to height, recent work shows that the length of the hip axis is related to fracture risk, with longer length increasing risk. Hip axis length has increased during the past few decades, an occurrence that may be related to better nutrition early in life.[117]

Geography

In developing countries, people may have greater exposure to sunlight and therefore higher vitamin D levels. Less exposure to hard (cement) surfaces may also contribute to the lower incidence of hip fracture in developing countries, as may the lack of slippery snow and ice in developing countries, which tend to have warmer climates. Better balance and the tendency to fall less often may also be a factor contributing to international differences in incidence of hip fracture.[118]

Physical Activity

Undoubtedly, this factor works in favor of those who live in developing countries, where physical activity is a normal part of daily life. More than 25 years ago, it was proposed that differences in physical activity may account for variations in the worldwide incidence of osteoporosis.[119] Researchers at the University of North Carolina suggest that exercise is more important for bone health than calcium and that exercise can compensate for a low calcium intake.[114]

The relationship of activity to bone health is easy to demonstrate. Hospitalized patients who are bedridden for long periods of time lose significant amounts of calcium.[120] Tennis players have bones that are a third thicker in the arm they use to play tennis than in their nondominant arm.[121] Recker et al,[122] based on results from a 5-year prospective study of young adult women, calculated that at a calcium intake of 800 mg active women experience 5- to 10-fold greater increases in spinal bone mineral density relative to sedentary women. Nelson et al[123] found that high-intensity exercise could even preserve bone mineral density, not just slow the loss of bone, in postmenopausal women. Even moderate exercise appears to be beneficial. In postmenopausal women, simply walking between 1.0 and 1.5 miles per day was associated with a reduced rate of bone loss.[124]

Caffeine

Caffeine increases bone loss;[42] in a recent study of postmenopausal women consuming an amount of caffeine contained in 2 to 3 cups of brewed coffee (five to seven servings of instant coffee) and 800 mg of calcium, bone loss was significantly increased.[125] One 6-oz serving of coffee causes a negative calcium balance of 4.6 mg/day. Approximately 40 mg of calcium are needed to offset the negative effect of one serving of coffee.[71]

Phosphorus

Studies in rats indicate that a high phosphorus intake relative to the amount of calcium in the diet may cause bone loss.[126] Phosphorus does not interfere with calcium absorption, however, and the adverse effects of high phosphorus intakes in animals have not been directly observed in human studies.[127,128] Nevertheless, when a high-phosphorus, low-calcium diet was fed to teenage girls, serum parathyroid hormone and urinary hydroxyproline levels increased, which suggests increased bone demineralization.[129] Furthermore, in a case-control study involving young Mexican children, individuals with low serum calcium levels (below 2.2 mmol/L) were five times more likely to drink large amounts of soft drinks (at least 1.5 L/week) than children with normal calcium levels (2.2 to 3.0 mmol/L).[130] The phosphorus content of Coca-Cola and Pepsi-Cola is 19.7 and 16.1 mg/dL, respectively.[131]

Vitamin D

Vitamin D significantly impacts bone health. See the discussion in Chapter 6.

CONCLUSION

Most lacto-ovo vegetarians will have little difficulty in meeting calcium needs. Indeed, calcium content tends to be high in these diets. In fact, the dietitian may wish to help clients avoid overemphasis on dairy products in the diet because these foods can displace fiber-rich plant foods. Therefore, it is appropriate to instruct all vegetarian clients in identifying plant sources of calcium (see Table 4–5 and Exhibit 4–1).

Dietary protein appears to have a significant impact on calcium balance. Diets high in protein probably raise calcium needs. Vegans are likely to need less calcium than omnivores because the vegan diet is moderate in protein compared with omnivore diets. Where vegans make considerable use of legumes, which are relatively low in sulfur amino acids, calcium balance may further be improved. Protein represents only one factor affecting calcium balance, however. Vegetarians who consume low-salt diets will also likely require less calcium. Another factor that may work to the advantage of vegetarians is their relatively higher potassium intake (Appendix H), since potassium itself, or when present as an alkali, salt may reduce calcium excretion.[132]

Because plant-based diets are often associated worldwide with lower hip fracture rates, many vegan clients may not give adequate thought to calcium sources in the diet. It is helpful to stress the importance of the role of total life style in supporting bone health. For example, populations in agrarian societies in developing countries may consume low-sodium diets and be much more physically active than Western vegans. They may also have more sun exposure and therefore higher blood levels of vitamin D. All these

Table 4–5 Plant Sources of Calcium

Food	Calcium Content (mg)	Food	Calcium Content (mg)
Legumes (1 cup, cooked)		**Vegetables** (½ cup, cooked)	
Chick peas	78	Bok choy	79
Great Northern beans	121	Broccoli	89
Kidney beans	50	Collard greens	178
Lentils	37	Kale	90
Lima beans	52	Mustard greens	75
Navy beans	128	Butternut squash	42
Pinto beans	82	Sweet potato	35
Black beans	103	Turnip greens	125
Vegetarian baked beans	128	**Fruits**	
Soyfoods		Dried figs (5)	258
Soybeans (1 cup, cooked)	175	Orange	56
Tofu (½ cup)	120 to 350*	Raisins (⅔ cup)	53
Tempeh (½ cup)	77	Calcium-fortified orange juice	300
TVP (½ cup, rehydrated)	85	**Grains**	
Soymilk (1 cup)	84	Corn bread (2-oz piece)	133
Fortified soymilk (1 cup)	250–300	Corn tortilla	53
Soynuts	252	English muffin	92
Nuts and seeds (2 tbsp)		Pita bread (1 small pocket)	31
Almonds	50	**Other foods**	
Almond butter	86	Blackstrap molasses (1 tbsp)	187
Brazil nuts	50	Fortified Rice Dream (1 cup)	300
Sesame seeds	176	Vegelicious (1 cup)	300
Tahini	128	Take Care (1 cup)	300

Note: TVP is a trademark of Archer Daniels Midland Company and is a textured soy protein.
*Indicates a range of calcium found in different tofu products.
Source: Data from Bowes, *Church's Food Value of Portions Commonly Used.* 16th edition, by Pennington. Lippincott-Raven © 1994.

factors strongly favor bone health. Also, genetics plays an important role. For example, individuals of African descent have denser bones and excrete less calcium than whites. Therefore, some Western vegans will have higher calcium needs than people in other parts of the world. For this reason, it is suggested that vegans strive to meet the RDA for calcium until the actual calcium needs of Western vegans are determined. When counseling vegan clients on diet and bone health, the following points should be stressed:

- Engage in regular physical exercise.
- Ensure adequate sun exposure or use vitamin D-fortified foods.

Exhibit 4–1 Two Sample Vegan Menus Providing the Adult RDA for Calcium

MENU 1	**MENU 2**
Breakfast	**Breakfast**
4 oz scrambled tofu	1 cup corn flakes
1 sesame seed bagel	½ cup fortified rice milk
1 tsp margarine	Cinnamon raisin bagel with 2 tbsp
6 oz orange juice	almond butter
Lunch	**Lunch**
1 whole wheat pita	Miso soup with ½ cup bok choy and
½ cup hummus spread	¼ cup tofu chunks
Sliced tomato	Pasta tossed with ½ cup steamed
Dinner	broccoli, ¼ cup steamed carrots,
1 cup baked beans with 1 tbsp	seasoned with herbs
blackstrap molasses	1 slice bread
1 cup steamed collards	**Dinner**
1 cup brown rice	Black bean soft tacos:
1 piece corn bread	1 cup black beans with taco
Snacks	seasoning
Soymilk shake with 1 cup fortified	2 corn tortillas (processed with lime)
soymilk, ½ banana, ¼ cup	Chopped tomatoes and lettuce
strawberries	**Snack**
	½ cup roasted soynuts

- Avoid excesses of sodium in the diet by limiting added sodium to foods and limiting the intake of highly processed foods.
- Identify plant foods that are rich in calcium and that can be used regularly in the diet.

REFERENCES

1. Cooper C, Campion G, Melton LJ III. Hip fractures in the elderly: A worldwide projection. *Osteoporosis Int.* 1992;2:285–289.

2. Osteoporosis Consensus Panel. Osteoporosis. *JAMA.* 1984;252:799–802.

3. Sernbo I, Johnell O. Consequences of hip fracture: A prospective study over 1 year. *Osteoporosis Int.* 1993;3:148–153.

4. Cummings SR, Kelsey JL, Nevitt MC, O'Dowd KJ. Epidemiology of osteoporosis and osteoporotic fractures. *Epidemiol Rev.* 1985;7:178–208.

5. Green J. The physiochemical structure of bone: Cellular and noncellular elements. *Miner Electrolyte Metab.* 1994;20:7–15.

6. Nilas L. Calcium intake and osteoporosis. *World Rev Nutr Diet.* 1993;73:1–26.

7. McBean LD, Forgac T, Finn SC. Osteoporosis: Visions for care and prevention—A conference report. *J Am Diet Assoc*. 1994;94:668–671.

8. Heaney RP. Calcium, bone health, and osteoporosis. In: Peck WA, ed. *Bone and Mineral Research, Annual 4: A Yearly Survey of Developments in the Field of Bone and Mineral Metabolism*. Amsterdam, Holland: Elsevier; 19xx:255–301.

9. Committee on Diet and Health, Food and Nutrition Board, Commission on Life Sciences, National Research Council. *Diet and Health. Implications for Reducing Chronic Disease Risk*. Washington, DC: National Academy Press, 1989.

10. Lauritzen JB, McNair PA, Lund B. Risk factors for hip fractures. *Dan Med Bull*. 1993;40:479–485.

11. Ross PD, Davis JW, Wasnich RD. Bone mass and beyond: Risk factors for fractures. *Calcif Tissue Int*. 1993;53(suppl 1):S134–S138.

12. Heaney RP. Is there a role for bone quality in fragility fractures? *Calcif Tissue Int*. 1993;53 (suppl 1):S3–S6.

13. US Department of Agriculture. *Nationwide Food Consumption Survey. Continuing Survey of Food Intakes of Individuals. Women 19–50 Years and Their Children 1–5 Years, 4 Days, 1985* (report 85–4). Hyattsville, Md: Nutrition Monitoring Division, Human Nutrition Information Service; 1987.

14. US Department of Agriculture. *Nationwide Food Consumption Survey. Individuals in 48 States, Year 1977–78* (report 1–2). Hyattsville, Md: Consumer Nutrition Division, Human Nutrition Information Service; 1984.

15. Rowe PM. New US recommendations on calcium intake. *Lancet*. 1994;343:1559–1560.

16. Abelow BJ, Holford TR, Insogna KL. Cross-cultural association between dietary animal protein and hip fracture: A hypothesis. *Calcif Tissue Int*. 1992;50:14–18.

17. Barger-Lux MJ, Heaney RP. The role of calcium intake in preventing bone fragility, hypertension, and certain cancers. *J Nutr*. 1994;124:1406S–1411S.

18. National Research Council. *Recommended Dietary Allowances*. 10th ed. Washington, DC: National Academy Press; 1989.

19. Heaney RP, Saville PD, Recker RR. Calcium absorption as a function of calcium intake. *J Lab Clin Med*. 1975;85:881–890.

20. Heaney RP, Weaver CM, Fitzsimmons ML, Recker RR. Calcium absorptive consistency. *J Bone Miner Res*. 1990;5:1139–1142.

21. Recker RR. Calcium absorption and achlorhydria. *N Engl J Med*. 1985;313:70–73.

22. Heaney RP, Gallagher JC, Johnston CC, Neer R, Parfitt AM, Whedon GD. Calcium nutrition and bone health in the elderly. *Am J Clin Nutr*. 1982;36:986–1013.

23. Heaney RP, Recker RR, Weaver CM. Absorbability of calcium sources: The limited role of solubility. *Calcif Tissue Int*. 1990;46:300–304.

24. Knox TA, Kassarjian Z, Dawson-Hughes B, et al. Calcium absorption in elderly subjects on high- and low-fiber diets: Effect of gastric acidity. *Am J Clin Nutr*. 1991;53:1480–1486.

25. Weaver CM. Age related calcium requirements due to changes in absorption and utilization. *J Nutr*. 1994;124:1418S–1425S.

26. Anderson JJB. Nutritional biochemistry of calcium and phosphorus. *J Nutr Biochem*. 1991;2:300–307.

27. Dawson-Hughes B, Dallal GE, Krall EA, Harris S, Sokoll LJ, Falconer G. Effect of vitamin D supplementation on wintertime and overall bone loss in healthy postmenopausal women. *Ann Intern Med*. 1991;115:505–512.

28. Morris HA, Morrison GW, Burr M, Thomas DW, Nordin BEC. Vitamin D and femoral neck fractures in elderly South Australian women. *Med J Aust*. 1984;140:519–521.

29. Riggs BL, Jowsey J, Kelly PJ, Hoffman DL, Arnaud CD. Effects of oral therapy with calcium and vitamin D in primary osteoporosis. *J Clin Endocrinol Metab*. 1976;42:1139–1144.

30. Dawson-Hughes B, Jacques P, Shipp C. Dietary calcium intake and bone loss from the spine in healthy postmenopausal women. *Am J Clin Nutr*. 1987;46:685–687.

31. Prentice A. Calcium: The functional significance of trends in consumption. In: Pietrzik K, ed. *Modern Lifestyles, Lower Energy Intake and Micronutrient Status*. New York, NY: Springer-Verlag; 1989:139–153.

32. Leitch I, Aitken FC. The estimation of calcium requirement: A re-examination. *Nutr Abstr Rev*. 1959;29:393–411.

33. Adams ND, Gray RD, Lemann J Jr. The effects of oral CaCO2 loading and dietary calcium deprivation in plasma 1,25-dihydroxyvitamin D concentrations in healthy adults. *J Clin Endocrinol Metabol*. 1979;48:1008–1016.

34. Kanis JA, Passmore R. Calcium supplementation of the diet—II. *Br Med J*. 1989;298:205–208.

35. O'Brien KO, Allen LH, Quatronmoni P, et al. High fiber diets slow bone turnover in young men but have no effect of efficiency of intestinal calcium absorption. *J Nutr*. 1993;123:2122–2128.

36. Lemann J Jr, Adams ND, Gray RW. Urinary calcium excretion in human beings. *N Engl J Med*. 1979;301:535–541.

37. Heaney RP. Cofactors influencing the calcium requirement—Other nutrients. Presented at the NIH Consensus Development Conference on Optimal Calcium Intake; June 6–8, 1994; Bethesda, Md.

38. Wachman A, Bernstein DS. Diet and osteoporosis. *Lancet*. 1968;2:958–959.

39. Sherman HC. Calcium requirements of maintenance in man. *J Biol Chem*. 1920;44:21–27.

40. Linkswiler HM, Zemel MB, Hegsted M, Schuette S. Protein-induced hypercalciuria. *Fed Proc*. 1981;40:2429–2433.

41. Schuette SA, Linkswiler HM. Effects of Ca and P metabolism in humans by adding meat, meat plus milk, or purified proteins plus Ca and P to a low protein diet. *J Nutr*. 1982;112:338–349.

42. Heaney RP, Recker RR. Effects of nitrogen, phosphorus, and caffeine on calcium balance in women. *J Lab Clin Med*. 1982;99:46–55.

43. Remer T, Manz F. Estimation of the renal net acid excretion by adults consuming diets containing variable amounts of protein. *Am J Clin Nutr*. 1994;59:1356–1361.

44. Zhao XH, Chen XS. Diet and bone density among elderly Chinese. *Nutr Rev*. 1992;50:395–397.

45. Lemann J Jr, Litzow JR, Lennon EJ. Studies of the mechanism by which chronic metabolic acidosis augments urinary calcium excretion in man. *J Clin Invest*. 1967;46:1318–1328.

46. Zemel MB, Schuette SA, Hegsted M, Linkswiler HM. Role of the sulfur-containing amino acids in protein-induced hypercalciuria in men. *J Nutr*. 1981;111:545–552.

47. Trilok G, Draper HH. Sources of protein-induced endogenous acid production and excretion by human adults. *Calcif Tissue Int*. 1994;44:335–338.

48. Dwyer J, Foulkes E, Evans M, Ausman L. Acid/alkaline ash diets: Time for assessment and change. *J Am Diet Assoc*. 1985;85:841–845.

49. Hegsted M, Schuette SA, Zemel MB, Linkswiler HM. Urinary calcium and calcium balance in young men as affected by level of protein and phosphorus intake. *J Nutr.* 1981;111:553–562.

50. Kerstetter JE, Allen LH. Dietary protein increases urinary calcium. *J Nutr.* 1990;120:134–136.

51. Riggs BL, Kelly PJ, Kinney VR, Scholz DA, Bianco AJ. Calcium deficiency and osteoporosis. *J Bone Joint Surg [Am].* 1967;49:915–924.

52. Breslau NA, Brinkley L, Hill KD, Pak CYC. Relationship of animal protein-rich diet to kidney stone formation and calcium metabolism. *J Clin Endocrinol Metabol.* 1988;66:140–146.

53. Chan JCM. The influence of dietary intake on endogenous acid production: Theoretical and experimental background. *Nutr Metab.* 1974;16:1–9.

54. Gonick HC, Goldberg G, Mulcare D. Reexamination of the acid-ash content of several diets. *Am J Clin Nutr.* 1968;21:898–903.

55. Blatherwick NR. The specific role of foods in relation to the composition of urine. *Arch Intern Med.* 1914;14:409–450.

56. Spencer HL, Kramer I, Osis D. Do protein and phosphorus cause calcium loss? *J Nutr.* 1988;118:657–660.

57. Spencer H, Kramer L, Osis D, Norris C. Effect of a high protein (meat) intake on calcium metabolism in man. *Am J Clin Nutr.* 1978;31:2167–2180.

58. Heaney RP. Protein intake and the calcium economy. *J Am Diet Assoc.* 1993;93:1259–1260.

59. Matkovic V, Rich JZ, Andon MB, et al. Urinary calcium, sodium, and bone mass of young females. *Am J Clin Nutr.* 1995;62:417–425.

60. Munger RG, Cerhan J, Chiu B, Yang S, Allnutt K. Protein intake and risk of hip fracture in a cohort of older Iowa women. *Am J Clin Nutr.* 1995;61:894 (abstr 15).

61. Hunt JR, Gallagher SK, Johnson LK, Lykken GI. High- versus low-meat diets: Effects on zinc absorption, iron status, and calcium, copper, iron, magnesium, manganese, nitrogen, phosphorus, and zinc balance in postmenopausal women. *Am J Clin Nutr.* 1995;62:621–632.

62. Recker RR, Davies M, Hinders SM, Heaney RP, Stegman MR, Kimmel DB. Bone gain in young adult women. *JAMA.* 1992;268:2403–2408.

63. Carroll MD, Abraham S, Dresser CM. *Dietary Intake Source Data: US, 1976–1980.* Washington, DC. US Department of Health and Human Services; 1983. DHHS publication (PHS) 83-PHS.

64. MacGregor GA, Cappuccio FP. The kidney and essential hypertension: A link to osteoporosis? *J Hypertens.* 1993;11:781–785.

65. Intersalt Cooperative Research Group. Intersalt: An international study of electrolyte excretion and blood pressure. Results for a 24 hour urinary sodium and potassium excretion. *Br Med J.* 1988;297:319–328.

66. Devine A, Criddle RA, Dick IM, et al. A longitudinal study of the effect of sodium and calcium intakes on regional bone density in postmenopausal women. *Am J Clin Nutr.* 1995;62:740–745.

67. Matkovic V, Rich JZ, Andon MB, et al. Urinary calcium, sodium, and bone mass of young females. *Am J Clin Nutr.* 1995;62:417–425.

68. Chan EL-P, Swaminathan R. The effect of high protein intake and high salt intake for 4 months on calcium and hydroxyproline excretion in normal and oophrectomized rats. *J Lab Clin Med.* 1994;124:37–41.

69. Kok DJ, Iestra JA, Doorenbos CJ, Papapoulos SE. The effects of dietary excesses in animal protein and in sodium on the composition and the crystallization kinetics of calcium oxalate monohydrate in urines of healthy men. *J Clin Endocrinol Metabol.* 1990;71:861–867.

70. Nordin BEC, Need AG, Morris HA, Horowitz M. The nature and significance of the relationship between urinary sodium and phosphorus metabolism. *J Nutr.* 1993;123:1615–1622.

71. Barger-Lux MJ, Heaney RP. Caffeine and the calcium economy revisited. *Osteoporosis Int.* 1995;5:97–102.

72. Sanchez-Casillo CP, Warrender S, Whitehead TP, James WP. An assessment of the sources of dietary salt in a British population. *Clin Sci.* 1987;72:95–102.

73. Sanchez-Castillo CP, Branch WJ, James WP. A test of the validity of the lithium-marker technique for monitoring dietary sources for salt in men. *Clin Sci.* 1987;72:87–94.

74. McCarron DA, Henry HJ, Morris CD. Human nutrition and blood pressure regulation, an integrated approach. *Hypertension.* 1982;4(suppl 3):2–13.

75. Page LB. Nutritional determinants of hypertension. *Curr Concepts Nutr.* 1981;10:113–126.

76. Ellis FR, Holesh S, Ellis JW. Incidence of osteoporosis in vegetarians and omnivores. *Am J Clin Nutr.* 1972;25:555–558.

77. Ellis FR, Holesh S, Sanders TAB. Osteoporosis in British vegetarians and omnivores. *Am J Clin Nutr.* 1974;27:769–770.

78. Sanchez TV, Mickelson O, Marsh AG, Garn SM, Mayor GH. Bone mineral density in elderly vegetarian and omnivorous females. In: Mazeness RB, ed. *Proceedings of the 4th International Conference on Bone Mineral Measurements.* Bethesda, Md: National Institute of Arthritis, Metabolism, and Digestive Diseases; 1980:94–98.

79. Tylavsky FA, Anderson JJB. Dietary factors in bone health of elderly lactoovovegetarian and omnivorous women. *Am J Clin Nutr.* 1988;48:842–849.

80. Tesar R, Notelovitz M, Shim E, Kauwell G, Brown J. Axial and peripheral bone density and nutrient intakes of postmenopausal vegetarian and omnivorous women. *Am J Clin Nutr.* 1992;56:699–704.

81. Reed JA, Anderson JJB, Tylavsky FA, Gallagher PN Jr. Comparative changes in radial-bone density of elderly female lactoovovegetarians and omnivores. *Am J Clin Nutr.* 1994;59(suppl):1197S–1202S.

82. Marsh AG, Sanchez TV, Michesen O, Chaffee FL, Fagal SM. Vegetarian lifestyle and bone mineral density. *Am J Clin Nutr.* 1988;48:837–841.

83. Hu J-F, Zhao X-H, Jiu J-B, Parpia B, Campbell TC. Dietary calcium and bone density among middle-aged and elderly women in China. *Am J Clin Nutr.* 1993;58:219–227.

84. Kin K, Lee JHE, Kushida K, et al. Bone density and body composition on the Pacific Rim: A comparison between Japan-born and US born Japanese-American women. *J Bone Miner Res.* 1993;8:861–869.

85. Russell-Aulet M, Wang J, Thornton JC, Colt EWD, Pierson RN Jr. Bone mineral density and mass in a cross-sectional study of white and Asian women. *J Bone Miner Res.* 1993;8:575–582.

86. Nnakwe N, Kies C. Calcium and phosphorus utilization by omnivorous and lacto-ovo-vegetarians fed laboratory controlled lacto-ovo-vegetarian diets. *Nutr Rep Int.* 1985;31:1009–1014.

87. Fleming KH, Heimbach JT. Consumption of calcium in the US: Food sources and intake levels. *J Nutr.* 1994;124:1426S–1430S.

88. Montgomery RK, Buller HA, Rings EHH, Grand RJ. Lactose intolerance and the genetic regulation of intestinal-phlorizin hydrolase. *FASEB J.* 1991;5:2824–2832.

89. Simoons FJ. The geographic hypothesis and lactose malabsorption. *Dig Dis Sci.* 1989;23:963–980.

90. Johnson AO, Semenya JG, Buchowski MS, Enwonwu CO, Scrimshaw NS. Adaptation of lactose maldigesters to continued milk intakes. *Am J Clin Nutr.* 1993;58:879–881.

91. Suarez FL, Saviano DA, Levitt MD. A comparison of symptoms after the comsumption of milk or lactose-hydrolyzed milk with self-reported severe lactose intolerance. *N Engl J Med.* 1995;333:1–4.

92. Eaton SB, Nelson DA. Calcium in evolutionary perspective. *Am J Clin Nutr.* 1991;54:281S–287S.

93. Heaney R, Recker R. Distribution of calcium absorption in middle-aged women. *Am J Clin Nutr.* 1986;43:299–305.

94. Brune M, Rossander L, Hallberg L. Iron absorption: No intestinal adaptation to a high-phytate diet. *Am J Clin Nutr.* 1989;49:542–545.

95. Ellis R, Morris ER, Hill AD, Smith JC. Phytate:zinc molar ratio, mineral, and fiber content of three hospital diets. *J Am Diet Assoc.* 1982;81:26–29.

96. Ellis R, Kelsay JL, Reynolds RD, Morris ER, Moser PB, Frazier CW. Phytate:zinc and phytate X calcium:zinc millimolar ratios in self-selected diets of Americans, Asian Indians, and Nepalese. *J Am Diet Assoc.* 1987;87:1043–1047.

97. Weaver CM, Heaney RP, Martin BR, Fitzsimmons ML. Human calcium absorption from whole-wheat products. *J Nutr.* 1991;121:1769–1775.

98. Heaney RP. Optimal calcium intake. *J Am Med Assoc.* 1995;274:1012.

99. McCance RA, Widdowson EM. Mineral metabolism of healthy adults on white and brown bread dietaries. *J Physiol (London).* 1942;101:44–85.

100. Rattan J, Levin N, Graff E, Weizer N, Gilat T. A high-fiber diet does not cause mineral and nutrient deficiencies. *J Clin Gastroenterol.* 1981;3:389–393.

101. Spencer H, Norris C, Derler J, Osis D. Effect of oat bran muffins on calcium absorption and calcium, phosphorus, magnesium and zinc balance in men. *J Nutr.* 1991;121:1976–1983.

102. van Dokkum W. The relative significance of dietary fibre for human health. *Front Gastrointest Res.* 1988;14:135–145.

103. Knox TA, Kassarjian Z, Dawson-Hughes B, et al. Calcium absorption in elderly subjects on high- and low-fiber diets: Effect of gastric acidity. *Am J Clin Nutr.* 1991;53:1480–1486.

104. Sandstead HH. Fiber, phytates, and mineral nutrition. *Nutr Rev.* 1992;50:30–31.

105. Moynahan EJ. Nutritional hazards of high-fibre diet. *Lancet.* 1977;1:654–655.

106. Rosado JL, Lopez P, Morales M, Munoz E, Allen LH. Bioavailability of energy, nitrogen, fat, zinc, iron, and calcium from rural and urban Mexican diets. *Br J Nutr.* 1992;68:45–58.

107. Anderson H, Navert B, Bingham SA, Englyst HN, Cummings JH. The effects of breads containing similar amounts of phytate but different amounts of wheat bran on calcium, zinc, and iron balance in man. *Br J Nutr.* 1983;50:503–510.

108. Weaver CM, Martin BR, Heaney RP. Calcium absorption from foods. In: Burkhardt P, Heaney RP, eds. *Nutritional Aspects of Osteoporosis.* New York, NY: Raven; 1991;85:133–139.

109. Heaney RP, Weaver CM. Calcium absorption from kale. *Am J Clin Nutr.* 1991;51:656–657.

110. Weaver CM, Heaney RP, Martin BR, Fitzsimmons ML. Human calcium absorption from whole-wheat products. *J Nutr.* 1991;121:1769–1775.

111. Heaney RP, Weaver CM, Fitzsimmons ML. Soybean phytate content: Effect on calcium absorption. *Am J Clin Nutr.* 1991;53:745–747.

112. Bell NH, Yergey AL, Vieira NE, Oexmann MJ, Shary JR. Demonstration of a difference in urinary calcium, not calcium absorption, in black and white adolescents. *J Bone Miner Res.* 1993;8:1111–1115.

113. Pollitzer WS, Anderson JJB. Ethnic and genetic differences in bone mass: A review with a hereditary vs environmental perspective. *Am J Clin Nutr.* 1989;50:1244–1259.

114. Anderson JJB, Metz JA. Contributions of dietary calcium and physical activity to primary prevention of osteoporosis in females. *J Am Coll Nutr.* 1993;12:378–383.

115. Morrison NA, Qi JC, Tokita A, et al. Prediction of bone density from vitamin D receptor alleles. *Nature (London).* 1994;367:216–217.

116. Hemenway D, Azrael DR, Rimm EB, Feskanich D, Willet WC. Risk factors for hip fracture in US men aged 40–75 years. *Am J Public Health.* 1994;84:1843–1845.

117. Reid IR, Chin K, Evans MC, Jones JG. Relation between increase in length of hip axis in older women between the 1950s and 1990s and increase in age specific rates of hip fracture. *Br Med J.* 1994;309:508–509.

118. Lord SR, Sambrook PN, Gilbert C, et al. Postural stability, falls and fractures in the elderly: Results of the Dubbo Osteoporosis Epidemiologic Study. *Med J Aust.* 1994;160:684–691.

119. Chalmers J, Ho KC. Geographic variations in senile osteoporosis. The association with physical activity. *J Bone Joint Surg [Br].* 1970;52:667–675.

120. Schneider VS, LeBlanc A, Rambaut PC. Bone and mineral metabolism. In: Nicogossian AE, Huntoon CL, Pool SL, eds. *Space Physiology and Medicine.* Philadelphia, Pa: Lea & Febiger; 1989:214–221.

121. Jacobson PC, Beaver C, Grubb SA, Taft TN, Talmage RV. Bone density in women: College athletes and older athletic women. *J Orthop Res.* 1984;2:328–332.

122. Recker RR, Davies M, Hinders SM, Heaney RP, Stegman MR, Kimmel DB. Bone gain in young adult women. *JAMA.* 1992;268:2403–2408.

123. Nelson ME, Fiatarone MA, Morganti CM, Trice I, Greenberg RA, Evans WJ. Effects of high-intensity strength training on multiple risk factors for osteoporotic fractures. *JAMA.* 1994;272:1909–1914.

124. Krall EA, Dawson-Hughes B. Walking is related to bone density and rates of bone loss. *Am J Med.* 1994;96:20–26.

125. Harris SS, Dawson-Hughes B. Caffeine and bone loss in healthy postmenopausal women. *Am J Clin Nutr.* 1994;60:573–578.

126. Draper HH, Scythes CA. Calcium, phosphorus and osteoporosis. *Fed Proc.* 1981;40:2434–2438.

127. Barltrop D, Mole RH, Sutton A. Absorption and endogenous faecal excretion of calcium by low birthweight infants on feeds with varying contents of calcium and phosphate. *Arch Dis Child.* 1977;52:41–49.

128. Spencer H, Kramer L, Osis D, Norris C. Effect of phosphorus on the absorption of calcium and on the calcium balance. *J Nutr.* 1978;108:447–457.

129. Calvo MS, Kumar R, Heath H III. Persistently elevated parathyroid hormone secretion and action in young women after four weeks of ingesting high phosphorus, low calcium diets. *J Clin Endocrinol Metab.* 1990;70:1334–1340.

130. Mazarlegos-Ramos E, Guerrero-Romero F, Rodríguez-Morán M, Lazcano-Burciaga G, Panlagua R, Amato D. Consumption of soft drinks with phosphoric acid as a risk factor for the development of hypocalcemia in children: A case-control study. *J Pediatr.* 1995;126:940–942.

131. Massey LK, Strang MM. Soft drink consumption, phosphorus intake, and osteoporosis. *J Am Diet Assoc.* 1982;80:581–583.

132. Green TJ, Whiting SJ. Potassium bicarbonate reduces high protein-induced hypercalciuria in adult men. *Nutr Rev.* 1994;14:991–1002.

CHAPTER 5

Minerals

Most minerals are widely available in plant-based diets. Three minerals, however, have been the focus of much attention regarding their levels and/ or bioavailability in vegetarian diets: calcium, iron, and zinc. Most of the emphasis in this chapter is on iron and zinc (calcium is discussed in Chapter 4); the rest of the minerals are briefly discussed.

IRON

Iron deficiency is considered the most common nutritional deficiency; more than 500 million people are believed to be iron deficient worldwide.[1] In developing countries, the likelihood of developing iron deficiency is greatly enhanced because of iron loss resulting from parasitic infections and repeated pregnancies. In the United States, impaired iron status has been estimated to occur in 1% to 6% of the general population and in 5% to 14% of women aged 15 to 44. Iron intake is often inadequate during four periods of life: 6 months to 4 years, adolescence, during the female reproductive period, and during pregnancy.[2]

Approximately 40% of the iron in meat products is heme iron; 60% of the iron in meat and all the iron in plant foods is nonheme iron.[3,4] Because heme iron is better absorbed than nonheme iron, it is often suggested that vegetarians are at a marked increased risk of developing iron deficiency.[5] Most evidence suggests otherwise, however, and recent research shows that there may be some advantages to consuming iron mostly, or totally, in the form of nonheme iron.

Iron Requirements

The primary function of iron is to transport oxygen. On average, total body iron in men and women is about 4.0 g and 2.5 g, respectively, and approximately three fourths of this iron is contained in hemoglobin (65%) and myoglobin (10%). Although a small amount of iron is used by enzymes, the remaining 25% of total body iron is considered storage iron. The average man has about 1,000 mg of stored iron (enough for about 3 years), whereas women on average have only about 300 mg (enough for about 6 months).[6]

Men lose about 1.0 mg of iron per day, whereas premenopausal women lose about 1.5 mg/day. Although menstrual losses generally average 0.5 mg of iron per day, about 5% of the female population loses three times this much.[7] In men and postmenopausal women, iron loss comes primarily from small amounts of intestinal blood loss or sloughing off of intestinal cells. Some iron is also lost via the urine and skin.

The recommended dietary allowance (RDA) for iron for adult men and women is 10 mg and 15 mg, respectively. The iron requirement for women drops to 10 mg after menopause. Because humans have a limited ability to excrete iron, body levels are controlled primarily through absorption. About 10% to 15% of the dietary iron in populations in industrialized countries is absorbed.[8]

Iron Deficiency Anemia

When iron needs are not adequately met, iron stores begin to decrease. Once stores are depleted, serum iron levels will begin to decrease, and hemoglobin production will be depressed. Eventually, hemoglobin production decreases to a point where iron-deficiency anemia, characterized as microcytic hypochromic anemia, appears. Another indication of low iron levels is an increase in total iron binding capacity. Iron is transported in the blood by transferrin; normally, about one third of the available iron binding sites on transferrin are filled. When iron levels decrease, the number of available iron binding sites on transferrin increases.

Dietary Iron Intake in the United States

Although iron is one of the earth's most abundant elements and is widely distributed in food, it is relatively insoluble and consequently poorly absorbed. Since 1909, the availability of iron in the US food supply has increased by about 25%, mainly due to the enrichment of flour and other grain products beginning in the 1940s.[9] This has no doubt been a contributing factor to the decline in the prevalence of anemia that has been observed over the past 15 years in infants and children.[10] Anemia has also decreased in adult women.[11] Iron fortification of foods and the increased use of iron supplements and oral contraceptives may have also contributed to these lower rates.[11] The typical US diet, however, provides only 6 to 7 mg of iron per 1,000 calories. Consequently, many girls and women may experience difficulty in meeting iron requirements. Survey results indicate that iron intake of women 19 to 50 years old average only about 10 mg per day, or about two thirds of the RDA.[9]

Meat products provide about one third of the iron in the US diet, grains about one third, and fruits and vegetables about one sixth, with smaller amounts being derived from eggs and legumes.[9,12] In the typical US diet, heme iron contributes only about 10% to 15% of the total dietary iron.[13] Because heme iron is better absorbed than nonheme iron, however, it may contribute as much as one third of the total amount of iron absorbed.[14]

Natural, whole, unprocessed plant foods are rich in iron, as can be seen in Table 5–1. A diet that includes 1 cup of soybeans (5.4 mg), 2 cups of brown rice (1.6 mg), four slices of bread (3.2 mg), 1 cup of broccoli (1.4 mg), 1 oz of sunflower seeds (2.2 mg), and two oranges contains 15 mg of iron, enough to meet the RDA even for premenopausal women.[15]

Iron Absorption

Concerns over the iron status of vegetarians are generally not based on the iron content of vegetarian diets but rather on the bioavailability of the iron in vegetarian diets. In fact, vegetarian and plant-based diets generally contain as much or more iron than animal-based diets (see Appendix H). Vegan diets are generally higher in iron than lacto-ovo vegetarian diets because dairy foods contain relatively little iron (also, the iron from eggs in particular is poorly absorbed).[3] The absorption of iron can vary dramatically depending on a variety of factors. Nonheme iron is much more sensitive to these factors than heme iron.

The primary factor determining absorption is iron status.[16] Nonheme iron absorption has been shown to be 10 times higher (2.0% to 22.5%), and heme iron absorption 2 times higher (26% to 47%) in iron-deficient compared with iron-replete individuals.[16] The total amount of iron ingested at any one time also strongly influences the amount of iron absorbed. For example, when the nonheme iron content of a meal increased 4-fold from 1.5 mg to 6.0 mg, absorption decreased 3-fold from 18% to 6%; consequently, there was little difference in the actual amount of iron absorbed.[17] In contrast, 20% of the

Table 5–1 Iron Content of Foods

Food	Iron Content (mg)	Food	Iron Content (mg)
Breads, cereals, grains		Tomato juice, 1 cup	1.3
Bread, white, one slice	0.7	Turnip greens	1.5
Bread, whole wheat,		**Fruits**	
one slice	0.9	Apricots, ¼ cup dried	1.5
Bran flakes, 1 cup	11.0	Prunes, ¼ cup	0.9
Cream of Wheat, ½ cup	5.5	Prune juice, ½ cup	1.5
Oatmeal, instant, one		Raisins, ¼ cup	1.1
packet	6.3	**Legumes (½ cup cooked)**	
Barley, whole, ½ cup		Baked beans, vegetarian	0.7
cooked	1.6	Black beans	1.8
Pasta, enriched, ½ cup		Garbanzo beans	3.4
cooked	1.2	Kidney beans	1.5
Rice, brown, ½ cup cooked	0.5	Lentils	3.2
Wheat germ, 2 tbsp	1.2	Lima beans	2.2
Vegetables (½ cup cooked		Navy beans	2.5
unless otherwise indicated)		Pinto beans	2.2
Acorn squash	0.9	Soybeans	4.4
Avocado, ½ raw	1.0	Split peas	1.7
Beet greens	1.4	Tempeh	1.8
Brussels sprouts	0.9	Tofu	6.6
Collards	0.9	Textured vegetable protein	2.0
Peas	1.2	**Soymilk/vegetable milk**	
Pumpkin	1.7	Soymilk, 1 cup	1.4*
Sea vegetables		**Nuts/seeds (2 tbsp)**	
Alaria	18.1	Cashews	1.0
Dulse	33.1	Pumpkin seeds	2.5
Kelp	42.0	Tahini	1.2
Nori	20.9	Sunflower seeds	1.2
Spinach	1.5	**Other Foods**	
Swiss chard	1.9	Blackstrap molasses, 1 tbsp	3.3

*Varies by brand

Source: Data from *Bowes & Church's Food Value of Portions Commonly Used.* 16th ed., by J. Pennington, Lippincott-Raven, © 1994.

heme iron was absorbed regardless of whether 1.5 or 6.0 mg of iron was ingested.[17]

Depending on the composition of a meal, iron absorption can vary 20-fold.[18] Factors in meat enhance the absorption of nonheme iron but have little effect on heme iron.[3] Vitamin C, which is abundant in vegetarian diets, enhances absorption of nonheme iron. Five fluid ounces of orange juice containing 75 mg of vitamin C can enhance iron absorption from a meal by as much as a factor of 4.[19] In addition to vitamin C or ascorbic acid, fruits and vegetables contain small amounts of other organic acids that can also enhance iron absorption, and the effect of citric acid (which is found in citrus fruits) is additive to that produced by ascorbic acid alone.[20,21] To enhance absorption, the vitamin C source and iron must be consumed at about the same time.[22] Some research indicates, however, that the enhancing effect of vitamin C on iron absorption is much less when consumed as part of the daily diet than at a single meal.[23]

Inhibitors of Iron Absorption

There are also inhibitors of iron absorption; for example, tannic acids in tea can reduce nonheme iron absorption by as much as half.[24] Populations that have high tea consumption rates also frequently have a high incidence of anemia, although other factors may contribute to this.[25] Many Indian spices, such as turmeric, coriander, chilies, and tamarind, also contain tannins.[26] Coffee can also inhibit iron absorption, and adding milk to coffee exacerbates this effect.[27] The calcium in dairy products can markedly inhibit iron absorption.[28] The addition of modest amounts of milk or cheese to a meal of pizza or hamburger has been shown to reduce iron absorption by 50% to 60%.[28] However, recent data suggest the effect of calcium on iron absorption is an acute effect and may be less relevant over the long term.[29] Fiber can also interfere with iron absorption to some extent,[30,31] and vegetarians consume 50% to 100% more fiber than nonvegetarians (Appendix A).

A more important factor than fiber with respect to iron absorption is phytate. Phytate is a phosphorus-containing organic compound found in whole grains and legumes. Under experimental conditions, phytate can inhibit iron absorption by as much as 90%.[32] Many studies have found phytates to be potent inhibitors of iron absorption,[33,34] and there is no intestinal adaptation to these inhibitory effects.[33] Processing of whole grains can remove much of the phytate but also much of the iron. Refined grains are generally much lower in phytate than whole grains, and for this reason the phytate content of breakfast cereals varies quite a bit and can range from 25 to 150 mg in a single portion.[35]

Generally, as the phytate and fiber content of a food or diet increases, so does the iron content. Consequently, consuming foods high in these components will have less of an effect on iron status than one might expect. In one study, for example, when subjects were switched from a diet containing a low-fiber white bread to one containing whole wheat bread, daily iron intake increased from 8.3 to 12.2 mg, but iron status was unaffected. The higher iron intake compensated for poorer bioavailability.[36] Because vegetarians consume more grains and legumes than nonvegetarians, their diets are higher in phytates. Vegan diets may contain up to two to three times as much phytate as omnivore diets; lacto-ovo vegetarian diets contain an amount intermediate between these two diets.[32,37,38]

Vitamin C can largely counteract the effects of phytate.[18,35,39] For example, researchers found that nonheme iron absorption from a vegetarian meal high in phytate was increased by a factor of 2.5 just by the addition of about ½ cup of cauliflower, which is rich in vitamin C.[39] Also, considerate hydrolysis of phytate occurs during fermentation and the baking process such that iron bioavailability from leavened breads is much higher than from unleavened breads.

Most studies have looked at how factors affect the absorption of iron from a single meal, however. These effects appear to be less important when iron absorption from the overall diet is considered because mixed diets will contain an assortment of both iron inhibitors and iron enhancers.[23,40,41] These factors are likely to be much more important when the diet is limited in the type and number of foods consumed, which is often the case in developing countries.[42] Consequently, it is difficult to determine accurately the overall absorption of iron from any given diet. According to the World Health Organization, about 10% to 15% of the iron present in the diets of most industrialized countries is absorbed.[8] These diets contain a mixture of both heme iron and nonheme iron and an assortment of enhancers and inhibitors of iron absorption. The National Research Council, in calculating the RDA for iron, adopted an absorption figure of 10%.

For primarily vegetarian diets, however, it may be that only 5% to 10% of the iron is absorbed.[42,43] Of course, this will depend on the relative amount of iron enhancers (vitamin C, organic acids, etc) versus inhibitors of iron (tea, coffee, etc). Committees responsible for establishing recommendations for iron intake for the United States, the United Kingdom, and Australia all suggest that iron intake be increased and/or that enhancers of iron absorption, such as vitamin C, be increased in vegetarian diets.[44,45] The Dutch Nutrition Council assumes an absorption figure of 12% in setting the recommended iron intake for both men and women at 15 mg/day for individuals consuming a mixed diet with a ratio of heme to nonheme iron of about 1:3.[46] For a diet without meat, however, iron absorption is assumed to be only 8%, which means that the recommended intake increases to 22 mg/day for vegetarians. Similarly, researchers from the Indian Council of Medical Research in India concluded that, because of the lower availability of iron from the largely vegetarian Indian diet (Indian diets are high in phytates), at least 17 mg of iron is needed.[47]

Vegetarian Iron Intake and Status

Plant-based diets tend to be rather high in iron. For example, the diets of rural Chinese and Mexicans, which are almost completely vegan, were found to contain on average 34 mg[48] and more than 17 mg[49] of iron per day, respectively. Dutch researchers designed what they considered typical vegan, lacto vegetarian, and nonvegetarian diets and found them to contain 20.4, 17.4, and 13.6 mg of iron per day, respectively.[50] This agrees with a nationwide survey of the Dutch population, which found that vegetarians consumed as much or more than the general nonvegetarian population.[46] Typical vegetarian diets constructed by investigators from the Veterans Administration Hospital in Hines, Illinois, contained (at 2,600 calories) 19.2, 15.0, and 16.3 mg of iron for vegan, lacto, and lacto-ovo vegetarian diets, respectively.[51] Similarly, Indian researchers designed typical Indian vegetarian diets and found them to contain more than 38 mg of iron.[52] Finally, in an analysis of three hospital diets, iron content was 13.4, 14.3, and 24.4 mg/day for a nonvegetarian, lacto-ovo vegetarian, and soy-based vegetarian diet, respectively.[37]

Clearly, well-planned vegetarian diets can be quite high in iron. Dietary surveys of Western populations tend to reflect the differences in iron content between the vegetarian and nonvegetarian experimentally designed diets cited above; vegans tend to consume more iron than lacto-ovo vegetarians, and lacto-ovo vegetarians tend to consume about the same amount as omnivores (see Appendix H). This appears to be true even in the case of children, although the data are limited. In a study involving 23 British vegan preschool children, the average iron intake was 10 mg/day (which is the US RDA), and their diet was nearly twice as iron dense as diets of preschool omnivores.[52]

On the whole, research indicates that vegetarian dietary iron intake, particularly in the case of vegans, meets or exceeds the US RDA for iron. The key question, however, is not how much iron vegetarians consume but how much is absorbed and, consequently, whether the iron status of vegetarians is adequate. Typically, the amount of stored iron of vegetarians is within the normal range, although it is substantially lower than that of omnivores (Appendix I).[31,53–55] Several studies indicate that more vegetarians are likely to have iron stores considered to be deficient or very low in comparison to nonvegetarians,[43,54–58] although iron stores can vary significantly without any apparent impairment of iron status.[59] Male vegetarians often have iron stores that are closer to levels of premenopausal omnivorous women than to those of male omnivores[43,54] (Figure 5–1). Nevertheless, studies indicate that there is little difference, if any, between parameters of iron status (ie, hemoglobin, hematocrit, total iron binding capacity and serum iron levels) of vegetarians and nonvegetarians (Appendix I).[32,43,55,56,60–64]

With respect to children, the only published studies involve individuals consuming a restricted macrobiotic diet, where it was found that about 15% of the young macrobiotic children in Boston and the Netherlands had poor iron status even though iron intake was adequate.[65,66] In contrast, children aged 6 to 12 years who consumed vegetarian diets that were more varied and balanced had iron-related blood values that were not significantly different from those of similarly aged nonvegetarian children.[67]

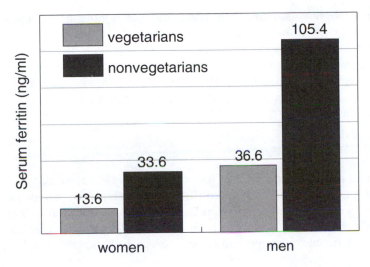

Figure 5–1 Iron stores in vegetarians and omnivores. Values are for 36 female and 14 male vegetarians and for equal numbers of nonvegetarians. Of the 36 female vegetarians, 31 were lacto-ovo vegetarians and 5 were vegans. Differences between the vegetarians and nonvegetarians were statistically significant for both men and women ($P < 0.01$, Mann-Whitney U test). The mean age of the female and male vegetarians was 26 and 28 years, respectively. The omnivorous controls were aged within 1 year of the vegetarians. *Source:* Data from Alexander D, Ball MJ, Mann J. Nutrient intake and haematological status of vegetarians and age-sex matched omnivores. *Eur J Clin Nutr.* 1994;48:538–546.

Iron Overload

A larger percentage of the population than previously thought has a gene(s) that can lead to hemochromatosis (excess iron storage).[68] Approximately 1 of every 250 people has the gene(s) that can make one susceptible to iron overload, which can have devastating consequences. For this reason, some researchers suggest that everyone should be tested for this condition.

Even in individuals without hemochromatosis, however, excess iron stores may have adverse effects, since iron is thought to be capable of generating free radicals *in vivo* and, although still speculative, may increase risk of heart disease[69,70] and cancer,[71,72] particularly colon cancer[72] but perhaps also breast cancer.[73] Additionally, heme iron may affect risks differently from nonheme iron. For example, in a study involving more than 50,000 male health professionals, heme iron intake but not nonheme iron intake was associated with an increased heart disease risk.[73] In this study, iron was a risk factor only in subjects who did not supplement their diet with vitamin E; the antioxidant properties of vitamin E were apparently able to negate the harmful effects of iron-generated free radicals. The lower but adequate iron stores of vegetarians and the intake of primarily nonheme iron may be the optimal situation.

ZINC

Animal products, and meat in particular,[75] provide 70% of the zinc in the typical American diet.[76] Vegetarian zinc intake is similar or somewhat lower than nonvegetarian intake (Appendix I), and the absorption of zinc from plants is somewhat lower than from animal products. The zinc RDA is a subject of debate, however, and some researchers believe that it may be higher than necessary.

Zinc Deficiency

In humans, outright zinc deficiency was first observed in Middle Eastern men and was associated with a condition called hypogonadism (small and underdeveloped testicles), which leads to dwarfism.[77] Turkish investigators have observed zinc deficiency in growth-stunted children who indulge in geophagia, the practice of eating clay.[78] Clay inhibits zinc absorption. Chinese investigators have reported that as many as 30% of Chinese children are stunted from zinc deficiency.[79]

There appear to be predisposing factors that contribute to zinc deficiency other than just inadequate zinc intake. For instance, zinc deficiency in school-age boys in some Middle East countries was associated with blood loss from parasitic infestations, geophagia, and excessive loss of zinc related to excessive perspiration.[77,80] Boys from the same population without these predisposing factors were not overtly zinc deficient.[81]

For North Americans, marginal zinc deficiency is more likely to occur than overt deficiency. Marginal or mild zinc deficiency has been observed in several studies of children and has been associated in many cases with poor appetite, suboptimal growth, and impaired taste acuity.[82,83] In a recent US survey, about 3% of the children between the ages of 3 and 8 years had low serum zinc levels.[84] The dietary zinc content of low-income children in the United States is particularly low.[85] Both children and pregnant women, because of increased needs, appear to be particularly vulnerable to zinc deficiency.

Body stores of zinc are not readily accessible and therefore cannot compensate for low zinc intakes. Consequently, and because of the specific functions that zinc has in the body, signs of zinc deficiency, at least in laboratory studies, appear quickly when zinc-deficient diets are fed.[86] Zinc is thought to be a cofactor for at least 60 different enzymes, but it is also involved in nonenzymatic reactions.[87] Zinc is particularly important for the synthesis and degradation of DNA.[88] Consequently, adequate zinc is needed for optimal cell growth, which explains why, in patients with low zinc levels, zinc supplements increase the rate of wound healing, a process involving rapid cell division.[89] Zinc also plays a role in protein synthesis and blood formation. In addition, zinc is involved in the immune system, and for this reason there is a concern that inadequate zinc intake impairs the immune response; zinc intake is lower in the elderly and may contribute to their impaired immunity.[90]

Zinc Intake and Dietary Requirements

The RDA for zinc should be viewed with some caution because of the difficulty in precisely determining zinc status. This problem is confounded because, as is the case for several nutrients, small amounts of zinc are better absorbed than large amounts and because people with low zinc status absorb more than those with adequate zinc status. The major route for zinc excretion is via the intestinal lumen through pancreatic and intestinal secretions. As discussed below, phytate can inhibit zinc absorption from foods but also the reabsorption of endogenously secreted zinc.

Zinc absorption increases in individuals with poor iron status and zinc losses can be reduced by as much as 80% in response to low zinc intakes.[91] Consequently, it takes little zinc to maintain a low zinc status and much more to maintain a high zinc status. The attainment of zinc balance, however, does not necessarily imply that normal zinc concentrations are maintained in all body tissues and fluids.[92] What is not known is to what extent a marginal zinc status hinders optimal health.

The adult US RDA for zinc is 15 mg for men and 12 mg for women. These values are viewed as somewhat controversial because in the healthy US population only a small percentage of individuals consume the recommended amount of zinc.[93] Thus it has been argued that if the population is healthy its dietary zinc requirement cannot be as high as currently recommended. The Canadian Bureau of Nutritional Sciences suggests that a much lower zinc intake is safe and adequate; their recommended nutrient intake is 9 mg for men and 8 mg for women.[94] Similarly, the World Health Organization recommends consuming anywhere from one third to three quarters of the USA RDA[95] (Table 5–2).

Differences between the Canadian and American recommendations for zinc intake, however, are based not on estimates of biologic zinc requirements but on absorption estimates; the US RDA uses a conservative value of 20% absorption, whereas the Canadian recommendation uses a value of 40% absorption

Table 5-2 Recommendations for Zinc Intake from Three Countries and the World Health Organization (WHO)

Population	Recommended Zinc Intake (mg)			
	United States	Canada	United Kingdom	WHO
Children	10	4–7	5–7	4
Adolescents	12–15	9–12	7–9.5	5.5–7
Adults	12–15	9–12	7–9.5	5.5
Pregnant women	15	15	7	7.5

Source: Data from World Health Organization Expert Committee on Trace Elements in Human Nutrition, *Trace Elements in Human Nutrition,* World Health Organization Technical Report Series 532, 1973.

less 5% for diets high in fiber (although the effect of fiber on zinc absorption is unclear) and phytate.[94] In typical US diets, high in meat and low in fiber and phytates, it is relatively certain that zinc absorption is relatively good. Less clear is how well zinc is absorbed from vegetarian diets. The World Health Organization has estimated that only 10% to 15% of the zinc is available in some diets, such as those consumed in poor Egyptian villages. In these diets, meat, poultry, and fish provide less than 10% of the zinc, whereas cereals provide more than 70%. A zinc absorption of 10% to 15%, at least in theory, indicates that overall intake would have to be increased markedly to meet biologic needs. The lower zinc absorption in Egyptian diets may have some relevance to vegetarians because this type of diet resembles that consumed by vegans more so than the typical American diet, although the use of unleavened bread (high in phytates) is common in Egypt.

Zinc Absorption

In the classic research first identifying human zinc deficiency in the Middle East, dietary zinc intake was adequate, but bioavailability was a problem. Zinc absorption from foods varies dramatically depending upon the type of meal consumed. For example, studies have shown that zinc absorption can vary fourfold, from as little as 8.2% to as high as 38.2%.[96,97] In these studies, the two most important factors affecting zinc absorption were animal protein and total zinc content, the former increasing relative absorption and the latter decreasing it.[96–99]

Phytate, which is found in whole grains and legumes, is a potent inhibitor of zinc absorption.[100] For example, zinc absorption from whole grain cereal meals with a high phytate content is only 5%.[101] When phytate levels are reduced by fermentation to about a third the initial level, however, absorption increases fourfold. Although phytate is likely to be a problem only when consumed in large amounts, the phytate content of plant-based diets can be high. Some reports have suggested that there is an intestinal adaptation to the inhibitory effects of phytate, but others have found this not to be the case.[32,38,100] There is, however, likely to be some hydrolysis of phytate by intestinal enzymes (only a minor role), intestinal bacteria, and plant phytases, thereby increasing zinc bioavailability.[102–104]

Fiber may also bind zinc.[105] The effect of fiber on mineral balance is controversial, however, because several studies have not shown any adverse effects.[106,107] Also, whole grain products are higher in zinc than refined ones, so that the absolute amount of zinc absorbed is often not compromised. For example, although relative zinc absorption was higher from refined white bread, total zinc absorbed was higher from whole wheat bread because of the higher zinc control.[108] Similarly, when subjects in one study were switched from a diet containing a low fiber white bread to one containing whole wheat bread, daily zinc intake increased from 9.0 to 12.7 mg, but zinc status was unaffected, indicating that the higher zinc intake compensated for the poorer bioavailability.[36]

The average phytate intake of omnivores ranges from between about 400 to 800 mg/day, a level that is unlikely to affect zinc absorption markedly.[37,109,110] Vegetarians, however, consume two to three times as much phytate as omnivores and also less zinc. It has been proposed that a phytate-to-zinc ratio of less than 10 (on a molar basis) would not hinder zinc absorption but that one of 20 and above would,[111,112] although there is some disagreement on this point.[113,114] Several studies have concluded that on this basis zinc bioavailability would be compromised on a vegetarian diet.[38,109,111,115]

Because calcium potentiates the inhibitory effects of phytate on zinc absorption,[116] however, it has been proposed that the amount of phytate and calcium relative to zinc is the key factor in determining zinc absorption.[38] This would work in favor of vegans but against lacto-ovo vegetarians because of their higher calcium intake.

Both phosphorus and protein raise zinc requirements. In one study, zinc requirements nearly doubled on a moderate-phosphorus, high-protein diet (100 g of protein per day) compared with a low-phosphorus, moderate-protein diet (60 g of protein per day), which is fairly typical of vegetarian, especially vegan, intake.[117]

Vegetarian Zinc Intake and Status

Canadian Seventh-day Adventist lacto-ovo vegetarian women with an average age of 50 years had a zinc intake of approximately 9 mg/day,[63] which is the Canadian RDA and similar to what older nonvegetarian Canadian[118] and American[119] women consume but still markedly below the US RDA. Similar results were found in two studies from the United Kingdom.[120,121]

Several other studies have found vegetarian zinc intake to be similar to or even slightly higher than nonvegetarians, but others have reported low intakes among vegetarians (Appendix H).

In one study of vegan preschool children, the zinc density of the diet (milligrams of zinc per 1,000 kcal) was identical to the average zinc density of the diet of nonvegetarian preschoolers.[53] Zinc intake among Canadian children aged 4 to 7 years was reported to be 8.5 mg/day,[122] and among Indian young adult lacto-ovo vegetarians it was found to be 9.3 mg/day.[123] Experimental diets designed to represent the typical intake of vegetarians found zinc levels to be about 10 mg in one case[51] and 17 mg in a second.[50] A typical Indian vegetarian diet designed by researchers contained more than 20 mg of zinc,[52] and vegetarian-designed hospital diets were found to contain 9.7 mg of zinc for lacto-ovo vegetarian diets and 15.0 mg for a vegan type diet in comparison to 12.2 mg for the nonvegetarian diet.[37]

These observations indicate that vegetarian diets can provide adequate zinc, although zinc intake seems to be lower than recommended in both US vegetarian and omnivore diets. As noted, however, both intake and bioavailability of zinc are important. Therefore, it may be more instructive to look at vegetarian status. Because there is no single accurate measure of zinc status, however, study results must be viewed cautiously.

Studies of pregnant women have found no difference in zinc status between vegetarians and nonvegetarians.[124–126] Levels of zinc in hair, saliva, and serum are in the normal range for vegetarians, although they are lower than in nonvegetarians.[113,127–129] Also, in some studies, greater numbers of vegetarians in comparison to nonvegetarians had very low blood zinc levels.[61,129]

The fact that zinc intake among vegetarians appears to be relatively similar to the intake of nonvegetarians but their zinc status is somewhat poorer appears to be due to poor absorption. It is possible that some adaptation to low zinc intake takes place, however. In one study, when omnivores and vegetarians were placed on identical vegetarian diets, zinc balance was better in the vegetarians.[126] In response to a high-fiber diet, vegetarians utilized zinc more efficiently than omnivores.[126] Ascorbic acid, which has a negative effect on zinc status, had a greater effect in omnivores than vegetarians.

Finally, two recent studies help provide some perspective about vegetarian diets and zinc. One found that zinc absorption from a lacto-ovo vegetarian diet was about 25% lower than from an omnivorous diet,[130] and the other found that young Chinese women, by greatly reducing fecal zinc losses, were able to maintain zinc balance when consuming just 5 mg of zinc per day.[131] Nevertheless, although overt zinc deficiency is typically not seen among vegetarians, because of the difficulty of determining zinc status and uncertainty over the effects of a marginally lower zinc status on overall health, it is appropriate for vegetarians to strive to meet the zinc RDA. This is especially true because of the

Table 5–3 Zinc Content of Foods

Food	Zinc Content (mg)	Food	Zinc Content (mg)
Bread, cereals, grains		Chick peas	1.3
Bran flakes, 1 cup	5.0	Cranberry beans	1.0
Granola, ¼ cup	0.7	Hyacinth beans	2.7
Grapenuts, ¼ cup	1.2	Kidney beans	1.0
Nutrigrain, ¾ cup	3.7	Lima beans	1.0
Oatmeal, instant, one packet	1.0	Lentils	1.2
Shredded wheat, 1 oz	0.9	Navy beans	0.9
Special K, 1⅓ cup	3.7	Pinto beans	0.9
Barley, whole, ½ cup cooked	1.2	Soybeans	1.0
Millet, ½ cup cooked	0.4	Split peas	1.0
Wheat germ, 2 tbsp	2.3	Tempeh	1.5
Vegetables (½ cup cooked)		Tofu	1.0
Asparagus	0.4	Textured vegetable protein	1.4
Collards	0.6	**Nuts/seeds (2 tbsp)**	
Corn	0.9	Brazil nuts	1.3
Mushrooms	0.7	Cashews	1.0
Okra	0.6	Peanut butter	1.0
Peas	1.0	Peanuts	1.8
Potato	0.4	Pumpkin/squash seeds	1.2
Sea vegetables		Sunflower seeds	0.9
Irish moss	2.0	Tahini	1.3
Kelp	1.2	**Animal products**	
Nori/laver	1.1	Milk, 1 cup	1.0
Spinach	0.7	Cheese	
Legumes (½ cup cooked)		Cheddar, 1 oz	0.9
Adzuki beans	2.0	Swiss, 1 oz	1.1
Black-eyed peas	1.1	Yogurt, 1 cup	1.8

Source: Data from *Bowes & Church's Food Value of Portions Commonly Used.* 16th ed., by J. Pennington, Lippincott-Raven, 1994.

lower zinc bioavailability of vegetarian diets,[49,95,126,132] although the lower protein intake of vegetarians may decrease zinc needs somewhat.

It is prudent for all vegetarians to include plenty of zinc-rich food in their diet (Table 5–3). Well-planned vegetarian menus can provide as much as 20 mg of zinc.[49,50,133] Whole grain cereals, mushrooms, peas, sea vegetables, beans, tofu, tempeh, textured vegetable protein, nuts, wheat germ, milk, and cheeses are all good choices.

SELENIUM

Selenium is a cofactor for the enzyme glutathione peroxidase, which is present in red blood cells and other tissues and helps prevent oxidative dam-

Table 5–4 Selenium Content of Foods

Food	Selenium Content (μg)	Food	Selenium Content (μg)
Bread, cereals, grains		Barley, whole, ½ cup cooked	0.03
Bread, white, one slice	7	Rice, white, ½ cup cooked	5
Bread, whole wheat,		**Legumes (½ cup cooked)**	
one slice	11	Lentils	10
English muffin, ½	8	Navy beans	10
Bran flakes, 1 cup	4	**Nuts/seeds**	
Oatmeal, ½ cup cooked	10	Brazil nuts, 2 tbsp	10
Barley, pearled, ½ cup		**Animal products**	
cooked	5	Egg, one large	12

Source: Data from *Bowes & Church's Food Value of Portions Commonly Used.* 16th ed., by J. Pennington, Lippincott-Raven, 1994.

age by neutralizing lipid hydroperoxides and hydrogen peroxides. It works closely in conjunction with vitamin E, another antioxidant. Glutathione peroxidase activity is the basis for establishing selenium status and requirements because blood selenium levels are not a good indicator of status.

The selenium content of foods varies widely (Table 5–4) and in plants it is largely dependent on the amount of selenium in the soil. In China, for example, in an area where human selenosis (excess selenium) occurs, the selenium concentration of corn, rice, and soybeans is 1,000 times higher than the selenium concentration of those crops grown in an area of China where selenium deficiency is common.[134] Variation in the selenium concentration of animal products is not nearly as great because animals can conserve selenium when intakes are low and excrete more selenium when intakes are high.

Selenium intake varies considerably among countries. In the United States, selenium intake is reported to be around 108 μg/day,[135] which compares favorably with the RDA of 70 and 55 μg for adult men and women, respectively. Although in many countries animal products are the most important sources of selenium, this tends to be the case only when dietary selenium content is low (generally as a result of low soil selenium), such as in many northern European countries.[136] This accounts for the low selenium intake of Swedish subjects placed on a lacto-ovo vegetarian diet[137] and reports showing Swedish vegetarian diets, particularly vegan diets, to be low in selenium.[138,139] This agrees with two recent studies conducted in Slovakia that found that parameters of selenium status (plasma levels of selenium and glutathione, and glutathione peroxidase activity) were lower in vegetarians compared with nonvegetarians.[140,141] The selenium content of soil in Slovakia is low relative to many other countries.

More relevant than these studies, however, is one showing that, when diets were designed to represent typical omnivorous, lacto-ovo vegetarian, and vegan diets consumed in the United States, selenium content was 92.7, 84.8, and 85.9 μg/day, all surpassing the RDA.[142] These results are similar to those reported by Gibson et al[143] for Canadian vegetarians. Cereals, which provided more than a third of the selenium intake of both vegetarians and nonvegetarians in this Canadian study, are much higher in selenium than cereals grown in many northern European countries. Interestingly, one study found that, although daily selenium intake did not differ between lactating lacto-ovo vegetarians and nonvegetarians (101 versus 106 μg), breast milk selenium concentration and glutathione peroxidase activity were significantly greater in vegetarians.[144] This may give added protection against oxidative damage to the infants of vegetarian mothers. However, other studies in the US and New Zealand indicate that although vegetarian intake is similar to omnivores, it is below the US RDA (Appendix I).

Selenium status is affected more by the selenium content of soil in a given region than by dietary pattern. Studies of North American vegetarians suggest there is little difference in selenium status between vegetarians and nonvegetarians.[144,145] In low selenium areas, all individuals, but particularly vegetarians, need to identify good sources of selenium.

COPPER

Copper has been used therapeutically since at least 400 BC, when Hippocrates prescribed copper compounds for pulmonary disorders and other diseases.[146] Currently, there are not enough data to establish an RDA for copper, but the estimated safe and adequate daily dietary intake is 1.5 to 3.0 mg/day. The average US diet supplies only about 1.0 mg/day.[147] Outright copper deficiency is rare, however, and generally occurs only in unusual circumstances.[148] There are a number of important copper-containing proteins and enzymes, some of which are essential for the proper utilization of iron.

The efficiency of copper absorption is better at lower intakes (eg, 56% absorption at an intake of 0.8 mg versus 12% absorption at 7.5 mg).[149] Some studies have found that ascorbic acid decreases copper absorption.[150] Also, higher vitamin C intakes (605 mg/day) were shown to decrease serum levels of ceruloplasmin, the protein that transports copper in the blood, although overall body copper status in this study was not adversely affected.[151]

One interesting theory about copper status involves the relationship between copper and zinc and the effect of this ratio on blood cholesterol levels. Epidemiologic data and studies in animals suggest a positive correlation between a higher zinc-to-copper ratio in the diet and the incidence of cardiovascular disease.[152] Vegetarians, particularly vegans, may benefit if this hypothesis is correct because their copper intakes are higher (particularly for vegans) than those of nonvegetarians and because zinc bioavailability is relatively lower on a vegetarian diet.

Some concerns have been raised about the bioavailability of copper on vegetarian diets. Several factors pertinent to vegetarian diets may positively affect copper absorption and/or requirements, however. Protein tends to decrease copper requirements, whereas zinc tends to increase it; thus for vegans, who consume relatively low amounts of zinc and protein, these factors might negate one another.[153,154] Conversely, high-fiber, high-phytate diets may depress copper absorption somewhat.[153,155,156] Nevertheless, some research indicates that vegetarians have lower serum copper levels[141] and that when shifting from an omnivorous diet to a vegetarian one, serum copper levels decrease.[137] Vegetarian diets tend to be higher in copper, however, which may override any concerns about absorption. Although data are limited, lacto-ovo vegetarians consume somewhat more copper, and vegans considerably more, than omnivores (Table 5–5, Appendix I).

Table 5–5 Copper Content of Foods

Food	Copper Content (µg)	Food	Copper Content (µg)
Breads, cereals, and grains		**Legumes (½ cup cooked)**	
Bread, whole wheat, one slice	0.09	Lentils	0.24
		Navy beans	0.24
Graham crackers, two whole	0.14	Soybeans	0.35
		Split peas	0.25
Bran flakes, 1 cup	0.29	Tempeh	0.55
Barley, whole, ½ cup cooked	0.22	Textured vegetable protein	0.33
		Tofu	0.23
Millet, ½ cup cooked	0.19	**Nuts/seeds (2 tbsp)**	
Vegetables (1/2 cup cooked unless otherwise indicated)		Almond butter	0.28
		Almonds	0.29
Avocado, ½	0.23	Brazil nuts	0.50
Mushrooms	0.24	Cashews	0.38
Peas	0.13	Peanuts	0.37
Potato	0.27	Pumpkin/squash seeds	0.23
Sweet potato	0.23	Sunflower seeds	0.30
Tomato juice, 1 cup	0.23	Tahini	0.45

Source: Data from *Bowes & Church's Food Value of Portions Commonly Used.* 16th ed., by J. Pennington, Lippincott-Raven, 1994.

MAGNESIUM

Magnesium may have a role in more diverse functions than any other single nutrient; more than 300 enzymes are thought to require magnesium for activation.[157] About half the body content of magnesium (about 25 g) is found in bone. The male and female adult RDA for magnesium is 350 and 280 mg, respectively, making this the nutrient with the third highest dietary requirement. Whole grains are extremely rich in magnesium. A slice of whole wheat bread, for example, contains 26 mg, but a slice of white bread contains only 5 mg. During refinement, more than 80% of the magnesium is lost by removal of the germ and outer layer of cereal grains.[158] The magnesium content of vegetarian type foods is generally higher than that of nonvegetarian type foods.[159]

In a recent study of nearly 600 omnivore men and women, about 40% of the men and about 50% of the women consumed less than two thirds of the RDA for magnesium.[160] Although outright dietary deficiency of magnesium has not been reported in people consuming natural diets, magnesium deficiency may result from a number of diseases, such as alcoholism.[161]

Recently, some research has suggested that magnesium supplementation may be useful in the treatment and/or prevention of coronary artery disease, preeclampsia, and asthma, although more research is needed before firm conclusions can be drawn. Supplemental magnesium has also been shown to decrease blood pressure.[162] Some evidence also suggests that additional magnesium can improve athletic performance,[158] and one area under study is the role of magnesium in bone health because magnesium may displace calcium in the bone when calcium levels are low.

Vegetarian diets are generally much higher in magnesium than nonvegetarian diets (Appendix H). In one study, when subjects were placed on a vegetarian diet, magnesium intake increased 34%.[163] Similarly, experimentally designed vegan diets were shown to contain more magnesium than lacto and lacto-ovo vegetarian diets.[51] In macrobiotic and nonmacrobiotic vegetarian children, magnesium intake was markedly higher than the RDA,[65] and in vegetarian macrobiotic adult women serum magnesium levels were about 10% higher.[164]

Although phytate and fiber, which are high in vegetarian diets, may reduce magnesium absorption somewhat,[165–167] absorption is still adequate.[136,168] The higher magnesium content of vegetarian diets should easily compensate for any lower absorption[49,141] (Table 5–6).

PHOSPHORUS

Approximately 85% of the total amount of phosphorus in the body (about 700 g) is in the bone in a 1:2 ratio with calcium. Although phosphorus has a

Table 5–6 Magnesium Content of Foods

Food	Magnesium Content (mg)	Food	Magnesium Content (mg)
Breads, cereals, grains		**Fruit**	
Bread, whole wheat,		Banana, one medium	33
one slice	26	Orange juice, 1 cup	24
Bran flakes, 1 cup	71	**Legumes (½ cup cooked)**	
Oatmeal, ½ cup cooked	28	Black-eyed peas	41
Barley, whole, ½ cup cooked	61	Kidney beans	40
Millet, ½ cup cooked	52	Navy beans	48
Pasta, whole wheat,		Pinto beans	47
½ cup cooked	21	Soybeans	74
Rice, brown, ½ cup cooked	43	Split peas	35
Wheat germ, 2 tbsp	45	Tempeh	52
Vegetables (1/2 cup cooked		Tofu	127
unless otherwise indicated)		**Nuts/seeds (2 tbsp)**	
Avocado, ½	35	Almond butter	96
Beet greens	49	Almonds	79
Beets	31	Brazil nuts	64
Lima beans	41	Cashews	44
Okra	45	Peanuts	52
Peas	31	Peanut butter	60
Potato	32	Pumpkin/squash seeds	92
Pumpkin	27	Sunflower seeds	63
Spinach	70	**Animal products**	
Swiss chard	75	Milk, 1 cup	34
Winter squash	43	Yogurt, 1 cup	43

Source: Data from *Bowes & Church's Food Value of Portions Commonly Used.* 16th ed., by J. Pennington, Lippincott-Raven, 1994.

critical role in bone development and maintenance, it has other functions as well. For example, the body stores and releases energy by breaking and making phosphate bonds via adenosine triphosphate (ATP).

The RDA for phosphorus for adult men and women is the same as for calcium, 800 mg, although intakes of phosphorus typically exceed those of calcium. Estimates are that nonvegetarian men and women consume approximately 1,500 mg[169] and 1,000 mg[170] of phosphorus per day, respectively. Intakes may actually be 15% to 20% higher than this because many food additives, which are not included in dietary surveys, contain phosphorus.[171] Diets based heavily on convenience foods may derive 20% to 30% of their phosphorus from food additives.[172]

Concerns over phosphorus intake center on the observation that intake may be too high, at least relative to the amount of calcium consumed. Studies in rats have shown that diets with low calcium-to-phosphorus ratios cause progressive bone loss.[173] When the dietary calcium-to-phosphorus ratio is too low (about 1:4), which would occur with the consumption of large amounts of meat but low amounts of calcium sources, bone health may be negatively affected.[174] This is likely to be the situation for as much as 20% of the US population.[175]

The finding that high-phosphorus, low-calcium diets might be harmful to bone health is of particular concern to young women, who tend to consume low levels of calcium but are often frequent consumers of soft drinks, which are high in phosphorus.[15] Animal protein is also high in phosphorus, and the absorption of phosphorus from typical Western diets is quite good; for example, about 70% of the phosphorus from meat is absorbed.[176]

In spite of these concerns, the adverse effects of high phosphorus intakes observed in animals have not been observed in human studies.[177,178] Nevertheless, when a high-phosphorus, low-calcium diet was fed to teenage girls, serum levels of parathyroid hormone and urinary levels of hydroxyproline were significantly increased, suggesting that this type of diet may in fact adversely affect bone health.[179] Furthermore, in a case-control study involving young Mexican children, individuals with low serum calcium levels (below 2.2 mmol/L) were five times more likely to drink large amounts of soft drinks (at least 1.5 L/week) than children with normal calcium levels (2.2 to 3.0 mmol/L).[180] The phosphorus content of Coca-Cola and Pepsi-Cola is 19.7 and 16.1 mg/dL, respectively.[181]

If there is in fact some disadvantage to consuming high phosphorus diets, then vegetarians may have a slight advantage in this regard because they do not consume animal flesh. Although the phosphorus intake of vegetarians (Appendix F) is similar to that of omnivores (cereals and beans can be quite high in phosphorus), the phosphorus in cereals is not as well absorbed as that in animal foods because it is in the form of phytate (inositol hexaphosphate).[182]

MANGANESE

Only two enzymes are known to require manganese specifically as a cofactor, pyruvate carboxylase and superoxide dismutase. Both are found in the mitochondria. Progress in the field of manganese nutrition has been hampered because of the lack of a practical method for assessing manganese status. Manganese deficiency has never been observed in noninstitutionalized human populations, however, because of the abundant supply of manganese in edible plant materials compared with the relatively low requirement.[183]

The recommended level of manganese for adults is 2 to 5 mg/day; mean daily intake in the United States for men and women was reported to be 2.7 and 2.2 mg, respectively.[147] Intakes of 8 to 9 mg/day, which nearly doubles the estimated safe and adequate daily dietary intake established by the Food and Nutrition Board, have not resulted in any apparent toxicity.[94]

Whole grains and cereal products are the richest dietary sources of manganese, but fruits and vegetables also are good sources (Table 5–7). Tea is also rich in manganese,[184] although some question has been raised about the bioavailability of manganese in tea.[185] Dairy products, meat, fish, and poultry are all low in manganese. Not surprising, although data are limited, manganese intake in vegetarians is as much as 50% to 100% higher than that in nonvegetarians (Appendix H).[143,186] In fact, Indian diets high in foods of plant origin supply a daily average intake of more than 8 mg, whereas highly refined hospital diets in the United States supply anywhere from less than 0.5 mg to about 2 mg.[187,188] Manganese absorption in general tends to be relatively low, but phytate appears to have relatively little effect on it.[189] In a study of college-age men consuming a vegetarian diet, manganese absorption was quite good.[190]

IODINE

Common table salt is fortified with iodine, so that it is rarely a concern in the diets of Americans. In other parts of the world, however, iodine deficiency, characterized by goiter and cretinism, is a major problem. In 1983, there were an estimated 400 million iodine-deficient individuals in less de-

Table 5–7 Manganese Content of Foods

Food	Manganese Content (mg)	Food	Manganese Content (mg)
Bread, cereal, grains		Sweet potato	0.63
Bran flakes, 1 cup	1.70	Turnip greens	0.39
Oatmeal, ½ cup cooked	0.68	**Fruits**	
Shredded wheat, 1 biscuit	0.75	Pineapple, ½ cup	0.82
Barley, whole, ½ cup cooked	0.89	Strawberries, ½ cup sliced	0.32
Pasta, whole wheat,		**Legumes (½ cup cooked)**	
½ cup cooked	0.96	Black-eyed peas	0.36
Rice, brown, ½ cup cooked	1.00	Lentils	0.48
Rice, white, ½ cup cooked	0.38	Pinto beans	0.47
Wheat germ, 2 tbsp	2.80	Soybeans	0.71
Vegetables (½ cup cooked)		Tempeh	1.10
Beet greens	0.37	Tofu	0.75
Carrots	0.33	Textured vegetable protein	0.65
Collards	0.56	**Nuts/seeds (2 tbsp)**	
Lima beans	0.48	Almond butter	0.75
Peas	0.42	Pumpkin/squash seeds	0.52
Spinach	0.96	Sunflower seeds	0.36

Source: Data from *Bowes & Church's Food Value of Portions Commonly Used.* 16th ed., by J. Pennington, Lippincott-Raven, 1994.

veloped parts of the world and an estimated 112 million in more developed countries.[191] Iodine is an integral part of the hormones thyroxine and triiodothyronine.

In the United States, the incidence of endemic goiter fell sharply after the introduction of iodized salt in 1924.[192] In other parts of the world, in addition to iodized salt, administration of iodized oil has been used quite successfully. Iodized walnut oil and iodized soybean oil have been in used in China since 1980.[193] Many populations are at risk of iodine deficiency because they live in an iodine-deficient environment characterized by soil from which iodine has been removed by glaciation, high rainfall, or flood. This situation occurs most often in mountainous areas, such as the Himalayan region, the Andean region, and the vast mountain ranges of China. Low-lying areas subject to flooding, however, as in the Ganges Valley in India and Bangladesh, are also severely iodine deficient. In addition to iodine deficiency, there are a number of food-borne compounds that interfere with utilization of iodine or with the functioning of the thyroid gland.[194]

The RDA for iodine for adult men and women is 150 μg. Intake (excluding iodized salt) in this country for men and women is 250 and 170 μg, respectively, quite a bit above the RDA.[147] In coastal areas, seafood, water, and iodine-containing mist from the ocean are important sources. Farther inland, the iodine content of plants is variable, depending on the geochemical environment and on fertilizing and food processing practices. Iodized salt is an excellent source of this nutrient, providing about 67 μg per quarter teaspoon. Additionally, iodates are still used as dough oxidizers in bread making, and dairy products accumulate iodine because iodine-containing disinfectants are used on cows, milking machines, and storage tanks.[195] Sea vegetables are also an especially good source of iodine. In fact, in the coastal regions of Hokkaido, the northern island of Japan, diets contain large amounts of seaweed, and daily iodine intakes are as high as 50,000 to 80,000 μg (more than 250 times the RDA).[196]

There are few data on the iodine intake of vegetarians, although studies of vegetarians in England and Sweden have shown iodine levels to be low.[138,197] Sweden is a low iodine area, however, and in the English study, the use of iodized salt was not considered. Finally, the US RDA has a considerable safety factor and may actually be twice what is required. Vegans not using iodized salt, however, should make sure that they are consuming reliable sources of iodine.

SODIUM

Sodium is the primary regulator of extracellular fluid volume but has several other important functions. It is involved in the regulation of acid-base balance and the membrane potential of cells. Excessive intake of sodium, at least in sensitive individuals, is linked with high blood pressure. It is estimated that 30% to 50% of hypertensives are sensitive to sodium.[198] Sodium increases urinary calcium loss and can therefore increase calcium requirements and adversely affect bone health (see Chapter 4). Sodium intake is difficult to quantify; a better measure of sodium intake is urinary sodium.

The average intake of sodium in the United States is anywhere from 2 to 5 g/day, well above the minimum requirement of 500 mg.[134] Actual needs may be even lower than this because the body can conserve sodium in response to low intakes. Although many agrarian societies whose diets are primarily vegetarian consume less sodium than Westerners, the sodium intake of vegetarians in industrialized countries is similar to that of omnivores (Appendix G). Estimates are that in Britain, only about 10% of sodium intake comes naturally from the food we eat, about 15% from salt added during cooking and at the table, and fully 75% from salt added during processing and manufacturing[196,197] (Figure 5–2). (Similar estimates exist for the U.S.) To reduce sodium intake substantially, a reduction in processed foods consumption is required.

CHLORIDE

Chloride plays a critical role in maintaining fluid and electrolyte balance, and it is a critical component of gastric juice. Because the intake of chloride from food as well as its loss from the body under normal conditions parallel those of sodium, the requirements specified for all age and sex groups (with the exception of infants) are similar to those for sodium. Dietary chloride

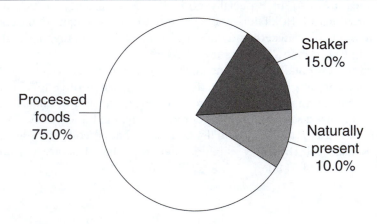

Figure 5–2 Sodium sources. Data are for the British population, based on references 199 and 200.

comes almost exclusively from the sodium chloride (ordinary salt). Chloride intake is similar between vegetarians and nonvegetarians, as determined from the limited direct dietary intake data and the similarity in sodium intake between these two groups.

POTASSIUM

Potassium is the principal intracellular cation; its concentration in cells is 30 times higher than that in blood. Potassium in the blood plays an important role in controlling skeletal muscle contractions and nerve impulses and in maintaining normal blood pressure.

Potassium is widely distributed in foods (Table 5–8). Fruits and vegetables are rich in this mineral; people who eat copious amounts of fruits and vegetables have high potassium intakes, as high as 11 g/day.[201] Vegetarians, particularly vegans, tend to consume somewhat more potassium than nonvegetarians (Appendix G). This may have health advantages because potassium intake has been linked with increased bone calcium retention and lower blood pressure.[202,203] Daily adult intake in the United States is about 2,500 mg;[135,203] the minimum recommended daily intake is 1,600 to 2,000 mg.

Table 5–8 Potassium Content of Foods

Food	Potassium Content (mg)	Food	Potassium Content (mg)
Bread, cereal, grains		Stewed tomatoes	304
Bran flakes, 1 cup	248	Tomato juice	521
Vegetables (½ cup cooked		**Legumes (½ cup cooked)**	
unless otherwise indicated)		Black-eyed peas	346
Avocado, ½	548	Chick peas	398
Asparagus	279	Kidney beans	329
Beet greens	659	Lentils	365
Beets	265	Navy beans	395
Parsnips	287	Pinto beans	400
Peas	217	Soybeans	443
Plantain	358	Split peas	296
Potato	498	**Nuts/seeds**	
Pumpkin	252	Almond butter, 2 tbsp	242
Spinach	305	**Animal products**	
Acorn squash	448	Milk, 1 cup	381
Sweet potato	397	Yogurt, 1 cup	590
Swiss chard	480		

Source: Data from *Bowes & Church's Food Value of Portions Commonly Used.* 16th ed., by J. Pennington, Lippincott-Raven, 1994.

FLUORIDE

The decline in dental caries in industrialized countries during the past 40 years is primarily attributed to the widespread use of fluoride. Through extensive epidemiologic studies of communities with naturally fluoridated water in the United States in the 1930s, the protective properties of fluoride in the prevention of dental caries were fully recognized. Although fluoride is best known for its prevention of tooth decay,[204] some evidence suggests that fluoride may promote bone health,[205] although there is some disagreement on this point.[206]

Although it is known that fluoride is beneficial for dental health, it is not officially classified as an essential nutrient because no specific deficiency due to a lack of fluoride has been identified. For adults, recommended intake is between 1.5 and 4.0 mg/day. Fluoridated drinking water is an important source of this mineral and accounts for much of the difference in fluoride intake among different areas of the U.S.[207] Rich sources of fluoride include tea and marine fish that are consumed with their bones.[208] Cooking with fluoridated water can increase the fluoride content of foods several times.[209] Even cooking with Teflon, which contains fluoride, can have a similar effect.[210]

Fluoride toxicity, referred to as fluorosis, adversely affects bone health, kidney function, and possibly muscle and nerve function. This condition occurs only after years of intake of 20 to 80 mg/day, however, which is greatly in excess of US intake. Mottling of teeth in children has been observed at 2 to 8 mg/kg concentrations of fluoride in the diet and drinking water. No published reports on the fluoride intake of vegetarians were identified, but because fluoridated water directly and indirectly accounts for most of the fluoride intake in the United States there is unlikely to be any difference between vegetarians and nonvegetarians.

CHROMIUM

Chromium is generally accepted as an essential nutrient that potentiates insulin action and thus influences overall metabolism, although the precise biologic manner in which this effect occurs is poorly understood. Chromium is considered an essential element of what is referred to as the glucose tolerance factor. It was first identified in Brewer's yeast and is not well characterized. Other components are thought to include nicotinic acid (niacin), glutamic acid, glycine, and a sulfur-containing amino acid.

For adults, the current estimated safe and adequate daily intake for chromium is 50 to 200 µg. There are considerable data suggesting that chromium intake is inadequate on typical Western diets.[211] This is consistent with the observation that in the majority of all chromium supplementation studies in the United States, at least half the subjects with impaired glucose tolerance improved upon chromium supplementation.[212]

Dairy products, fruits, and vegetables contain low amounts of chromium, whereas whole grain products, including ready-to-eat bran cereals, processed meats, and spices, are the best sources. Considerable amounts of chromium are lost when grains are refined.[213] Conversely, substantial amounts can be added to the food supply during processing and preparation because chromium can be leached from stainless steel containers, particularly when acidic juices are heated in them.[214] Some beers also contain significant amounts of chromium, although brands vary quite a bit in their content.[215]

Although chromium absorption is thought to be relatively poor, in a study of Indian vegetarian or largely vegetarian diets chromium intake was generally between 100 and 200 μg/day, and absorption was quite good.[168] There are some indications that pregnant women consume inadequate levels of chromium and that this contributes to glucose intolerance during pregnancy.[216] Athletes also may have higher needs for chromium than sedentary individuals.[217] The chromium intake of Western vegetarians has not been assessed.

MOLYBDENUM

Molybdenum functions as a constituent of several enzymes, including aldehyde oxidase, xanthine oxidase, and sulfite oxidase. Molybdenum may play an important role in the detoxification of foreign compounds. The estimated safe and adequate daily intake for molybdenum is 75 to 250 μg, and the diets of most Americans contain adequate levels of this mineral.[218,219] There may be a sizeable segment of the population for which this is not true, however. Vegetarian intake is likely to be adequate because the foods that contribute the most to molybdenum intake—milk, beans, breads, and cereals—are staples of many vegetarian diets.[218] Although molybdenum appears to be relatively non-toxic, it may have an adverse effect on copper status. Some research suggests that molybdenum increases urinary copper excretion when consumed at levels only twice the upper recommended range.[220] Extremely high intakes (40 times the upper safe limit), which can occur as a result of high environmental concentrations, were thought to be responsible for goutlike symptoms in humans living in a province of the former Soviet Union.

REFERENCES

1. DeMaeyer EM, Adiels-Tegman M. The prevalence of anemia in the world. *World Health Stat Q*. 1985;38:302–316.
2. Life Sciences Research Office. *Assessment of Iron Nutritional Status of the United States Population Based on Data Collected in the Second NHANES Survey, 1976–1980*. Bethesda, Md: Federation of American Societies for Experimental Biology; 1984.

3. Cook JD, Monsen ER. Food iron absorption in human subjects. III. Comparison of the effects of animal protein on nonheme iron absorption. *Am J Clin Nutr.* 1976;29:859–867.

4. Monsen ER, Hallberg L, Layrisse M, et al. Estimation of available dietary iron. *Am J Clin Nutr.* 1978;31:134–141.

5. Monsen ER. Iron nutrition and absorption: Dietary factors which impact iron bioavailability. *J Am Diet Assoc.* 1988;88:786–790.

6. Bothwell TH, Charlton RW, Cook JD, Finch CA. *Iron Metabolism in Man.* Oxford, England: Blackwell Scientific; 1979.

7. Hallberg L, Hogdahl A-M, Nilsson I, Rybo G. Menstrual blood loss—A population study. Variation at different ages and attempts to define normality. *Acta Obstet Gynecol Scand.* 1966;45:320–351.

8. Food and Agriculture Organization (FAO). *Requirements of Vitamin A, Iron, Folate, and Vitamin B12. Report of a Joint FAO/World Health Organization Expert Consultation* (FAO Food and Nutrition Series 23). Rome, Italy: Food and Agriculture Organization; 1988.

9. Committee on Diet and Health, Food and Nutrition Board, Commission on Life Sciences, National Research Council. *Diet and Health.* Washington, DC: National Academy Press; 1989.

10. Yip R, Walsh KM, Goldfarb MG, Binkin NV. Declining prevalence of anemia in childhood in a middle class setting: A pediatric success story? *Pediatrics.* 1987;80:330–334.

11. Dallman PR, Yip R, Johnson C. Prevalence and causes of anemia in the United States, 1976–1980. *Am J Clin Nutr.* 1984;39:437–445.

12. Murphy SP, Calloway DH. Nutrients intakes of women in NHANES II emphasizing trace minerals, fiber, and phytate. *J Am Diet Assoc.* 1986;86:1366–1372.

13. Raper NR, Rosenthal JC, Woteki CE. Estimates of available iron in diets of individuals 1 year old and older in the Nationwide Food Consumption Survey. *J Am Diet Assoc.* 1984;84:783–787.

14. Bjorn-Rasmussen E, Hallberg L, Isaksson B, Arvidsson B. Food iron absorption in man. Applications of two-pool extrinsic tag method to measure heme and nonheme iron absorption from the whole diet. *J Clin Invest.* 1974;53:247–255.

15. Pennington JAT. *Bowes and Church's Food Values of Portions Commonly Used.* 15th ed. New York: Harper & Row; 1989.

16. Cook JD. Adaptation in iron metabolism. *Am J Clin Nutr.* 1990;51:301–308.

17. Bezwoda WR, Bothwell TH, Charlton RW, et al. The relative dietary importance of haem and non-haem iron. *S Afr Med J.* 1983;64:552–556.

18. Hallberg L, Rossander L. Absorption of iron from Western-type lunch and dinner meals. *Am J Clin Nutr.* 1982;35:502–509.

19. Monsen ER, Balintfy JL. Calculating dietary iron bioavailability: Refinement and computerization. *J Am Diet Assoc.* 1982;80:307–311.

20. Gillbooly M, Bothwell TH, Torrance JD, et al. The effects of organic acids, phytates, and polyphenols on the absorption of iron from vegetables. *Br J Nutr.* 1983;49:311–342.

21. Ballot D, Baynes RD, Bothwell TH, et al. The effects of fruit juices and fruits on the absorption of iron from a rice meal. *Br J Nutr.* 1987;57:331–343.

22. Cook JD, Monsen ER. Vitamin C, the common cold, and iron absorption in man. *Am J Clin Nutr.* 1977;30:234–241.

23. Hunt JR, Gallagher SK, Johnson LK. Effect of ascorbic acid on apparent iron absorption by women with low iron stores. *Am J Clin Nutr.* 1994;59:1381–1385.

24. Rossander L, Hallberg L, Bjorn-Rasmussen E. Absorption of iron from breakfast meals. *Am J Clin Nutr.* 1979;32:2484–2489.

25. Disler PB, Lynch SR, Charlton RW, et al. The effect of tea on iron absorption. *Gut.* 1975;16:193–200.

26. Narasinga RBS, Prabhavathi T. Tannin content of foods commonly consumed in India and its influence on ionizable iron. *J Sci Food Agric.* 1982;33:89–96.

27. Morck TA, Lynch SR, Cook JD. Inhibition of food iron absorption by coffee. *Am J Clin Nutr.* 1983;37:416–420.

28. Hallberg L, Rossander-Hultén, Brune M, Gleerup A. Calcium and iron absorption: Mechanism of action and nutritional importance. *Eur J Clin Nutr.* 1991;46:317–327.

29. Tidehag P, Sandberg A-S, Hallmans G, et al. Effect of milk and fermented milk on iron absorption in ileostomy subjects. *Am J Clin Nutr.* 1995;62:1234–1238.

30. Reinhold JG, Ismail-Beigi F, Faradji B. Fiber vs phytate as a determinant of the availability of calcium, zinc, and iron of breadstuffs. *Nutr Rep Int.* 1975;12:75–85.

31. Cook JD, Noble NL, Morck TA, Lynch SR, Petersburg SJ. Effect of fiber on nonheme iron absorption. *Gastroenterology.* 1983;85:1354–1358.

32. Brune M, Rossander L, Hallberg L. Iron absorption: No intestinal adaptation to a high-phytate diet. *Am J Clin Nutr.* 1989;49:542–545.

33. Hurrell RF, Juillerat M-A, Reddy MB, Lynch SR, Dassenko SA, Cook JD. Soy protein, phytate, and iron absorption in humans. *Am J Clin Nutr.* 1992;56:573–578.

34. Hallberg L, Rossander L, Skanberg A. Phytates and the inhibitory effect of bran on iron absorption in man. *Am J Clin Nutr.* 1987;45:988–996.

35. Hallberg L, Brune M, Rossander L. Iron absorption in man: Ascorbic acid and dose-dependent inhibition by phytate. *Am J Clin Nutr.* 1989;49:140–144.

36. van Dokkum W, Wesstra A, Schippers FA. Physiological effects of fibre-rich types of bread. *Br J Nutr.* 1982;47:451–460.

37. Ellis R, Morris ER, Hill AD, Smith JC. Phytate:zinc molar ratio, mineral, and fiber content of three hospital diets. *J Am Diet Assoc.* 1982;81:26–29.

38. Ellis R, Kelsay JL, Reynolds RD, Morris ER, Moser PB, Frazier CW. Phytate:zinc and phytate X calcium:zinc millimolar ratios in self-selected diets of Americans, Asian Indians, and Nepalese. *J Am Diet Assoc.* 1987;87:1043–1047.

39. Soegemberg D, Baynes RD, Bothwell TH, et al. Ascorbic acid prevents the dose-dependent inhibitory effects of polyphenols and phytates on nonheme-iron absorption. *Am J Clin Nutr.* 1991;53:537–541.

40. Cook JD, Dassenko SA, Lynch SR. Assessment of the role of nonheme-iron availability in iron balance. *Am J Clin Nutr.* 1991;54:717–722.

41. Cook JD, Watson SS, Simpson KM, Lipschitz DA, Skikne BS. The effect of high ascorbic acid supplementation on body iron stores. *Blood.* 1984;64:721–726.

42. Joint Food and Agriculture Organization (FAO)/World Health Organization Expert Consultation. *Requirements of Vitamin A, Iron, Folate and B₁₂*. Rome, Italy: FAO; 1988.

43. Shaw N-S, Chin C-J, Pan W-H. A vegetarian diet rich in soybean products compromises iron status in young students. *J Nutr.* 1995;125:212–219.

44. Panel on Dietary Reference Values of the Committee on Medical Aspects of Food Policy, Department of Health. *Dietary Reference Values for Food, Energy and Nutrients for the United Kingdom*. London, England: Her Majesty's Stationery Office; 1990.

45. Dreosti IE. Recommended dietary intakes of iron, zinc, and other inorganic nutrients and their chemical form and bioavailability. *Nutrition*. 1993;9:542–545.

46. van Dokkum W. Significance of iron bioavailability for iron recommendations. *Biol Trace Elem Res*. 1992;35:1–11.

47. Apte SV, Venkatachalam PS. Iron absorption in human volunteers using high phytate cereal diet. *Indian J Med Res*. 1962;50:516–520.

48. Campbell TC, Chen J. Diet and chronic degenerative diseases: Perspectives from China. *Am J Clin Nutr*. 1994;59(suppl):1153S–1161S.

49. Rosado JL, Lopez P, Morales M, Munoz E, Allen LH. Bioavailability of energy, nitrogen, fat, zinc, iron, and calcium from rural and urban Mexican diets. *Br J Nutr*. 1992;68:45–58.

50. van Dokkum W, Wesstra JA, Schippers FA. Effect of lactovegetarian, vegan and mixed diets on mineral utilization. Presented at the 5th International Symposium on Trace Elements in Man and Animals; 1986; Zeist, The Netherlands.

51. Kramer LB, Osis D, Coffey J, Spencer H. Mineral and trace element content of vegetarian diets. *J Am Coll Nutr*. 1984;3:3–11.

52. Couzy F, Kastenmayer P, Mansourian R, Guinchard S, Munoz-Box R, Dirren H. Zinc absorption in healthy elderly humans and the effect of diet. *Am J Clin Nutr*. 1993;58:690–694.

53. Sanders TAB, Purves R. An anthropometric and dietary assessment of the nutritional status of vegan preschool children. *J Hum Nutr*. 1981;35:349–357.

54. Alexander D, Ball MJ, Mann J. Nutrient intake and haematological status of vegetarians and age–sex matched omnivores. *Eur J Clin Nutr*. 1994;48:538–546.

55. Worthington-Roberts BS, Breskin MW, Monsen ER. Iron status of premenopausal women in a university community and its relationship to habitual dietary sources of protein intake. *Am J Clin Nutr*. 1988;47:275–279.

56. Reddy S, Sanders TAB. Haematological studies on pre-menopausal Indian and caucasian vegetarians compared with caucasian omnivores. *Br J Nutr*. 1990;64:331–338.

57. Brants HAM, Lowik MRH, Westenbrink S, Hulshof KFAM, Kistemaker C. Adequacy of a vegetarian diet at old age (Dutch Nutrition Surveillance System). *J Am Coll Nutr*. 1990;9:292–302.

58. Helman AD, Darnton-Hill I. Vitamin and iron status in new vegetarians. *Am J Clin Nutr*. 1987;45:785–789.

59. Dallman PR. Biochemical basis for the manifestations of iron deficiency. *Annu Rev Nutr*. 1986;6:13–40.

60. Donovan UM, Gibson RS. Iron and zinc intake of young women aged 14 to 19 years consuming vegetarian and omnivorous diets. *J Am Coll Nutr*. 1995;14:463–472.

61. Latta D, Liebman M. Iron and zinc status of nonvegetarian males. *Nutr Rep Int*. 1984;30:141–149.

62. Tungtronochitr R, Pongpaew P, Prayurahong B, et al. Vitamin B12, folic acid and haematological status of 132 Thai vegetarians. *Int J Vitam Nutr Res*. 1992;63:201–207.

63. Anderson BM, Gibson RS, Sabry JH. The iron and zinc status of long-term vegetarian women. *Am J Clin Nutr*. 1981;34:1042–1048.

64. Armstrong BA, Davis RE, Nicol DJ, van Merwyk AJ, Larwood CJ. Hematological, vitamin B12, and folate studies on Seventh-Day Adventist vegetarians. *Am J Clin Nutr*. 1974;27:712–718.

65. Dangnelie PC, van Staveren WA, Vergote FJVRA, Dingjan PG, van den Berg H, Hautvast JGAJ. Increased risk of vitamin B12 and iron deficiency in infants on macrobiotic diets. *Am J Clin Nutr*. 1989;50:818–824.

66. Dwyer JT, Dietz WH, Andrews EM, Sistind RM. Nutritional status of vegetarian children. *Am J Clin Nutr.* 1982;35:204–216.

67. Kim YC. *The Effect of a Vegterian Diet on the Iron and Zinc Status of School-Age Children.* Amherst, Mass: University of Massachusetts; 1988. Thesis.

68. Herbert V. Everyone should be tested for iron disorders. *J Am Diet Assoc.* 1992;92:1502–1509.

69. Salonen JT, Nyyssonen K, Korpela H, et al. High stored iron levels are associated with excess risk of myocardial infarction in eastern Finnish men. *Circulation.* 1992;86:803–811.

70. Lauffer RB. Iron stores and the international variation in mortality from coronary artery disease. *Med Hypotheses.* 1990;35:96–102.

71. Knekt P, Reunanen A, Takkunen H, Aroma A, Heliovaara M, Hakulinen T. Body iron stores and risk of cancer. *Int J Cancer.* 1994;56:379–382.

72. Nelson RL. Dietary iron and colorectal cancer risk. *Free Radical Biol Med.* 1992;13:161–168.

73. Thompson HJ, Kennedy K, Witt M, Juzefyk J. Effect of dietary iron deficiency or excess on the induction of mammary carcinogenesis by 1-methyl-1-nitrosourea. *Carcinogenesis.* 1991;12:111–114.

74. Ascherio A, Willet WC, Rimm EB, Giovannucci EL, Stampler MJ. Dietary iron intake and risk of coronary disease among men. *Circulation.* 1994;89:969–974.

75. Welsh SO, Marston RM. Zinc levels of the US food supply; 1909–1980. *Food Technol.* 1982;36:70–76.

76. US Department of Agriculture, Food and Consumer Services. *Nutrition Monitoring in the United States: A Progress Report from the Joint Nutrition Monitoring Evaluation Committee.* Hyattsville, Md: Department of Health and Human Services, Public Health Service; 1986. National Center for Health Statistics, Human Nutrition Information Service publication PHS 1255.

77. Prasad AS, Miale A Jr, Sandstead HH, Schulert AR. Zinc metabolism in patients with syndrome of iron deficiency anemia, hepatosplenomegaly, dwarfism, and hypogonadism. *J Lab Clin Med.* 1961;61:537–549.

78. Arcasoy A, Cavdar AO, Babacan E. Decreased iron and zinc absorption in Turkish children with iron deficiency and geophagia. *Acta Haematol.* 1978;60:76–84.

79. Xue-Cun C, Tai-An Y, Jin-Sheng H, Gui-Yan M, Zhi-Min H, Li-Xiang L. Low levels of zinc in hair and blood, pica, anorexia and poor growth in Chinese preschool children. *Am J Clin Nutr.* 1985;42:694–700.

80. Prasad AS, Schulert AR, Sandstead HH. Zinc and iron deficiencies in male subjects with dwarfism but without ancylostomiasis, schistosomiasis, or severe anemia. *Am J Clin Nutr.* 1963;12:437–444.

81. Ronaghy HA, Reinhold JG, Mahloudji M, Ghavami P, Fox MRS, Halsted JA. Zinc supplementation of malnourished schoolboys in Iran: Increased growth and other effects. *Am J Clin Nutr.* 1974;27:112–121.

82. Gibson RS, Vanderkooy PDS, MacDonald AC, Goldman A, Ryan BA, Berry M. A growth-limiting mild zinc deficiency syndrome in some southern Ontario boys with low height percentiles. *Am J Clin Nutr.* 1989;45:1266–1277.

83. Vanderkooy PDS, Gibson RS. Food consumption patterns of Canadian preschool children in relation to zinc and growth status. *Am J Clin Nutr.* 1987;45:609–616.

84. Pilch SM, Senti FR. Analysis of zinc data from the Second National Health and Nutrition Examination Survey (NHANES II). *J Nutr.* 1985;115:1393–1397.

85. Hambridge KM, Walravens PA, White S, Anthony ML, Roth ML. Zinc nutrition of preschool children in the Denver Head Start Program. *Am J Clin Nutr.* 1976;29:734–744.

86. Chesters JK. Metabolism and biochemistry of zinc. In: Prasad AS, ed. *Current Topics in Nutrition and Disease.* New York, NY: Liss; 1982;6:221–238.

87. Cousins RJ, Hempe JM. *Present Knowledge in Nutrition.* Washington, DC: International Life Sciences Institute Nutrition Foundation; 1990.

88. Duerre JA, Ford KM, Sandstead HH. Effects of zinc deficiency on protein synthesis in brain and liver of suckling rats. *J Nutr.* 1977;107:1082–1093.

89. Pories WJ, Mansour EG, Plecha FR, Flynn A, Strain WH. Metabolic factors affecting zinc metabolism in the surgical patient. In: Prasad AS, ed. *Trace Elements in Health and Disease.* New York, NY: Academic Press; 1976;1:115–141.

90. Greger JL. Potential for trace mineral deficiencies and toxicities in the elderly. In: Bales CW, ed. *Current Topics in Nutrition and Disease.* New York, NY: 1982;21:171–200.

91. Johnson PE, Hunt CD, Milne DB, Mullen LK. Homeostatic control of zinc metabolism in men: Zinc excretion in men fed diets low in zinc. *Am J Clin Nutr.* 1993;57:557–565.

92. King JC. Assessment of techniques for determining zinc requirements. *J Am Diet Assoc.* 1986;86:1523–1528.

93. Sandstead HH. Zinc nutrition in the United States. *Am J Clin Nutr.* 1973;26:1251–1260.

94. Health and Welfare Canada Committee. *Nutrition Recommendations.* Ottawa, Ontario: Department of National Health and Welfare; 1990.

95. World Health Organization (WHO) Expert Committee on Trace Elements in Human Nutrition. *Trace Elements in Human Nutrition* (WHO Technical Report 532). Geneva, Switzerland: WHO; 1973.

96. Sandstrom B, Arvidsson B, Cederblad A, Bjorn-Rasmussen E. Zinc absorption from composite meals. I. The significance of wheat extraction rate, zinc, calcium, and protein content in meals based on bread. *Am J Clin Nutr.* 1980;33:739–745.

97. Sandstrom B, Cederblad A. Zinc absorption from composite meals. II. Influence of the main protein source. *Am J Clin Nutr.* 1980;33:1778–1783.

98. Sandstrom B, Almegren A, Kivisto B, Cederblad A. Effect of protein level and protein source on zinc absorption in humans. *J Nutr.* 1989;119:48–53.

99. Zheng J-J, Mason JB, Rosenberg IH, Wood RJ. Measurement of zinc bioavailability from beef and a ready-to-eat high-fiber breakfast cereal in humans: Application of a whole-gut lavage technique. *Am J Clin Nutr.* 1993;58:902–907.

100. Reinhold JG, Nasr K, Lahimgarzadeh A, Hedayati H. Effects of purified phytate and phytate-rich bread upon metabolism of zinc, calcium, phosphorus, and nitrogen in man. *Lancet.* 1973;1:283–288.

101. Navert B, Sandstrom B, Cederblad A. Reduction of the phytate content of bran by leavening in bread and its effect on zinc absorption in man. *Br J Nutr.* 1985;53:47–53.

102. Cooper JR, Gowing HS. Mammalian small intestinal phytase (EC 3.1.3.8). *Br J Nutr.* 1983;50:673–678.

103. Cosgrove DJ. *Inositol Phosphates—Their Chemistry, Biochemistry and Physiology.* New York, NY: Elsevier; 1980.

104. Sandberg AS, Andersson H. Effect of dietary phytase on the digestion of phytate in the stomach and small intestine of humans. *J Nutr.* 1988;118:469–473.

105. Wisker E, Nagel R, Tanudjaja TK, Feldheim W. Calcium, magnesium, zinc, and iron balances in young women: Effects of low-phytate barley-fiber concentrate. *Am J Clin Nutr.* 1991;54:553–559.

106. Spencer H, Norris C, Derler J, Osis D. Effect of oat bran muffins on calcium absorption and calcium, phosphorus, magnesium and zinc balance in men. *J Nutr.* 1991;121:1976–1983.

107. Behall KM, Scholfield DJ, Lee K, Powell AS, Moser PB. Mineral balance in adult men: Effect of four refined fibers. *Am J Clin Nutr.* 1987;46:307–314.

108. Sandstrom B, Arvidsson B, Cederblad A, Bjorn-Rasmussen E. Zinc absorption from composite meals. I. The significance of wheat extraction rate, zinc, calcium, and protein content in meals based on bread. *Am J Clin Nutr.* 1980;33:739–745.

109. Harland BF, Peterson M. Nutritional status of lacto-ovo-vegetarian Trappist monks. *J Am Diet Assoc.* 1978;72:259–264.

110. Murphy SP, Calloway DH. Dietary correlates of trace element status for young women in NHANES II. *Fed Proc.* 1985;44:757.

111. Oberleas D, Harland BF. Phytate content of foods: Effect on dietary zinc bioavailability. *J Am Diet Assoc.* 1981;79:433–436.

112. Davies NT, Olpin SE. Studies on the phytate:zinc molar contents in diets as a determinant of zinc availability to young rats. *Br J Nutr.* 1979;41:591–603.

113. Morris ER, Ellis R, Hill AD, et al. Apparent zinc and iron balance of adult men consuming three levels of phytate. *Fed Proc.* 1986;45:819.

114. Ferguson EL, Gibson RS, Thompson LU, Ounpuu S. The dietary calcium, phytate and zinc intakes, and the calcium, phytate and zinc molar ratios of a selected group of East African children. *Am J Clin Nutr.* 1989;50:1450–1456.

115. Bindra GS, Gibson RS, Thompson LU. (Phytate)(calcium)/(zinc) ratios in Asian immigrant lacto-ovo vegetarian diets and their relationship to zinc nutriture. *Nutr Res.* 1986;6:475–483.

116. Morris ER, Ellis R. Bioavailability of dietary calcium: Effect of phytate on adult men consuming non-vegetarian diets. In: Kies C, ed. *Nutritional Bioavailability of Calcium.* Washington, DC: American Chemical Society; 1985:63–72.

117. Sandstead HH. Availability of zinc and its requirement in human subjects. In: Prasad AS, ed. *Clinical, Biochemical, and Nutritional Aspects of Trace Elements.* New York, NY: Liss; 1982:83–101.

118. Nutrition Canada. *Food Consumption Patterns Report.* Ottawa, Ontario: Bureau of Nutritional Sciences, Department of National Health and Welfare; 1977.

119. Greger JL, Sciscoe BS. Zinc nutriture of elderly participants in an urban feeding program. *J Am Diet Assoc.* 1977;70:37–41.

120. Davies GJ, Crowder M, Dickerson JWT. Dietary fibre intakes of individuals with different eating patterns. *Human Nutr: Appl Nutr.* 1985;39A:139–148.

121. Draper A, Lewis J, Malhotra N, Wheeler E. The energy and nutrient intakes of different types of vegetarian: A case for supplements. *Br J Nutr.* 1993;69:3–19.

122. Gibson RS. Content and bioavailability of trace elements in vegetarian diets. *Am J Clin Nutr.* 1994;59(suppl):1223–1232.

123. Bhattacharya RD, Patel TS, Pandya CB. Copper and zinc level in biological samples from healthy subjects of vegetarian food habit in reference to community environment. *Chronobiology.* 1985;12:145–153.

124. King JC, Stein T, Doyle M. Effect of vegetarianism on the zinc status of pregnant women. *Am J Clin Nutr.* 1981;34:1049–1055.

125. Abu-Assal MJ, Craig WJ. The zinc status of pregnant vegetarian women. *Nutr Rep Int.* 1984;29:485–494.

126. Campbell-Brown M, Ward RJ, Haines AP, North WRS, Abraham R, McFadyen IR. Zinc and copper in Asian pregnancies—Is there evidence for a nutritional deficiency? *Br J Obstet Gynaecol.* 1985;92:875–885.

127. Kies C, Young E, McEndree L. Zinc bioavailability from vegetarian diets. Influence of dietary fiber, ascorbic acid, and past dietary practices. In: Inglett GE, ed. *Nutritional Bioavailability of Zinc* (American Chemical Society Symposium Series 210B). Washington, DC: American Chemical Society; 1983:115–126.

128. Freeland-Graves JH, Bodzy PW, Epright MA. Zinc status of vegetarians. *J Am Diet Assoc.* 1980;77:655–661.

129. Srikumar TS, Ockerman PA, Akesson B. Trace element status in vegetarians from southern India. *Nutr Res.* 1992;12:187–198.

130. Hunt JR, Matthys LA, Lykken GI. Reduced zinc absorption from a lacto-ovo-vegetarian diet. *Am J Clin Nutr.* 1995;61:908. Abstract.

131. Lei S, Mingyan X, Miller LV, Krebs NF, Tong L, Hambidge KM. Zinc (Zn) homeostasis in young Chinese women with a marginal Zn intake. *Am J Clin Nutr.* 1995;61:908. Abstract.

132. Pecoud A, Donzel P, Schelling JL. Effect of foodstuffs on the absorption of zinc sulfate. *Clin Pharmacol Ther.* 1975;17:469–473.

133. Agte V, Chiplonkar S, Joshi N, Paknikar K. Apparent absorption of copper and zinc from composite vegetarian diets in young Indian men. *Ann Nutr Metab.* 1994;38:13–19.

134. Yang GQ, Wang S, Zhou R, Sun S. Endemic selenium intoxification of humans in China. *Am J Clin Nutr.* 1983;37:872–881.

135. Pennington JAT, Wilson DB, Newell RF, Harland BF, Johnson RD, Vanderveen JE. Selected minerals in foods surveys, 1974–1981/1982. *J Am Diet Assoc.* 1984;84:771–780.

136. Gissel-Nielsen G, Gupta UC, Lamand M, Westermarck T. Selenium in soils and plants and its importance in livestock and human nutrition. *Adv Agron.* 1984;37:397–464.

137. Srikumar TS, Johansson GK, Ockerman P-A, Gustafsson J-A, Akesson B. Trace element status in healthy subjects switching from a mixed to a lactovegetarian diet for 12 mo. *Am J Clin Nutr.* 1992;55:586–590.

138. Abdulla M, Andersson I, Asp N-G, et al. Nutrient intake and health status of vegans. Chemical analyses of diets using the duplicate portion sampling technique. *Am J Clin Nutr.* 1981;34:2464–2477.

139. Abdulla M, Aly K-O, Andersson I, et al. Nutrient intake and health status of lactovegetarians: Chemical analysis of diets using duplicate portion sampling technique. *Am J Clin Nutr.* 1984;40:325–338.

140. Nagyova A, Ginter E, Kovacikova. Low glutathione levels and decreased glutathione peroxidase activity in the blood of vegetarians. *Internat J Vit Nutr Res.* 1995;65:221.

141. Kadrabova J, Madaric A, Kováčová Z, Ginter E. Selenium status, plasma zinc, copper, and magnesium in vegetarians. *Biological Trace Element Res.* 1995;50:13–24.

142. Ganapathy SN, Dhandra R. Selenium content of omnivorous and vegetarian diets. *Indian J Nutr Diet.* 1980;17:53–59.

143. Gibson RS, Anderson BM, Sabry JH. The trace metal status of a group of postmenopausal vegetarians. *J Am Diet Assoc.* 1983;82:246–250.

144. Debski B, Finley DA, Picciano MF, Lonnerdal B, Milner J. Selenium content and glutathione peroxidase activity of milk from vegetarian and nonvegetarian women. *J Nutr.* 1989;119:215–220.

145. Shultz TD, Leklem JE. Selenium status of vegetarians, nonvegetarians, and hormone-dependent cancer subjects. *Am J Clin Nutr.* 1983;37:114–118.

146. Mason KE. A conspectus of research on copper metabolism and requirements of man. *J Nutr.* 1979;109:1979–2066.

147. Pennington JAT, Young BE, Wilson DB. Nutritional elements in US diets: Results from the Total Diet Study, 1982–1986. *J Am Diet Assoc.* 1989;89:659–664.

148. Atkinson RL, Dahms WT, Bray GA, Jacob R, Sandstead HH. Plasma zinc and copper in obesity and after intestinal bypass. *Ann Intern Med.* 1978;89:491–493.

149. Turnland JR, Keyes WR, Anderson HL, Acord LL. Copper absorption and retention in young men at three levels of dietary copper using the stable isotope ^{65}Cu. *Am J Clin Nutr.* 1989;49:870–878.

150. Cook JD. Absorption of food iron. *Fed Proc.* 1977;36:2028–2032.

151. Jacob RA, Skala JH, Omaye ST, Turnland JR. Effect of varying ascorbic acid intakes on copper absorption and ceruloplasmin levels of young men. *J Nutr.* 1987;117:2109–2115.

152. Klevay LM, Inman L, Johnson K, et al. Increased cholesterol in plasma in a young man during experimental copper depletion. *Metabolism.* 1984;33:1112–1118.

153. Sandstead HH. Copper bioavailability and requirements. *Am J Clin Nutr.* 1982;35:809–814.

154. Greger JL, Snedeker SM. Effect of dietary protein and phosphorus levels on the utilization of zinc, copper, manganese by adult males. *J Nutr.* 1980;110:2243–2253.

155. Cheryan M. Phytic acid interaction in food systems. *CRC Crit Rev Food Sci Nutr.* 1980;13:297–335.

156. Brewer GJ, Yuzbasiyan-Gurkan V, Dick R, Wang Y, Johnson V. Does a vegetarian diet control Wilson's disease? *J Am Coll Nutr.* 1993;12:527–530.

157. Garfinkel L, Garfinkel D. Magnesium regulation of the glycolytic pathway and the enzymes involved. *Magnesium.* 1985;4:60–72.

158. Marier JR. Magnesium content of the food supply in the modern-day world. *Magnesium.* 1986;5:1–8.

159. McNeill DA, Ali PS, Song YS. Mineral analyses of vegetarian, health, and conventional foods: Magnesium, zinc, copper, and manganese content. *J Am Diet Assoc.* 1985;85:569–572.

160. Hallfrisch J, Muller DC. Does diet provide adequate amounts of calcium, iron, magnesium, and zinc in a well-educated adult population? *Exp Gerontol.* 1993;28:473–483.

161. Shils ME. Magnesium in health and disease. *Annu Rev Nutr.* 1988;8:429–460.

162. Karppanen H, Tanskanen A, Tuomilehto J, et al. Safety and effects of potassium- and magnesium-containing low-sodium salt mixtures. *J Cardiovasc Pharmacol.* 1984;6:S236–S243.

163. Rouse IL, Armstrong BK, Beilin LJ, Vandongen R. Vegetarian diet, blood pressure and cardiovascular disease risk. *Aust NZ J Med.* 1984;14:439–443.

164. Specker BL, Tsang RC, Mo M, Miller D. Effect of vegetarian diet on serum 1,25-dihydroxyvitamin D concentrations during lactation. *Obstet Gynecol.* 1987;70:870–874.

165. Kelsay JL, Behall KM, Prather ES. Effect of fiber from fruits and vegetables on metabolic responses of human subjects. II. Calcium, magnesium, iron and silicon balances. *Am J Clin Nutr.* 1979;32:1876–1880.

166. Reinhold JB, Faradji B, Abadi P, Ismail-Beigi F. Decreased absorption of calcium, magnesium, zinc, and phosphorus by humans due to increased fiber and phosphorus consumption as wheat bread. *J Nutr.* 1976;106:493–503.

167. Schwartz R, Spencer H, Welsh JJ. Magnesium absorption in humans from leafy vegetables, intrinsically labeled with stable ^{26}Mg. *Am J Clin Nutr.* 1984;39:571–576.

168. Rao CN, Rao BSN. Absorption and retention of magnesium and some trace elements by man from typical Indian diets. *Nutr Metab.* 1980;24:244–254.

169. US Department of Agriculture. *Nationwide Food Consumption Survey. Continuing Survey of Food Intakes by Individuals. Men 19–50 Years, 1 Day, 1988* (Report 85-3). Hyattsville, Md: Nutrition Monitoring Division, Human Nutrition Information Service, US Department of Agriculture; 1986.

170. US Department of Agriculture. *Nationwide Food Consumption Survey. Continuing Survey of Food Intakes by Individuals. Women 19–50 Years and Their Children 1–5 Years, 4 Days, 1985* (Report 85-4). Hyattsville, Md: Nutrition Monitoring Division, Human Nutrition Information Service, US Department of Agriculture; 1987.

171. Oenning LL, Vogel J, Calvo MS. Accuracy of methods estimating calcium and phosphorus intake in daily diets. *J Am Diet Assoc.* 1988;88:1076–1078.

172. Greger JL, Krystofiak M. Phosphorus intake of Americans. *Food Technol.* 1982;36:78–84.

173. Draper HH, Scythes CA. Calcium, phosphorus and osteoporosis. *Fed Proc.* 1981;40:2434–2438.

174. Anderson JJB. Nutritional biochemistry of calcium and phosphorus. *J Nutr Biochem.* 1991;2:300–307.

175. Carroll MD, Abraham S, Dresser CM. *Dietary Intake Source Data: US, 1976–1980.* Washington, DC: US Department of Health and Human Services; 1983. Dept of Health and Human Services publication (PHS) 83–PHS.

176. Schuette S, Linkswiler H. Effects on Ca and P metabolism in humans by adding meat, meat plus milk, or purified proteins plus Ca and P to a low protein diet. *J Nutr.* 1982;112:338–349.

177. Barltrop D, Mole RH, Sutton A. Absorption and endogenous faecal excretion of calcium by low birthweight infants on feeds with varying contents of calcium and phosphate. *Arch Dis Child.* 1977;52:41–49.

178. Spencer H, Kramer L, Osis D, Norris C. Effect of phosphorus on the absorption of calcium and on the calcium balance. *J Nutr.* 1978;108:447–457.

179. Calvo MS, Kumar R, Health H III. Persistently elevated parathyroid hormone secretion and action in young women after four weeks of ingesting high phosphorus, low calcium diets. *J Clin Endocrinol Metab.* 1990;70:1334–1340.

180. Mazarlegos-Ramos E, Guerrero-Romero F, Rodríguez-Morán M, Lazcano-Burciaga G, Panlagua R, Amato D. Consumption of soft drinks with phosphoric acid as a risk factor for the development of hypocalcemia in children: A case-control study. *J Pediatr.* 1995;126:940–942.

181. Massey LK, Strang MM. Soft drink consumption, phosphorus intake, and osteoporosis. *J Am Diet Assoc.* 1982;80:581–583.

182. Ketaren PP, Batterham ES, Dettman B. Phosphorus studies in pigs. *Br J Nutr.* 1993;70:289–311.

183. Underwood EJ. The incidence of trace element deficiency diseases. *Philos Trans R Soc London Ser B.* 1981;294:3–8.

184. Gibson RS, Scythes CA. Trace element status of women. *Br J Nutr.* 1982;48:241–248.

185. Kies C, Aldrich KD, Johnson JM, Crepes C, Kowalski C, Wang RH. Manganese availability for humans. Effect of selected dietary factors. In: Kies C, ed. *Nutritional Bioavailability of Manganese*. Washington, DC: American Chemical Society; 1987:136–145.

186. Kelsay JL, Frasier CW, Prather ES, Canary JJ, Clark WM, Powell AS. Impact of variation in carbohydrate intake on mineral utilization by vegetarians. *Am J Clin Nutr*. 1988;48:875–879.

187. Bindra GS, Gibson RS. Mineral intakes of predominantly lacto-ovo vegetarian east Indian adults. *Biol Trace Elem*. 1986;10:223–234.

188. Nielsen FH. Ultratrace minerals. In: Shils ME, Olson JA, Shike M. *Modern Nutrition and Health and Disease*. 8th ed. Philadelphia, Pa: Lea & Febiger; 1994:269–286.

189. Bales CW, Freeland-Graves JH, Lin P-H, Stone J, Dougherty V. Plasma uptake of manganese: Response to dose and dietary factors. In: Kies C, ed. *Nutritional Bioavailability of Manganese*. Washington, DC: American Chemical Society; 1987:112–122.

190. Lang VM, North BB, Morse LM. Manganese metabolism in college men consuming vegetarian diets. *J Nutr*. 1965;85:132–138.

191. Matovinovic J. Endemic goiter and cretinism at the dawn of the third millenium. *Annu Rev Nutr*. 1983;3:341–412.

192. Brush BE, Altland JK. Goiter prevention with iodized salt: Results of a thirty-year study. *J Clin Endocrinol Metab*. 1952;12:1380–1388.

193. Dunn JT. Iodized oil in the treatment and prophylaxis of IDD. In: Hetzel BS, Dunn JT, Stanbury JB, eds. *The Prevention and Control of Iodine Deficiency Disorders*. Amsterdam, Holland: Elsevier; 1987:127–134.

194. Tookey GL, Van Etten CH, Daxenbichler MD. Glucosinolates. In: Liener IE, ed. *Toxic Constituents of Plant Feedstuffs*. 2nd ed. New York, NY: Academic Press, 1980:103–142.

195. Hemken RW. Factors that influence the iodine content of milk and meat: A review. *J Anim Sci*. 1979;48:981–985.

196. Suzuki H. Etiology of endemic goiter and iodide excess. In: Stanbury JB, Hertzel BS, eds. *Endemic Goiter and Endemic Cretinism*. New York, NY: Wiley; 1980:237–253.

197. Draper A, Lewis J, Malhotra N, Wheeler E. The energy and nutrient intakes of different types of vegetarian: A case for supplements? *Br J Nutr*. 1993;69:3–19.

198. Sullivan JM, Prewitt RL, Ratts TE. Sodium sensitivity in normotensive and borderline hypertensive humans. *Am J Med Sci*. 1988;295:370–377.

199. Sanchez-Casillo CP, Warrender S, Whitehead TP, James WP. An assessment of the sources of dietary salt in a British population. *Clin Sci*. 1987;72:95–102.

200. Sanchez-Castillo CP, Branch WJ, James WP. A test of the validity of the lithium-marker technique for monitoring dietary sources for salt in men. *Clin Sci*. 1987;72:87–94.

201. National Research Council. *Diet and Health: Implications for Reducing Chronic Disease Risk. Report of the Committee on Diet and Health, Food and Nutrition Board*. Washington, DC: National Academy Press; 1989.

202. Lemann J Jr, Pleuss JA, Gray RW. Potassium causes calcium retention in healthy adults. *J Nutr*. 1993;123:1623–1626.

203. Khaw KT, Barrett-Connor E. Dietary potassium and stroke-associated mortality. A 12-year prospective population study. *N Engl J Med*. 1987;316:235–240.

204. Burt BA. The epidemiologic basis for water fluoridation in the prevention of dental caries. *J Public Health*. 1982;3:391–407.

205. Kroger H, Alhava E, Honkanen R, Tuppurainen M, Saarikoski S. The effect of fluoridated drinking water on axial bone mineral density—A population-based study. *Bone Miner.* 1994;27:33–41.

206. Riggs BL, Hodgson SF, O'Fallon WM, et al. Effect of fluoride treatment on the fracture rate in postmenopausal women with osteoporosis. *N Engl J Med.* 1990;322:802–809.

207. Singer L, Ophang RH, Harland BF. Flouride intake of young male adults in the United States. *Am J Clin Nutr.* 1980;33:328–332.

208. Kumpulainen J, Koivistoinen P. Flourine in foods. *Residue Rev.* 1977;68:37–57.

209. Marier JR, Rose D. The flouride content of some food and beverages—A brief survey using a modified Zr-SPADNS method. *J Food Sci.* 1966;31:941–946.

210. Full CA, Parkins FM. Effect of cooking vessel composition on flouride. *J Dent Res.* 1975;54:192.

211. Anderson RA, Kozlovsky AS. Chromium intake, absorption, and excretion of subjects consuming self-selected diets. *Am J Clin Nutr.* 1985;41:1177–1183.

212. Anderson RA, Polansky MM, Bryden NA, Roginski EE, Mertz W, Glinsmann WH. Chromium supplementation of human subjects: Effects on glucose, insulin, and lipid variables. *Metabolism.* 1983;32:894–899.

213. Schroeder HA. Losses of vitamins and trace minerals resulting from processing and preparation of foods. *Am J Clin Nutr.* 1971;24:562–573.

214. Offenbacher EG, Pi-Sunyer FX. Temperature and pH effects on the release of chromium from stainless steel into water and fruit juices. *J Agric Food Chem.* 1983;31:89–92.

215. Anderson R, Bryden NA. Concentration, insulin potentiation, and absorption of chromium in beer. *J Agric Food Chem.* 1983;31:308–311.

216. Davidson IWF, Burt RL. Physiologic changes in plasma chromium of normal and pregnant women: Effect of a glucose load. *Am J Obstet Gynecol.* 1973;116:601–608.

217. Campbell WW, Anderson RA. Effects of aerobic exercise and training on the trace minerals chromium, zinc, and copper. *Sports Med.* 1987;4:9–16.

218. Tsongas TA, Meglen RR, Walravens PA, Chappel WR. Molybdenum in the diet; An estimate of average daily intake in the United States. *Am J Clin Nutr.* 1980;33:1103–1107.

219. Pennington JAT, Jones JW. Molybdenum, nickel, cobalt, vanadium, and strontium in total diets. *J Am Diet Assoc.* 1987;87:1644–1650.

220. Deosthale YG, Goplan C. The effect of molybdenum levels in sorghum (*Sorghum vulgare Pers*) on uric acid and copper excretion in man. *Br J Nutr.* 1974;31:351–355.

CHAPTER 6

Vitamins

Lacto-ovo vegetarian diets tend to be adequate in all the vitamins. Vegan diets may be lacking in vitamin B_{12} and vitamin D, and there is also some debate about the status of riboflavin in these diets. Consequently, most of the discussion in this chapter will focus on these three nutrients.

VITAMIN B_{12} (COBALAMIN)

All the vitamin B_{12} in nature is produced by microorganisms, bacteria, fungi, and algae; plants and animals cannot synthesize vitamin B_{12}. Animal foods are sources of this vitamin because animals ingest vitamin B_{12}-containing microorganisms or because they absorb some of the vitamin B_{12} produced by their intestinal bacteria. Plant foods may contain some vitamin B_{12} if they are contaminated with vitamin B_{12}-producing bacteria. In the United States and other developed countries, it is likely that most or all of this B_{12} is removed when the food is cleaned.

Concerns over the vitamin B_{12} status of vegetarians have precipitated much discussion within the professional and vegetarian communities. Because plant foods do not naturally contain vitamin B_{12}, unsupplemented vegan diets are theoretically completely lacking in this nutrient. Surprisingly, however, symptomatic vitamin B_{12} deficiency is relatively rare within vegan populations.

Terminology

It is worthwhile to discuss some terminology related to the structure of vitamin B_{12}, because some foods contain vitamin B_{12} analogues. Not only do these analogues not possess any biologic activity, but they can actually impair the utilization of vitamin B_{12} by blocking its absorption and may even accelerate nerve damage in vitamin B_{12}-deficiency states. Recent work indicates that in many "vitamin B_{12}-rich foods," between 5% and 30% of the vitamin B_{12} is analogue.[1] In some foods, the B_{12} is nearly all analogue.[1]

The core structure of vitamin B_{12} is a macrocyclic ring designated as corrin, which comprises four reduced pyrrole rings linked together. Compounds containing this ring are designated as corrinoids. Cobalt is at the center of the corrin structure. All molecules containing the corrin ring with attached cobalt are considered cobalamins. A number of chemical constituents may be attached to the cobalt. In active vitamin B_{12} either a methyl group or 5'-deoxyadenosyl is attached to form either methylcobalamin or 5'-deoxyadenosyl cobalamin. These are the only two active forms of vitamin B_{12}.

Commercially available vitamin B_{12} supplements contain cyanocobalamin, which has a cyanide molecule attached to cobalt that stabilizes the vitamin. This form is converted to metabolically active vitamin B_{12} in the body by removal of the cyanide. There is a rare genetic disorder, however, wherein infants are unable to remove the cyanide and thus are unable to use this type of vitamin B_{12} preparation.[2]

Virtually all the vitamin B_{12} within cells is bound to the only two vitamin B_{12}-dependent enzymes. Methylmalonyl coenzyme A mutase uses vitamin B_{12} for the metabolism of certain amino acids and odd-chain fatty acids. Methionine synthase requires vitamin B_{12} to convert homocysteine to methionine.

Vitamin B_{12} Digestion and Absorption

Vitamin B_{12} digestion begins in the stomach, where gastric secretions and proteases split vitamin B_{12} from the peptides to which it is attached in foods. Vitamin B_{12} is then free to bind to R factor, which is present in many bodily fluids. Pancreatic secretions then partially degrade the R factor, and vitamin B_{12} becomes bound by intrinsic factor (IF), which is secreted by the gastric parietal cells. IF binds to specific receptors on the ileal brush border (the lower small intestine) and facilitates absorption of vitamin B_{12}. Vitamin B_{12} is one of those few nutrients absorbed primarily from the lower half of the small bowel. The formation of the vitamin B_{12}-IF complex protects vitamin B_{12} against bacterial degradation and against the hydrolytic action of pepsin and chymotrypsin.

Vitamin B_{12} is transported in the plasma bound to the protein transcobalamin and eventually is transferred to R proteins. In contrast to the situation with other B vitamins, considerable amounts of vitamin B_{12} relative to need are stored. Approximately 60% of the total body vitamin B_{12} is stored in the liver, and about 30% is stored in the muscles.

Small amounts of vitamin B_{12} are excreted in the urine, but the primary mode of excretion is in the bile and, ultimately, the feces. Only about 0.1% to 0.2% of total body reserves (2 to 5 µg) is excreted into the bile each day, however, regardless of the amount stored. About 65% to 75% percent of the vitamin B_{12} excreted into the bile is actually reabsorbed as a result of an extremely efficient enterohepatic circulation. This helps explain why the recommended dietary allowance (RDA) for vitamin B_{12} is so low and why deficiency symptoms do not develop for many years in people who consume no vitamin B_{12}, but develop very quickly in people who cannot reabsorb this vitamin. Interestingly, vitamin B_{12} analogues seem to be preferentially excreted, whereas cobalamins are largely reabsorbed.[3]

Vitamin B_{12} Deficiency

Vitamin B_{12} deficiency causes red blood cells to increase in size because cell division is inhibited but the cell itself continues to grow. This same type of megaloblastic anemia is seen in folate deficiency. Vitamin B_{12} deficiency is also associated with demyelinization of peripheral nerves, the spinal cord, the cranial nerves, and the brain, however, resulting in nerve damage and neuropsychiatric abnormalities. Symptoms include decreased sensation, difficulty in walking, loss of control of bowel and bladder, optic atrophy, memory loss, dementia, depression, general weakness, and psychosis.[4] Nerve damage due to B_{12} deficiency can be irreversible.

Although neuropsychiatric symptoms are clearly associated with vitamin B_{12} deficiency, the biologic explanation for why this is so is unclear. It has recently been proposed that perhaps a deficiency of a third enzyme that requires vitamin B_{12}, or a combined deficiency of the two known vitamin B_{12}-requiring enzymes along with some other genetic or environmental factor, is responsible.

High levels of folate can mask B_{12} deficiency to some degree, since normal red blood cells continue to be produced even in the presence of B_{12} deficiency. In this case, anemia, an early and reversible symptom of B_{12} deficiency, is not apparent, so that the B_{12} deficiency may not be detected until the more serious and irreversible nerve damage is observed. This may be of some concern for vegans because their intake of vitamin B_{12} may be low and their intake of folate is generally quite high.

Assessing Vitamin B_{12} Status

Disagreements over the vitamin B_{12} status of vegans exist in part because there is no gold standard for assessing status. A number of hematologic indices that are not specific to vitamin B_{12} deficiency, including hemoglobin measures, are sometimes used. Blood levels of vitamin B_{12} can be measured using microbiologic or radiodilution methods. In some of these assays, both active vitamin B_{12} and analogue levels are included in the measure, so that levels of active vitamin B_{12} can be overestimated.[5] In fact, as much as 30% of the vitamin B_{12} in serum may be analogue.[1] This same problem exists when the amount of B_{12} in foods is assessed. Other tests of vitamin B_{12} status include measurement of serum holotranscobalamin II, urinary or serum methylmalonic acid (MMA), total homocysteine levels, and the deoxyuridine suppression test.

Evidence indicates that serum holo transcobalamin II (the protein that transports vitamin B_{12} in serum) levels fall to low values in vitamin B_{12} deficiency.[6] Tests for this protein will identify low vitamin B_{12} status even before total serum vitamin B_{12} levels begin to drop.[7] A functional test of vitamin B_{12} status is the measurement of MMA in serum or urine because the vitamin B_{12}–requiring enzyme methylmalonyl coenzyme A mutase is necessary for the normal metabolism of MMA. In B_{12} deficiency, MMA levels increase. This may be one of the better means of assessing B_{12} deficiency because it detects early stages of the problem.[8] Each test has advantages and disadvantages.

Vegetarians and Vitamin B_{12} Status

Approximately 95% of the known cases of vitamin B_{12} deficiency occur in individuals who are not able to absorb this vitamin because of the lack of IF or because of a reduction in gastric acid or in the gastric enzymes required to cleave vitamin B_{12} from the proteins in food.[9] Reported cases of symptomatic vitamin B_{12} deficiency due to inadequate intake are rare, although they do exist.

There are several possible explanations for the scarcity of published observations of vitamin B_{12} deficiency among vegans, a population that consumes no natural sources of this vitamin. First, there have been relatively few studies of long-term vegans who do not use supplements or fortified foods. For example, Sanders et al[10] studied 34 vegans and found no signs of vitamin B_{12} deficiency, but most of the subjects had followed their vegan diet for less than 5 years. Second, food and drinking water contaminated with vitamin B_{12}–producing bacteria may contribute significant B_{12}, particularly in developing countries. It is likely, however, that all Western vegans consuming unsupplemented diets will eventually develop vitamin B_{12} deficiency, although it may take decades for this to occur.

Although overt symptoms of deficiency are infrequently observed, plasma levels of vitamin B_{12} tend to be much lower in both vegans[10–13] and lacto-ovo vegetarians[13-15] than in the general population (Figure 6–1). Ellis and Montegriffo[12] studied 26 vegans, 7 of whom did not take vitamin B_{12} supplements, and found no blood abnormalities related to vitamin B_{12} deficiency. Serum vitamin B_{12} levels were low, however, and three subjects had vitamin B_{12} levels indicative of deficiency (30, 50, and 60 pg/mL). Interestingly, 4 vegans who had been on this diet for 13 years and longer without supplements had normal vitamin B_{12} levels. A study of Thai vegetarians, however, illustrates the effect of duration of vegetarian diet on serum vitamin B_{12} levels (Figure 6–2).

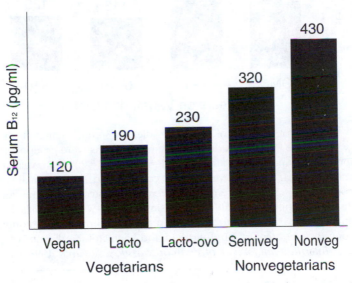

Figure 6–1 Serum vitamin B_{12} levels in five dietary groups (values are in picograms per milliliter). Subjects were recruited from the American Natural Hygiene Society and included a mixture of men and women with an approximate age range of 30 to 60 years. These vegetarians were atypical in that their dietary intake included few grains and legumes and mostly raw fruits, vegetables, nuts, and seeds. Values for men and women were averaged for each group and included 13 vegans, 28 lacto vegetarians, 15 lacto-ovo vegetarians, 10 semivegetarians, and 4 omnivores. Vegetarians had been vegetarians for, on average, between 10 and 17 years. None of the 70 subjects reported taking vitamin B_{12} supplements. Serum vitamin B_{12} levels were determined using a radioassay. Normal levels for this assay are between 200 and 900 pg/mL. Values among the five dietary groups were statistically significant at the 1% level (*F* ratio = 12.1). Subjects with values below 100 pg/mL were considered deficient in vitamin B_{12}. *Source:* Data from Dong A, Scott SC. Serum vitamin B_{12} and blood cell values in vegetarians. *Annals of Nutrition Metabolism.* 1970;23:249–255.

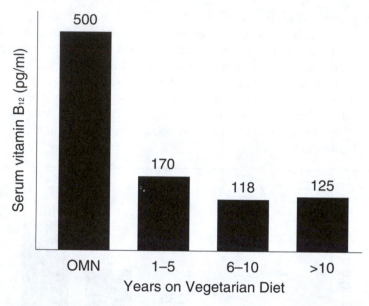

Figure 6–2 Effects of duration of vegetarian diet on serum vitamin B₁₂ levels. All subjects were female lacto vegetarians. Vegetarian subjects were grouped according to duration of consuming a vegetarian diet; 1–5 years (N = 22), 6–10 years (N = 29), and more than 10 years (N = 17), values were compared to a group female omnivore (OMN) controls (N = 22). Differences between the omnivores and the vegetarians were statistically significant (P value <0.05 using Kruskal-Wallis analysis of variance and multiple comparison). *Source:* Data from Tungtrongchitr R, Pongpaew P, Prayurahong B, et al. Vitamin B₁₂, folic acid and haematological status of 132 Thai vegetarians. *International Journal of Vitamin Nutrition Research.* 1993;63:201–207.

In an Israeli study, 4 vegans with low blood levels of vitamin B₁₂ had no hematologic abnormalities but complained of weakness, fatigue, and poor mental concentration, symptoms often associated with neurologic disturbances stemming from a lack of vitamin B₁₂. Upon administration of B₁₂, their blood levels increased and, most important, their symptoms improved.[11]

In another study of Thai vegetarians, vitamin B₁₂ blood level values were one tenth those of the omnivores, although all the vegans appeared healthy, and none displayed any symptoms of vitamin B₁₂ deficiency anemia.[16] This was also the case in an Indian study, where it was found that, although lacto vegetarians had low vitamin B₁₂ blood levels (121 versus 366 pg/mL for omnivores), none of the vegetarians had any apparent signs or symptoms of vitamin B₁₂ deficiency.[17] Studies of macrobiotics reveal low levels of vitamin B₁₂ in this population.[18,19] In a study of vegans, among those who did not use supplements, vitamin B_{12} levels tended to be lower the longer the subjects had followed a vegan diet.[20] Finally, in what may be considered to be the most definitive study conducted to date, Crane et al investigated vitamin B_{12} levels in individuals who had been vegans for between 12 and 340 months and who reported not consuming vitamin B_{12} supplements or fortified foods for at least one year prior to the study (see Figure 6–3). Of the 78 vegans, 60% had vitamin B_{12} levels below 200 pg/mL (normal values are considered to be above 200) and 46% had levels below 160 pg/mL. In comparison, the mean serum vitamin B_{12} level of vegans (N = 12) who used soymilk fortified

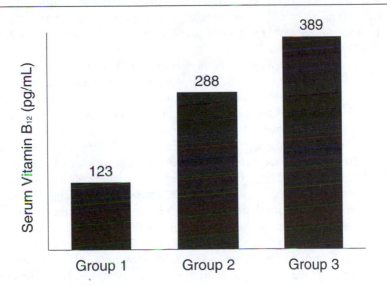

Figure 6–3 Effect of vegan diet on serum vitamin B_{12} levels. Subjects were primarily residents of the Weimer Institute in California, and had consumed a vegan diet for 12–340 months avoiding not only eggs and milk, but added free fats and sugars. After analysis of the data, subjects were divided into groups. Individuals in groups 1 and 2 were placed in their respective groups according to whether their serum B_{12} levels were below the value considered to be normal, 200 pg/mL (group 1) or above 200 pg/mL (group 2). Groups 1 (25 males and 22 females) and 2 (16 males and 15 females) consist of individuals who did not use vitamin B_{12} fortified foods or B_{12} supplements for one year prior to the study, whereas individuals in group 3 (6 males and 6 females) used vitamin B_{12} fortified soymilk. In another study by these authors, when subjects consuming a lacto-ovo vegetarian diet adopted a strict vegan diet, serum vitamin B_{12} levels decreased from a mean of 417 to 268 pg/mL after 2 months, and remained at about that level (276 pg/mL) for the 5 months of the study. *Source:* Crane MG, Sample C, Patchett S, Register UD. Vitamin B_{12} studies in total vegetarians (vegans). *Journal of Nutrition Medicine*. 1994;4:419–430.

with B_{12} was 389 pg/mL. Four vegans in the unsupplemented group had a mean corpuscular volume above 100 (normal values, 79–100 fl), an indication of abnormal red cell blood synthesis.

Nonanimal Sources of Vitamin B_{12}: Fact or Fantasy?

The standard assay for determining B_{12} content does not distinguish between biologically active forms of vitamin B_{12} and analogues.[1] This has caused considerable confusion about the presence of vitamin B_{12} in plant foods.

Foods that have been reported to contain vitamin B_{12} include fermented foods (such as tempeh), sea vegetables, algae and spirulina, various greens, grains, and legumes.[21–28] Even rainwater has been reported to be a source of vitamin B_{12}[29] (Exhibit 6–1).

In an analysis of 40 plant foods, however, van den Berg et al[25] found that most did not contain vitamin B_{12}. Using an assay specific for active vitamin B_{12}, the investigators determined that none of the fermented soy products tested, which included tempeh, shoyu, tamari, rice miso, and barley miso, and none of the fermented nonsoy products, such as amesake rice and umeboshi plums, contained any. Neither did tofu. Tiny amounts (0.02 to 0.50 μg/100 g) were found in barley malt syrup, sourdough bread, parsley, and shiitake mushrooms. Only the algae nori (*Porphyra tenera*) and spirulina contained appreciable amounts. Herbert et al[30] and Herbert and Drivas,[31] however, reported that the vitamin B_{12} in spirulina is mostly analogue, and Dagnelie et al[32] reported that the consumption of nori, spirulina, kombu, whole-meal sourdough bread, and barley malt syrup did not improve mean corpuscular volume or mean corpuscular hemoglobin mass despite an increase in vitamin B_{12} plasma volume. This suggests that the vitamin B_{12} in these prod-

---

Exhibit 6–1 Foods Reported in the Popular Literature To Be Good Sources of Vitamin B_{12} but Shown by Analysis To Contain Either No Vitamin B_{12} or Only Analogue

Tempeh	Amaranth	Tamari
Sea vegetables (arame, wasake, kombu)*	Spinach	Miso
	Turnip greens	Umeboshi plums
Algae	Legumes	Tofu
Spirulina	Peanuts	Barley malt syrup
Comfrey	Soybeans	Sourdough bread
Alfalfa	Rainwater	Shiitake mushrooms
	Shoyu	

*Recent studies indicate that some sea vegetables may contain some active vitamin B_{12}.

ucts is also mostly analogue. It has been reported, however, that the consumption of sea vegetables (arame, wakame, and kombu) by a lactating woman led to an improvement in the vitamin B_{12} status of her breastfed infant.[19] The consumption of nori and chlorella sea vegetables was also associated with higher serum B_{12} levels in subjects adhering to a raw foods vegan diet, although serum levels of B_{12} were low among all of the subjects. These studies suggest that sea vegetables may in fact provide some active vitamin B_{12}, although the levels in these foods, when consumed in reasonable amounts, is not sufficient to meet vitamin B_{12} needs.[33] The presence of analogues is a particularly important issue because some reports have found that high levels of cobalamin analogs are associated with neurologic abnormalities in cases of cobalamin deficiency.[34]

Some plant foods may be contaminated with vitamin B_{12}-producing bacteria, the value of which was demonstrated many years ago. Iranian vegans maintain normal B_{12} status by consuming vegetables that were grown in night soil (human manure) and are not thoroughly washed before eaten.[35] This demonstrates not only the potential contribution of bacterial contamination but also the fact the human feces contains active vitamin B_{12}, a point discussed below.

Legumes, such as soybeans, possess root nodules that can be inhabited by bacteria. These bacteria may produce small amounts of both active B_{12} and analogue. US Department of Agriculture data indicate, however, that soybeans and other legumes contain no vitamin B_{12}. These foods should not be considered a reliable source of this vitamin.

Bacteria in the digestive tract of humans produce considerable amounts of active vitamin B_{12}, but the extent to which this is available for absorption is unclear. Most of this B_{12} is produced too far down in the colon to be absorbed,[36] and most of it ends up in the feces.[1] Smaller amounts of vitamin B_{12} may be produced in the small intestine, and there is evidence that some of this could be absorbed.[37,38]

Intestinal synthesis of B_{12} has been proposed as one explanation for why vitamin B_{12} deficiency is uncommon among the largely vegetarian population of India.[39] Vegetarian diets may modify the types of bacteria in the gut; Indian vegetarians reportedly have a larger growth of microflora than nonvegetarians.[39] The extent to which bacteria in the small intestines contribute to vitamin B_{12} status is still poorly understood, however. Indian immigrants to the United Kingdom experience a higher incidence of vitamin B_{12} deficiency, which theoretically could be due to changes in the microecology of the gut but is more likely due to improved hygiene and a reduced intake of food and water contaminated with vitamin B_{12}-producing bacteria.[40]

Finally, the oral cavity does produce vitamin B_{12}, although only in small amounts.[41] Studies demonstrating this did not distinguish between active B_{12} and analogue, however. Nevertheless, the quantity of vitamin B_{12} produced is not sufficient to meet daily requirements, although it might contribute to intake.

Vitamin B$_{12}$ Deficiency in Vegan Infants

There have been many reports of vitamin B$_{12}$ deficiency in breastfed infants of vegan mothers,[19,42–54] although many of these are findings from macrobiotic populations, in which infant feeding practices differ markedly from those in the general vegan population. The fetus obtains its initial store of B$_{12}$ via the placenta. Under normal conditions, full-term infants will have enough stored vitamin B$_{12}$ to last 6 months to 1 year.[55] Newborn vitamin B$_{12}$ stores are normally about 14.7 to 18.4 nmol. In contrast, neonates of deficient mothers can have stores as low as 1.5 to 3.7 nmol.[56] At birth, however, these infants have much higher serum vitamin B$_{12}$ levels than their mothers,[56,57] and in most instances they show no signs of B$_{12}$ deficiency.

Serum vitamin B$_{12}$ levels of normal infants decrease progressively and reach a nadir at 6 months.[49] This decrease is probably accentuated in breastfed infants of vitamin B$_{12}$-deficient mothers because the vitamin B$_{12}$ content of the milk reflects maternal serum levels and because these infants will have smaller storage levels. Lactation also can decrease vitamin B$_{12}$ stores in mothers. In repeated pregnancies, infants may be at risk.[58] Interestingly, in numerous reports of nutritional vitamin B$_{12}$ deficiency in infants, the mothers had no clinical manifestation or hematologic abnormality.[43,50,59–61] Some studies have shown improvement when deficient infants are given vitamin B$_{12}$, but questions remain about the long-term neurologic consequences of nutritional vitamin B$_{12}$ deficiency during infancy.[47,61]

One study involving poor vitamin B$_{12}$ status in infants found that infant MMA levels were not related to the length of time the mother had been practicing a vegetarian diet, even though women who had been vegetarian the longest had the lowest serum levels of vitamin B$_{12}$.[19] This suggests, as was proposed some time ago, that it is only newly absorbed vitamin B$_{12}$ that is transported readily across the placenta or is present in human milk.[62] In contrast, a more recent study found that vitamin B$_{12}$ concentration in breast milk decreased with increasing time on a vegetarian diet, suggesting that vitamin B$_{12}$ stores may in fact contribute to vitamin B$_{12}$ levels in human milk.[49] When maternal serum vitamin B$_{12}$ levels are low, breast milk vitamin B$_{12}$ levels will also be low, resulting in inadequate vitamin intake in infants.[49,63,64]

Counseling Vegan Clients

The biologic need for vitamin B$_{12}$ is about 1.0 μg/day or less; in fact, as little as 0.1 μg/day may be enough to satisfy the requirements of most people.[3] The World Health Organization recommends a daily intake of 1.0 µg. Although the RDA for this nutrient was lowered from 3.0 to 2.0 µg in the 1989 version of the RDAs, it is still well above biologic needs.

A strict vegan diet is theoretically devoid of this nutrient. Although some foods may be contaminated with this nutrient, this is unreliable. Therefore, all vegans need a regular, reliable source of B_{12} in their diet, either in fortified foods or as a vitamin supplement. In counseling vegans about dietary sources of vitamin B_{12}, it is important that they understand the difference between the active vitamin and its analogues. There is a great deal of misinformation in the popular vegetarian literature about foods that are purported to contain vitamin B_{12} but actually contain only analogue. Exhibit 6–1 lists a number of these foods.

Many foods that are acceptable to vegans are excellent sources of vitamin B_{12} (Table 6-1). Nutritional yeast is one of the best. Only nutritional yeast that has been grown on a vitamin B_{12}-rich medium is a good source of this vitamin, however. Red Star brand nutritional yeast T6635 is one that is reliably high in vitamin B_{12}. A tablespoon provides 4 µg.

Table 6–1 Vitamin B_{12} Content of Foods

Food	Vitamin B_{12} Content (µg)	Food	Vitamin B_{12} Content (µg)
Breads, cereals, grains		**Fortified soymilk/vegetable**	
Kellogg's Corn Flakes, ¾ cup	1.5	**milks** (8 oz)	
Grapenuts, ¼ cup	1.5	Better Than Milk (soymilk)	0.6
Nutrigrain, ⅔ cup	1.5	Edensoy Extra	3.0
Product 19, ¾ cup	6.0	Sno E (soymilk)	1.2
Raisin Bran, ¾ cup	1.5	Soyagen	1.5
Total 1 cup	6.2	Take Care (soymilk)	0.9
Meat analogue (servings sizes		Vegelicious (vegetable milk)	0.6
are one burger or one serving		**Animal products**	
according to package)		Milk, 1 cup	0.9
Loma Linda "Chicken" Nuggets	3.0	Yogurt, plain, nonfat, 1 cup	0.6
Morningstar Farms Grillers	6.7	Egg, one large	0.6
Loma Linda Sizzle Franks	2.0	**Other**	
Worthington Stakelets	5.2	Nutritional yeast (Red Star	
		brand T6635), 1 tbsp	4.0

Note: Fortification of commercial products can change over time, so that it is always a good idea to check the label.
Source: Data from *Bowes & Church's Food Value of Portions Commonly Used.* 16th ed., by J. Pennington, Lippincott-Raven, 1994, and package information.

Most commercial soymilk companies have been slow to fortify their products with vitamin B_{12}. Brands that contain B_{12} include Better Than Milk, Soyagen, and Edensoy Extra. Vegelicious, a vegetable-based milk, is also vitamin B_{12}-fortified, but it is not vegan because it contains honey. Some meat analogues are also good sources of vitamin B_{12}. Finally, many commercial breakfast cereals are rich in vitamin B_{12}, although fortification varies among brands and in the same brand over time.

Although vitamin B_{12} is an important issue in vegan nutrition, it is an easily resolved one. Regular use of fortified foods provides adequate B_{12} for vegans. Some vegans may be suspicious of fortification, however, because nutrients may be derived from animal products and would not be considered vegan. In this case, a supplement may be the best choice. Dietitians should be able to provide suggestions for brand names of B_{12} supplements that are vegan.

Some B_{12} supplements provide as much as 500 µg per dose. At these high levels of intake, however, vitamin B_{12} absorption efficiency decreases markedly. Therefore, clients should be counseled to take supplements several times a week in smaller doses even though it may appear that one vitamin pill will provide enough B_{12} for several weeks. Most importantly, recent research indicates that for B_{12} to be absorbed, B_{12} pills need to be chewed before swallowing. This allows for the vitamin to combine with the R factor.

Summary

There have been relatively few cases of frank vitamin B_{12} deficiency among vegans. There may be a number of explanations for this:

- Few studies of long-term vegans have been conducted.
- Vitamin B_{12} requirements are small, and storage capacity for this vitamin is considerable, so that deficiency can take many years to manifest.
- The body conserves vitamin B_{12} through an efficient enterohepatic circulation, so that little vitamin B_{12} is excreted.
- Plant foods that are not thoroughly cleaned may be contaminated with vitamin B_{12}-producing bacteria. This may be especially relevant in countries where food and water supplies are not completely sterile.
- Vitamin B_{12} production in the human digestive tract (oral cavity and intestines) may make a minor contribution to B_{12} intake.

Although all these factors may contribute to the B_{12} status of vegans, none is sufficiently reliable to promote adequate vitamin B_{12} status. It is likely that all Western vegans whose diets are unsupplemented will eventually develop vitamin B_{12} deficiency.

Also, although vitamin B_{12}-related anemia is rare in vegans, studies consistently show that vegans have low serum levels of vitamin B_{12} and that many have levels that are considered inadequate and/or marginally deficient. Furthermore, at least among elderly, serum levels of vitamin B_{12} have been shown to underestimate the prevalence of deficiency.[65] This appears to be the case even in individuals without anemia who are apparently healthy. There are two concerns related to these findings. One is that individuals with such low levels will be ill equipped to adapt sufficiently during times when vitamin B_{12} needs are increased (eg, during aging or in the presence of infection). In fact, it has been suggested that some of the vitamin B_{12} deficiency in older vegans may be due to a subtle vitamin B_{12} malabsorption in combination with a marginal intake of vitamin B_{12}.

Much more important, however, anemia is not by any means the only clinical consequence of low vitamin B_{12}. Vitamin B_{12} deficiency even in the absence of anemia may have deleterious effects on the nervous system.[66,67] It is possible that subtle neurologic damage could be occurring even though anemia is not evident. This possibility is increased in vegans because they consume more folate than nonvegetarians. Folate delays or prevents vitamin B_{12}-related anemia and thus could prevent early detection of B_{12} deficiency.

Low vitamin B_{12} levels in the elderly have also been linked to elevated homocysteine concentrations,[68] which may be an important risk factor for cerebral, coronary, and peripheral vascular disease.[69,70] More research is needed to establish whether this is due to inadequate intake and/or absorption or whether there is some biologic defect that occurs with aging that increased vitamin B_{12} intake will not remedy.

Some individuals have suggested that the lack of vitamin B_{12} in the vegan diet implies that this is not a natural or recommended way of eating. Actually, the evidence suggests that humans evolved to function on a small intake of vitamin B_{12}. It seems reasonable to speculate that the original diet of humans contained only the smallest amounts of B_{12} because the body conserves it so carefully. It is likely that, until recently, vitamin B_{12} needs could be met entirely through consumption of foods contaminated with bacteria or contaminated drinking water. It is only as our food supply has become more hygienic that additional sources of this vitamin have become necessary.

RIBOFLAVIN

Riboflavin, commonly called vitamin B_2, is a yellow fluorescent compound that is quite widely distributed among the plant and animal kingdom. Although green leafy vegetables are rich in riboflavin, meats and dairy products supply about half the riboflavin intake in the typical American diet. Cheese is a particularly rich source. Consequently, some concerns have been raised about the ability of strict vegans to obtain adequate amounts of riboflavin, particularly those who are not consuming whole or enriched grains.

Riboflavin forms part of the coenzymes flavin mononucleotide (FMN) and flavin adenine dinucleotide (FAD), both of which are required by many enzymes involved primarily in oxidation and reduction reactions. Riboflavin status is assessed by measuring urinary levels or measuring the activity of glutathione reductase, an enzyme that requires FAD as a coenzyme. Overt deficiency of riboflavin is uncommon in Western countries. Deficiency signs include cheilosis, angular stomatitis, glossitis, hyperemia and edema of the oral mucosa, seborrheic dermatitis around the nose and mouth and scrotum/vulva, and normocytic normochromic anemia.

The adult RDA for riboflavin is 1.3 mg for women and 1.7 mg for men. Most Americans meet or exceed these requirements.[71,72] There is some debate over the actual riboflavin requirement; however, some experts believe it to be too high. A survey of different populations in the People's Republic of China found intake to vary greatly among different regions, but the average intake was only 0.8 mg/day, or about half the US RDA.[73] There were no outright clinical signs of riboflavin deficiency, however. Early clinical studies, in which dietary riboflavin intake was well below the RDA, reported that signs of deficiency rarely if ever resulted.[74,75] The RDA value allows for greater reserves of riboflavin and greater variability among individuals, however, and even without clinical signs of deficiency, riboflavin status can still be subnormal and may result in impaired function.[76,77]

Lacto-ovo vegetarians generally have little difficulty meeting the RDA for riboflavin (Appendix H). Far fewer studies have examined the riboflavin intake of vegans. Limited data suggest intake of this group is similar to or only slightly lower than that of lacto-ovo vegetarians and omnivores (Appendix H), and clinical signs of riboflavin deficiency have not been observed in vegan subjects.[78–81]

Riboflavin is stable to heat but not to sunlight (irradiation); exposure of milk to sunlight can result in the destruction of more than half the riboflavin content within just 1 day, so that most milk is now sold in opaque containers. Also, substantial amounts of riboflavin can be lost via the water used to boil vegetables. Riboflavin from plants appears to be somewhat less well absorbed than the riboflavin from animal products.

About half the riboflavin in whole grain rice, and more than a third of that of whole wheat, is lost when these grains are milled (riboflavin is located in the germ and the bran). When refined grains are enriched, the riboflavin content can be twice that of the whole grain. Enriched white rice does not contain riboflavin because the yellow tinge it provides is considered undesirable. Parboiled (converted) rice contains most of the riboflavin of the parent grain.

A varied vegan diet should provide adequate amounts of riboflavin (Table 6–2). Although whole grains are a relatively poor source of riboflavin, generous use of these foods can make a substantial contribution to riboflavin intake. In the United States, refined grains supply about 25% of the RDA.[82] Vegetables, such as broccoli and many leafy green vegetables, are reasonably good sources of riboflavin. Legumes provide moderate amounts of riboflavin, about 0.1 mg per cup. Soybeans are an excellent source, providing 0.49 mg of riboflavin per cup.

Table 6–2 Riboflavin Content of Foods

Food	Riboflavin Content (mg)	Food	Riboflavin Content (mg)
Bread, cereals, grains		Spinach	0.17
Pumpernickel bread,		Sweet potatoes	0.14
one slice	0.17	**Fruit**	
Bran flakes, 1 cup	0.60	Banana, one medium	0.11
Cheerios, 1¼ cup	0.42	**Legumes (½ cup cooked)**	
Corn flakes, 1¼ cup	0.40	Kidney beans	0.09
Granola, ¼ cup	0.42	Soybeans	0.24
Grapenuts, ¼ cup	0.42	Split peas	0.09
Nutrigrain, ¾ cup	0.40	**Soymilks/vegetable milks (1 cup)**	
Rice krispies, 1 cup	0.40	Edensoy	0.06
Wheaties, 1 cup	0.42	Edensoy Extra	0.10
Barley, whole, ½ cup	0.13	Soyagen	0.17
Pasta, enriched, ½ cup	0.18	Sno E	0.17
Pasta, whole wheat, ½ cup	0.03	Take Care	0.42
Vegetables (½ cup cooked)		Vitasoy Original	0.17
Asparagus	0.10	Westsoy Plus	0.42
Beet greens	0.21	Vegelicious	0.17
Collards	0.09	**Nuts/seeds (2 tbsp)**	
Mushrooms	0.14	Almonds	0.25
Peas	0.12	Almond butter	0.19
Sea vegetables		Peanuts	0.12
Alaria	2.73	**Animal products**	
Dulse	1.91	Egg, one large	0.25
Kelp	2.48	Milk, 1 cup	0.40
Nori (laver)	2.93	Yogurt, 1 cup	0.59

Source: Data from *Bowes & Church's Food Value of Portions Commonly Used.* 16th ed., by J. Pennington, Lippincott-Raven, 1994, and package information.

Sea vegetables are especially rich in this nutrient and can provide significant amounts of riboflavin in vegetarian diets. This can be especially important in the diets of macrobiotics, who make considerable use of these foods. Other vegetables, including asparagus, greens, mushrooms, and sweet potatoes, are good sources of riboflavin. Nutritional yeast that is grown on a riboflavin-rich medium contains more than twice the RDI for riboflavin in 1 tbsp. Many ready-to-eat cereals and many brands of soymilk are fortified with this nutrient, so that a meal of cereal with soymilk can provide between 33% and 150% of the RDI for riboflavin, depending on the brands used.

VITAMIN D

Although vitamin D is classified as a fat-soluble vitamin, it is not an essential nutrient. With sufficient exposure to sunlight, endogenous synthesis can adequately meet biologic requirements for vitamin D. There are many circumstances under which people do not make adequate vitamin D, however, in which case a dietary source becomes necessary.

In children, inadequate vitamin D leads to rickets, characterized by bowed legs, knock-knees, curvatures of the upper and/or lower arms, swollen joints, and/or enlarged heads. Rickets is associated with urbanization and industrialization and was the scourge of the cities in northern Europe and the United States until the early part of the 20th century. In fact, around the turn of the 19th century, estimates were that nearly 80% of the children in London had rickets, and for that reason rickets became known as the English disease. Rickets was also common in other European countries at this time. For example, in the Netherlands autopsies of young children revealed that 80% to 90% had residual evidence of rickets. Rickets was rare or nonexistent in southern Europe, however.

In adults, vitamin D deficiency leads to undermineralization of the bone matrix osteoid, which can result in excessive bone loss and osteomalacia. The symptoms of osteomalacia are typically more generalized than those of rickets and include muscular weakness and bone tenderness.

Cod liver oil was long used as an effective medicine to prevent rickets. It was not until the early part of the 20th century, however, that the antirachitic factor vitamin D was actually discovered. Soon thereafter, it was shown that skin is fully capable of making vitamin D upon exposure to ultraviolet light. As early as 1822, the importance of exposure to the outdoors and sunlight for the prevention and cure of rickets had been recognized by at least some of the clinical community.

The primary function associated with vitamin D is calcium regulation or homeostasis. Vitamin D stimulates the absorption of phosphorus and calcium (particularly at low levels of calcium intake), decreases urinary calcium excretion, and causes bone demineralization, thereby releasing calcium into the bloodstream. This last action is done in conjunction with parathyroid hormone. All three actions of vitamin D work to increase blood calcium levels.

It appears that physiologic effects of vitamin D are manifest in a wide range of tissues and organs, including the immune system, the skin, and the pancreas. In fact, there are more than 30 tissues that possess a nuclear receptor for 1,25-dihydroxyvitamin D.[83] Vitamin D may also have a role in cancer prevention and treatment.[84]

Vitamin D Requirements

In 1969, on the basis of observed vitamin D deficiency in seven patients, several of whom were vegetarians and consumed no natural sources of vitamin D, the daily requirement for vitamin D was estimated to be 2.5 μg.[85] The current RDA for adults is 5.0 μg. This is considered a generous amount, however, and it is readily acknowledged that because vitamin D is synthesized endogenously vitamin D dietary requirements are difficult to determine.[86] In the United States, the average daily vitamin D intake is between 1.25 and 1.75 μg, but nutritional osteomalacia is rare, presumably because of regular exposure to sunlight, at least during the summer months.[87]

Based on studies of vitamin D synthesis in infants, it is estimated that adults need 10 to 15 minutes of exposure to sunlight during the summer months on the hands and face two to three times per week to ensure adequate vitamin D levels.[88] Brief exposure to sunlight is thought to be the same as ingesting 5 μg of vitamin D.[89] Because so many factors affect vitamin D synthesis, however, it is unwise to depend entirely on endogenous synthesis to meet vitamin D requirements unless sun exposure is routine. Also, the elderly and dark-skinned people require longer sun exposure to meet vitamin D needs.

Unless vitamin D is regularly included in the diet, sufficient stores must be achieved during summertime sun exposure to last through the winter months. In fact, variation in circulating vitamin D levels is usually attributed to seasonal changes. In most people, even in the winter the concentration of vitamin D in the serum is not determined by current vitamin D intake but rather by the amount of exposure to solar radiation the previous summer.[90] Vitamin D levels tend to be lowest in the winter months. In one study of lacto vegetarians, for example, serum values of 25-hydroxyvitamin D_3 in January, March, May, and August were 10.1, 11.9, 18.0, and 27.9 μg/L, respectively (Figure 6–4).[91]

Factors Affecting Vitamin D Synthesis

Both season and latitude affect vitamin D synthesis. This was clearly illustrated by a study conducted in Boston, Massachusetts, that used foreskin

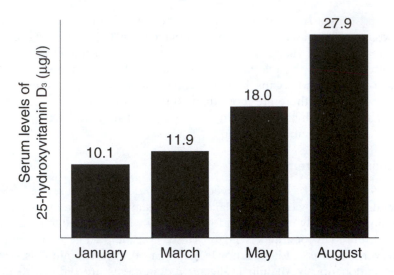

Figure 6–4 Effects of season on vitamin D levels in Finnish lacto vegetarians. Serum vitamin D (25-hydroxyvitamin D₃) values are for 17 lacto vegetarians who were not taking supplements. Values for May and August were significantly different ($P < 0.05$) from January and March. *Source:* Data from Kumpusalo E, Karinpää A, Jauhiainen M, Laitinen Lappeteläinen R, Mäenpää PH. Multivitamin supplementation of adult omnivores and lactovegetarians: Circulating levels of vitamin A, D, and E, lipids, apolipoproteins and selenium. *International Journal of Vitamin Nutrition Research.* 1989;60:58–66.

taken from circumcised infants to monitor vitamin D synthesis. When exposed to sunlight (cloudless days) for 3 hours 1 day per month, skin was able to synthesize vitamin D during the months of April through October but was unable to do so during the winter months of November and February.[92] Synthesis also took place during the months of November through March in Los Angeles and Puerto Rico but not in Edmonton, Canada, demonstrating the importance of latitude. This experiment utilized skin cultures to evaluate the ability of the skin to synthesize vitamin D; other observations suggest, however, that infants can synthesize vitamin D during the winter months.[93] Also, although in northern latitudes 25-hydroxyvitamin D₃ levels vary according to time of year, the active form of the vitamin, 1,25-dihydroxyvitamin D₃ does not.[94]

Vitamin D synthesis is poorer in dark skin.[95] Six times the amount of simulated solar irradiation was shown to be required in individuals with dark skin to raise serum levels of vitamin D₃ to the same extent as in light-skinned individuals.[95] Air pollution and sunscreen also block ultraviolet light and inhibit vitamin D synthesis. In fact, it has been shown that topical application of a sunscreen with a sun protection factor of 8 can completely block the photosynthesis of vitamin D in the skin.[96]

Vegetarians and Vitamin D

Vitamin D deficiency is rare in the general population. For example, of 100,000 pediatric admissions in the 266 teaching hospitals in the United States between 1956 and 1960, only 0.4% of cases were reported as being due to rickets. These results are consistent with two other large US surveys involving thousands of subjects, where it was found that between 0.1% and 0.2% of the children had signs of rickets. Similarly, in Oslo, Norway, no cases of rickets were reported in the pediatric departments between 1967 and 1974.[97] Vitamin D deficiency has been reported in vegetarians, however, particularly Asian vegetarians.[98-100] Lower circulating levels of vitamin D have also been seen in Asian vegetarians.[101-104] In some studies, though, dietary intake of vitamin D was actually higher than in omnivore populations, suggesting that problems with vitamin D nutriture were a result of inadequate sun exposure rather than a low level of vitamin D intake. The darker skin of Asians reduces their ability to synthesize vitamin D in comparison with light-skinned people. Consistent with this hypothesis, Henderson et al[104] found that the prevalence of rickets in Asians residing in England rose from south to north and that the incidence of rickets was inversely associated with daylight outdoor exposure.

Findings indicate that exposure to sunlight is the dominant factor affecting risk of rickets and that, in an environment where exposure is limited, dietary factors play a pivotal role. Dietary fiber may decrease vitamin D absorption[105] or increase its excretion.[106] This may be especially relevant for vegetarians when sun exposure is poor and vitamin D dietary intake is marginal, given their higher intake of fiber.

Vitamin D deficiency has also been reported in macrobiotic children in the United States. Vitamin D, calcium, and phosphorus intakes in macrobiotic preschoolers were marginal and were much less than those of other vegetarians.[107] Instances of rickets have also been reported in macrobiotics in other countries, such as England[108] and the Netherlands.[109] In the Netherlands study, between 25% and 50% of the infants examined showed signs of rickets. In addition to the low levels of vitamin D, low availability of calcium was an independent risk factor for rickets.[110] Over a 6-year period, several cases of rickets in vegetarians, thought to be due to low vitamin D intake, were identified in Norway.[97] The lower sunlight exposure in Norway may predispose to rickets. Vitamin D intake has been found to be lower in both vegans and lacto-ovo vegetarians than in omnivores (see Appendix I), although in several studies serum levels of vitamin D were similar among the groups.[12,91]

Vitamin D Fortification/Supplementation and Hypervitaminosis D

Because vitamin D is poorly supplied in foods, endogenous vitamin D synthesis may have met most or all of the vitamin D needs throughout history. Modern humans, however, have less sun exposure as a result of urbanization, smog, greater population density at northern latitudes, and less time spent outdoors. Thus a regular source of vitamin D in the diet is good insurance for all people. Except under ideal circumstances, endogenous synthesis by itself should not be viewed as an adequate means of meeting vitamin D needs. Because there are few natural food sources of vitamin D, fortified foods (Table 6–3) are nearly always relied upon to provide dietary vitamin D. Vitamin D is not present in any plant foods.

Fortification with vitamin D needs to be monitored because vitamin D is potentially toxic, especially in young children. The effects of excessive vitamin D, intake include hypercalcemia and hypercalciuria, which lead to the deposition of calcium in soft tissues and irreversible renal and cardiovascular damage. Elevated vitamin D levels have also been associated with bone resorption.[111] Vitamin D increases aluminum absorption, and excessive amounts of aluminum may be linked to Alzheimer's disease risk.[112,113]

Table 6–3 Vitamin D Content of Foods

Food	Vitamin D Content (μg)	Food	Vitamin D Content (μg)
Bread, cereals, grains		Take Care	2.5
Bran flakes, 1 cup	1.8	Vegelicious	1.0
Corn flakes, 1 cup	1.8	Vitamite*	2.5
Granola, ¼ cup	1.8	Westsoy Plus	2.5
Grapenuts, ¼ cup	2.4	**Animal products**	
Fortified soymilk or		Milk, 1 cup	2.5
vegetable milk (1 cup)		Egg, one large	0.7
Edensoy Extra	1.0	**Other**	
Rice Dream	2.5	Margarine, 1 tsp	0.5
Soyagen	2.5		

*Contains milk protein.
Source: Data from Bowes & Church's Food Value of Portions Commonly Used. 16th ed., by J. Pennington, Lippincott-Raven, 1994, and package information.

Although the toxic level of vitamin D has not been established for all age groups, consumption of as little as 45 µg of vitamin D[3] per day in young children has been associated with signs of hypervitaminosis D.[114] This is only four to five times the RDA and represents a narrow range of safety. Because of this and the evidence that sunlight-stimulated production of the vitamin is active throughout the warm months, dietary supplements should be used with caution, especially where children may already be consuming vitamin D–fortified cow's milk.

In the United States, milk has been fortified with vitamin D since the 1930s; according to federal regulations, it should contain 400 IU (10 µg) of vitamin D per quart.[115] Fortification was also common in Great Britain, but as a result of toxicity problems this practice has been halted.[116,117] Recently, in the United States hypervitaminosis D in eight individuals was linked to consumption of milk, which in some cases contained vitamin D at concentrations 500 times higher than regulations permit.[118] Because vitamin D is added to large volumes of milk at one time, there is some concern that it is not thoroughly mixed. As a result, vitamin D content of individual samples of milk can vary significantly. Prolonged exposure to sun will not result in vitamin D toxicity because the vitamin D is converted into two biologically inert and harmless isomers.[119]

Although fortified milk is traditionally viewed as the most important dietary source of vitamin D, a variety of foods are actually fortified with this vitamin. Many commercial cereals are good sources. Both soymilk and rice milk are also often fortified.

VITAMIN B[6]

Vitamin B[6] comprises three compounds—pyridoxol, pyridoxal, and pyridoxamine—all of which are converted to pyridoxal phosphate and pyridoxamine, the active forms of the vitamin. Vitamin B[6] functions as a coenzyme for more than 60 enzymes, most of which are involved in amino acid metabolism. It is not surprising that vitamin B[6] needs are closely linked to protein intake. Recommended intakes are 0.016 mg of vitamin B[6] per gram of protein consumed. The adult RDA of 1.6 mg for women and 2.0 mg for men assumes a protein intake of 100 g and 126 g for women and men, respectively. Average vitamin B[6] intake in the United States is actually a bit below the RDA, but protein intake appears to be slightly lower than assumed also.[71,72] Thus the ratio of vitamin B[6] to protein appears to be adequate, although a recent study indicated that this ratio may be a bit low.[120] In typical US diets, about 40% of vitamin B[6] comes from meat, poultry, and fish; about 23% comes from fruits and vegetables, and about 19% comes from grains.[121] Vitamin B[6] participates in the conversaion of homocysteine to cystathionine. Low serum levels of vitamin B6 have been associated with increased levels of homocysteine,[122] which increases heart disease risk. Vitamin B6 supplementation has been associated with protection against myocardial infarction.[123]

Vitamin B6 in Vegetarian Diets

Because vegetarians consume less total protein than omnivores, they need less vitamin B6. The ratio of vitamin B6 to protein in plant foods is actually superior to that in animal foods.[124] Consequently, vitamin B6 intake of vegetarians is likely to be appropriate to their needs. There has been some debate, however, over whether vitamin B6 needs are affected differently by plant and animal protein.

Some animal work has suggested that low-quality proteins increase vitamin B6 requirements, but other studies suggest that B6 from plant foods may meet needs more efficiently. One study found that in men vitamin B6 status correlated inversely with both total protein intake and animal protein intake but not with the intake of plant protein.[125] Consistent with this finding, a 1982 study reported that female subjects depleted of vitamin B6 required 25% more vitamin B6 to return B6 status to normal when protein from animal foods was consumed in comparison with plant proteins (2.0 mg versus 1.5 mg of vitamin B6).[126] Recent research from this same group of investigators indicated, however, that the amount of vitamin B6 required to replete vitamin B6–depleted women was the same whether they were fed a high–animal protein or a high–plant protein diet.[127] They did find, though, that the current RDA of 0.016 mg per gram of protein may not provide for an adequate margin of safety.

Although vegetarians, because of their lower protein intake, need less vitamin B6 than nonvegetarians, some concerns have been raised about the bioavailability of B6 from plant foods.[128,129] This is probably of little significance in the diets of vegetarians, however. Vitamin B6 in plant foods is most often in the form of glycosides. Although initial research suggested that this form is poorly absorbed,[129,130] more recent studies show that glycosylated vitamin B6 appears to be well absorbed.[131,132]

The high fiber content of plant foods may also be a factor in vitamin B6 bioavailability because this vitamin was shown to be more poorly absorbed from whole wheat bread than from white bread, although blood levels of vitamin B6 were not affected.[133] In one study, the addition of bran to diets did reduce the absorption of vitamin B6, but only by 17%.[134] Any adverse effect of fiber may be offset by the fact that fiber-rich foods tend also to be rich in vitamin B6, however. In most populations a high fiber intake does not seem to interfere with B6 status.[125,135]

Some concerns have been expressed about the effects of processing on vitamin B6 bioavailability. The vitamin can form complexes with amino acids during food processing, cooking, and digestion, which can reduce utilization. Vitamin B6 is stable under acidic conditions but not neutral or alkaline ones, particularly when exposed to heat or light. Of the several forms of the vitamin, however, the kind found most often found in plant foods (pyridoxine) is more stable than the forms found in animal foods.

Vitamin B6 in Vegetarians

Studies have generally shown that both intake of vitamin B6[77,125,135] and vitamin B6 status[15,125,135,136] of vegetarians are adequate and similar to nonvegetarians (Appendix H). One study did find that the vitamin B6 intake of elderly vegetarians (65 to 97 years old) was below recommended levels, but because of their relatively low protein intake, vitamin intake was thought to be adequate.[137] Similarly, a study of Seventh-day Adventist vegetarians revealed that the average vitamin B6 intake of both men and women was similar to that of nonvegetarians, although because of the lower protein intake of male vegetarians their ratio of vitamin B6 to protein was much better.[138] Not surprising, less information is available about the vitamin B6 intake of vegans. Vegan adults and children were both found to consume adequate amounts of vitamin B6, however, and given their lower protein intake they are actually likely to have a favorable ratio of vitamin B6 to protein.[78,81,139]

Vitamin B6 is well distributed among different groups of plant foods (Table 6–4). Good sources include many ready-to-eat cereals, potatoes, bananas, figs, chickpeas, soybeans, and brewer's yeast.

VITAMIN B1 (THIAMIN)

Thiamin, as thiamin pyrophosphate, is a coenzyme required for the metabolism of carbohydrates. Recommendations for thiamin intake are based largely on caloric intake. It is thought that 0.5 mg of thiamin per 1,000 kcal is adequate to meet the needs of the general healthy population, although an intake of at least 1.0 mg is recommended by the National Research Council even for individuals consuming less than 2,000 cal/day. For men between the ages of 19 and 50, the RDA is 1.5 mg, whereas for women the RDA is 1.1. mg. The RDA for older men and women (51 years and older) is 1.2 and 1.0 mg, respectively, reflecting their somewhat lower energy intake.

Thiamin is widely distributed in foods (Table 6–5), but most foods contain only low concentrations of this vitamin. Yeasts (eg, dried brewer's yeast and baker's yeast) are particularly good sources, but cereals represent the most

Table 6–4 Vitamin B₆ Content of Foods

Food	Vitamin B₆ Content (mg)	Food	Vitamin B₆ Content (mg)
Breads, cereals, grains		Figs, 10	0.42
Bran flakes, 1 cup	0.70	Orange juice, 1 cup	0.22
Cheerios, 1¼ cup	0.50	Prune juice, ½ cup	0.28
Corn flakes, 1¼ cup	0.50	Raisins, ⅔ cup	0.32
Cream of Wheat, instant,		Watermelon, 1 cup cubes	0.23
one packet	0.50	**Legumes (½ cup cooked)**	
Granola, ¼ cup	0.50	Chickpeas	0.57
Grapenuts, ¼ cup	0.50	Kidney beans	0.10
Oatmeal, instant, one packet	0.70	Lentils	0.17
Rice, brown ½ cup	0.15	Lima beans	0.11
Vegetables (½ cup cooked		Meat analogues, 3–4 oz	0.30–0.70
unless otherwise indicated)		Navy beans	0.15
Asparagus	0.12	Pinto beans	0.15
Avocado, ½ raw	0.24	Soybeans	0.20
Nori	0.16	Soynuts	0.19
Okra	0.15	Tempeh	0.25
Peas	0.17	Vegetarian baked beans	0.17
Plantains	0.18	**Soymilk**	
Potatoes	0.38	Soymilk, plain, 1 cup	0.12
Spinach	0.14	**Nuts/seeds**	
Sweet potato, one medium	0.28	Sunflower seeds, 2 tbsp	0.22
Tomato juice, 1 cup	0.26	**Animal products**	
Winter squash	0.14–0.20	Egg, one large	0.06
Fruits		**Other**	
Banana, one medium	0.66	Brewer's yeast, 1 tbsp	0.20
Elderberries, 1 cup	0.33		

Source: Data from *Bowes & Church's Food Value of Portions Commonly Used.* 16th ed., by J. Pennington, Lippincott-Raven, 1994.

important dietary sources of thiamin in most diets. In omnivore diets, about 42% of the thiamin comes from grains and about 24% from meat, fish, and poultry.[121]

Interestingly, there are a number of heat-stable thiamin antagonists in food, such as polyphenols (caffeic acid, chlorogenic acid, and tannic acid) and flavonoids (quercitin and rutin), that can inhibit thiamin absorption. Also, some foods, such as raw fish, tea, betel nuts, blueberries, and red cabbage, contain thiaminases, which are enzymes that can inactivate thiamin by altering its structure.[140] Excessive reliance on these foods could contribute to thiamin deficiency.[141]

The average daily thiamin intake of adult men and women in the United States is reported to be 1.75 mg (0.68 mg/1,000 kcal)[71] and 1.05 mg (0.69

Table 6–5 Thiamin Content of Foods

Food	Thiamin Content (mg)	Food	Thiamin Content (mg)
Breads, cereals, grains		Winter squash	0.17
Bagel, one whole	0.21	**Fruit**	
Corn bread, one 2-oz piece	0.10	Figs, 10	0.13
English muffin, one whole	0.26	Orange, one medium	0.12
Pita bread, one 6-inch pocket	0.18	Orange juice, 1 cup	0.20
Rye bread, one slice	0.10	Pineapple, 1 cup chunks	0.14
White bread, one slice	0.11	Watermelon, 1 cup cubes	0.13
Whole wheat bread, one slice	0.09	**Legumes (½ cup cooked)**	
Bran flakes, 1 cup	0.50	Kidney beans	0.14
Cheerios, 1¼ cups	0.37	Lentils	0.16
Cream of Wheat, ½ cup	0.12	Lima beans	0.15
Grapenuts, ¼ cup	0.37	Navy beans	0.13
Grits, enriched, ½ cup	0.12	Pinto beans	0.15
Instant oatmeal, 1 packet	0.53	Soybeans	0.13
Oatmeal, regular ⅔ cup	0.19	Soymilk	0.15
Barley, whole, ½ cup	0.29	Split peas	0.15
Millet, ½ cup	0.13	**Nuts/seeds (2 tbsp)**	
Pasta, enriched, ½ cup	0.10	Brazil nuts	0.23
Pasta, whole wheat, ½ cup	0.07	Peanuts	0.28
Rice, brown, ½ cup	0.10	Sunflower seeds	0.40
Rice, white, ½ cup	0.17	Tahini	0.40
Wheat germ, 2 tbsp	0.24	**Other**	
Vegetables (½ cup cooked)		Brewer's yeast, 1 tbsp	1.25
Peas	0.20	Nutritional yeast, 1 tbsp	5.0
Potatoes	0.13		

Source: Data from *Bowes & Church's Food Value of Portions Commonly Used.* 16th ed., by J. Pennington, Lippincott-Raven, 1994.

mg/1,000 kcal), respectively.[72] The intake of thiamin has increased fairly substantially (by about 25%) since the early part of this century, despite a decrease in grain consumption, because of enrichment of refined flours and cereals. With few exceptions, studies indicate that vegetarians consume adequate thiamin and that their thiamin status is good.[12,13] This applies to adult vegans as well as to young vegetarian children (Appendix H).[140,142,143]

NIACIN

Niacin functions as part of the coenzymes nicotinamide adenine dinucleotide (NAD) and nicotinamide adenine dinucleotide phosphate (NADP), which are used in many metabolic reactions, including the metabolism of glucose and fatty acids and in tissue respiration. Pellagra is the deficiency disease most closely associated with niacin; its symptoms include dermatitis, diarrhea, and dementia. Often, pellagra occurs in individuals suffering from a deficiency of several B vitamins.

Niacin is somewhat different from the other vitamins in that a substantial part of the daily requirement is met by consumption of the amino acid tryptophan. Sixty milligrams of tryptophan yields 1 mg of niacin, which is quite significant considering that adults consume approximately 50 to 100 g of protein per day and approximately 1% of that is tryptophan (500 to 1,000 mg; animal products are somewhat higher and plant products somewhat lower). For this reason, the RDA is actually expressed as niacin equivalents (NEs); for adult men and women the RDA is 19 and 15 mg NE, respectively. One NE is equal to 1 mg of niacin or 60 mg of tryptophan. In the United States, niacin intake (including both tryptophan and preformed niacin) is about 42 mg NE for men and 28 mg NE for women.

Niacin in grains is poorly absorbed because it is present in covalently bound complexes with small peptides and carbohydrates.[144] Diets based on corn, in particular, can be problematic because the niacin in corn is largely unavailable for absorption and because corn is low in tryptophan. A common practice in Latin American cultures, however, where corn products are frequently consumed, is to soak corn in lime-treated water (specifically for preparation of corn tortillas), which makes the niacin available for absorption and also greatly increases the calcium content.[145] Also, synthetic niacin added to refined grains is well absorbed.

In the United States, meat, fish, and poultry supply the largest amount of preformed niacin (about 44%), whereas grains supply about 25% to 40%.[121] Both vegan and lacto-ovo vegetarian niacin intake is adequate (Table 6–6 and Appendix G).

FOLATE

Folate functions in the body as a coenzyme that participates in the transfer of single carbon fragments. This function is particularly important in the metabolism of amino acids and in the synthesis of nucleic acids. In prolonged deficiency, the impaired DNA synthesis will result in macrocytic anemia. Folate and vitamin B_{12} function together in the synthesis of DNA. As discussed previously, large amounts of folate replace the need for vitamin B_{12} in the synthesis of nucleic acids and thereby prevent vitamin B_{12} deficiency anemia. Nevertheless, folate cannot substitute for vitamin B_{12} in its role in the nervous system. More recent research has focused on the role of folate in preventing neural tube defects and in maintaining normal levels of

Table 6–6 Niacin Content of Foods

Food	Niacin Content (mg)	Food	Niacin Content (mg)
Breads, cereals, grains		Rice, brown, ½ cup cooked	1.3
Bran flakes, fortified, 1 cup	5.0	Rice, white, ½ cup cooked	1.8
Cheerios, 1¼ cup	5.0	**Vegetables (½ cup cooked**	
Corn flakes, 1 cup	5.0	**unless otherwise indicated)**	
Granola, ¼ cup	4.9	Avocado, ½ raw	1.6
Grapenuts, ¼ cup	4.9	Corn	1.0
Rice Krispies, 1 cup	5.0	Mushrooms	2.1
Shredded wheat, one		Peas	1.6
biscuit	1.1	Potatoes	1.7
Bread, white, one slice	0.9	**Nuts/seeds (2 tbsp)**	
Bread, whole wheat, one		Peanuts	3.3
slice	1.0	Peanut butter	4.6
Corn tortillas (enriched),		Tahini	1.5
one	1.5	**Legumes**	
Barley, pearled, ½ cup	1.6	Soybeans, green,	
Barley, whole, ½ cup	2.1	immature, ½ cup	1.1
Bulgur, ½ cup	1.6	Tempeh, ½ cup	3.8
Millet, ½ cup	1.5	**Other**	
Pasta, whole wheat, ½ cup	0.5	Brewer's yeast, 1 tbsp	2.9

Source: Data from *Bowes & Church's Food Value of Portions Commonly Used.* 16th ed., by J. Pennington, Lippincott-Raven, 1994.

---

homocysteine. Increased homocysteine levels are an independent risk factor for heart disease.

Folate is widely distributed in foods (Table 6–7). There are methodologic problems with accurately determining folate, and current food values may actually underestimate folate content.[146] Much of the folate in foods, however, may be destroyed during household preparation, food processing, and storage. Average daily intakes for men and women in the United States are reported to be 305 µg and 189 µg, respectively.[71,147] Reported intakes of folate and the lack of apparent folate deficiency were used as a partial basis for decreasing the folate RDA from the 1980 value of 400 µg to the current value of 200 µg for men and 180 µg for women.

Folate absorption varies significantly, although it appears to be somewhat better absorbed from animal foods than plant foods. Adequate iron and vitamin C status is necessary for proper folate absorption. In general, folate intakes and folate status of vegetarians are equal to or superior to those of

Table 6–7 Folate Content of Foods

Food	Folate Content (µg)	Food	Folate Content (µg)
Breads, cereals, grains		Turnip greens	32
Bran flakes, ¾ cup	100	Tomato juice, 1 cup	47
Corn flakes, 1¼ cup	100	**Fruits**	
Granola, ¼ cup	99	Banana, one medium	21
Most, ⅔ cup	400	Cantaloupe, 1 cup chunks	27
Nutrigrain, ¾ cup	100	Grapefruit, ½ pink or red	15
Oatmeal, instant, one package	150	Orange juice, 1 cup	109
Oatmeal, quick or regular,		Orange, one medium	39
⅔ cup cooked	29	Strawberries, ½ cup sliced	20
Rice Krispies, 1 cup	100	**Legumes (½ cup cooked)**	
Wheat germ, 2 tbsp	49	Black beans	128
Vegetables (½ cup cooked		Black-eyed peas	86
unless otherwise indicated)		Kidney beans	63
Acorn squash	11	Lentils	179
Asparagus	88	Lima beans	78
Avocado, ½ raw	56	Pinto beans	147
Beets	45	Soybeans	46
Broccoli	38	Split peas	64
Brussels sprouts	46	Tempeh	43
Cauliflower	32	**Nuts/seeds (2 tbsp)**	
Collards	64	Peanuts	35
Endive, ½ cup raw	36	Peanut butter	25
Mustard greens	51	Sunflower seeds	40
Parsnips	45	Tahini	27
Spinach	110	**Animal products**	
Sweet potato	25	Yogurt, 1 cup	27

Source: Data from *Bowes & Church's Food Value of Portions Commonly Used.* 16th ed., by J. Pennington, Lippincott-Raven, 1994.

nonvegetarians. Adult lacto-ovo vegetarians and vegans typically consume 25% to 50% more folate than omnivores (see Appendix H).

BIOTIN

Although biotin is an essential nutrient, there is no established RDA. The estimated safe and adequate daily dietary intake is 30 to 100 µg. Biotin can be synthesized in the large intestine, although the amount of this biotin that is absorbed is uncertain. Biotin serves as a coenzyme for enzymes involved in the synthesis of glucose and fatty acids and the metabolism of amino acids. Symptoms of biotin deficiency, which occurs only rarely in humans, include anorexia, nausea, vomiting, glossitis, and mental depression, among others. One way of producing biotin deficiency is by ingesting avidin, which is a biotin binding protein found only in raw egg white.[148]

There is relatively little information about biotin with respect to dietary intake in either vegetarians or nonvegetarians. One study of Seventh-day Adventists found that vegetarians had higher plasma blood levels of biotin than nonvegetarians and that vegans had higher levels than lacto-ovo vegetarians.[149] Good sources of this vitamin include egg yolk, soy flour, and cereals, but there is as much as a 10-fold variation in the amount of biotin found in different cereals. Fruit and meat are poor sources. Brewer's yeast is rich in biotin (Table 6–8).

The bioavailability of biotin is an area that needs additional research. Some reports suggest, for example, that on average about 50% of the biotin is available for absorption. The biotin in corn is completely available, whereas only 20% to 30% in most other grains is available, and none in wheat is available.

PANTOTHENIC ACID

Pantothenic acid is widely distributed in nature and is abundant in many foods. Some synthesis by intestinal bacteria may also occur. Pantothenic acid plays a role as a coenzyme in the release of energy from carbohydrates, in the synthesis of glucose, and in the synthesis and degradation of fatty acids; it has many other functions as well. The estimated safe and adequate daily dietary intake is 4 to 7 mg.

Table 6–8 Biotin Content of Foods

Food	Biotin Content (µg)	Food	Biotin Content (µg)
Breads, cereals, grains		**Legumes (½ cup cooked)**	
Oat bran, ½ cup cooked	7.0	Black-eyed peas	10.7
Oatmeal, instant, one packet	7.0	Lentils	13.0
Barley, pearled, ½ cup		Textured vegetable protein	17.5
cooked	3.0	**Nuts/seeds (2 tbsp)**	
Vegetables (½ cup cooked)		Almonds	23.0
Corn	4.9	Peanut butter	12.8
Mushrooms	7.6	**Animal products**	
Spinach	7.2	Egg, one medium	11.0

Source: Data from *Bowes & Church's Food Value of Portions Commonly Used.* 16th ed., by J. Pennington, Lippincott-Raven, 1994.

Not surprising, because pantothenic acid is so widely distributed in food, deficiencies in free-living populations have not been reliably documented. The average intake in the United States is reported to be around 6 mg/day, which appears to be quite adequate.[150,151] Because plant foods are rich in this vitamin, vegetarians should have no problem meeting requirements for pantothenic acid. In one study, however, lacto vegetarians consumed only about 4 mg of pantothenic acid per day, slightly less than the suggested intake. Conversely, vegans consumed more than 5 mg/day, slightly more than the omnivores in that study.[81]

VITAMIN C (ASCORBIC ACID)

Dietary deficiency of vitamin C leads to scurvy, a serious disorder that is characterized by weakening of collagen. Vitamin C has many diverse functions in the body, some of which are only partly understood. It is used as a cosubstrate for the formation of collagen, but it also appears to be involved in reactions affecting the immune system. Although the value of vitamin C against the common cold is still under debate, a recent review of more than 21 studies conducted since 1971 found that, even though vitamin C does not decrease the incidence of the common cold, it does appear to reduce the duration of episodes and the severity of the symptoms by an average of 23%.[152]

Vegetables and fruits, such as green peppers, broccoli, tomatoes, and oranges, contain high concentrations of vitamin C (Table 6-9). Grains, meat (except for organ meats and meats processed with sodium ascorbate), fish, poultry, and dairy products, however, contain essentially none. A recent survey found that 38% of the vitamin C in the diets of Americans was provided by citrus fruits, 16% by potatoes, and 32% from other vegetable sources.[153] The average vitamin C intake is reported to be around 100 mg/day, which is well above the RDA of 60 mg for adults.[71] Vegetarians consume more than this, generally around 150 mg/day, although findings vary. Most studies show vitamin C intake among vegetarians to be higher than among omnivores and vegan intake to be higher than that of lacto-ovo vegetarians (Appendix H).

VITAMIN A

Night blindness, as well as several other eye ailments, were treated by the ancient Egyptians with the topical application of juice squeezed from cooked liver or by prescribing liver in the diet, illustrating an early use of vitamin A long before the actual vitamin was identified.[154]

Preformed vitamin A is found only in animal products. Vitamin A can be synthesized from the provitamin carotenoids, however, which are widely distributed in many fruits and vegetables (Table 6–10). There are as many as

Table 6–9 Vitamin C Content of Foods

Food	Vitamin C Content (mg)	Food	Vitamin C Content (mg)
Breads, cereals, grains		Watermelon, 1 cup chunks	15
Cheerios, 1¼ cup	15	**Vegetables (½ cup cooked**	
Corn flakes, 1 cup	15	**unless otherwise indicated)**	
Most, ⅔ cup	60	Acorn squash	11
Nutrigrain, ¾ cup	15	Asparagus	24
Rice Krispies, 1 cup	15	Beet greens	18
Special K, 1⅓ cups	15	Broccoli	58
Wheaties, 1 cup	15	Brussels sprouts	48
Fruits		Butternut squash	15
Banana, one medium	10	Cabbage	17
Blackberries, ½ cup	15	Cauliflower	36
Blueberries, ½ cup	19	Collards	22
Cantaloupe, 1 cup chunks	68	Hubbard squash	10
Elderberries, ½ cup	26	Kale	27
Grapefruit, ½ medium	47	Kohlrabi	44
Grapefruit juice, 6 oz	70	Mustard greens	18
Guava, one medium	165	Okra	13
Honeydew melon,		Nori	39
1 cup chunks	92	Parsnips	10
Kiwi, one medium	75	Peas	11
Lychees, 10 medium	72	Pepper (sweet bell)	76
Mano, one medium	57	Potatoes	16
Orange, one medium	69	Rutabaga	19
Orange juice, 6 oz	62	Spinach	12
Papaya, one medium	188	Sweet potato	28
Persimmon, one medium	17	Swiss chard	15
Pineapple, 1 cup chunks	24	Tomato, one medium	22
Raspberries, ½ cup	15	Tomato juice, 6 oz	30
Strawberries, ½ cup sliced	42	Turnips	9
Tangerine, one medium	26	Turnip greens	17

Source: Data from *Bowes & Church's Food Value of Portions Commonly Used.* 16th ed., by J. Pennington, Lippincott-Raven, 1994.

600 carotenoids in nature, and about 50 of these can be converted into vitamin A. The best known and most active is β-carotene.[155] The carotenoids are yellow-orange pigments, but the color of fruits and vegetables is not necessarily an indicator of the concentration of provitamin A.

Vitamin A refers to a group of compounds—retinol, retinaldehyde, and retinoic acid—that are essential for vision, growth, cellular differentiation and proliferation, reproduction, and the integrity of the immune system. Although rare in the United States, vitamin A deficiency is a major nutritional problem in some parts of the world, causing a number of the more than

Table 6–10 Vitamin A Content of Foods

Food	Vitamin A Content (µg)	Food	Vitamin A Content (µg)
Vegetables (½ cup cooked unless otherwise indicated)		Tomato, one medium	1399
		Tomato juice, 6 oz	101
Beet greens	367	Tomato puree, ½ cup	170
Broccoli	110	Turnips	396
Bok choy	218	Vegetable juice cocktail, 6 oz	213
Butternut squash	714	**Fruits**	
Carrots, one raw	2025	Apricots, three raw	277
½ cup cooked	1915	Cantaloupe, 1 cup chunks	516
Chicory greens, ½ cup raw	360	Mango, one medium	806
Collards	422	Nectarine, one medium	100
Dandelion greens	608	Papaya, one medium	612
Hubbard squash	616	Persimmon, one medium	364
Kale	481	Plantain, 1 cup cooked	140
Mustard greens	212	Prunes, 10 medium	167
Pumpkin	2691	**Animal products**	
Nori	520	Milk	
Spinach	737	Skim, 1 cup	149
Sweet potato	2797	Whole, 1 cup	76
Swiss chard	276	Cheese, cheddar, 1 oz	86

Source: Data from Bowes & Church's Food Value of Portions Commonly Used. 16th ed., by J. Pennington, Lippincott-Raven, 1994.

500,000 new cases of active corneal lesions that occur annually in children.[156] Vitamin A deficiency is found most commonly in children under the age of 5 years. More recently, much research has also focused on the possible role that vitamin A and the retinoids (synthetic compounds related to retinol) have in cancer prevention and treatment.

The RDA for vitamin A is expressed as micrograms of retinol equivalents (REs). Men and women need 1,000 and 800 µg of RE per day, respectively. This is a bit confusing because the older terminology for vitamin A was in international units and because the provitamin A activity of the carotenoids has to be converted into REs. These relationships are expressed as follows:

$$1 \text{ RE} = 1 \text{ µg of all-}trans \text{ retinol}$$
$$6 \text{ µg of all-}trans \text{ β-carotene}$$
$$12 \text{ µg of other provitamin A carotenoids}$$
$$1 \text{ IU} = 0.30 \text{ µg of all-}trans \text{ retinol or } 0.60 \text{ µg of all-}trans \text{ β-carotene}$$
$$1 \text{ RE} = 3.3 \text{ IU (if vitamin A from animal sources [retinol])}$$
$$10 \text{ IU (if vitamin A from plants [β-carotene])}$$

About one third of the β-carotene in foods is absorbed, and only about half that is actually converted into retinol. The other provitamin A carotenoids are only about half as active as β-carotene. The international unit measures of vitamin A did not consider absorption rates.

One cautionary note about the relationship between the β-carotene content of vegetables and vitamin A status warrants mention. A recent study found that, although a β-carotene–enriched wafer when fed to women markedly improved serum retinol levels, a similar amount of β-carotene when fed in the form of green leafy vegetables had no effect.[157] The authors speculated that the β-carotene in some vegetables and perhaps fruits is not readily available for absorption.

In the United States, approximately 75% of REs are derived from preformed vitamin A and about 25% from provitamin A carotenoids.[158] In lacto-ovo vegetarians, this ratio decreases; for example, among Hindu vegetarians approximately 50% comes from carotene and 50% from retinol.[159] In vegans, all the vitamin A comes from carotenoids. Not surprising, carotenoid intake[160,161] and serum carotenoid levels are about twice as high in vegetarians as in nonvegetarians.[12,136,162,163] Most studies, but not all, indicate that the intake of total milligrams of REs is also higher in vegetarians. Thus vegetarians have no trouble meeting vitamin A needs by consuming plant foods. Also, vegetarians may have some advantage in their higher consumption of carotenoids.

Many of the carotenoids, such as β-carotene and lycopene, are excellent antioxidants. Retinol, or preformed vitamin A, has no antioxidant activity.[164,165] Carotenoids may reduce cancer risk,[166] help prevent the development of cataracts,[167] and inhibit the oxidation of lipoproteins, thereby reducing heart disease risk.[168] There also appear to be potentially important synergistic effects between β-carotene and vitamin E.[169] Finally, even in vitamin A–sufficient animals, carotenoids, both with and without provitamin A activity, enhance the immune system.[170] Consequently, there seems to be considerable advantage to meeting vitamin A needs via the carotenoids.

Although vitamin A is toxic in large amounts, the carotenoids are not.[171] For acute toxicity to occur, however, vitamin A consumption must be at least 100 times the RDA or 10 times the RDA over a period of many weeks.[172] There is a benign condition called hypercarotenosis, characterized by a jaundicelike yellowing of the skin and high plasma carotenoid concentrations, that can occur when large amounts of carotene-rich foods are ingested.[173] This condition, however, which is harmless, is most likely to occur only when juices made from carotenoid-rich foods or dietary supplements are consumed.

VITAMIN E

Vitamin E was not recognized formally by the National Research Council as an essential nutrient until 1968. Vitamin E deficiency tends to occur in only two situations: in premature, very low–birthweight infants or in individuals who do not absorb fat normally. In adults, it may take 5 to 10 years of malabsorption for deficiency symptoms, which are primarily neurologic, to appear.

The RDA for vitamin E is expressed in terms of milligrams of α-tocopherol equivalents (TEs). Adult men and women need 10 and 8 mg of TEs per day, respectively. There are two main forms of vitamin E found in foods: tocopherol and tocotrienols. Within each main group there are four members, each with differing amounts of vitamin E activity. The most active form of vitamin E is alpha tocopherol; this is the form against which all other forms are measured.[139] The relative vitamin E activity for the main forms of vitamin E are:

α-tocopherol = 100%
β-tocopherol = 25–50%
γ-tocopherol = 10–35%
α-tocotrienol = 30%

Estimates of total alpha-TE activity of mixed diets can be calculated by multiplying milligrams of β-tocopherol by 0.5, milligrams of γ-tocopherol by 0.1, and milligrams of α-tocotrienols by 0.3. A number of different forms of α-tocopherol are found in chemically synthesized vitamins that do not occur naturally in foods. The chemically synthesized form has 74% the vitamin activity of natural α-tocopherol.

The primary and best understood function of vitamin E is as an antioxidant. Vitamin E is found in cellular membranes in association with polyunsaturated fatty acids (PUFAs). Vitamin E traps free radicals, thereby preventing the oxidation of PUFAs, which are susceptible to oxidation. Increased amounts of free radicals are associated with many diseases, most notably heart disease and cancer but also cataracts and arthritis; they may even hasten the aging process.[174] One symptom of a lack of vitamin E is the hemolysis of erythrocytes: The membranes of red blood cells become more fragile without the protection of vitamin E.

Recently, two studies involving more than 87,000 female and about 40,000 male health professionals[175,176] found that people who consumed the largest amounts of vitamin E had about a 33% reduced risk of coronary heart disease. Vitamin E is thought to exert this protective effect by inhibiting low-density lipoprotein cholesterol oxidation. Because vitamin E protects PUFAs from oxidation, the biologic requirements for vitamin E are based on the relative amount of dietary PUFA consumed. It is thought that 0.4 mg of RRR-α-tocopherol is needed for every gram of PUFA consumed.[177] In extreme situations, the need for α-tocopherol may vary by as much as a factor of 4 depending on the type of diet consumed. Not surprising, vegetarians tend to consume more polyunsaturated fat than saturated fat. But their absolute intake of PUFA in many studies is similar to omnivores due to their overall lower fat intake (Appendix A). In other studies, however, PUFA intake is as much as 50% higher than nonvegetarians.

The US population consumes 7.4 mg of TE/day, less than the RDA.[178] Most studies show that vegetarians consume about 50% to 100% more vitamin E than omnivores (Appendix H). Therefore, although vegetarians may need more vitamin E because of their higher PUFA intake, in most instances, the vitamin E to PUFA dietary intake ratio is higher among vegetarians than nonvegetarians, providing greater protection against the potentially harmful effects of free radicals.

Foods that are high in PUFA are also high in vitamin E. Thus vegetable oils are rich sources, but many oils, such as soybean oil, corn oil, and rapeseed oil, have excessive amounts of PUFAs relative to their vitamin E content.[179] On the basis of ratios of vitamin E to PUFA, olive oil and sunflower oil are good sources of vitamin E, whereas soybean oil, corn oil, and rapeseed oil are not. Some vegetables are also rich in vitamin E. One sweet potato contains 5.0 mg of vitamin E, and 1/2 cup of cabbage, spinach, turnip greens, or parsnips contains about 0.5 mg (Table 6–11).

Because of their higher vitamin E intake and lower serum cholesterol levels, most studies, but not all, indicate that vegetarians have higher serum ratios of vitamin E to cholesterol,[91,163,180–182] suggesting that their low-density lipoprotein cholesterol will be more resistant to oxidation. Vitamin C levels are also higher in vegetarians, and vitamin C, vitamin E, and perhaps β-carotene may work together to inhibit oxidation. Although all the fat-soluble vitamins can cause toxic effects when consumed in excessive amounts, vitamin E is relatively nontoxic even when consumed at levels more than 50 times the RDA.[183]

VITAMIN K

Compounds with vitamin K activity are essential for the formation of prothrombin and at least five other proteins involved in the regulation of blood clotting. Vitamin K deficiency results in defective coagulation. Vitamin K is also required for the synthesis of other proteins found in plasma, bone, and kidney. There are two different forms of vitamin K: phyloquinone (vitamin K_1), which is the only form found in plants, and menaquinone (vitamin K_2), which is made by bacteria. Animal foods contain both types of vitamin K.

Table 6–11 Vitamin E Content of Foods

Food	Vitamin E Content (mg)	Food	Vitamin E Content (mg)
Breads, cereals, grains		**Nuts/seeds (2 tbsp)**	
Wheat germ, 2 tbsp	1.9	Almond butter	2.9
Vegetables (½ cup cooked		Almonds	1.5
unless otherwise indicated)		Brazil nuts	2.1
Avocado, ½ raw	1.8	Hazelnuts	6.7
Asparagus	1.7	Peanuts	2.1
Cabbage	1.2	Peanut butter	6.0
Kohlrabi	1.3	Sunflower seeds	8.9
Mustard greens	1.4	**Vegetable oils (1 tbsp)**	
Parsnips	0.8	Corn oil	1.9
Pumpkin	1.2	Olive oil	1.6
Kelp	0.9	Peanut oil	1.6
Sweet potato	5.2	Safflower oil	4.6
Swiss chard	1.3	Sesame oil	0.2
Stewed tomatoes	0.9	Soybean oil	1.5
Fruits		Sunflower oil	6.1
Apple	0.8	Wheat germ oil	20.3
Mango	2.3	Mayonnaise	3.0–11.0
Pear	0.8		(varies by brand)
Pomegranate	0.8	Margarine, 1 tsp	0.1–8.0
Legumes			(varies by brand)
Soybeans, ½ cup	1.6		

Source: Data from *Bowes & Church's Food Value of Portions Commonly Used.* 16th ed., by J. Pennington, Lippincott-Raven, 1994.

Although stores of vitamin K are relatively small, vitamin K deficiency in adults is rare for at least three reasons. First, vitamin K is widely distributed in plants and animals. Second, the body tends to conserve this vitamin. Third, human colon bacteria synthesize significant quantities of vitamin K, although the extent to which bacterial synthesis contributes to vitamin K nutriture is unclear. Some reports suggest that it plays a key role,[184] whereas others suggest only a minor role, if any.[185]

For these reasons, only adults treated chronically with broad-spectrum antibiotics (which reduces bacterial synthesis of vitamin K) or people who suffer from malabsorption are at risk of vitamin K deficiency. Many older hospitalized patients do have low blood levels of vitamin K and do respond to vitamin K administration.[186] These findings in the elderly may be particularly important because new insight into the biologic functions of vitamin K suggest that it may have an important role in bone health. Recent research, for example, has shown that elderly women with hip fractures have much lower serum levels of vitamin K than elderly women without hip fracture.[187] Impaired synthesis of some vitamin K-dependent proteins, some of which may be required for optimal bone health, may be far more prevalent in the human population than coagulation assays alone indicate.[188]

Although outright vitamin K deficiency is rare in adults, vitamin K deficiency in breastfed newborn infants remains a major worldwide cause of infant morbidity and mortality.[189] In the United States, injections of vitamin K for newborn infants are standard procedure.

The RDA for adult men and women is 80 and 65 µg, respectively. The average daily vitamin K intake of adults in the United States has been estimated to be 300 to 500 µg, quite a bit above the RDA, but more recent data suggest that is an overestimate.[190] Until recently, there were few reliable data on the vitamin K content of foods, but the US Department of Agriculture recently released a provisional table on the vitamin K content of foods. It is clear from this table that green leafy vegetables are the major source of vitamin K and that animal products, fruits, and grains are extremely poor sources (Table 6–12). For example, just one serving of kale provides more than five times the RDA for vitamin K.[191] Soybean oil is another good source of vitamin K; 1 tbsp provides about a third of the RDA. Vegetarians should easily be able to meet their vitamin K needs; very limited data suggest this is the case.[192]

Vitamin K is generally not toxic. Even large amounts ingested over an extended period of time do not produce any overt signs of toxicity.[193] Ad-

Table 6–12 Vitamin K Content of Foods

Food	Vitamin K Content (mg)	Food	Vitamin K Content (mg)
Vegetables (½ cup cooked)		**Legumes (½ cup cooked)**	
Asparagus	35	Black-eyed peas	23
Broccoli	119	Lentils	261
Cabbage	90	Split peas	81
Kale	179	**Animal products**	
Lettuce, 1 cup raw	56	Milk, 1 cup	10
Pumpkin	18	Egg, one large	25
Spinach	141	**Vegetable oil**	
Turnip greens	53	Soybean oil, 1 tbsp	77

Source: Data from US Department of Agriculture, provisional table on the vitamin K content of foods. Hyattsville, Md: US Department of Agriculture, 1994.

ministration of the synthetic vitamin K menadione can be toxic, however.[193] Also, the vitamin K status of patients receiving anticoagulant drugs (which inhibit the clotting action of vitamin K) should be carefully monitored.

REFERENCES

1. Herbert V, Drivas G, Manusselis C, Mackler B, Eng J, Schwartz E. Are colon bacteria a major source of cobalamin analogues in human tissues? 24 hr human stool contains only about 5 µg of cobalamin but about 100 µg of apparent analogue (and 200 µg of folate). *Trans Assoc Am Physicians*. 1984;97:382. Letter.

2. Cooper B, Rosenblatt D. Inherited defects of vitamin B_{12} metabolism. *Annu Rev Nutr*. 1987;7:291–320.

3. Herbert V. Recommended dietary intakes (RDA) of vitamin B_{12} in humans. *Am J Clin Nutr*. 1987;45:671–678.

4. Allen RH, Stabler SP, Savage DG, Lindenbaum J. Metabolic abnormalities in cobalamin (vitamin B_{12}) and folate deficiency. *FASEB J*. 1993;7:1344–1353.

5. Herbert V. The 1986 Herman Award Lecture. Nutrition science as a continuing unfolding story, the folate and vitamin B_{12} paradigm. *Am J Clin Nutr*. 1987;46:387–402.

6. Herbert V, Colman N, Palat D, et al. Is there a "gold standard" for human serum vitamin B_{12} assay? *J Lab Clin Med*. 1984;104:829–841.

7. Herzlich B, Herbert V. Depletion of serum holotranscobalamin II: An early sign of negative vitamin B_{12} balance. *Lab Invest*. 1988;58:332–337.

8. Norman EJ. Detection of cobalamin deficiency using the urinary methylmalonic acid test by gas chromatography mass spectrometry. *J Clin Pathol*. 1992;45:382.

9. Herbert V. Vitamin B_{12}. In: Brown ML, ed. *Present Knowledge in Nutrition*. 5th ed. Washington, DC: Nutrition Foundation; 1984:347–364.

10. Sanders TAB, Ellis FR, Dickerson JWT. Haematological studies on vegans. *Br J Nutr*. 1978;40:9–15.

11. Bar-Sella P, Rakover Y, Ratner D. Vitamin B_{12} and folate levels in long-term vegans. *Isr J Med Sci*. 1990;26:309–312.

12. Ellis FR, Montegriffo VME. Veganism, clinical findings and investigations. *Am J Clin Nutr*. 1970;23:249–255.

13. Dong A, Scott SC. Serum vitamin B_{12} and blood cell values in vegetarians. *Ann Nutr Metab*. 1982;26:209–216.

14. Millet P, Guilland JC, Fuchs F, Klepping J. Nutrient intake and vitamin status of healthy French vegetarians and nonvegetarians. *Am J Clin Nutr*. 1989;50:718–727.

15. Helman AD, Darnton-Hill I. Vitamin and iron status in new vegetarians. *Am J Clin Nutr*. 1987;45:785–789.

16. Areekul S, Churdchu K, Pungpapong V. Serum folate, vitamin B_{12} and vitamin B_{12} binding protein in vegetarians. *J Med Assoc Thai*. (May 1988):253–257.

17. Mehta BM, Rege DV, Satoskar RS. Serum vitamin B_{12}, and folic acid activity in lactovegetarians and nonvegetarian healthy adult Indians. *Am J Clin Nutr*. 1964;15:77–84.

18. Miller DR, Specker BL, Ho ML, Norman EJ. Vitamin B_{12} status in a macrobiotic community. *Am J Clin Nutr*. 1991;53:524–529.

19. Specker BL, Miller D, Norman EJ, Greene H, Hayes KC. Increased urinary methylmalonic acid excretion in breast-fed infants of vegetarian mothers and identification of an acceptable dietary source of vitamin B_{12}. *Am J Clin Nutr*. 1988;47:89–92.

20. Sanders TAB, Ellis FR, Dickerson JWT. Studies of vegans: The fatty acid composition of plasma choline phosphoglycerides, erythrocytes, adipose tissue, and breast milk, and some indicators of susceptibility to ischemic heart disease in vegans and omnivore controls. *Am J Clin Nutr*. 1978;31:805–813.

21. Hesseltime CW, Smith M, Bradle R, Djien KS. Investigations of tempeh, an Indonesian food. *Dev Indian Microbiol*. 1963;4:275–280.

22. Van Veen AG, Steinkraus KH. Nutritive values and wholesomeness of fermented foods. *J Agric Food Chem*. 1970;18:576–579.

23. Truesdell DD, Green NR, Acosta PB. Vitamin B_{12} activity in miso and tempeh. *J Food Sci*. 1977;52:493–494.

24. Areekul S, Cheeramakara C, Nitavapabskoon S, Pattanamatum S, Churdchue K, Chongsanguan M. The source and content of vitamin B_{12} in the tempehs. *J Med Assoc Thailand*. 1990;73:153–156.

25. van den Berg H, Dagnelie PC, van Staveren WA. Vitamin B_{12} and seaweed. *Lancet*. 1988;1:242–243.

26. Long A. Vitamin B_{12} for vegans. *Br Med J*. 1977;2:191. Letter.

27. Jathar VS, Desphande LV, Kulkarni PR, Satoskar RS, Rege DV. Vitamin B_{12} like activity in leafy vegetables. *Indian J Biochem Biophys*. 1974;11:71–73.

28. Gray LF, Daniel IJ. Studies of vitamin B_{12} in turnip greens. *J Nutr*. 1958;67:623–634.

29. Parker BC. Rain as a source of vitamin B_{12}. *Nature (London)*. 1968;219:617–618.

30. Herbert V, Drivas G, Ghu M, Levitt D, Cooper B. Differential radioassays better measure cobalamin content of vitamins and "health foods" than do macrobiologic assays. Some products sold to vegetarians as rich vitamin B_{12} sources are not. The official United States Pharmacopeia (USP) method (*L leichmanii*) and *E gracilis* assay as vitamin B_{12} non-cobalamin corrinoids. *Blood*. 1983;62:(suppl 1):37A.

31. Herbert V, Drivas G. Spirulina and vitamin B_{12}. *JAMA*. 1982;248:3096–3097.

32. Dagnelie PC, van Staveren WA, van den Berg H. Vitamin B_{12} from algae appears not to be bioavailable. *Am J Clin Nutr*. 1991;53:695–697.

33. Rauma A-L, Törrönen, O Hänneninen, H Mykkänen. Vitamin B_{12} status of long-term adherents of a strict uncooked vegan diet ("living food diet") is compromised. *J Nutr*. 1995;125:2511–2515.

34. Carmel R, Karnaze DS, Weiner JM. Neurologic abnormalities in cobalamin deficiency are associated with higher cobalamin "analogue" values than are hematologic abnormalities. *J Lab Clin Med*. 1989;3:57–62.

35. Halsted JA, Carroll J, Robert S. Serum and tissue concentration of vitamin B_{12} in certain pathologic states. *N Engl J Med*. 1959;260:575–580.

36. Armstrong BK. Absorption of vitamin B_{12} from the human colon. *Am J Clin Nutr*. 1968;21:298–299.

37. Alberts MJ, Mathan VI, Baker SJ. Vitamin B_{12} synthesis by human small intestinal bacteria. *Nature (London)*. 1980;283:781–782.

38. Kapadia CR, Mathan VI, Baker SJ. Free intrinsic factor in the small intestine in man. *Gastroenterology*. 1976;70:704–706.

39. Bhat P, Shantakumari S, Rajan D, et al. Bacterial flora of the gastrointestinal tract in southern Indian control subjects and patients with tropical sprue. *Gastroenterology.* 1972;62:11–21.

40. Rose M. Vitamin B12 deficiency in Asian immigrants. *Lancet.* 1976;2:681. Letter.

41. Hardinge MG, Gibb DS, Oakley SD, Hardinge MO, Register UD. New dietary source of vitamin B12. *Fed Proc.* 1974;33:665. Abstract.

42. Lampkin BC, Saunders EF. Nutritional vitamin B12 deficiency in an infant. *J Pediatr.* 1969;75:1053–1055.

43. Higginbottom MC, Sweetman L, Nyhan Wl. A syndrome of methylmalonic aciduria, homocysteinura, megaloblastic anemia and neurologic abnormalities in a vitamin B12-deficient breast-fed infant of a strict vegetarian. *N Engl J Med.* 1978;299:317–323.

44. Davis JR, Goldenring J, Lubin BH. Nutritional vitamin B12 deficiency in infants. *Am J Dis Child.* 1981;135:566–567.

45. Wrighton MC, Manson JL, Speed I, Robertson E, Chapman E. Brain damage in infancy and dietary vitamin B12 deficiency. *Med J Aust.* 1979;2:1–3.

46. Gambon RC, Lentze MJ, Rossi E. Megaloblastic anaemia in one of monozygous twins breast fed by their vegetarian mother. *Eur J Pediatr.* 1986;145:570–571.

47. Grahamn SM, Arvela OM, Wise GA. Long-term neurologic consequences of nutritional vitamin B12 deficiency in infants. *J Pediatr.* 1992;121:710–714.

48. Sklar R. Nutritional vitamin B12 deficiency in a breast-fed infant of a vegan-diet mother. *Clin Pediatr.* 1986;25:219–221.

49. Specker BL, Black A, Allen L, Morrow F. Vitamin B12: Low milk concentrations are related to low serum concentrations in vegetarian women and to methylmalonic aciduria in their infants. *Am J Clin Nutr.* 1990;52:1073–1076.

50. MacPhee AJ, Davidson GP, Leahy M, Beare T. Vitamin B12 deficiency in a breast-fed infant. *Arch Dis Child.* 1988;63:921–923.

51. Frader J, Reibman B, Turkewitz D. Vitamin B12 deficiency in strict vegetarians. *N Engl J Med.* 1978;29:1319–1320.

52. Zmora D, Gorodischer R, Bar-Ziv J. Multiple nutritional deficiencies in infants from a strict vegetarian community. *Am J Dis Child.* 1979;133:141–144.

53. Ashkenazi S, Weitz R, Varsano I, Mimouni M. Vitamin B12 deficiency due to a strictly vegetarian diet in adolescence. *Clin Pediatr.* 1987;26:662–663.

54. Shinwell ED, Gorodischer R. Totally vegetarian diets and infant nutrition. *Pediatrics.* 1982;70:582–586.

55. Lubby AL, Cooperman JM, Stone ML, Slobody LB. Physiology of vitamin B12 in pregnancy, the placenta, and the newborn. *Am J Dis Child.* 1961;102:753–754.

56. Baker SJ, Jacob E, Rajan KT, Swaminathan SP. Vitamin B12 deficiency in pregnancy and the puerperium. *Br Med J.* 1962;16:1658–1661.

57. Gingliani ERJ, Jorge SM, Goncalves AL. Serum vitamin B12 levels in parturients, in the intervillous space of the placenta and in full-term newborns and their interrelationships with folate levels. *Am J Clin Nutr.* 1985;41:330–335.

58. Allen LH, Rosado JL, Casterline JE, et al. Vitamin B12 deficiency and malabsorption are highly prevalent in rural Mexican communities. *Am J Clin Nutr.* 1995;62:1013–1019.

59. Danielson L, Enecksson E, Hagenfeldt L, Rasmussen EB, Tillberg E. Failure to thrive due to subclinical maternal pernicious anemia. *Acta Paediatr Scand.* 1988;77:310–311.

60. Johnson RP, Roloff JS. Vitamin B12 deficiency in an infant strictly breastfed by a mother with latent pernicious anemia. *J Pediatr.* 1982;100:917–919.

61. Carmel R. Pernicous anemia: The expected findings of very low serum cobalamin levels, anemia, and macrocytosis are often lacking. *Arch Intern Med.* 1988;148:1712–1714.

62. Lubby AL, Cooperman JM, Donnfeld AM, et al. Observations on transfer of vitamin B_{12} from mother to fetus and newborn. *Am J Dis Child.* 1958;96:532–533.

63. Black AK, Allen LH, Pelto GH, de Mata MP, Chavez A. Iron, vitamin B_{12} and folate status in men and women and during pregnancy and lactation. *J Nutr.* 1994;124:1179–1188.

64. Kuhne T, Bubl R, Baumgartner R. Maternal vegan diet causing a serious infantile neurological disorder due to vitamin B_{12} deficiency. *Eur J Pediatr.* 1991;150:205–208.

65. Joosten E, van den Berg A, Riezler R, et al. Metabolic evidence that deficiencies of vitamin B_{12} (cobalamin), folate, and vitamin B_6 occur commonly in elderly people. *Am J Clin Nutr.* 1993;58:468–476.

66. Lindenbaum J, Healton EB, Savage DG, et al. Neuropsychiatric disorders caused by cobalamin deficiency in the absence of anemia or macrocytosis. *N Engl J Med.* 1988;318:1720–1728.

67. Healton EB, Savage DG, Brust JCM, Garrett TJ, Lindenbaum J. Neurologic aspects of cobalamin deficiency. *Medicine.* 1991;70:229–245.

68. Selhub J, Jacques PF, Wilson PWF, Rush D, Rosenberg IH. Vitamin status and intake as primary determinants of homocysteinemia in an elderly population. *JAMA.* 1993;27:2693–2698.

69. Kang SS, Wong PWK, Malinow MR. Hyperhomocyst(e)inemia as a risk factor for occlusive vascular disease. *Annu Rev Nutr.* 1992;12:279–298.

70. Clark R, Daly L, Robinson K, et al. Hyperhomocysteinemia: An independent risk factor for vascular disease. *N Engl J Med.* 1991;324:1149–1155.

71. US Department of Agriculture. *Nationwide Food Consumption Survey. Continuing Survey of Food Intakes by Individuals: Women 19–50 Years and Their Children 1–5 Years, 4 Days, 1985* (report 85.4). Hyattsville, Md: Nutrition Monitoring Division, Human Nutrition Information Service, US Department of Agriculture; 1986.

72. US Department of Agriculture. *Nationwide Food Consumption Survey. Continuing Survey of Food Intakes by Individuals: Men 19–50 Years, 1 Day, 1985* (report 85-3). Hyattsville, Md: Nutrition Monitoring Division, Human Nutrition Information Service, US Department of Agriculture; 1987.

73. Campbell TC, Brun T, Junshi C, Zulin F, Parpia B. Questioning riboflavin recommendations on the basis of a survey in China. *Am J Clin Nutr.* 1990;51:436–445.

74. Keys A, Henschel AF, Mickelson O, Brozak JM, Crawford JH. Physiological and biochemical functions in normal young men on a diet restricted in riboflavin. *J Nutr.* 1944;27:165–178.

75. Horwitt MK, Harvey CC, Hills OW, Liebert E. Correlation of urinary excretion of riboflavin with dietary intake and symptoms of ariboflavinosis. *J Nutr.* 1950;41:247–264.

76. Sterner RT, Price WR. Restricted riboflavin: Within-subject behavioral effects in humans. *Am J Clin Nutr.* 1973;26:150–160.

77. Prasad PA, Bamji MS, Lakshmi AV, Satyanarayana K. Functional impact of riboflavin supplementation in urban school children. *Nutr Res.* 1990;10:275–281.

78. Draper A, Lewis J, Malhotra N, Wheeler E. The energy and nutrient intakes of different types of vegetarian: A case for supplements. *Br J Nutr.* 1993;69:3–19.

79. Carlson E, Kipps M, Lockie A, Thomson J. A comparative evaluation of vegan, vegetarian and omnivore diets. *J Plant Foods.* 1985;6:89–100.

80. Hughes J, Sanders TAB. Riboflavin levels in the diet and breast milk of vegans and omnivores. *Proc Nutr Soc.* 1979;38:95A.

81. Janelle KC, Barr SI. Nutrient intakes and eating behavior scores of vegetarian and nonvegetarian women. *J Am Diet Assoc.* 1995;95:180–186.

82. Cook DA, Welsh SO. The effect of enriched and fortified grain products on nutrient intake. *Cereal Foods World.* 1987;32:191–196.

83. Norman AW. The vitamin D endocrine system: Identification of another piece of the puzzle. *Endocrinology.* 1994;134:1601A–1601C. Editorial.

84. Lipkin M, Newmark H, Boone CW, Kelloff GJ. Calcium, vitamin D, and colon cancer. *Cancer Res.* 1991;51:3069–3070.

85. Dent CE, Smith R. Nutritional osteomalacia. *Q J Med.* 1969;38:195–209.

86. National Research Council. *Recommended Dietary Allowances.* Washington, DC: National Academy Press; 1989.

87. US Department of Agriculture. *Nationwide Food Consumption Survey of Food 1977–78. Food Intakes: Individuals in 48 States, Year 1977–78* (report 1-1). Hyattsville, Md: Consumer Nutrition Division, Human Nutrition Information Service, US Department of Agriculture; 1983.

88. Specker BL, Valanis B, Hertzberg V, et al. Sunshine exposure and serum 25-hydroxyvitamin D concentrations in exclusively breast-fed infants. *J Pediatr.* 1985;107:372–376.

89. Haddad JG. Vitamin D—Solar rays, the milky way, or both. *N Engl J Med.* 1992;326:1213–1215.

90. Poskit EME, Cole TJ, Lawson DEM. Diet, sunlight, and 25-hydroxyvitamin D in healthy children and adults. *Br Med J.* 1979;1:221–223.

91. Kumpusalo E, Karinpää A, Jauhiainen M, Laitinen Lappeteläinen R, Mäenpää PH. Multivitamin supplementation of adult omnivores and lactovegetarians: Circulating levels of vitamin A, D, and E, lipids, apolipoproteins and selenium. *Int J Vitam Nutr Res.* 1989;60:58–66.

92. Webb AR, Kline L, Holick MF. Influence of season and latitude on the cutaneous synthesis of vitamin D_3: Exposure to winter sunlight in Boston and Edmonton will not promote vitamin D_3 synthesis in human skin. *J Clin Endocrinol Metabol.* 1988;67:373–378.

93. Specker BL. Do North American women need supplemental vitamin D during pregnancy or lactation? *Am J Clin Nutr.* 1994;59 (suppl):484S–491S.

94. Landin-Wilhelmsen K, Wilhelmsen L, Wilske J, et al. Sunlight increases serum 25(OH) vitamin D concentration whereas $1,25(OH)_2D_3$ is unaffected. Results from a general population study in Goteborg, Sweden (The WHO MONICA Project). *Eur J Clin Nutr.* 1995;49:400–407.

95. Clemens TL, Henderson SL, Adams JS, Holick MF. Increased skin pigment reduces capacity of skin to synthesize vitamin D_3. *Lancet.* 1982;1:74–76.

96. Matsuoka LY, Ide L, Wortsman J, et al. Sunscreen suppress cutaneous vitamin D_3 synthesis. *J Clin Endocrinol Metab.* 1987;64:1165–1168.

97. Hellebostad M, Markestad T, Seeger Halvorsen K. Vitamin D deficiency rickets and vitamin B_{12} deficiency in vegetarian children. *Acta Paediatr Scand.* 1985;74:191–195.

98. Iq-bal SJ. Evidence of continuing deprivational vitamin D deficiency in Asians in the UK. *J Hum Nutr Diet.* 1994;7:47–52.

99. Dent CE, Round JM, Bowe DJF, et al. Effects of chappatia and ultraviolet irradiation on nutritional rickets in an Indian immigrant. *Lancet.* 1973;1:1282–1284.

100. Cooks WT, Asquith P, Ruck N, et al. Rickets, growth and alkaline phosphatase in urban adolescents. *Br Med J.* 1974;2:293–297.

101. Hunt SP, O'Riordon JLH, Windo J, Truswell S. Vitamin D status in different subgroups of British Asians. *Br Med J.* 1976;2:1351–1354.

102. Dandona P, Mohiuddin J, Weerakoon JW, Freedman DB, Fonseca V, Healey T. Persistence of parathyroid hypersecretion after vitamin D treatment in Asian vegetarians. *J Clin Endocrinol Metab.* 1984;59:535–537.

103. Dent CE, Gupta MM. Plasma 25-hydroxyvitamin-D levels during pregnancy in caucasians and in vegetarian and non-vegetarian Asians. *Lancet.* 1975;2:1057–1060.

104. Henderson JB, Dunnigan MG, McIntosh WB, Abdul-Motaal AA, Gettinby G, Glekin BM. The importance of limited exposure to ultraviolet radiation and dietary factors in the aetiology of Asian rickets: A rick-factor model. *Q J Med.* 1987;63:413–425.

105. Robertson I, Fords JA, McIntosh WB, Dunnigan MG. The role of cereals in the aetiology of nutritional rickets: The lesson from the Irish National Nutrition Survey 1943–8. *Br J Nutr.* 1981;45:17–22.

106. Batchelor AJ, Compston JE. Reduced plasma half-life of radiolabelled 25-hydroxyvitamin D in subjects receiving a high-fibre diet. *Br J Nutr.* 1983;49:213–216.

107. Dwyer JT, Dietz W, Hass G, Suskind R. Risk of nutritional rickets among vegetarian children. *Am J Dis Child.* 1979;133:134–140.

108. Roberts IF, West RJ, Dillon MJ. Malnutrition in infants receiving cult diets: A form of child abuse. *Br Med J.* 1979;1:296–298.

109. Dagnelie PC, Vergote FJVRA, van Staveren WA, van den Berg H, Dingjan PG, Hautvast JGAG. High prevalence of rickets in infants on macrobiotic diets. *Am J Clin Nutr.* 1990;51:202–208.

110. Lamberg-Allardt C, Karkkainen M, Sepanen R, Bistrom H. Low serum 25-hydroxyvitamin D concentrations and secondary hyperparathyroidism in middle-aged white strict vegetarians. *Am J Clin Nutr.* 1993;58:684–689.

111. Maierhofer WJ, Gray RW, Cheung HS, Lemann J Jr. Bone resorption stimulated by elevated serum 1,25-$(OH)_2$-vitamin D concentrations in healthy men. *Kidney Int.* 1983;24:555–560.

112. Colussi G, Rombola G, De Ferrari ME et al. Vitamin D treatment: A hidden risk factor for aluminum bone toxicity? *Nephron.* 1987;47:78–80.

113. Moon J, Davison A, Bandy B. Vitamin D and aluminum absorption. *Can Med Assoc J.* 1992;147:1308–1309.

114. American Academy of Pediatrics. The prophylactic requirement and the toxicity of vitamin D. *Pediatrics.* 1963;31:512–525.

115. Department of Health and Human Services. Grade "A" pasteurized milk ordinance. 21 CFR 131.110, 1989, 243.

116. Lightwood R. Idiopathic hypercalcaemia with failure to thrive: Nephrocalcinosis. *Proc R Soc Med.* 1952;45:401.

117. Clemens TL, O'Riordan JLH. Vitamin D. In: Becker KL, ed. *Principles and Practice of Endocrinology and Metabolism.* Philadelphia, Pa: Lippincott; 1990:417–423.

118. Jacobus CH, Holick MF, Shao Q, et al. Hypervitaminosis D associated with drinking milk. *N Engl J Med.* 1992;326:1173–1177.

119. Holick MF, MacLaughlin JA, Doppelt SH. Factors that influence the cutaneous photosynthesis of previtamin D_3. *Science.* 1981;211:590–593.

120. Kretsch MJ, Sauberlich HE, Skala JH, Johnson HL. Vitamin B_6 requirement and status assessment: Young women fed a depletion diet followed by a plant or animal protein diet with graded amounts of vitamin B_6. *Am J Clin Nutr.* 1995;61:1091–1101.

121. US Department of Agriculture. *Nationwide Food Consumption Survey. Nutrient Intakes: Individuals in 48 States, Year 1977–78* (report 1-2). Hyattsville, Md: Consumer Nutrition Division, Human Nutrition Information Service, US Department of Agriculture; 1984.

122. Dalery K, Lussier-Cacan S, Selhub J, et al. Homocysteine and coronary artery disease in French Canadian subjects: Relation with vitamins B_{12}, B_6, pyridoxal phosphate, and folate. *Am J Cardiol.* 1995;75:1107–1111.

123. Ellis JM, McCully KS. Prevention of myocardial infarction by vitamin B_6. *Res Comm Molec Pathol Pharmacol.* 1995;89:208–220.

124. Brubacher G, Hornig D, Ritzel G. Food patterns in modern society and their consequences on nutrition. *Biblthca Nutr Dieta.* 1981;30:90–99.

125. Löwik MRH, Schrijver J, van den Berg, Hulshof KFAM, Wedel M, Ockhuizen T. Effect of dietary fiber on the vitamin B_6 status among vegetarian and nonvegetarian elderly (Dutch Nutrition Surveillance System). *J Am Coll Nutr.* 1990;9:241–249.

126. Kretsch MJ, Sauberlich HE, Johnson HL, Skala JH. Effect of animal or plant protein composition on the vitamin B_6 requirement of young women. *Fed Proc.* 1982;21:227. Abstract.

127. Kretsch MJ, Sauberlich HE, Skala JH, Johnson HL. Vitamin B_6 and status assessment: Young women fed a depletion diet followed by a plant- or animal-protein diet with graded amounts of vitamin B_6. *Am J Clin Nutr.* 1994;61:1091–1101.

128. Leklem JE, Shultz TD, Miller LT. Comparative bioavailability of vitamin B_6 from soybeans and beef. *Fed Proc.* 1980;39:558. Abstract.

129. Reynolds RD. Bioavailability of vitamin B_6 from plant foods. *Am J Clin Nutr.* 1988;48:863–867.

130. Kabir H, Leklem JF, Miller LT. Relationship of the glycosylated vitamin B_6 content of foods to vitamin B-6 bioavailability in humans. *Nutr Rep Int.* 1983;28:709–716.

131. Trumbo PR, Gregory JF III, Sartain DB, Toth JP, Bailey LB, Cerda JJ. Bioavailability of pyridoxine-β-glucoside in rats and humans. *FASEB J.* 1988;2:1086. Abstract.

132. Andon MB, Reynolds RD, Moser-Veillon PB, Howard MP. Dietary intake of total and glycosylated vitamin B_6 and the vitamin B_6 nutritional status of unsupplemented lactating women and their infants. *Am J Clin Nutr.* 1989;50:1050–1058.

133. Leklem JE, Miller LT, Perera AD, Peffers DE. Bioavailability of vitamin B_6 from whole wheat bread in humans. *J Nutr.* 1980;110:1819–1828.

134. Lindberg AS, Leklem JE, Miller LT. The effect of wheat bran on the bioavailability of vitamin B_6 in young men. *J Nutr.* 1983;113:2578–2583.

135. Shultz TD, Leklem JE. Vitamin B6 status and bioavailability in vegetarian women. *Am J Clin Nutr.* 1987;46:647–651.

136. Löwik MRH, Schrijver J, Odink J, van den Berg H, Wedel M. Long-term effects of a vegetarian diet on the nutritional status of elderly people (Dutch Nutrition Surveillance System). *J Am Coll Nutr.* 1990;9:600–609.

137. Brants HAM, Lowik MRH, Westenbrink S, Hulshof KFAM, Kistemaker C. Adequacy of a vegetarian diet at old age (Dutch Nutrition Surveillance System). *J Am Coll Nutr.* 1990;9:292–302.

138. Shultz TD, Leklem JE. Dietary status of Seventh-Day Adventists and nonvegetarians. *J Am Diet Assoc.* 1983;83:27–33.

139. Dwyer JT, Dietz WH Jr, Andrews EM, Suskind RM. Nutritional status of vegetarian children. *Am J Clin Nutr.* 1982;35:204–216.

140. Hilker DM, Somogyi JC. Antithiamines of plant origin: Their chemical nature and mode of action. *Ann NY Acad Sci*. 1982;378:137–145.

141. Vimokesant S, Kunjara S, Rungruangask K, et al. Beriberi caused by antithiamine factors in food and its prevention. *Ann NY Acad Sci*. 1982;378:123–136.

142. Tayter M, Stanek KL. Anthropometric and dietary assessment of omnivore and lacto-ovo-vegetarian children. *J Am Diet Assoc*. 1989;89:1661–1663.

143. Hardinge MG, Stare FJ. Nutritional studies of vegetarians. *J Clin Nutr*. 1954;2:73–82.

144. Carter EGA, Carpenter KJ. The bioavailability for humans of bound niacin from wheat bran. *Am J Clin Nutr*. 1982;36:855–861.

145. Goldsmith GA. Experimental niacin deficiency. *J Am Diet Assoc*. 1956;32:312–316.

146. Phillips DR, Wright AJA. Studies on the response of *Lactobacillus casei* to folate vitamin in foods. *Br J Nutr*. 1983;49:181–186.

147. US Department of Agriculture. *Nationwide Food Consumption Survey. Continuing Survey of Food Intakes of Individuals: Low-Income Women 19–50 Years and Their Children 1–5 Years, 1 Day, 1986* (report 86-2). Hyattsville, Md: Nutrition Monitoring Division, Human Nutrition Information Service, US Department of Agriculture; 1987.

148. Baugh CM, Malone JW, Butterworth CE Jr. Human biotin deficiency. A case of biotin deficiency induced by raw egg consumption in a cirrhotic patient. *Am J Clin Nutr*. 1968;21:173–182.

149. Lombard KA, Mock DM. Biotin nutritional status of vegans, lactoovovegetarians, and nonvegetarians. *Am J Clin Nutr*. 1989;50:486–490.

150. Tarr JB, Tamura T, Stokstad ELR. Availability of vitamin B6 and pantothenate in an average American diet in man. *Am J Clin Nutr*. 1981;34:1328–1337.

151. Srinivasan V, Christensen N, Wyse BW, Hansen RG. Pantothenic acid nutritional status in the elderly—Institutionalized and noninstitutionalized. *Am J Clin Nutr*. 1981;34:1736–1742.

152. Hemilä H. Does vitamin C alleviate the symptoms of the common cold?—A review of current evidence. *Scand J Infect Dis*. 1994;26:1–6.

153. Marston R, Raper N. Nutrient content of the US food supply. *Natl Food Rev*. 1987;36:18–23.

154. Wolf G. A historical note on the mode of vitamin A for the cure of night blindness. *Am J Clin Nutr*. 1978;31:290–292.

155. Krinsky NI. Antioxidant functions of carotenoids. *Free Radical Biol Med*. 1989;7:617–635.

156. Food and Agriculture Organization (FAO). *Requirements of Vitamin A, Iron, Folate, and Vitamin B12. Report of a Joint FAO/World Health Organization Expert Consultation*. (FAO Food and Nutrition Series 23.) Rome, Italy: FAO; 1988.

157. de Pee S, West CE, Muhilal, Karyadi D, Hautvast JGAJ. Lack of improvement in vitamin A status with increased consumption of dark-green leafy vegetables. *Lancet*. 1995;344:75–81.

158. Olson JA. Recommended dietary intakes (RDI) of vitamin A in humans. *Am J Clin Nutr*. 1987;45:704–716.

159. Abraham R, Brown C, North WRS, McFayden IR. Diets of Asian pregnant women in Harrow: Iron and vitamins. *Hum Nutr Appl Nutr*. 1987;41A:164–173.

160. Alexander D, Ball MJ, Mann J. Nutrient intake and haematological status of vegetarians and age-sex matched omnivores. *Eur J Clin Nutr*. 1994;48:538–546.

161. Rana SK, Sanders TAB. Taurine concentrations in the diet, plasma, urine and breast milk of vegans compared with omnivores. *Br J Nutr*. 1986;56:17–27.

162. Rider AA, Arthur RS, Calkins BM, Nair PP. Diet, nutrition intake, and metabolism in populations at high and low risk for colon cancer. *Am J Clin Nutr.* 1984;40:917–920.

163. Malter M, Schreiver G, Eilber U. Natural killer cells, vitamins, and other blood components of vegetarian and omnivorous men. *Nutr Cancer.* 1989;12:271–278.

164. Krinsky NI. Antioxidant functions of carotenoids. *Free Rad Biol Med.* 1989;7:617–635.

165. Di Mascio P, Kaiser S, Sies H. Lycopene as the most efficient biological carotenoid single oxygen quencher. *Arch Biochem Biophys.* 1989;274:532–538.

166. van Poppel G. Carotenoids and cancer: An update with emphasis on human intervention studies. *Eur J Cancer.* 1993;29A:1335–1344.

167. Hankinson SE, Stampfer MJ, Seddon JM, et al. Nutrient intake and cataract extraction in women: A prospective study. *Br Med J.* 1992;305:335–339.

168. Naruszewica M, Selinger E, Davignon J. Oxidative modification of lipoprotein(a) and the effect of β-carotene. *Metabolism.* 1992;41:1215–1224.

169. Palozza P, Krinsky NI. β-Carotene and α-tocopherol are synergistic antioxidants. *Arch Biochem Biophys.* 1992;297:184–187.

170. Bendich A. Carotenoids and the immune response. *J Nutr.* 1989;119:112–115.

171. Miller RK, Brown K, Cordero J, et al. Position paper by the Teratology Society: Vitamin A during pregnancy. *Teratology.* 1987;35:267–275.

172. Bauernfeind JC. *The safe use of vitamin A.* Washington, DC: International Vitamin A Consultative Group, Nutrition Foundation.

173. Micozzi MS, Brown ED, Taylor PR, Wolfe E. Carotenodermia in men with elevated carotenoid intake from foods and β-carotene supplements. *Am J Clin Nutr.* 1988;46:1061–1064.

174. Cross CE. Oxygen radicals and human disease. *Ann Intern Med.* 1987;107:526–545.

175. Stampfer MJ, Hennekens CH, Manson JE, Colditz GA, Rosner B, Willet WC. Vitamin E consumption and the risk of coronary disease in women. *N Engl J Med.* 1993;328:1444–1449.

176. Rimm EB, Stampfer MJ, Ascherio A, Giovannucci E, Colditz GA, Willet WC. Vitamin E consumption and the risk of coronary heart disease in men. *N Engl J Med.* 1993;328:1450–1456.

177. Witting LA, Lee I. Dietary levels of vitamin E and polyunsaturated fatty acids and plasma vitamin E. *Am J Clin Nutr.* 1975;28:571–576.

178. Murphy SP, Subar AF, Block G. Vitamin E intakes and sources in the United States. *Am J Clin Nutr.* 1990;52:361–367.

179. Gey KF. Extra vitamin E beyond PUFA-dependent vitamin E requirement is supplied by olive oil and sunflower oil but not by soybean oil and other oils with insufficient α-tocopherol/PUFA ratio. *Int J Vitam Nutr Res.* 1995;65:61–64.

180. Pronczuk A, Kipervarg Y, Hayes KC. Vegetarians have higher plasma α-tocopherol relative to cholesterol than do nonvegetarians. *J Am Coll Nutr.* 1992;11:50–55.

181. Reddy S, Sanders TAB. Lipoprotein risk factors in vegetarian women of Indian descent are unrelated to dietary intake. *Atherosclerosis.* 1992;95:223–229.

182. Sanders TAB, Roshanai F. Platelet phospholipid fatty acid composition and function in vegans compared with age- and sex-matched omnivore controls. *Eur J Clin Nutr.* 1992;46:823–831.

183. Bendich A, Machlin IJ. Safety of oral intake of vitamin E. *Am J Clin Nutr.* 1988;48:612–619.

184. Lipsky JJ. Nutritional sources of vitamin K. *Mayo Clin Proc*. 1994;69:462–466.

185. Morley JE, Mooradian AD, Silver AJ, Heber D, Alfin-Slater RB. Nutrition in the elderly. *Ann Intern Med*. 1988;109:890–894.

186. Hasell K, Baloch KH. Vitamin K deficiency in the elderly. *Gerontol Clin*. 1970;12:10–17.

187. Hodges SJ, Akesson K, Vergnaud P, Obrant K, Delmas PD. Circulating levels of vitamin K_1 and K_2 decreased in elderly women with hip fracture. *J Bone Miner Res*. 1993;8:1241–1245.

188. Price PA. Vitamin K nutrition and postmenopausal osteoporosis. *J Clin Invest*. 1994;91:1268.

189. Lane PA, Hathaway WE. Vitamin K in infancy. *J Pediatr*. 1985;106:351–359.

190. Suttie JW, Mummah-Schendel LL, Shah DV, Lyle BJ, Gregor JL. Vitamin K deficiency from dietary vitamin K restriction in humans. *Am J Clin Nutr*. 1988;47:475–480.

191. US Department of Agriculture. *Provisional Table on the Vitamin K Content of Foods*. Hyattsville, Md: US Department of Agriculture; 1994.

192. Lloyd T, Schaeffer JM, Walker MA, Demers L. Urinary hormonal concentrations and spinal bone densities of premenopausal vegetarian and nonvegetarian women. *Am J Clin Nutr*. 1991;54:1005–1010.

193. Owen CA Jr. Pharmacology and toxicology of the vitamin K group. In: Sebrell WH, Harris RS, eds. *The Vitamins*. New York, NY: Academic Press; 1971;3:492–509.

CHAPTER 7

Food Guides for Vegetarians

A HISTORY OF FOOD GUIDES

The first food guide, introduced by the US Department of Agriculture (USDA) in 1916, included five groups: vegetables and fruits; meat, fish, and milk; cereals; simple sweets; and butter and wholesome fats. Although there was limited knowledge about the newly discovered vitamins at this time, nutritionists well understood the importance of these new nutrients. In 1918, McCollum coined the phrase *protective foods* for foods rich in calcium, vitamin A, and ascorbic acid. He suggested that daily food habits should address the consumption of these nutrients specifically and recommended daily consumption of a quart of milk, a large serving of greens or potherbs, and at least two salads with raw fruits and vegetables. There was little concern about harmful effects of overnutrition, as was evident in McCollum's advice to "Eat what you want after you have eaten what you should."[1(p22)]

The first recommended dietary allowances (RDAs) were announced over the radio in 1941. With this kind of specific information about nutrient needs available, several new food guides were developed by various government agencies. Eating well and keeping fit were viewed as patriotic duties. The Office of Defense, Health and Welfare Services introduced eight new food groups in 1942 and attached a wartime slogan to the new guide: "US Needs Us Strong—Eat Nutritional Food." The objective of the new nutritional program was to seek "full health returns from the nation's food resources . . . for victory."[2] Indeed, the link between nutrition and the war effort was a real one because a report published at the time noted that "a third of all men rejected by Selective Service were disqualified for reasons of physical disability and defects related to malnutrition."[3] This food guide also gave special consideration to the food shortages brought on by the war by including alternative choices in certain groups.

The guide that was to become the standard until the mid-1950s was introduced in 1943 and billed as the National Wartime Nutrition Guide.[1] It was based on seven food groups: leafy green and yellow vegetables; citrus fruits; potatoes and other vegetables; milk and milk products; meat, poultry, fish, eggs, dried beans, and peanuts; cereals, breads, and flours; and butter and margarine. This food guide was presented via a Wheel of Good Eating to indicate that no group was more important than any other. This was the nation's nutrition education model until 1955.

The guide that is most recognizable today to several generations of Americans is the Basic Four Food Groups. Introduced in 1956, it was widely embraced for its simplicity and ease of use and was employed with relatively few changes by nutrition educators until the Food Guide Pyramid was introduced in 1992. Foods were grouped as follows: meat, milk, vegetables and fruits, and breads and cereals. In 1979 the guide was revised into the Daily Food Guide, which used the same groups but expanded the number of servings of grains, fruits, and vegetables and added a group that included fats, sweets, and alcohol. In view of the increasing body of data on the harmful effects of dietary overconsumption, however, the Daily Food Guide became a nutritional anachronism long before it was discarded. Criticisms included the fact that meat and dairy foods were visually overemphasized in the guide and that it allowed, or even encouraged, the consumption of too much fat and cholesterol. The Daily Food Guide continued in use even though other government guidelines (the Dietary Guidelines) were urging Americans to reduce consumption of fat and cholesterol.

Both the Basic Four Food Groups and the Daily Food Guide were somewhat adaptable to lacto-ovo vegetarian diets. Vegetarians could use the guide exactly as it was, choosing "alternatives" from the meat, fish, and poultry group. One problem was that the alternative choices were limited. They included eggs, beans, and peanut butter. Also, serving sizes were too large. For example, a 3-oz piece of chicken could be replaced by 1½ cups of cooked beans, providing significantly greater food volume and more calories. Because there were no alternatives to dairy foods in the milk group, neither the Basic Four Food Groups nor the Daily Food Guide was usable by vegans.

In 1992, the USDA released its latest food guide for Americans: the Food Guide Pyramid. Although its release was steeped in controversy, it was largely hailed by the nutrition profession as a marked improvement over former plans. The pyramid visually reinforced the idea that plant foods need to be emphasized in a healthy diet. It also promoted the consumption of animal foods in amounts that may be greater than is advised for optimal health, however. Guidelines allow as much as 9 oz of meat and three servings of milk per day. Although the guide does emphasize plant foods, it is not particularly useful to vegetarians. As was true for the Basic Four Food Groups, serving sizes of legumes are excessive, and the variety of foods that might be typical in a vegetarian diet is limited. Again, the pyramid does not allow for vegan eating patterns.

DEVELOPING FOOD GUIDES FOR VEGETARIANS

Government meal-planning guidelines have always focused on meat- and dairy-based diets and have limited use in counseling vegetarian clients. Over the past several decades, however, a number of meal-planning tools aimed directly at vegetarians have been developed. With changes in our understanding of nutrition, some have become obsolete. A number of the guides are especially useful, however, and the best choices are presented in Appendix 7-A.

Ideally, a food guide will steer its user toward choosing a diet that meets or comes close to meeting the RDAs for all nutrients without excesses of fat, cholesterol, and calories. One point of controversy that is bound to affect the way vegetarian food guides are viewed is the issue of nutrient needs of vegetarians. For example, there is evidence that vegans, particularly those who exercise regularly and consume diets low in sodium, have lower calcium needs than omnivores. Vegetarians may also have lower vitamin B_6 needs because of their lower protein intake. Conversely, their need for protein and iron may be slightly higher than that of omnivores. There have been no studies to determine the exact nutritional requirements of either lacto-ovo vegetarians or vegans, however. Therefore, dietitians should employ food guides that help all vegetarians meet the current RDAs.

Vegan diets represent a fairly dramatic departure from standard American eating habits. In addition to the fact that vegans avoid foods that make up a considerable proportion of the usual American diet, many use foods that are not a part of typical American eating patterns. For this reason, there has been some concern among health professionals that vegan diets planned without benefit of individual counseling by a dietitian may be deficient.

With appropriate guidelines, however, vegan clients should be able to plan nutritious diets with minimal knowledge about nutrients in foods. In a 1981 issue of the *Journal of Nutrition Education,* Food and Drug Administration nutritionist Jean Pennington wrote "A food guide is an instrument which converts the professional's scientific knowledge of food composition and nutrient requirements for health into a practical plan for food selection by those without training in nutrition."[4(p53)]

Challenges in developing such a guide exist for any type of dietary pattern. For example, food guides for omnivores have not been completely successful in guaranteeing diets that fall within recommendations for fat, cholesterol, and fiber intake. No food guide is completely reliable. At best, a food guide can only provide general guidelines to increase the likelihood that a consumer will choose a healthy diet. Individual diets will differ in quality depending on individual food preferences, habits, and choices within food groups. A food guide cannot act as a foolproof means of ensuring adequate nutrient intake and of avoiding dietary excesses.

The challenge in developing guidelines for vegans is that this pattern of eating is foreign to many American consumers as well as American health professionals. Nevertheless, there is no greater difficulty in planning healthy meals for vegans than for lacto-ovo vegetarians or omnivores. Although attention to certain nutrients in the vegan diet is warranted, these diets are likely to be lower in fat and higher in fiber than diets of those eating a more traditional diet. They frequently come closer to meeting the dietary guidelines than nonvegetarian diets. Vegans are no more or less likely to benefit from individual counseling than those following nonvegetarian diets as long as vegans have access to appropriate general guidelines for menu planning.

It is important to recognize that there are many patterns of meal planning for vegetarians that will support good health. The easiest and most common approach to menu planning is to classify foods into groups based on similar nutrient content. It is assumed that choosing a certain number of foods from each group every day will increase the probability of consuming a balanced diet.

Foods typically used in vegetarian diets generally fall into the following 12 categories. Note that most food guides do not treat each of these groups separately. In nearly all cases some of these categories are combined, but different food guides combine them in different ways. As a starting point for looking at food guides for vegetarians, we will look first at the ways in which vegetarian foods are classified or grouped.

Grains

In all food guides, vegetarian or otherwise, grains form the backbone of the diet. Usually whole grains are emphasized, although most of the guides also include refined grains. Refined grains can play an important role in the diets of children or others who may have difficulty meeting calorie needs.

Foods included are all breads (including bagels, English muffins, pita, Indian breads such as poori and chapati, rolls, and biscuits), corn and flour tortillas, dry cereals, cooked cereals, rice, bulgur, couscous, millet, quinoa, pasta, polenta, wheat berries, popcorn, wheat germ, and bran; crackers such as melba toast, rice cakes, and matzo; and pancakes, waffles, corn bread, bread stuffing, and chow mein noodles. Some guides may include the starchy vegetables, such as corn, potatoes, and winter squash, in this group. Some guides may also include low-fat, low-sugar cookies and snacks, such as graham crackers, some oatmeal cookies, ginger snaps, vanilla wafers, and animal crackers.

Foods from this group contribute fiber, protein, iron, B vitamins, and, when whole grains are used, some trace nutrients. These foods tend to be low in fat, but this is not always the case. It is clear that the extent to which these foods contribute nutrients and are low fat will vary considerably depending on the choices made within the group. Clients need to be guided toward using more cereal grains and breads and fewer prepared foods such as pancakes and crackers. Also, fortified dry cereals, if they are acceptable to the client, can make significant contributions to nutrient intake because many of these cereals are fortified with vitamin D, vitamin B_{12}, calcium, iron, and other nutrients. Breakfast cereals can also be high in sugar and fat, however. Exhibit 7–1 lists some breakfast cereals that are good choices because they are low in fat and nutrient dense. It is a good idea to suggest to vegetarians that they read labels of cereals for further nutrition information, however, because fortification can change over time and different brands of similar cereals contain different nutrients.

Vegetables

This group comprises all vegetables including those that are botanically fruits (eg, avocado and plantain). The starchy vegetables, such as potatoes,

---

Exhibit 7–1 Commercial Breakfast Cereals Typically Fortified with Vitamin D and Vitamin B_{12}

Bran Flakes, Kelloggs	Nutrigrain, Kelloggs
Cheerios, General Mills	Post Toasties, Post
Corn Bran, Quaker	Product 19, Kelloggs
Corn Chex, Ralston Purina	Raisin Bran, Kelloggs
Fortified Oat Flakes, Post	Rice Chex, Ralston Purina
Fruit'n Fiber, Post	Sun Flakes, Ralston Purina
Grapenuts, Post	Team, Nabisco
Hearty Granola, Post	Total, General Mills
Kix, General Mills	Wheat Chex, Ralston Purina
Most, Kelloggs	Wheaties, General Mills

might be included in this group in some guides, or they might be placed in the grains group. In many cases, food guides will further divide this group to include separate categories for leafy green vegetables (beet greens, kale, collards, mustard greens, turnip greens, Swiss chard, spinach, dandelion greens, bok choy, and sometimes broccoli) or vegetables that are particularly rich in vitamin A (squash, carrots, pumpkin, sweet potatoes, tomatoes, and leafy greens). Leafy greens will nearly always be mentioned in a food guide for vegans because of their high calcium content. Although vegans can reasonably meet their calcium needs without consuming leafy greens, these vegetables are so nutrient dense that they probably should be emphasized. Most guides specify a serving of these foods each day. Although they are somewhat common in the cuisine of southern Americans and African Americans, leafy green vegetables, excepting spinach, have not been an especially popular vegetable choice in this country. When counseling new vegetarians, it can be helpful to be able to provide recipes or cooking hints for these vegetables. See Chapter 13 for ideas on preparing leafy green vegetables.

An ideal vegetarian food guide will include sea vegetables (alaria, dulse, kelp, nori, and wakame) because these are especially rich sources of calcium, iron, and trace nutrients. Again, these vegetables, which are common in the cuisine of some Asian countries, are still considered an unusual food choice in this country. Because macrobiotic diets make wide use of sea vegetables, macrobiotic cookbooks can serve as good resources for ways to incorporate more of these foods into the diet. These foods contribute fiber, protein, and a variety of micronutrients depending on choices within the group (eg, calcium, vitamin A, vitamin C, iron, and trace minerals).

Fruits

This group includes all whole fresh fruits, fruit juices, dried fruits, and canned or frozen fruits. Some foods are botanically fruits (avocado, plantain, tomatoes, and peppers), but because of their nutrient composition and the fact that they are traditionally viewed as vegetables, they are most often placed in the vegetable group. Fruits contribute vitamins C and A and some B vitamins and minerals. Dried fruits can contribute significant iron.

Legumes

Legumes are botanically vegetables, but their nutrient content and cultural use differ markedly from those of the foods we typically place in the vegetable group. Legumes are used extensively in many parts of the world and are common to a number of international cuisines that are increasingly popular, including Indian, Latin American, and African cooking. They play a minor role in the diets of most Americans, however, and are generally served as baked beans or in bean soups. In vegetarian diets legumes tend to play an important supporting role in the diet.

Foods included in this group are all cooked dried beans (the most common are adzuki, anasazi, black turtle beans, blackeyed peas, brown beans, cannellini, chickpeas, cranberry beans, great northern beans, kidney beans, lentils, lima beans, navy beans, pinto beans, soybeans, and split peas) and all soy products, including tofu, tempeh, and textured vegetable protein.

Meat Analogues

These are simulated meat products, most frequently made from soy protein or gluten (wheat protein) but sometimes from other legumes or from vegetables. A growing number of these products are appearing in grocery stores. They often have tastes, textures, and appearances similar to those of hamburgers, hot dogs, sausages, chicken patties, beef chunks, or ground beef. The nutrient content of these products varies greatly. They tend to be high in protein, and until recently most have been high in fat. New reduced-fat and nonfat versions of these products are increasingly available. Meat analogues have been produced by a few large companies since the early part of the century. Many of these more traditional products are heavily fortified with a number of nutrients, including vitamin B_{12}, making them a good choice for vegans.

Milk and Dairy

Traditionally, the milk group includes all forms of cow's milk (whole, low fat, nonfat, and buttermilk) and its derivatives (yogurt, kefir, and cheese). Foods in this group contribute significant amounts of calcium, protein, vitamin D, and riboflavin. These foods can also contribute considerable amounts of fat and saturated fat.

Soymilk and Other Vegetable Milks

These foods are likely to be found in either the legume group or the milk group as a milk alternative. Unlike cow's milk, soymilk from different manufacturers varies dramatically in nutrient content (Table 7–1). First, it is important to differentiate between regular and fortified soymilk because their nutrient content differs significantly. Regular soymilk is a good source of

Table 7–1 Comparison of the Nutrient Content of Selected Milks (All Examples Are for 1 Cup Plain Milk unless Otherwise Indicated)

Milk	Calories	Protein (grams)	Fat (grams)	Calcium	Iron	Ribo-flavin	Vitamin D	Vitamin B_{12}
						RDI (%)		
Edensoy Extra	140	10	4	20	10	6	10	150
Soy Moo	110	6	0	40	8		100	0
Pacific Ultra Plus	160	6	5	30	15	30	30	
Solait	110	5	3	30	8		0	0
Westsoy Low-Fat Concentrate	100	4	2	20	2		25	0
Sno E	90	2	5	50	0	10	10	20
Vegelicious	100	2	2	30	<2	10	10	50
Rice Dream (fortified, vanilla)	130	1	2	30	0		25	0
Soyagen	130	6	6	15	10	10	25	25
Cow's milk, nonfat	86	8.4	0.4	37	<2	20	25	50
Cow's milk, low fat	121	8.1	5	37	<2	20	25	50

protein and B vitamins and provides some iron and calcium. Fortified soymilk is generally higher in calcium and can also provide significant vitamin D, riboflavin, and vitamin B_{12}. Fortification varies considerably, however, and there are few brands of soymilk that are good sources of all these nutrients. Soymilks also are available in different flavors and have various fat contents. Traditionally, soymilk is made by expressing the liquid from soaked mature soybeans.

Because of concerns about allergies to both soymilk and cow's milk protein, and in an effort to broaden the range of products available to vegans, there are a number of other vegetable milks on the market. Vegelicious is a powdered milk made from potatoes. It also includes some soy protein and is not suitable for clients who prefer to avoid soy. This product is lower in fat than many soymilks and is fortified with vitamin D, calcium, vitamin B_{12}, and riboflavin, making it an excellent source of all these nutrients. It is considerably lower in protein than either soymilk or cow's milk and may not be a suitable substitute for children.

Rice milk is also a popular choice among vegetarians. A few are fortified with both calcium and vitamin D; all are considerably lower in protein than either soymilk or cow's milk. Unless these foods are supplemented, they make minimal contributions to nutrient intake.

Nuts and Seeds

This food group includes all nuts and seeds as well as nut butters (peanut butter and almond butter) and tahini (sesame seed butter). Although peanuts are legumes, they are nearly always grouped with nuts because of their fat content. These foods contribute protein, fiber, iron, calcium, and trace minerals.

Often, nuts and seeds are placed in a larger food group along with legumes because these are all protein-rich foods. Nuts and seeds are quite high in fat compared with most legumes, however. Although these foods provide excellent nutrition and can be especially important in the diets of vegan children, they need to be limited in the diets of most adults because of their fat content.

Fats

Although not essential in the diet, fats are generally included in food guides as an option for adults and as an important contributor of calories for children. In vegetarian food guides, fats usually include vegetable oils, mayonnaise, salad dressings, margarine, butter, soy or dairy cream cheese, and sour cream. These foods contribute calories to the diet and can contribute vitamin E and essential fatty acids, but should be limited in the diets of adults.

Other

In most food guides, the "other group" is a catchall for foods that are not nutrient dense, are high in fat and/or sugar, but are typically part of Western diets. Foods usually included are snack items (chips), sweets (candy and soft drinks), frozen desserts (ice cream and sorbet), and baked desserts (cakes, cookies, and pies). The USDA Food Guide Pyramid combines the fats and other groups, as do many vegetarian food guides. In all food guides, foods from this group are considered optional because they are not necessary for optimal health.

Eggs

Eggs present a special problem in vegetarian food guides. In guides for omnivores, they are placed in the meat group. Because they are high in fat and protein and lack fiber, this is an appropriate food grouping. In vegetarian guides, however, there seems to be no place for eggs. In some guides, all the protein-rich foods (legumes, nuts, seeds, and eggs) are grouped together. In others, eggs are given a separate group or are relegated to the other group because of their high fat content. Eggs can contribute protein and B vitamins to the diet, but lacto-ovo vegetarians should be counseled to limit them in their diet because they are rich in both cholesterol and saturated fat.

Supplemental Foods

Some food items do not fit into the food grouping system but are often mentioned in vegetarian meal-planning guides because they contribute significantly to nutrient intake. These can be placed in a group called supplemental foods.

Blackstrap molasses is a valuable addition to the vegan diet in particular because it is rich in calcium. One level tablespoon contains 187 mg of calcium. It is also rich in iron, providing 3.3 mg per tablespoon. Nutritional yeast is an inactive yeast grown on a nutrient-rich culture. The actual nutrient content of the yeast will depend on the culture. Nutritional yeast that is grown on a vitamin B_{12}–rich culture is especially valuable in the diets of vegans. The brand that is most likely to be a reliable source of B_{12} is Red Star brand T6635. This nutritional yeast is also a good source of other B vitamins, iron, and potassium.

VEGETARIAN FOOD GUIDES

An important feature of any food guide is that it should be adaptable to the needs of children and of pregnant and lactating women. Presenting completely different sets of guidelines for different family members can be confusing. Children can follow the same menu-planning guidelines as adults; the difference is that their meals will emphasize different foods within the groups, and of course serving sizes will be different. Food guides for pregnant women and children can be found in Chapters 8 and 10.

We recently developed a new set of guidelines for vegetarians[5] (Appendix 7-A). Our goal was to produce a guide that is usable by both lacto-ovo vegetarians and vegans, is adaptable to all age groups, and allows but does not require consumption of either cow's milk or vegetable milks. Cow's milk, soymilk, and other vegetable milks are all found along with legumes, nuts, and seeds in a food group that provides a variety of sources of protein, calcium, and other minerals. An upper limit is placed on the number of milk servings for adults (to encourage consumption of a variety of foods from this group), but there is no minimum requirement for them. In addition, all calcium-rich foods throughout the guide are printed in bold type to encourage both vegans and lacto-ovo vegetarians to choose a variety of calcium sources rather than depend on one food group to provide these foods.

In this guide, both eggs and cheese are placed in the "other group." Although both can contribute significant nutrients to the diet, they do so at the expense of a high saturated fat and cholesterol content. Placing these foods in the "other group" is one way to discourage lacto-ovo vegetarians from overemphasizing these foods in the diet, a practice that is often common with new vegetarians. Nonsoy vegetable milks that are not fortified are also placed in the "other group." These foods provide negligible nutrition. Because they are usually low in fat, it is not necessary to discourage their use. They may displace other, more nutrient-dense foods from meals, however, and therefore some moderation should be exercised in their use.

A number of other food plans for vegetarians have been published in both the popular and the professional literature (Appendix 7-A). Any of these can be useful in counseling vegetarians.

REFERENCES

1. Hertzler AA, Anderson HL. Food guides in the United States. *J Am Diet Assoc.* 1974;64:19–28.

2. Office of Defense, Health and Welfare Services. *US Needs Us Strong—Eat Nutritional Food.* Washington, DC: Government Printing Office; Office of Defense, Health and Welfare Services publication 0–457183.

3. Office of Defense, Health and Welfare Services. *How Industry Can Cooperate With the National Nutrition Plan.* Washington, DC: Information Services; 1943.

4. Pennington JT. Considerations for a new food guide. *J Nutr Educ.* 1981;13:53–55.

5. Messina VK, Messina MJ. *The Vegetarian Way.* New York, NY: Harmony Books. In press.

6. Chaij-Rhys S. A diet pattern for total vegetarians. *Adventist Rev.* 1980 (August 14):6–7.

7. Haddad EH. Development of a vegetarian food guide. *Am J Clin Nutr.* 1994;59(suppl): 1248S–1254S.

8. American Dietetic Association (ADA). *Eating Well the Vegetarian Way.* Chicago, Ill: ADA; 1992.

9. Health Connection. *The Vegetarian Food Pyramid.* Hagerstown, Md: Health Connection; 1994.

10. New York Medical College. *New York Medical College Vegetarian Pyramid.* Valhalla, NY: New York Medical College; 1994.

11. Kushi M, Kushi A. *Macrobiotic Diet.* New York, NY: Japan Publications; 1985.

Food Guides for Vegetarians

FOOD GUIDE FOR LACTO-OVO VEGETARIANS AND VEGANS

Type of vegetarian diet: Lacto-ovo or vegan
Developed by: Virginia Messina, MPH, RD, and Mark Messina, PhD, Nutrition Matters, Port Townsend, Washington.[5]

Food Group	Foods Included	Number of Servings	Serving Sizes
Grains	Breads, muffins, crackers, cereals, pasta, tortillas; whole grains such as amaranth, barley, bulgur, kasha, kamut, oats, quinoa, rice, wheat berries	Eight	½ cup grain or cereal; one slice bread, one 6-inch tortilla, one pancake, one small muffin, 2 cups popcorn, 1/2 cup pasta
Vegetables	Asparagus, beets, **bok choy, broccoli,** Brussels sprouts, cabbage, carrots, cauliflower, chard, **collards,** corn, eggplant, **greens,** jicama, **kale,** leeks, lettuce, mushrooms, okra, peas, peppers,	Four (include at least one serving per day of broccoli, kale, collards, or other dark green leafy vegetables)	½ cup cooked or 1 cup raw

Note: Foods printed in bold type are good sources of calcium.

Food Group	Foods Included	Number of Servings	Serving Sizes
	potatoes, rutabaga, **sea vegetables (dulse, kelp, nori, wakame),** spinach, squash, sweet potatoes, tomatoes, turnips, any other vegetable		
Fruits	Apples, apricots, bananas, berries, cantaloupe, dates, **figs,** grapefruit, grapes, honeydew, kiwifruit, oranges, papaya, peaches, pears, persimmons, pineapple, plums, prunes, raisins, strawberries, water-melon, all fruit juices	Three	One piece fresh fruit, one wedge melon, ½ cup cooked or canned fruit, ¾ cup fruit juice, ¼ cup dried fruit
Legumes, nuts, seeds, milks		Five	
Legumes	Adzuki, **black beans,** black-eyed peas, **chickpeas, great northern beans,** kidney beans, lentils, lima beans, mung beans, **navy beans, pinto beans, soybeans,** split peas, **vegetarian baked beans, tempeh, textured vegetable protein, tofu,** meat analogues		½ cup cooked beans, tofu, tempeh, textured vegetable protein; 3 oz meat analogues
Nuts/seeds	**Almonds,** cashews, Brazil nuts, pecans, pine nuts, pistachios, walnuts, coconut, **almond butter,**		2 tbsp nuts, nut butter, seeds

Food Group	Foods Included	Number of Servings	Serving Sizes
	peanut butter, **tahini,** pumpkin seeds, **sesame seeds,** sunflower seeds		
Milks	**Soymilk, fortified soymilk**		1 cup fluid milk or yogurt
Fats	Vegetable oils, marga-rine, butter, salad dressing	Two to three	1 tsp oil, margarine, butter; 2 tsp salad dressing
Other	Soy cheese, **cow's milk cheese,** eggs, baked sweets, snack chips	Limit to one per day	1 oz cheese, one egg, 1 oz snack chips, 2 oz cookies or baked goods

SAMPLE MENU

Meal	Vegan	Lacto-Ovo Vegetarian
Breakfast	½ cup scrambled tofu, two slices oatmeal bread toast, 6 oz grapefruit juice	1 cup seven-grain cereal, 1 cup nonfat milk, ½ cup sliced peaches, one slice rye toast, 1 tsp margarine
Lunch	1½ cups pasta and great northern bean soup, 1½ cup spinach salad with ½ cup broccoli florets and 1 tbsp oil and vinegar dressing, two whole wheat dinner rolls, ½ mango	Bean spread sandwich (pureed navy beans with lemon, basil, and chopped sun-dried tomatoes) with lettuce, 1 cup vegetable soup (carrots, green beans, potatoes, tomatoes)
Dinner	One bean burrito (½ cup refried pinto beans, one flour tortilla, salsa, chopped lettuce and tomatoes), ½ cup steamed collards with ginger and chili powder, ½ cup Spanish rice, ½ cup corn	½ cup mixed quinoa and amaranth, 1 cup steamed broccoli, one nonfat veggieburger, whole wheat hamburger roll, ½ cup fresh fruit salad
Snacks	Soymilk shake (1 cup fortified soymilk, ½ banana, ½ cup strawberries), bagel with 2 tbsp almond butter	1 cup nonfat yogurt with ½ cup raspberries, ½ cup roasted soynuts

THE 1-2-3-4-5 VEGETARIAN FOOD GUIDE

Type of vegetarian diet: Vegan
Developed by: Selma Chaij Rhys, PhD, RD, Andrews University, Hinsdale, Illinois.[6]

Food Group	Number of Servings	Serving Sizes
Nuts/seeds/legumes	One	½ cup beans, 2 tbsp nuts/seeds
Vitamin B12-fortified soymilk/fortified meat analogues	Two	One slice meat analogue, 1 cup soymilk
Vegetables	Three	½ cup
Fruits	Four	One fresh fruit, 2 tbsp dried fruit, ½ cup juice
Grains	Five	½ cup cooked grain or pasta, one slice bread

SAMPLE MENU

Meal	Vegan
Breakfast	1¼ cup Cheerios, 1 cup fortified soymilk, ½ grapefruit, one slice whole wheat toast
Lunch	One small pita pocket, ½ cup seasoned broiled tofu, one banana, carrot sticks
Dinner	½ cup barley with mushrooms and seasoned with herbs, one nonfat veggie burger, ½ cup steamed broccoli, tossed salad with nonfat dressing, ½ cup strawberries
Snacks	Orange, ½ bagel with fruit spread

HADDAD VEGETARIAN FOOD GUIDE

Type of vegetarian diet: Lacto-ovo or vegan
Developed by: Ella Haddad, PhD, RD, Loma Linda University, Loma Linda, California.[7]
Comments: This guide is unusual in that it includes a group devoted to sugars to maintain adequate calorie levels for vegans. It also groups tofu not with legumes but with milk and milk alternatives. Haddad offers several different plans to meet different calorie levels as well as an adapted guide for children. The servings listed here are for 1,600 cal.

Food Group	Number of Servings	Serving Sizes
Grains	Eight	One slice bread; ¾–1 cup dry cereal, ½ cup cooked grain or cereal
Legumes	One	½ cup cooked beans or tofu
Vegetables	Four	½ cup cooked vegetables, 1 cup raw vegetables; includes two servings leafy green vegetables
Fruit	Two	One medium fresh fruit, 1/2 cup chopped or canned fruit, ¼ cup dried fruit/¾ cup juice
Nuts/seeds	One	¼ to ⅓ cup nuts or seeds, 2 tbsp nut or seed butter
Milk/milk alternatives/tofu	Two to three	1 cup cow's or fortified vegetable milk, 1 cup tofu
Fats	Two	1 tsp oil, mayonnaise, margarine; 2 tsp salad dressing
Sugar	3 tsp	1 tsp sugar, jam, jelly, syrup, honey

SAMPLE MENU

Meal	Vegan	Lacto-Ovo Vegetarian
Breakfast	Soymilk shake (1 cup fortified soymilk, ¼ cup dates, ½ cup banana slices), cinnamon raisin bagel with 2 tbsp almond butter	1¼ cup Cherrios, 1 cup 2% milk, bagel with 1 tsp soy margarine, 6 oz orange juice
Lunch	"Missing egg salad" sandwich (two slices seven-grain bread, ½ cup tofu chunks, 1 tbsp tofu mayonnaise), 1 cup spinach salad with tomato, pear	1 cup cream of broccoli soup, baked sweet potato with margarine and brown sugar, two oat bran rolls
Dinner	½ cup dal (curried lentils) cooked in vegetable oil, ½ cup braised collards, 1 cup basmati rice, ½ cup steamed carrots	1 cup quiona, ½ cup corn, ½ cup chickpeas with lemon and dill, ½ cup steamed kale
Snacks	One English muffin with 1 tbsp apricot jam	One slice whole wheat bread with 2 tbsp peanut butter, 1 cup cantaloupe balls

AMERICAN DIETETIC ASSOCIATION'S VEGETARIAN FOOD GUIDE

Type of vegetarian diet: Lacto-ovo or vegan
Developed by: American Dietetic Association,[8] Chicago, Illinois.

Food Group	Number of Servings	Serving Sizes
Breads, cereals, rice, pasta	Six or more	One slice bread, ½ cup cooked cereal or grain, 1 oz dry cereal
Vegetables	Four or more	½ cup cooked, 1 cup raw
Legumes and other meat substitutes	Two to three	½ cup cooked beans, tofu, or tempeh; 8 oz soymilk; 2 tbsp nuts or seeds
Fruits	Three or more	One piece fresh fruit, ¾ cup juice, ½ cup canned fruit
Dairy products	Optional: up to three per day	1 cup low-fat or skim milk, 1 cup yogurt, 1½ oz low-fat cheese
Eggs	Optional: three to four yolks per week	One egg or two egg whites
Fats, sweets, alcohol	Sparingly	

SAMPLE MENU

Meal	Vegan	Lacto-Ovo Vegetarian
Breakfast	One package instant oatmeal, ½ cup strawberries, one slice whole wheat toast with fruit spread	Two pancakes, ½ cup applesauce, 2 tbsp maple syrup, two vegetarian sausage links
Lunch	Tempeh burger on hamburger roll with tomato and lettuce, 1 cup pineapple chunks	Cheese sandwich (1 oz American cheese, sliced tomato, sprouts), peach, carrot sticks
Dinner	Cream of broccoli soup (1 cup soymilk, ½ cup cooked broccoli, ½ cup potatoes), ½ cup steamed carrots, two whole wheat rolls	1 cup pasta with 1 cup spaghetti sauce made with ½ cup textured soy protein, tossed salad with nonfat dressing
Snacks	½ bagel with 2 tbsp almond butter, 1 cup watermelon chunks	1 cup nonfat yogurt with ½ cup frozen blueberries

THE VEGETARIAN FOOD PYRAMID

Type of vegetarian diet: Lacto-ovo or vegan
Developed by: The Health Connection, Hagerstown, Maryland[9] (see Figure 7A–1).
Comments: Legumes are found in both the grains group and the legume group in this guide.

Food Group	Number of Servings	Serving Sizes
Grains and legumes	6–11	One slice bread, ½ cup cooked cereal or grain, ¾ cup dry cereal, ½ cup cooked beans
Vegetables	3–5	½ cup cooked, 1 cup raw
Fruits	2–4	One medium whole fruit, ½ cup canned fruit, ¼ cup dried fruit, 1 cup berries, ¾ cup fruit juice
Low-fat/nonfat cow's milk or fortified milk alternatives	2–3	1 cup cow's milk or soymilk, ¾ cup low-fat cottage cheese, ½ cup soy cheese, 1½ oz cheese, 1 cup low-fat or soy yogurt
Legumes, nuts, seeds, and meat alternatives	2–3	½ cup cooked beans or tofu, ⅓ cup nuts, 2 tbsp nut butter, ¼ cup seeds, ¼ cup meat alternative; two egg whites
Fats, oils, sweets	Eat sparingly	

SAMPLE MENU

Meal	Vegan	Lacto-Ovo Vegetarian
Breakfast	One package instant oatmeal, 1 cup fortified soymilk, 6 oz grapefruit juice, one slice whole wheat toast	1 cup Rice Krispies, 1 cup nonfat milk, one slice pumpernickel toast, ½ cup sliced banana
Lunch	1½ cup black bean soup, one whole wheat roll, 1 cup steamed broccoli and cauliflower	½ cheese sandwich (1 oz Swiss cheese, one slice whole wheat bread, sliced tomato, nonfat mayonnaise), tossed salad with 1 cup romaine lettuce, ½ tomato, 2 tbsp sunflower seeds
Dinner	Chinese stir-fry (1 cup brown rice, ½ cup bok choy, ¼ cup carrots, ¼ cup water chestnuts)	½ cup vegetarian baked beans, ½ cup mashed potatoes, one slice sourdough bread, ½ cup steamed green beans, one kiwifruit
Snacks	½ bagel with 2 tbsp almond butter, soymilk shake (1 cup fortified soymilk, ½ banana, ½ cup blueberries)	1 English muffin with fruit spread

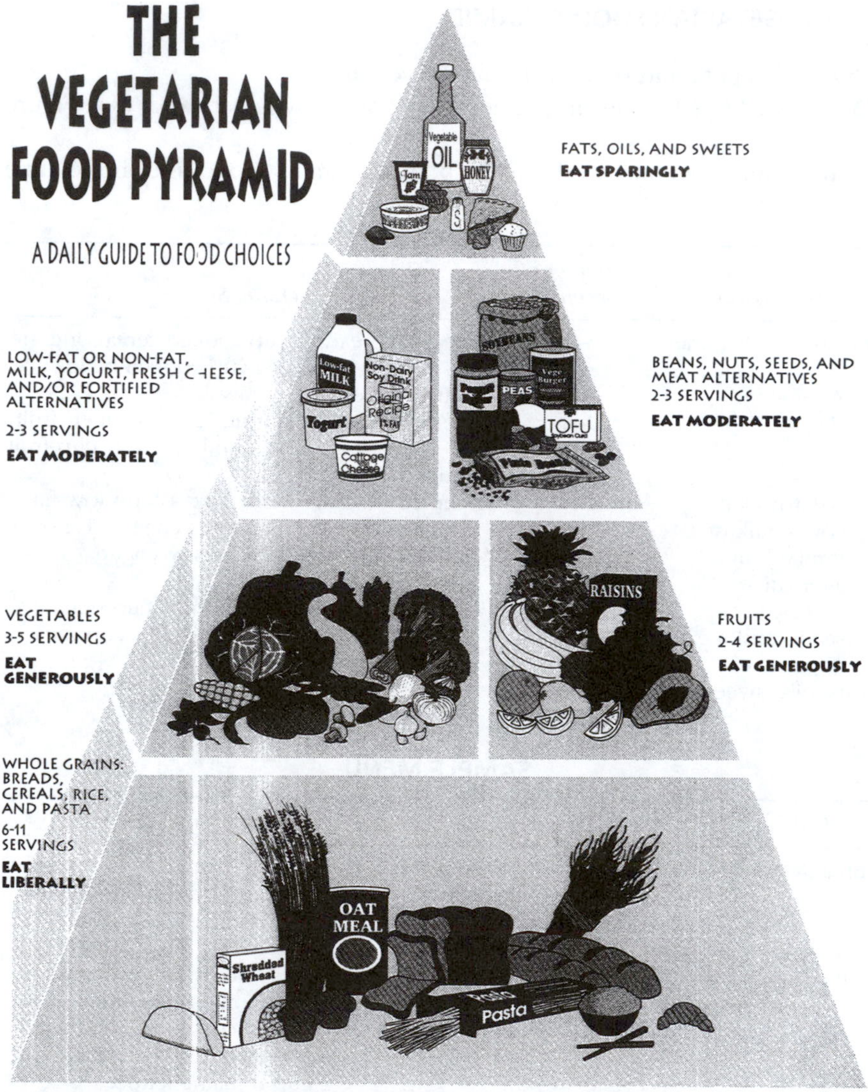

THE VEGETARIAN FOOD PYRAMID

A DAILY GUIDE TO FOOD CHOICES

FATS, OILS, AND SWEETS
EAT SPARINGLY

Vegetable OIL

Jam HONEY S

LOW-FAT OR NON-FAT,
MILK, YOGURT, FRESH CHEESE,
AND/OR FORTIFIED
ALTERNATIVES

2-3 SERVINGS

EAT MODERATELY

Low-fat MILK Non-Dairy Soy Drink Original Recipe 1% FAT

Yogurt

Cottage Cheese

BEANS, NUTS, SEEDS, AND
MEAT ALTERNATIVES
2-3 SERVINGS

EAT MODERATELY

SOYBEANS PEAS Vege Burger TOFU

VEGETABLES
3-5 SERVINGS

EAT GENEROUSLY

RAISINS

FRUITS
2-4 SERVINGS

EAT GENEROUSLY

WHOLE GRAINS:
BREADS,
CEREALS, RICE,
AND PASTA

6-11 SERVINGS

EAT LIBERALLY

OAT MEAL

Shredded Wheat

Pasta

Figure 7A–1 Vegetarian Food Pyramid. A daily guide to food choices. *Source:* Reprinted with permission from General Conference Nutrition Council. The Health Connection. Illustration by Merle Poirier.

THE VEGETARIAN PYRAMID

Type of vegetarian diet: Lacto-ovo or vegan
Developed by: New York Medical College, Valhalla, New York[10] (see Figure 7A–2).
Comments: This guide differs from most others in that the serving sizes of legumes, nuts, and tofu are twice as large as those specified by most other plans. The allowance for ½ cup nuts per day may result in eating patterns that are too high in fat and calories. Also, note that starchy vegetables appear in the same group with grains.

Food Group	Number of Servings	Serving Size
Grains and starchy vegetables	6–11	½ cup cooked grain or starchy vegetable, 1 cup dry cereal, one slice bread
Vegetables	3 or more	½ cup cooked, 1 cup raw
Fruits	2–4	1 fresh fruit, ½ cup canned, ¾ cup juice
Meat/fish substitutes	2–3	1 cup cooked beans or tofu, ½ cup nuts
Milk and milk substitutes	2	1 cup cow's or vegetable milk
Suggestions for vegans		1 tbsp fortified brewer's yeast, 1 tbsp blackstrap molasses, 1 tbsp vegetable oil

SAMPLE MENU

Meal	Vegan	Lacto-Ovo Vegetarian
Breakfast	½ cup scrambled tofu with 1 nutritional yeast, two slices whole wheat toast, one sliced kiwifruit	1 cup nonfat yogurt, ½ cup sliced strawberries, one low-fat bran muffin
Lunch	1½ cup vegetable soup (potatoes, carrots, green beans, tomato broth), one whole wheat roll, ½ cup fresh fruit salad	1½ cups tomato soup made with 2% milk, two slices whole wheat toast, 1 cup tossed lettuce salad with nonfat dressing, orange
Dinner	½ cup baked beans with 1 tbsp blackstrap molasses, 1 cup bulgur, ½ cup steamed collards	Bean burritos (½ cup refried pinto beans, two flour tortillas, chopped lettuce and tomato)
Snacks	2 cups popcorn, soymilk shake (1 cup fortified soymilk, ½ banana, ½ cup strawberries)	½ English muffin with 2 tbsp peanut butter, apple

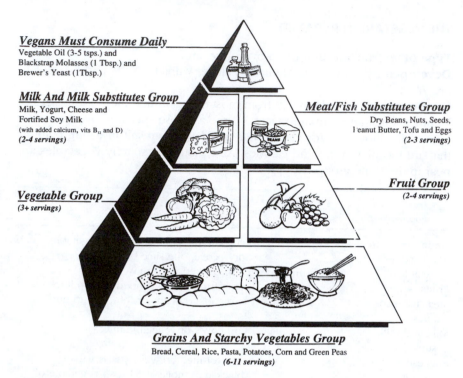

Vegans Must Consume Daily
Vegetable Oil (3-5 tsps.) and
Blackstrap Molasses (1 Tbsp.) and
Brewer's Yeast (1Tbsp.)

Milk And Milk Substitutes Group
Milk, Yogurt, Cheese and
Fortified Soy Milk
(with added calcium, vits B$_{12}$ and D)
(2-4 servings)

Meat/Fish Substitutes Group
Dry Beans, Nuts, Seeds,
Peanut Butter, Tofu and Eggs
(2-3 servings)

Vegetable Group
(3+ servings)

Fruit Group
(2-4 servings)

Grains And Starchy Vegetables Group
Bread, Cereal, Rice, Pasta, Potatoes, Corn and Green Peas
(6-11 servings)

Figure 7A–2 New York Medical College Vegetarian Food Pyramid. *Source:* Reprinted with permission from New York Medical College, Valhalla, New York. Copyright © 1994 New York Medical College.

MACROBIOTIC FOOD GUIDE

Type of vegetarian diet: Macrobiotic
Developed by: Based on general guidelines for macrobiotic diets presented by Michio and Aveline Kushi, *Macrobiotic Diet,* Japan Publications, Inc., New York, New York, 1985.[11]
Comments: Guidelines for macrobiotic meals tend to be fairly general and are not presented in terms of specific servings from food groups. We have adapted the guidelines presented in a popular book on macrobiotics to fit them to the food group model.

Food Group	Number of Servings	Serving Sizes
Grains	10	½ cup cooked grain
Vegetables	7	½ cup cooked, 1 cup raw
Sea vegetables	1–2	½ cup cooked
Miso soup	2	1 cup (2 tbsp miso)
Legumes	1	½ cup cooked beans or tofu
Pickles	1	¼ cup homemade pickled vegetables
Nuts/seeds/fruits	1	Foods from this group are all consumed infrequently in macrobiotic diets; 1 serving a day of either nuts, seeds (¼ cup), or fruit (one fresh fruit) might be typical

SAMPLE MENU

Meal	Macrobiotic
Breakfast	1 cup oatmeal with 1 tbsp sesame seeds, grain coffee
Lunch	1 cup miso soup with ½ cup wakame, 2 cups mixed barley and brown rice seasoned with tamari and grated fresh ginger root, 1 cup steamed broccoli, 1 cup baked carrots
Dinner	1 cup miso soup with ½ cup adzuki beans and ½ cup mixed carrots, onions, bok choy; 1 cup steamed kale seasoned with brown rice vinegar; 2 cups mixed brown rice and wheat berries seasoned with umeboshi plum; ¼ cup pickled cabbage

PART III

Vegetarian Diets throughout the Life Cycle

CHAPTER 8

Pregnancy and Lactation

The requirements for all nutrients increase with pregnancy. Energy needs increase also but to a lesser extent, so that some attention to dietary needs and food choices that highlight nutrient-dense foods is important for all pregnant women.

WEIGHT GAIN AND CALORIE NEEDS IN PREGNANCY

Estimates of the energy cost of pregnancy range from 45,000 to 110,000 kcal over the 280 days of pregnancy.[1] The World Health Organization[2] and the National Research Council[3] both assume an average energy cost of 80,000 kcal. Assuming no increase in calorie intake during the first month of pregnancy, an additional 300 cal/day for the remaining 250 days of pregnancy should meet energy needs. This represents only a 13% increase over average daily kilocalorie needs of nonpregnant women. The increased need for some individual nutrients is much greater than this, however. For example, the recommended dietary allowances (RDAs) for pregnant women for folate, iron, vitamin D, and calcium are 120%, 100%, 100%, and 50% higher, respectively, than for nonpregnant women. Therefore, when pregnant women eat to appetite, they may easily meet energy needs but will not necessarily meet nutrient needs unless some attention is given to choosing nutrient-dense foods.

The RDAs specify calorie needs for normal, healthy adult women who are at ideal weight. Weight gain recommendations vary, however, depending on the needs of the woman, and therefore energy requirements will vary as well. Current weight gain recommendations for white women are as follows; African American women should strive for weight gains at the upper end of these ranges:

- normal weight woman: 25 to 35 lb
- underweight woman (<90% of desirable): 28 to 40 lb
- overweight woman (>120% of desirable): 15 to 25 lb
- obese woman (>135% desirable): 15 lb
- adolescent: 30 to 45 lb
- normal weight woman carrying twins: 35 to 45 lb

In healthy, normal weight women, weight gain ideally follows a pattern of only 2 to 4 lb in total for the first trimester of pregnancy and then 1 to 1½ lb per week thereafter. Clearly, however, there is a great deal of variation within the above groups, and weight gain goals (for both total and weekly weight gains) for adolescents or for overweight or underweight women must be determined on an individual basis.

Appropriate weight gain during pregnancy will support both the fetus and the placenta as well as growth in maternal tissues that support the pregnancy and provide stored energy for lactation. Table 8–1 illustrates the average weight of the products of pregnancy.

WEIGHT GAIN IN PREGNANT VEGETARIANS

Because of the low-fat, high-fiber content of vegetarian diets, the energy density (kilocalories per gram) of vegetarian diets is lower than that of omnivore diets. Weight gain of pregnant vegan and lacto-ovo vegetarians is generally adequate, however, and infants of vegetarian women are of normal weight. For example, average weight gain in vegan women living on the Farm, a vegetarian community in western Tennessee, was 5 lb greater than

---

Table 8–1 Average Weights of the Products of Pregnancy

Product	Weight (lb)
Fetus	7.6
Placenta	1.5
Amniotic fluid	1.8
Uterus	2.2
Breast tissue	1.0
Blood volume	2.8
Extracellular fluid	5.6
Maternal fat stores	1.5–8.5
Total	24–31

Source: Brown JE. Weight gain during pregnancy: What is "optimal"? *Clin Nutr.* 1988;7:181.

for the reference population.[4] Interestingly, the longer a woman had been on a vegan diet, the greater her weight gain. Similarly, in a British study, although weight gain during pregnancy was not reported, birth weights of infants born to vegan mothers were almost identical to those of infants of nonvegetarian mothers.[5] A study comparing Asian vegetarian and nonvegetarian women living in India and in England showed no differences in maternal weight gain or in infant birth weight.[6] Finally, two studies in the United States found that birth weights of infants born to lacto-ovo vegetarian women were similar to those of infants born to nonvegetarian mothers;[7,8] maternal weight gain was also similar in the one study in which those values were reported.[7]

In contrast to these findings, inadequate weight gain resulting in small offspring has been seen in some macrobiotic populations and has been attributed to low energy intake.[9,10] Macrobiotics often eat a diet that is much more restrictive than that of nonmacrobiotic vegetarians. Consistent with this, Shull et al[11] found that, although overall birth weight of infants of vegetarian mothers was similar to that of the reference population, macrobiotic vegetarian mothers gave birth to low–birth weight infants.

For women who have difficulty meeting calorie needs and sustaining an ideal weight gain, it is important to identify foods that are calorie rich but high in nutrients. Because adequate calories are of paramount importance, however, judicious use of added fats, even where they do not add nutritional value to the diet, can be appropriate. Therefore, use of salad dressings, spreads such as margarine, or small amounts of oil for cooking can be encouraged. Foods that are rich in both calories and nutrients include soy products, nuts, seeds, nut and seed butters, avocados, and legumes. Because the high fiber content of vegetarian diets can produce satiety on fewer calories, using some refined products such as fruit juices and refined enriched grains can help meet energy needs.

MEETING NUTRIENT NEEDS OF PREGNANCY ON A VEGETARIAN DIET

Table 8–2 compares the RDAs for protein, vitamins, and minerals for nonpregnant, pregnant, and lactating women.

Protein

Protein synthesis increases during pregnancy to support expansion of the maternal blood volume, uterus, and breasts and to produce fetal and placental proteins. The net result is an average deposition of 454 g (1 lb) of protein in the fetus and 470 g of protein in the maternal tissues. There is some

Table 8–2 Comparison of RDAs for Nonpregnant, Pregnant, and Lactating Women

Nutrient	Nonpregnant (25 to 50 years)	Pregnant	Lactating
Protein (g)	50	60	62–65
Vitamin A (retinol equivalents)	800	800	1,200–1,300
Vitamin D (μg)	5	10	10
Vitamin E (mg)	8	10	11–12
Vitamin K (μg)	60	65	65
Vitamin C (mg)	60	70	90–95
Folic acid (μg)	180	400	260–280
Niacin (mg)	15	17	20
Riboflavin (mg)	1.3	1.6	1.7–1.8
Thiamin (mg)	1.1	1.5	1.6
Vitamin B6 (mg)	1.6	2.2	2.1
Vitamin B12 (μg)	2.0	2.2	2.6
Calcium (mg)	800	1,200	1,200
Phosphorus (mg)	800	1,200	1,200
Iodine (μg)	150	175	200
Iron (mg)	15	30	15
Magnesium (mg)	280	320	355–340
Zinc (mg)	12	15	16–19
Selenium (μg)	55	65	75

debate over whether protein needs increase over time during pregnancy or whether they remain fairly constant throughout the three trimesters. Another issue of debate is whether low protein intake increases risk for pregnancy-induced hypertension (PIH).[12–16] Conversely, some researchers suggest that excess protein intake during pregnancy may be linked to premature delivery and neonatal death.[17,18]

The RDA of 60 g of protein represents an additional 10 g of protein per day for pregnant women, or a 20% increase over nonpregnant needs. Because the average protein intake of nonpregnant women in the United States is about 70 g, most women will meet protein needs with no change in dietary habits. Lacto-ovo vegetarian women consume diets comprising between 12% and 14% protein; therefore, if adequate calories are consumed, protein needs will easily be met. Vegans consume diets comprising between 10% and 12% protein. These diets would still be adequate to meet the RDA, but the lower range of that intake would be close to the RDA. The RDA does include a generous margin of safety, so that it is actually higher than what most pregnant women need. Menus based on the food guides in Appendix 8-A will provide protein intakes that are somewhat in excess of the RDA.

Iron

In pregnancy, iron is needed for the manufacture of hemoglobin in maternal and fetal red blood cells. A full-term infant has about 246 mg of iron in its blood and stores. An additional 134 mg is found in the placenta, and about 290 mg is necessary for expansion of the mother's blood volume.

Infants born to iron-deficient mothers are unlikely to be anemic. The most common cause of iron deficiency is premature birth because the fetus accumulates most of its iron during the last trimester. The effects of maternal iron-deficiency anemia on the fetus are not clear, however. Low maternal blood levels of iron are associated with low birth weight in infants and infant mortality. Low iron levels are most often seen in high-risk populations, however, such as low-income women. Poor pregnancy outcome is more common among such populations for a myriad of reasons, so that it is difficult to establish whether low birth weight or infant mortality can be directly linked to iron deficiency.

Several factors promote iron sufficiency in pregnancy. Lack of menstruation saves about 120 mg of iron over the 36 weeks of pregnancy. Iron absorption also increases dramatically, to as much as 50% compared with 10% to 20% in nonpregnant women. The iron requirement of pregnancy is still high enough, however, that the diet needs to be especially iron rich.

Iron supplements are commonly prescribed for pregnant women. Because iron recommendations double in pregnancy and iron deficiency is a relatively common nutritional deficiency among pregnant women, conventional wisdom has been that supplements are nearly always indicated. This practice has recently been questioned, however, because of the lack of convincing evidence that using iron supplements improves pregnancy outcome.[19]

One study of lacto-ovo vegetarians showed iron intake without supplements to be more than 90% of the RDA.[20] In a study of Tennessee vegan women, rates of anemia among pregnant women who were not using supplements were low; in fact, the incidence of anemia actually increased when supplements were used.[4] Although iron deficiency is somewhat common among pregnant women, it does not appear to be any more common among pregnant vegetarians.[21] Iron stores are lower in vegetarians, however, which may make them theoretically more vulnerable during pregnancy.

Although the need for iron supplements is debated, there is evidence that it takes several years to build iron stores to prepregnancy levels after delivery when supplements are not used. Whether or not iron supplements are used, it is important to stress the inclusion of iron-rich foods in the diets of all pregnant women. Vegetarian women should include a wide variety of whole and enriched grains, legumes, soy products, nuts, seeds, dried fruits, and vegetables in their diet. Consuming a source of vitamin C with each meal can improve iron absorption.[22]

Calcium

Recommendations for calcium intake during pregnancy vary widely among countries, although there is universal agreement that these needs are significantly elevated over nonpregnant needs. There is no evidence that low calcium intake jeopardizes infant health, however, and the life-long consequences to maternal bone health are unclear. Data on the effect of pregnancy and lactation on bone health are inconsistent.[23] As noted in Chapter 4, vegetarians may need less calcium than omnivores by virtue of their lower intake of total protein and also perhaps because of their lower intake of animal foods. Nevertheless, because of the complexity of bone health and the myriad of factors that affect it, in the absence of better data it is prudent for Western pregnant vegetarians to meet the current RDA of 1,200 mg of calcium.

Western cultures stress the use of dairy foods to meet calcium needs, especially in conditions where the calcium requirement is elevated. So pervasive is the emphasis on dairy that other equally valid means of meeting calcium requirements are often viewed as overly difficult or inferior. Chapter 4 discusses in some detail how calcium needs can be met with plant foods.

Despite the high calcium content of many plant foods, the calcium intake of vegans is substantially lower than that of omnivores and lacto-ovo vegetarians. Therefore, when calcium needs are elevated, as they are in pregnancy and lactation, it is important that vegan women be able to identify several good sources of calcium that can be included in their diet on a daily basis. Many practitioners suggest daily use of fortified soymilk as a convenient way to meet calcium needs. Where clients prefer not to use soymilk or do not use it daily, a list of calcium-rich foods can help in planning diets that meet needs. The food guides in Appendix 8-A will not automatically produce diets that are adequate in calcium unless appropriate choices are made within the groups. Therefore, it is helpful if clients have an understanding of which foods are rich in calcium.

It is also important to remember that calcium absorption from some plant foods is superior to that from milk. Therefore, the amount of calcium absorbed may meet biologic needs even when total calcium consumed is lower than the RDA. If only foods with poorly absorbed calcium are chosen, the opposite may be true.

Vitamin D

Historically, severe osteomalacia has caused pelvic deformities significant enough to prevent normal delivery, but it was not until the 1920s that vitamin D deficiency was found to be the cause.[24,25] Although severe cases of osteomalacia are now rare, women with inadequate vitamin D status can give birth to infants with tetany and congenital rickets.[26]

Vitamin D deficiency has been reported in vegetarians, particularly Asian vegetarians,[27-31] and in comparison with omnivores vitamin D intake is lower in vegans and is somewhat lower in lacto-ovo vegetarians.[32-36] Also, lower circulating levels of vitamin D have been seen in Asian vegetarians,[27,37-43] although in some cases where vegetarian vitamin D intake was lower than in nonvegetarians no differences in serum levels of vitamin D were observed.[44,45] In most people, even in the winter, the concentration of vitamin D in the serum is not determined by current vitamin D intake but rather by the amount of exposure to solar radiation during the previous summer.[46]

Vitamin D recommendations are 100% higher (10 µg) for pregnant than for nonpregnant women. It is possible to meet vitamin D requirements through sun exposure, but this may not be a realistic option for many women, so that exogenous sources of the vitamin are sometimes required. Vitamin D is poorly supplied by foods, so that fortified foods are nearly always the best way to provide dietary vitamin D. For vegetarians, fortified foods can include some brands of soymilk, cow's milk, some cheeses, some cereals, and some meat analogues. Chapter 6 includes a list of fortified foods. Vitamin D supplements should be used with caution because vitamin D intake that is only a few times the RDA can be toxic. Vitamin D toxicity can cause fetal abnormalities.

Vitamin B12

Fetal vitamin B12 requirements are small, just 0.1 to 0.2 µg/day. The National Research Council notes that infant needs can generally be met through the mother's stores. Some research suggests, however, that stored vitamin B12 is not available to the fetus or to the breastfeeding infant.[47,48] Specker et al[48] reported that in infants breastfed by vegetarian mothers levels of methylmalonic acid (MMA) were not related to the length of time that the mother had been a vegetarian, although maternal levels of serum vitamin B12 decreased the longer she had been a vegetarian. MMA levels increase in response to a deficiency of vitamin B12 because the vitamin B12–requiring enzyme methymalonyl coenzyme A mutase is required for the normal metabolism of MMA.[49] Consequently, it was suggested that only newly absorbed vitamin B_{12} is transported across the placenta or into breast milk. In contrast, however, a later study by Specker et al[50] found that breast milk vitamin B_{12} levels decreased the longer a woman had followed a vegetarian diet. This suggests that, for breastfeeding at least, storage forms of B_{12} do pass into breast milk. Other studies have shown that, when maternal serum vitamin B_{12} levels are low, breast milk vitamin B_{12} levels will also be low, resulting in inadequate vitamin intake in infants.[51,52] Furthermore, infants may be born with low stores of vitamin B_{12} if maternal B_{12} levels are low. Lactation may also deplete maternal vitamin B_{12} stores.[53]

As long as the availability of vitamin B_{12} from maternal stores remains controversial, it is prudent to recommend that all pregnant vegetarians consume a regular source of vitamin B_{12} throughout pregnancy. Milk and eggs can provide considerable amounts of vitamin B_{12} in the diets of lacto-ovo vegetarians. Vegans can meet needs easily if fortified foods or supplements are used.

Zinc

Because body stores of zinc are not readily accessible[54] and dietary zinc requirements increase by 50% during pregnancy, concern has been expressed over vegetarian zinc status during pregnancy. Poor maternal zinc status has been associated with low birth weight and infant growth retardation.[55,56] Also, the use of folate and iron supplements, which are common in pregnancy, can adversely affect zinc status.[57,58] In one study of pregnant women, vegetarians consumed slightly less zinc than omnivores, although there were no differences in plasma, urine, and hair zinc levels.[7] Another study of pregnant women reported that vegetarian zinc intake was similar to that of nonvegetarians.[8] Finally, although Hindu lacto-ovo vegetarians had low zinc intakes, even in the few subjects who consumed less than 5 mg/day the birth weights of infants were normal.[59]

Zinc intake is generally quite a bit lower than the RDA among Western pregnant women, whether or not they are vegetarians. Zinc absorption is likely to be lower from a vegetarian diet; therefore, pregnant women, but especially pregnant vegetarians, need to emphasize zinc-rich foods in the diet. Chapter 5 provides a list of vegetarian foods that are rich in zinc.

MEAL-PLANNING GUIDELINES

A number of food guides have been developed to help pregnant vegetarians meet nutrient needs. As is true at all stages of the life cycle, these can serve only as a general guide. Calorie needs will vary among women depending on many factors.

A meal pattern of three meals and several snacks per day can help many women meet their calorie needs. As the third trimester progresses, many women will feel some discomfort after large meals, so that frequent small meals are advised. This may be especially valuable for vegetarians, whose diets are higher in fiber and therefore produce a greater feeling of fullness.

Although a woman experiencing a first-time pregnancy may have the time and energy to prepare a variety of meals throughout the day, women with small children and/or those who work full time outside of the home may have little time and energy for meal preparation. Dietitians can help pregnant clients plan meals and snacks that take little time and should encourage clients to use convenience foods if time is a factor. There are many that are suitable for vegetarians. Exhibit 8–1 provides some ideas for fast meals and snacks.

ADOLESCENT PREGNANCY

The frequency of perinatal complications is higher among adolescents than among adult women. Good nutrition, proper prenatal care, and improved health habits can all serve to reduce the risk of complications in adolescent pregnancy.[60] Because the average age of menarche in the United States is 12 to 13 years and growth usually continues for 4 years after menarche, pregnant adolescents younger than 17 years need to meet the high nutritional needs of both pregnancy and their own growth and development.

Estimated energy requirements for adolescent girls are between 2,500 and 2,700 kcal/day. An additional 300 kcal/day are needed for pregnancy. Energy needs are somewhat difficult to determine, however, because growth

---

Exhibit 8–1 Suggestions for Fast Meals and Snacks

- Bagel with almond butter and a piece of fruit
- Canned vegetable soup, salad, bread
- Rice pilaf using a packaged mix tossed with steamed frozen mixed vegetables
- Cereal with soymilk or cow's milk and sliced fresh fruit
- Bran muffin and fruit juice
- Trail mix and fruit juice
- Spaghetti with prepared sauce
- Textured vegetable protein with Sloppy Joe sauce served over hamburger buns
- Bean burritos using canned or dehydrated beans and chopped tomatoes

rates and calorie needs vary considerably throughout adolescence. It is more helpful to monitor weight gain during the pregnancy. In determining weight gain goals for the adolescent, it is necessary to remember that total gain must account for the needs of pregnancy as well as the normal weight gain that would take place in a nonpregnant adolescent. Table 8–3 shows approximate weight gains for nonpregnant teenage girls over a 9-month period based on postmenarcheal year. Weight gain goals for pregnant adolescents can be determined by adding normal 9-month weight increases to the desired weight gain for an adult pregnant woman. In some cases, if the teenager is underweight, goals for weight gain can be as high as 40 lb.

Nutrient requirements can be estimated by adding the increase in RDAs for pregnancy to the RDAs for nonpregnant adolescent girls. For example, the RDA for calcium increases by 400 mg in pregnancy. When 400 mg is added to the adolescent calcium RDA of 1,200 mg, the suggested intake for pregnant adolescents would be 1,600 mg/day.

Exhibit 8–2 illustrates the increased nutrient needs of adolescent pregnancy. Because the RDAs have considerable safety margins, however (with the exception of calories), this summing of the needs of adolescence and pregnancy may yield numbers that are quite a bit higher than necessary. Also, growth is erratic during adolescence, and both energy and nutrient needs will vary among pregnant teens accordingly. For these reasons, the nutrient needs of pregnant adolescents are poorly understood. An appropriate approach is to plan diets to meet the RDAs of pregnant adults with caloric adjustments for teenagers. By meeting energy needs with a variety of nutrient-dense foods, a nutrient intake adequate for pregnant teens should be achieved. Because teenage girls commonly do not meet the RDA for iron, supplements are probably advised for all pregnant teens.

It is likely that dietitians who counsel pregnant women will have occasion to work with pregnant teenagers who are vegetarians. Pregnancy is on the

---

Table 8–3 Approximate 9-Month Weight Gains for Postmenarcheal Women

Postmenarcheal Year	Weight Gain (lb)
1	8.0
2	5.0
3	2.0
4	1.3

Source: Worthington BS. Human milk composition and infant growth and development. In: Worthington-Roberts B, Rodwell-Williams S, eds, *Nutrition in Pregnancy and Lactation,* 5th ed. St. Louis: Mosby; 1978: 347–401.

Exhibit 8–2 Suggested Rate of Weight Gain for Adolescents (in Second and Third Trimesters)

Normal weight: 0.529 kg/week (1.6 lbs/week)
Underweight: 0.588 kg/week (1.30 lbs/week)
Overweight: 0.386 kg/week (0.850 lbs/week)

Source: Data from Institute of Medicine, National Academy of Sciences, *Nutritional during Pregnancy.* National Academy Press: Washington, DC; 1990.

---

rise among the adolescent population, and vegetarianism is increasingly popular with this age group as well. Lacto-ovo vegetarian diets can meet the calorie and nutrient needs of pregnant adolescents with ease. Vegan diets can also supply all the nutrients to support a healthy pregnancy. The satiety value of the high-fiber vegan diet and the lower fat content, however, may require that some attention be given to meeting energy and nutrient needs.

There are no data on the pregnancy outcome of pregnant vegetarian teens. Pregnancy outcome in well-nourished vegetarian adult women is at least as good as in nonvegetarian adult women, however, and growth of nonpregnant vegetarian teens is comparable to that of omnivore teens. Based on these relationships, it is a fair assumption that pregnancy outcome among vegetarian adolescents should be comparable to that of nonvegetarian adolescents.

POTENTIAL COMPLICATIONS OF PREGNANCY

Pregnancy Induced Hypertension (PIH)

PIH, also referred to as preeclampsia, is a set of symptoms that include elevated blood pressure and proteinuria. One early sign is rapid weight gain due to edema. Women who are especially at risk include adolescents, older women, and low-income women. If preeclampsia progresses to eclampsia or toxemia of pregnancy, the result can be convulsions, coma, and fetal death.

The etiology of preeclampsia remains elusive. It is more likely to occur in women who had hypertension before pregnancy as well as women with diabetes and kidney disease. It has been suggested that inadequate protein or calcium intake is linked to an increased risk.[12] There is also evidence that increased intake of antioxidants, which are abundant in plant foods, may reduce risk.[18] Interestingly, one study has shown a remarkable reduction in risk among vegetarians. Of 775 vegan pregnancies, there was only one case of preeclampsia.[4] Because preeclampsia occurs in about 5% to 10% of all pregnancies in the general population, the rate among these vegans was about 2% of the rate seen in the general population.[61] In a smaller study, however, there were no differences in the incidence of PIH between vegans and controls.[5]

Gestational Diabetes

Gestational diabetes is a temporary condition that occurs during pregnancy and generally disappears after delivery. It occurs in 3% to 12% of pregnant women, generally around week 25 of pregnancy.[62] Gestational diabetes is a more extreme case of the insulin resistance that is typical in pregnancy, which is due to activity of placental hormones. Complications of gestational diabetes include macrosomia, hypoglycemia in the newborn, respiratory distress syndrome in the newborn, preeclampsia, and urinary tract infections in the mother.

Adequate weight gain and an even, steady pace of gain is important for women with gestational diabetes. Small, frequent meals can help control blood glucose levels. Dietary guidelines for women with gestational diabetes combine the general principles for treating diabetes discussed in Chapter 14 with the increased nutrient needs of pregnancy. If exogenous insulin therapy is needed, the dietitian will need to work closely with the client to ensure that distribution of caloric intake is appropriate to the insulin schedule being followed.

There are no data to suggest that vegetarian women are at greater or lesser risk for gestational diabetes. Once the physician and dietitian have determined the appropriate caloric intake and the distribution of macronutrients, the exchange lists in Chapter 14 can be used to plan a vegetarian diet that meets the needs of the client with gestational diabetes.

COMMON CONDITIONS OF PREGNANCY

Dietitians are frequently called upon to help clients manage temporary conditions of pregnancy.

Nausea

Commonly referred to as morning sickness, nausea of early pregnancy can occur at any time of the day. It can be exacerbated by an empty stomach, so that many women will experience it first thing in the morning. Although nausea typically disappears by the end of the fourth month of pregnancy, it can persist throughout pregnancy. Nausea of pregnancy is linked to the presence of progesterone and estrogens in the stomach.

In addition to the discomfort of the mother, the most serious consequence of nausea of pregnancy is that women will often not feel like eating, or the variety of foods that they are comfortable eating may be limited. The dietitian can help clients plan food intake in such a way that it will ease the symptoms of morning sickness and maximize the nutritional quality of the diet to the greatest extent possible under the circumstances. The following suggestions may be helpful:

- *Avoid an empty stomach.* Increased acid in the stomach and the possibility of low blood glucose can exacerbate nausea. Frequent small meals will help the pregnant woman keep something in her stomach and maintain normal levels of blood glucose.

- *Keep food near the bed.* Eating immediately upon waking may stave off morning sickness in some women. Dry foods such as crackers or bread may be best tolerated.

- *Eat healthy foods that are well tolerated.* The pregnant woman may experience many food aversions, so that the number of foods tolerated may be limited, but by concentrating on the foods that she is able to tolerate it is often possible to plan a diet that will meet both calorie and nutrient needs. Many women will find starchy, sweet, and salty foods to be best tolerated. Good suggestions in these categories include whole grain breads, bagels, crackers, muffins, stewed fruits, dried fruits, vegetable juices, dry cereals, miso broth, and mashed potatoes. Although some foods tend to be tolerated better than others, this can vary considerably among women. Conventional wisdom can aid the dietitian in generating a list of suggested foods, but it is important to listen to the client's own ideas about what appeals to her. Many foods that are staples in some vegetarian diets, such as soymilk, leafy green vegetables, and legumes, may not appeal to the woman with morning sickness. The consumption of these foods should be encouraged on the days when the woman does feel good, and more acceptable ways in which they can be included in the diet should be considered. For example, although a serving of steamed kale may not be tolerated, a small amount of kale in a cup of miso broth may be acceptable.

- *Avoid liquids with meals.* The mixture of solid foods with liquids can increase nausea in some women.

Constipation

Constipation is common in the last trimester of pregnancy but can occur at any time. It is partly due to increased levels of the hormone progesterone, which slows muscle contractions. Also, the pressure of the growing uterus on the intestines can interfere with elimination. The constipating effects of iron supplements and, in some women, reduced physical activity as pregnancy progresses also contribute to constipation. Vegetarians may have an advantage because they eat high-fiber diets. Other ways to relieve constipation include moderate exercise (such as walking) and drinking plenty of liquids.

Heartburn

Heartburn results when stomach acid is released into the esophagus. It is common in pregnancy for two reasons. First, progesterone causes the esophageal sphincter to relax, allowing acid to pass into the esophagus more easily. Second, as the uterus presses on the stomach, it creates pressure, allowing more acid to pass into the esophagus. The following strategies can help ease heartburn in pregnancy:

- Eat smaller, more frequent meals to avoid feelings of overfullness.
- Remain upright after eating.
- Engage in moderate exercise, such as walking, after a meal.
- Avoid fatty foods, carbonated beverages, and acidic foods.
- Eat slowly.

VEGETARIANS AND LACTATION

Nutritional needs of lactating women are similar to those of pregnant women. The nutritional cost of milk synthesis and of providing nutrients for a growing infant, however, means that breastfeeding women require more calories. Energy requirements are about 500 calories above the needs of a nonpregnant, nonbreastfeeding woman or about 200 kcal/day more than for pregnancy. Requirements are also higher for protein, vitamin E, vitamin C, thiamin, riboflavin, niacin, vitamin B_{12}, magnesium, zinc, iodine, and selenium. Iron, vitamin B_6, and folate requirements decrease, and the needs for calcium, vitamin D, phosphorus, and vitamin K are the same as for pregnant women.

The nutritional composition of milk is affected by the woman's diet to variable degrees. Nutrients that are most sensitive to the mother's intake are most of the B vitamins and vitamins A, C, and D.[63] The levels of other nutrients, including vitamin K, folate, sodium, calcium, phosphorus, magnesium, iron, zinc, and copper, remain constant regardless of the mother's diet. Concentrations of fluoride, iodine, and selenium show geographic variations in cow's milk and may do the same in human milk, although the data to support this are not available[63] (Table 8–4).

The fat content of milk varies widely depending on maternal diet.[64,65] Generally, breast milk is about 51% fat, but in undernourished women the fat content can be considerably lower than this.[66] The total fat content of the milk of vegetarian mothers is similar to that of omnivores.[67] Fatty acid content varies according to the type of dietary fat consumed, however.[68–70] The saturated fat content of vegetarians' milk reflects the lower saturated fat content of the maternal diet.[67] A study of four British vegans found that their breast milk contained less eicosapentaenoic acid (EPA) and saturated fat and more linoleic and linolenic acid than that of the general population.[71] The milk of macrobiotic vegans is also higher in linoleic and linolenic acid than that of omnivores[72] (Table 8–5).

Fat composition will vary only to a limited degree, however. There appears to be an upper limit to how much fat can be removed from the mother's blood and passed into milk; above this level, the primary source of fatty acids is mammary synthesis.[67] The cholesterol content of breast milk is not sensitive to maternal diet and ranges from 10 to 20 mg/dL; daily infant consumption is about 100 mg.

The milk of vegetarian mothers is nutritionally adequate, and breastfed infants of well-nourished vegetarian women grow and develop normally.[73,74] An analysis of the milk of a group of macrobiotic women showed slightly decreased levels of calcium, magnesium, and vitamin B_{12} but no differences

Table 8–4 Effects of Maternal Dietary Changes on Nutrient Composition of Breast Milk

Nutrient Levels That Change with Changes in Maternal Diet	Nutrient Levels That Do Not Change with Changes in Maternal Diet	Nutrients for Which Effects of Changes in Maternal Diet Are Unknown
Thiamin	Folate	Pyridoxine
Riboflavin	Vitamin K	Biotin
Niacin	Sodium	Vitamin E
Pantothenic acid	Calcium	Selenium
Vitamin B_{12}	Phosphorus	
Vitamin C	Magnesium	
Vitamin A	Iron	
Vitamin D	Zinc	
Manganese	Copper	
Iodine	Fluoride	

Table 8–5 Mean Breast Milk Fatty Acid Concentration in Vegans and Nonvegetarians (mg/g Total Methyl Esters)

Methyl Esters	Vegans	Controls
Lauric	39	33
Myristic	68	80
Palmitic	166	276
Stearic	52	108
Palmitoleic	12	36
Oleic	313	353
Linoleic	317	69
Linolenic	15	8

Source: Sander TAB et al. Studies of vegans: The fatty acid composition of plasma choline phospho-glycerides, erythrocytes, adipose tissue and breast milk and some indicators of susceptibility to ischemic heart disease in vegans and omnivore controls. *American Journal of Clinical Nutrition.* 1978; 31:805.

in energy or protein levels.[75] Several of these women did have increased levels of lactose in their milk, however; elevated lactose in milk has been associated with maternal undernutrition[76] (Table 8–6).

Vitamin D content of milk varies with maternal diet or sun exposure.[77,78] Cord levels of vitamin D in a group of Asian, largely vegetarian women were only about half those of the Caucasian nonvegetarian women in this study, although cord levels were not related to birth weight.[79] Supplemental vitamin D is commonly prescribed for all breastfed infants and decreases in bone mineral content have been found in unsupplemented infants.[80,81]

The milk of vegans is lower in the amino acid taurine compared with the milk of omnivores,[82] but levels are still approximately 30 times greater than in cow's milk infant formula.[83] Selenium levels and glutathione peroxidase activity were significantly greater in the breast milk of vegetarians in com-

Table 8–6 Content of Selected Nutrients in Breast Milk of Well-Nourished and Poorly Nourished Women

Population	Fat (g/100 mL)	Lactose (g/100 mL)	Protein (g/100 mL)	Calcium (mg/100 mL)
United States	4.50	6.80	1.10	34.0
England	4.78	6.95	1.16	29.9
South Africa (Black)	3.90	7.10	1.35	28.7
Nigeria	4.05	7.67	1.22	not reported
Wuppertal, Germany (after World War II)	3.59	not reported	1.20	not reported

parison to that of nonvegetarians in one study, which may provide the infant with an extra measure of protection against free radical–induced oxidative damage.[84]

Generally, the mineral content of milk does not vary with maternal diet.[63] Specifically, no differences were reported in levels of iron, copper, zinc, sodium, potassium, calcium, magnesium, and lactose or in total fat in the milk of vegetarians and omnivores, although in this study both groups used supplements.[85]

One observed difference between the milk of vegetarians and omnivores is in the level of environmental contaminants (Figure 8–1). The passage of certain contaminants into breast milk has been noted since 1951.[86] The substances of most concern are those that are soluble in fat and are toxic. These include the pesticides DDT, chlordane, heptachlor, and dieldrin and industrial compounds or byproducts, such as polychlorinated biphenyls (PCBs)

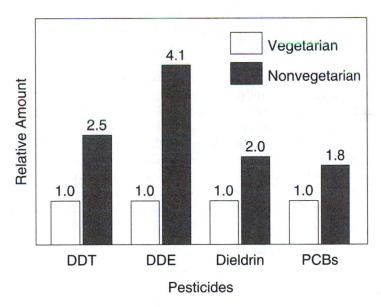

Figure 8–1 Relative levels of pesticides in breast milk from two sisters with different dietary habits. For purposes of the graph, concentrations of pesticides and PCBs in the nonvegetarian sister (age, 32 years) are expressed as a percentage relative to the lactovegetarian (age, 33 years). Actual values for the nonvegetarian sister for DDT, DDE, dieldrin, and PCBs were 0.50, 1.60, 0.025, and 0.80 mg/kg milk fat, respectively. Values for the vegetarian sister for DDT, DDE, dieldrin, and PCBs were 0.20, 0.39, 0.012, and 0.44 mg/kg milk fat, respectively. *Source:* Data from reference 91.

and polychlorinated dibenzodioxins. It is estimated that 30% of breast milk contains higher than allowable levels (as determined by the Food and Drug Administration and the World Health Organization) of some of these compounds.[87] Potentially toxic environmental pollutants are commonly found in human milk at levels that would prevent its sale as a commercial food for infants.[88]

Studies of vegetarians show lower levels of these compounds in their breast milk. In an analysis of breast milk of Tennessee vegans, levels of 17 chemicals were markedly lower than in the general population.[89] The highest vegan value was lower than the lowest value seen in breast milk samples from the general population. In most cases, levels were only 1% to 2% of those in the samples from the general population. Similar results were seen in the breast milk of macrobiotic women.[75] Frequency of consumption of meat, dairy, and fish was directly related to milk contamination.[75] Contaminant levels were much higher in the milk of women with a high consumption of meat and animal fat than in the milk of vegetarians who shopped at health food stores.[90] Finally, levels of DDT, DDE, and PCBs were lowest in the milk of lacto-ovo vegetarians and highest in the milk of women who ate fatty fish from the Baltic Sea. Women on conventional diets fell somewhere in the middle.[91]

Breastfeeding vegetarian mothers can follow the same general meal-planning guidelines as pregnant women with slight increases in intake to meet the slightly elevated energy and nutritional requirements of lactation (see Appendix 8-A). An additional serving each of legumes, grains and vegetables per day can provide the necessary calories and nutrients. In addition, lactating women should be encouraged to drink plenty of fluids, although women who drink to satisfy the increased thirst that is typical in breastfeeding seem to meet fluid needs. There does not appear to be any advantage to forcing fluids. Small reductions in calories can aid in gradual weight loss without compromising milk output. Severe caloric restriction should be avoided, however, because it can reduce milk volume.

REFERENCES

1. Hytten RE, Leitch I. *The Physiology of Human Pregnancy*. 2nd ed. Oxford, England: Blackwell Scientific; 1971.

2. World Health Organization (WHO). *Energy and Protein Requirements. Report of a Joint Food and Agriculture Organization/WHO/United Nations University Expert Consultation* (Technical Report Series 724). Geneva, Switzerland: WHO; 1985.

3. National Research Council. *Recommended Dietary Allowances*. 10th ed. Washington, DC: National Academy Press; 1989.

4. Carter JP, Furman T, Hutcheson HR. Preeclampsia and reproductive performance in a community of vegans. *South Med J.* 1987;80:692–697.

5. Thomas J, Ellis FR. The health of vegans during pregnancy. *Proc Nutr Soc.* 1977;36:46A.

6. Ward RJ, Abraham R, McFadyen IR, et al. Assessment of trace metal intake and status in a Gujerati pregnant Asian population and their influence on the outcome of pregnancy. *Br J Obstet Gynaecol.* 1988;95:676–682.

7. King JC, Stein T, Doyle M. Effect of vegetarianism on the zinc status of pregnant women. *Am J Clin Nutr.* 1981;34:1049–1055.

8. Abu-Assal MJ, Craig WJ. The zinc status of pregnant women. *Nutr Rep Int.* 1984;29:485–494.

9. Dagnelie PC, van Staveren WA, van Klaveren JD, Burema J. Do children on macrobiotic diets show catch-up growth? *Eur J Clin Nutr.* 1988;42:1007–1016.

10. Dagnelie PC, van Staveren WA, Vergote FJVRA, et al. Nutritional status of infants aged 4 to 18 months on macrobiotic diets and matched omnivorous control infants: A population-based mixed-longitudinal study. II. Growth and psychomotor development. *Eur J Clin Nutr.* 1989;43:325–328.

11. Shull MW, Reed RB, Valadian I, Palombo R, Thorne H, Dwyer JT. Velocities of growth in vegetarian preschool children. *Pediatrics.* 1977;60:410–417.

12. Brewer T. Role of malnutrition in pre-eclampsia and eclampsia. *Am J Obstet Gynecol.* 1977;125:281–282.

13. Osofsky HJ. Relationships between prenatal medical and nutritional measures, pregnancy outcome and early infant development in an urban poverty setting. *Am J Obstet Gynecol.* 1975;123:682–690.

14. Grieve JF. Prevention of gestational failure by high protein diet. *J Reprod Med.* 1974;13:170–174.

15. Williams C, Highley W, Ma EH, et al. Protein, amino acid and caloric intakes of selected pregnant women. *J Am Diet Assoc.* 1981;78:28–35.

16. Johnstone FD, Campbell DM, MacGillivary I. Nitrogen balance studies in human pregnancy. *J Nutr.* 1981;111:1884–1893.

17. Rush D, Stein Z, Susser M. Controlled trial of prenatal nutrition supplementation defended. *Pediatrics.* 1980;66:656–658.

18. Rush D, Stein Z, Susser M. *Diet in Pregnancy: A Randomized Controlled Trial of Nutritional Supplements.* New York, NY: Liss; 1980.

19. US Preventive Services Task Force. Routine iron supplementation during pregnancy: Policy statement. *JAMA.* 1993;270:2846–2854.

20. Finley DA, Dewey KG, Lonnerdal B, Grivetti LE. Food choices of vegetarians and nonvegetarians during pregnancy and lactation. *J Am Diet Assoc.* 1985;85:678–685.

21. Hubel CA. Lipid peroxidation in pregnancy: New perspectives on preeclampsia. *Am J Obstet Gynecol.* 1989;161:1025–1034.

22. Monsen ER, Balintfy JL. Calculating dietary iron bioavailability: Refinement and computerization. *J Am Diet Assoc.* 1982;80:307–311.

23. Sowers MR, Galuska DA. Epidemiology of bone mass in premenopausal women. *Epidemiol Rev.* 1993;16:374–398.

24. Maxwell JP, Miles LMJ. *J Obstet Gynecol.* 1925;32:433.

25. Maxwell JP. *Proc R Soc Med.* 1935;28:265.

26. Ford JA, Davidson DC, McIntosh WB, Fyfe WM, Donningan MG. *Br Med J.* 1973;3:211.

27. Iq-bal SJ, Garrick DP, Howl A. Evidence of continuing "deprivational" vitamin D deficiency in Asians in the UK. *J Hum Nutr Diet.* 1994;7:47–52.

28. Ford JA, Calhoun EM, McIntosh WB, et al. Biochemical response of late rickets and osteomalacia to a chupatty-free diet. *Br Med J.* 1972;3:446–447.

29. Stadler VG, Schmid R, Held U, et al. Serological and radiological improvement of vitamin D-deficiency rickets on treatment with vitamin D in spite of a calcium-free diet. *Ann Pediatr.* 1962;199:215–225.

30. Dent CE, Round JM, Bowe DJF, et al. Effects of chappatia and ultraviolet irradiation on nutritional rickets in an Indian immigrant. *Lancet.* 1973;2:1282–1284.

31. Cooks WT, Asquith P, Ruck N, et al. Rickets, growth and alkaline phosphatase in urban adolescents. *Br Med J.* 1974;2:293–297.

32. Carlson E, Kipps M, Lockie A, Thomson J. A comparative evaluation of vegan, vegetarian and omnivore diets. *J Plant Foods.* 1985;6:89–100.

33. Lamberg-Allardt C, Karkkainen M, Sepanen R, Bistrom H. Low serum 25-hydroxyvitamin D concentrations and secondary hyperparathyroidism in middle-aged white strict vegetarians. *Am J Clin Nutr.* 1993;58:684–689.

34. Lloyd T, Schaeffer JM, Walker MA, Demers LM. Urinary hormonal concentrations and spinal bone densities of premenopausal vegetarian and nonvegetarian women. *Am J Clin Nutr.* 1991;54:1005–1010.

35. Nieman DC, Underwood BC, Sherman KM, et al. Dietary status of Seventh-Day Adventist vegetarian and non-vegetarian elderly women. *J Am Diet Assoc.* 1989;89:1763–1769.

36. Alexander D, Ball MJ, Mann J. Nutrient intake and haematological status of vegetarians and age-sex matched omnivores. *Eur J Clin Nutr.* 1994;48:538–546.

37. Preece MA, Tomlinson S, Ribot CA, et al. Studies of vitamin D deficiency in man. *Q J Med.* 1975;44:575–579.

38. Hunt SP, O'Riordon JLH, Windo J, Truswell S. Vitamin D status in different subgroups of British Asians. *Br Med J.* 1976;2:1351–1354.

39. Wilmana PF, Brodie MJ, Mucklow JC, et al. Reduction of circulating 25-hydroxyvitamin D by antipyrine. *Br J Clin Pharmacol.* 1979;8:523–528.

40. Dandona P, Mohiuddin J, Weerakoon JW, Freedman DB, Fonseca V, Healey T. Persistence of parathyroid hypersecretion after vitamin D treatment in Asian vegetarians. *J Clin Endocrinol Metab.* 1984;59:535–537.

41. Isenberg DA, Newham D, Edwards RHT, Wiles CM, Young A. Muscle strength and pre-osteomalacia in vegetarian and Asian women. *Lancet.* 1982;1:55.

42. Dent CE, Gupta MM. Plasma 25-hydroxyvitamin-D levels during pregnancy in Caucasians and in vegetarian and non-vegetarian Asians. *Lancet.* 1975;2:1057–1060.

43. Henderson JB, Dunnigan MG, McIntosh WB, Abdul-Motaal AA, Gettinby G, Glekin BM. The importance of limited exposure to ultraviolet radiation and dietary factors in the aetiology of Asian rickets: A risk-factor model. *Q J Med.* 1987;63:413–425.

44. Kumpusalo E, Karinpää A, Jauhiainen M, Laitinen Lappeteläinen R, Mäenpää PH. Multivitamin supplementation of adult omnivores and lactovegetarians: Circulating levels of vitamin A, D, and E, lipids, apolipoproteins and selenium. *Int J Vitam Nutr Res.* 1989;60:58–66.

45. Ellis FR, Montegriffo VME. Veganism, clinical findings and investigations. *Am J Clin Nutr.* 1970;23:249–255.

46. Poskit EME, Cole TJ, Lawson DEM. Diet, sunlight, and 25-hydroxyvitamin D in healthy children and adults. *Br Med J.* 1979;1:221–223.

47. Lubby AL, Cooperman JM, Donnfeld AM, et al. Observations on transfer of vitamin B12 from mother to fetus and newborn. *Am J Dis Child.* 1958;96:532–533.

48. Specker BL, Miller D, Norman EJ, Greene H, Hayes KC. Increased urinary methylmalonic acid excretion in breast-fed infants of vegetarian mothers and identification of an acceptable dietary source of vitamin B12. *Am J Clin Nutr.* 1988;47:89–92.

49. Norman EJ. Detection of cobalamin deficiency using the urinary methylmalonic acid test by gas chromatography mass spectrometry. *J Clin Pathol.* 1992;45:382.

50. Specker BL, Black A, Allen L, Morrow F. Vitamin B12: Low milk concentrations are related to low serum concentrations in vegetarian women and to methylmalonic aciduria in their infants. *Am J Clin Nutr.* 1990;52:1073–1076.

51. Kuhne T, Bubl R, Baumgartner R. Maternal vegan diet causing a serious infantile neurological disorder due to vitamin B12 deficiency. *Eur J Pediatr.* 1991;150:205–208.

52. Black AK, Allen LH, Pelto GH, de Mata MP, Chavez A. Iron, vitamin B12 and folate status in men and women and during pregnancy and lactation. *J Nutr.* 1994;124:1179–1188.

53. Allen LH, Rosado JL, Casterline JE, et al. Vitamin B12 deficiency and malabsorption are highly prevalent in rural Mexican communities. *Am J Clin Nutr.* 1995;62:1013–1019.

54. Chesters JK. Metabolism and biochemistry of zinc. In: Prasad AS, ed. *Current Topics in Nutrition and Disease.* New York, NY: Liss; 1982;6:221–238.

55. Neggers YH, Cutter GR, Action RT, et al. A positive association between maternal serum zinc concentration and birth weight. *Am J Clin Nutr.* 1990;51:678–684.

56. Wells HL, James DK, Luxton R, Rennock CA. Maternal leukocyte zinc deficiency at start of third trimester as a predictor of fetal growth retardation. *Br Med J.* 1987;294:1054–1056.

57. Meadows NJ, Grainger SL, Ruse W, Keeling PWN, Thompson RPH. Oral iron and the bioavailability of zinc. *Br Med J.* 1983;287:1013–1014.

58. Milne DB, Canfield WK, Mahalko JR, Sandstead HH. Effect of oral folic acid supplements on zinc, copper and iron absorption and excretion. *Am J Clin Nutr.* 1984;39:535–539.

59. Campbell-Brown M, Ward RJ, Haines AP, North WRS, Abraham R, McFadyen IR. Zinc and copper in Asian pregnancies—Is there evidence for a nutritional deficiency? *Br J Obstet Gynaecol.* 1985;92:875–885.

60. Committee on Adolescence, American Academy of Pediatrics. Statement on teenage pregnancy. *Pediatrics.* 1979;63:795–797.

61. Institute of Medicine Subcommittee on Nutritional Status and Weight Gain during Pregnancy. *Nutrition during Pregnancy.* Washington, DC: National Academy Press; 1990.

62. Braveman P, et al. Evaluating outcomes of pregnancy in diabetic women, epidemiologic considerations and recommended indicators. *Diabetes Care.* 1985;6:365.

63. Worthington BS. Human milk composition and infant growth and development. In: Worthington-Roberts B, Rodwell-Williams S, eds. *Nutrition in Pregnancy and Lactation.* 5th ed. St Louis, Mo: Mosby; 1978:347–401.

64. Jensen RG, Clark RM, Ferris AM. Composition of the lipids in human milk: A review. *Lipids.* 1980;15:345–355.

65. Jensen RG, Hagerty MH, MaMahon KE. Lipids of human milk and infant formulas: A review. *Am J Clin Nutr.* 1980;31:990–1016.

66. Jelliffe DB, Jelliffe EFP. The volume and composition of human milk in poorly nourished communities. A review. *Am J Clin Nutr.* 1978;31:492–515.

67. Finley DA, Lonnerdal B, Dewey KG, Grivetti LE. Breast milk composition: Fat content and fatty acid composition in vegetarians and non-vegetarians. *Am J Clin Nutr.* 1985;41:787–800.

68. Emery WB III, Canolty NL, Atchison JM, Dunkley WL. Effects of sampling and dietary fat on gross and fatty acid composition of human milk. *Nutr Rep Int.* 1978;17:63–70.

69. Kramer M, Szoke K, Lindner K, Tarjan R. The effect of different factors on the composition of human milk and its variations. III. Effect of dietary fats on lipid composition of human milk. *Nutr Diet.* 1965;7:71–79.

70. Mellies MJ, Ishikawa TT, Gartside PS, et al. Effects of varying maternal dietary fatty acids in lactating women and their infants. *Am J Clin Nutr.* 1979;32:299–303.

71. Sanders TAB, Ellis FR, Dickerson JWT. Studies of vegans: The fatty acid composition of plasma choline phosphoglycerides, erythrocytes, adipose tissue, and breast milk, and some indicators of susceptibility to ischemic heart disease in vegans and omnivore controls. *Am J Clin Nutr.* 1978;31:805–813.

72. Specker BL, Wey HE, Miller D. Differences in fatty acid composition of human milk in vegetarian and nonvegetarian women: Long term effect of diet. *J Pediatr Gastroenterol Nutr.* 1987;6:764–768.

73. American Dietetic Association. Position of the American Dietetic Association: Vegetarian diets. *J Am Diet Assoc.* 1988;88:351–355.

74. Johnston P. Counseling the pregnant vegetarian. *Am J Clin Nutr.* 1988;48:901–905.

75. Dagnelie PC, van Staveren WA, Roos AH, Tuinstra LGMT, Burema J. Nutrients and contaminants in human milk from mothers on macrobiotic and omnivorous diets. *Eur J Clin Nutr.* 1992;46:355–366.

76. Grindler J, Nwankwo MU, Omene JA, Roberts IM, LaRocca GM, Glew RH. Breast-milk composition and bile salt-stimulated lipase in well-nourished and undernourished Nigerian mothers. *Eur J Pediatr.* 1987;146:184–186.

77. Specker BL, Tsang RC. Effect of race and diet on human-milk vitamin D and 25-hydroxyvitamin D. *Am J Dis Child.* 1985;139:1134–1137.

78. Specker BL, Tsang RC. Cyclical serum 25-hydroxyvitamin D concentrations paralleling sunshine exposure in exclusively breast-fed infants. *J Pediatr.* 1987;110:744–747.

79. Abraham R, Brown C, North WRS, McFayden IR. Diets of Asian pregnant women in Harrow: Iron and vitamins. *Hum Nutr Appl Nutr.* 1987;41A:164–173.

80. Greer FR, et al. Bone mineral content and serum 25-hydroxyvitamin D concentrations in breast-fed infants with and without supplemental vitamin D. *J Pediatr.* 1981;98:696–701.

81. Greer FR, Searcy JE, Levin RS, et al. Bone mineral content and serum 25-hydroxyvitamin D concentrations in breast-fed infants with and without supplemental vitamin D: One year follow-up. *J Pediatr.* 1982;100:919–962.

82. Rana SK, Sanders TAB. Taurine concentrations in the diet, plasma, and urine and breast milk of vegans compared with omnivores. *Br J Nutr.* 1986;56:17–27.

83. Rassin DK, Sturman JA, Gaull GE. Taurine in developing rat brain, subcellular distribution and association with synaptic vesicles of [35S] taruine in maternal, fetal and neonatal rat brain. *J Neurochem.* 1977;28:41–50.

84. Debski B, Finley DA, Picciano MF, Lonnerdal B, Milner J. Selenium content and glutathionine peroxidase activity of milk from vegetarian and nonvegetarian women. *J Nutr.* 1989;119:215–220.

85. Finley DA, Lonnerdal B, Dewey KG, Grivetti LE. Inorganic constituents of breast milk from vegetarian and nonvegetarian women: Relationships with each other and with organic constituents. *J Nutr.* 1985;115:772–781.

86. Laug EP, Kunze FM, Prickett CS. Occurrence of DDT in human fat and milk. *Arch Ind Hyg Occup Med*. 1951;3:245–246.

87. Rogan WJ, Bagniewska A, Damstra T. Pollutants in breast milk. *N Engl J Med*. 1980;302:1450–1453.

88. Rogan WJ, Blanton PJ, Portier CJ, Stallard E. Should the presence of carcinogens in breast milk discourage breast feeding? *Regul Toxicol Pharmacol*. 1991;13:228–240.

89. Hergenrather J, Hlady G, Wallace B, Savage E. Pollutants in breast milk of vegetarians. *N Engl J Med*. 1981;304:792.

90. Centinkaya M, Gabel B, Podbielski A, Thiemann W. Untersuchung uber den Zusammenhang Zwischen Ernahrung und Lebensumstanden stillender Mutter und der Kontamination der Muttermilch mit schwerfluchtigen Organochlorverbindungen. *Akt Ernaehr*. 1984;9:157–162.

91. Noren K. Levels of organochlorine contaminants in human milk in relation to the dietary habits of the mothers. *Acta Paediatr Scand*. 1983;72:811–816.

Food Guides for Pregnant and Breastfeeding Vegetarians

FOOD GUIDE 1

	Number of Servings per Day*	
Food Group	Pregnant Women	Breastfeeding Women
Legumes, Nuts, Seeds	3	4
Milk or Milk Alternatives	4	4
Grains	6	7
Fruits	4	4
Vegetables	4	5

FOOD GUIDE II

	Number of Servings per Day*	
Food Group	Pregnant Women	Breastfeeding Women
Legumes, Nuts, Seeds, Milks	5	6
Grains	7	8
Vegetables	4	5
Fruits	4	4

*Suggested minimum number of servings. Some women may need additional servings and/or added fats to maintain adequate weight gain.

CHAPTER 9

Vegetarian Diets in Infancy

All infants begin life as vegetarians. Meats are generally not introduced into an infant's diet until 6 or 7 months of age. Until that time, infants consume breast milk, cow's milk formula, or soymilk formula. First solid foods are preferably infant cereals, vegetables, and fruits. Adapting the diet of older infants (6 to 12 months) to a vegetarian meal plan is a fairly simple matter achieved by substituting vegetable proteins, such as pureed beans or tofu, for strained meats.

GROWTH IN VEGETARIAN INFANTS

The birth weights of infants born to vegetarian mothers are similar to birth weight norms and those of infants born to nonvegetarian women.[1-4] In some macrobiotic populations, birth weights have been low and have been attributed to low weight gain in the mother during pregnancy.[5,6]

Vegetarian infants grow normally during the first 6 months of life.[1,2,7] This is expected because typically infants in both vegetarian and nonvegetarian families consume similar diets during this time. A slightly slower rate of growth among vegetarian infants that is still within the normal range may be attributed to the fact that vegetarian mothers are more likely to breastfeed.[2,8-10] Breastfed infants grow more slowly than formula-fed infants.[11] Energy intake that is too low may be a problem in some macrobiotic populations, however.[1,6,12] There is some evidence of poor growth in macrobiotic infants that has been attributed to inadequate quantities of milk in the diet.[6] When vegetarian infants receive adequate breast milk or formula and good sources of iron, vitamin B_{12}, and vitamin D, however, they grow well throughout infancy.[13] Soy formula has been shown to be adequate for supporting normal growth in infants.[14]

There are few data on the growth and development of nonmacrobiotic vegan infants. Older studies show, however, that restrictive food patterns among some vegetarian groups, coupled with erroneous ideas about what constitutes an appropriate diet for infancy, have led to nutritional deficiencies in some vegetarian infants, particularly those in macrobiotic families. Observations of rickets, iron deficiency anemia, and vitamin B_{12} deficiency in some vegan infants have led to concerns about the advisability of such diets for infants.[15,16] It is important to note that these deficiencies are linked to unusually restrictive diets that do not conform to appropriate guidelines for feeding vegan infants. Such diets cannot be used as an argument against the use of well-balanced vegan or lacto-ovo vegetarian diets in infancy. Poorly planned diets are dangerous for infants regardless of the dietary beliefs of the parents.

Although such findings do raise concerns about the appropriateness of macrobiotic diets for infants, they do not necessarily rule out macrobiotics for infants and young children. With some adjustments in the emphasis given to the different food groups in the macrobiotic diet, it is possible to plan appropriate macrobiotic diets for infants. Recently, macrobiotic teachers in the United States have liberalized some of their guidelines for children.[16]

Healthy vegan diets can be planned easily for infants. Today's vegetarian parents are somewhat more likely to be mainstream than those in years past and to have better access to information about vegetarian diets. When parents are educated about appropriate infant feeding, both lacto-ovo and vegan feeding patterns are safe and appropriate. Dietitians who counsel parents of vegan infants need to be knowledgeable and positive about this eating pattern for infants.

VEGETARIAN DIETS DURING THE FIRST 6 MONTHS OF INFANCY

Breastfed Infants

Breastfeeding is a wise option for all infants. Nevertheless, the number of breastfed infants has fallen off somewhat in recent years.[17] Today, about 50% of all infants are breastfed compared with 60% in the mid-1980s. The number of vegetarian mothers who breastfeed is considerably higher than the average in the general population.[2] Breastfeeding has the following advantages over formula feeding:

- superior nutritional composition[18,19]
- immunologic components[19,20]
- lower cost

- perceived enhanced maternal-infant bonding[21]
- fewer respiratory and gastrointestinal infections[22]
- less likelihood of allergies[23]
- reduced risk of developing non-insulin-dependent diabetes mellitus[24–26]

Appropriate diets for lactating women are discussed in Chapter 8. Infants of both lacto-ovo vegetarian mothers and vegan mothers thrive, and the breast milk of vegetarian women is adequate in nutrients.[1,3,12,27,28] Vegan women need to be certain that they are consuming foods fortified with vitamin B12 or should use a supplement or their infants should receive a supplement (Table 9–1). There is some evidence that vitamin B12 from a woman's stores does not appear in her milk and that only B12 consumed during lactation will be available to her infant,[29] although more recent evidence suggests that this may not be the case.[30] If there is any question about adequate vitamin B12 in a woman's diet, a B12 supplement is recommended for her breastfed infant.

Light-skinned infants can make adequate vitamin D if hands and face are exposed to the sun three times a week for 20 to 30 minutes each time.[31] The need for vitamin D supplements in breastfed infants is controversial. Most experts recommend vitamin D supplements of 10 µg/day, particularly in infants who are at risk for vitamin D deficiency.[32,33] At-risk infants include those who are dark skinned because greater sun exposure is needed in these infants; those who live in northern, smoggy areas; those who are kept covered because of cultural practices; and those whose mothers have inadequate vitamin D intake and sun exposure. Vegan mothers who do not have

---

Table 9–1 Recommended Supplements for Vegetarian Infants

Nutrient	Breastfed Infants	Formula-Fed Infants
Vitamin K	Single dose at birth: 0.5–1.0 mg intramuscularly 1.0–2.0 mg orally	Single dose at birth: 0.5–1.0 mg intramuscularly 1.0–2.0 mg orally
Vitamin D	10 µg for at-risk infants	Infant formulas contain vitamin D
Iron	1 mg/kg/day beginning at 4–6 months	Use iron-fortified infant formula
Fluoride	0.25 mg/day by 2 weeks if water supply is not fluoridated	0.25 mg/day if water is not fluoridated or if ready-to-feed formula is used
Vitamin B12	0.1–0.3 µg	

adequate sun exposure, who are dark skinned, or who live in northern areas may not make adequate vitamin D. If they also do not include fortified foods in their diet, supplementation with vitamin D for their breastfed infants is advised.

Breast milk is generally low in iron, regardless of the mother's intake. Nevertheless, the bioavailability of this iron is high; approximately 50% is absorbed.[34] It appears that healthy, full-term infants can obtain adequate iron from breast milk for the first 9 to 12 months of life,[35] but recommendations are for iron supplementation beginning by 4 to 6 months.[32,36,37] Supplementation can be in the form of iron drops or through introduction of iron-fortified infant formula.

Fluoride in the mother's diet does not appear in her milk; therefore, where water is not fluoridated, all infants should receive fluoride supplements. Finally, both breastfed and formula-fed infants receive a one-time supplement of vitamin K at birth.

Formula-Fed Infants

Commercial infant formula is recommended for infants who are not breastfed or who are weaned before 1 year of age. There are several types of formulas available.

Standard Formulas

These are the most commonly used infant formulas. They are based on cow's milk that is modified by removal of the butter fat, addition of vegetable oils and carbohydrate, and reduction of protein content. The addition of whey to some of these standard formulas results in a better approximation of the ratio of whey to casein in breast milk. Standard formulas are low in iron unless they are iron fortified. Newborn infants can be started on unfortified standard formulas and then switched to iron-fortified ones at 4 months of age, when iron supplementation to the diet is indicated. Some pediatricians recommend using iron-fortified formulas right from the beginning, however, so that parents do not forget to switch later.

Soy Formulas

Soy formulas contain methionine-fortified soy protein isolate, vegetable oil, and carbohydrate. They are lactose free. Some are also corn free and sucrose free. Infants who are fed exclusively soy formula grow and develop normally.[14] These formulas are a common option when an infant exhibits an allergy to cow's milk protein, is lactose intolerant, or has galactosemia. They are also the only choice for infants in vegan families who are not breastfed. There are currently four commercial soy formulas on the market: Nursoy,

Prosobee, Isomil, and Soyalac. Nursoy is not an appropriate choice when parents wish to provide a vegan diet because it contains animal-derived fats.

When parents choose soy formula, it is crucial to make sure that they understand the difference between soy infant formulas and commercial soy beverages. The latter are not appropriate food for infants.

Protein Hydrolysates

Bottle-fed infants who are allergic to both cow's milk protein and soy protein are often placed on formulas that contain casein hydrolysate. Vegan parents may not be willing to feed these formulas to their infants because they contain cow's milk protein. For vegan infants who show intolerance to soy formulas, there are no commercial vegan formula options. This represents a strong argument in favor of breastfeeding in vegan families.

Follow-Up Formulas

These formulas are marketed for older infants who are eating some solid foods. The two available follow-up formulas both contain cow's milk protein. According to the American Academy of Pediatrics, there is no advantage to using such formulas for older infants.[38]

Other Milk Feedings

Homemade formula based on evaporated milk is sometimes chosen as a lower cost alternative to commercial infant formulas. Although these are a better choice than plain cow's milk, they are not recommended. These formulas contain poorly digested fat, inadequate iron and vitamin C, and excessive amounts of phosphorus and sodium. There are no available recipes for homemade infant soy formulas. Infants fed soy formula must use a commercial product. In some macrobiotic populations, milks made from rice have been used. These milks are not adequate nutrition for infants and should not be used. When families cannot afford to purchase commercial infant formula a referral to the Women, Infants, and Children Supplemental Food Program is appropriate.

Infants should receive breast milk or infant formula for the first 12 months of life. Introduction of unmodified cow's milk (whole, low fat, or nonfat), goat's milk, commercial soy beverages, or other vegetable milks is not recommended during infancy.[39] Unmodified cow's milk is high in protein and minerals and is lacking or low in vitamin C, vitamin E, iron, and essential fatty acids. Early introduction of cow's milk, particularly before 6 months of age, is associated with a greater risk of milk protein allergy, gastrointestinal blood loss, and poor iron status.[40] Cow's milk should definitely not be introduced before 6 months and preferably not before 12 months. If it is introduced during the second half of infancy, only whole cow's milk should be used, not low fat or nonfat.

Commercial soy beverages do not provide adequate nutrition for infants and should not be used during the first year. The same is true for other vegetable milks, such as commercial rice and almond milks, or the grain preparations described in some macrobiotic books.

SOLID FOODS FOR VEGETARIAN INFANTS

The introduction of solid foods into an infant's diet is usually viewed by parents as a happy milestone. For this reason, there is often a tendency to start infants on solid foods before they are ready. Parents may erroneously believe that breast milk or formula is not adequate nutrition for their infant. It is also commonly, and mistakenly, believed that introducing solids will help an infant sleep through the night.

Either breast milk or commercial formula (based on soymilk or cow's milk) is adequate nutrition for most infants for the first 4 to 6 months of life (Table 9–2) as long as appropriate supplements are offered. Age is a poor indicator of readiness for solid foods. Rather, eating habits and physical

Table 9–2 Guidelines for Feeding Vegetarian Infants*

First 4–6 months	4–6 months	6–7 months	7–8 months	8–9 months	10–12 months
Breast milk or infant formula	Breast milk or infant formula	Breast milk or infant formula	Breast milk or infant formula	Breast milk or infant formula	Breast milk or infant formula
	Introduce iron-fortified cereal	Iron-fortified infant cereal	Iron-fortified infant cereal	Iron-fortified infant cereal	Iron-fortified infant cereal
		Mashed or pureed fruits and vegetables	Mashed or pureed fruits and vegetables	Mashed or pureed fruits and vegetables	Soft chopped fruits, vegetables, and protein foods
			Protein foods	Protein foods	Soft finger foods
			Juice from a cup	Juice from a cup	Milk or juice in a cup at mealtimes
				Soft finger foods	

*Overlap in age groups accounts for the variation in infant developmental rates.

preparedness provide better cues to whether solid foods are indicated. One developmental sign of readiness for solid foods is the disappearance of the tongue extrusion reflex. The extrusion reflex allows infants to swallow only liquid foods. As long as this reflex persists, infants will push solids out of the mouth with their tongue, so that feeding such foods will be difficult. Between 4 and 6 months of age, the infant is able to move food from the front to the back of the mouth, where it can be swallowed more easily. Another developmental sign of readiness is the ability to sit independently and maintain balance. This allows the infant to express both hunger and satiety by either leaning forward to receive food or pulling back and turning away. Most often, other signs of readiness will occur at roughly the same time that these become evident. These include doubling of the infant's weight since birth (or about 13 lb), breastfed infants demanding to be fed more than 8 to 10 times in 24 hours, or bottle-fed infants drinking more than 1 qt of formula per day.

Although solid foods are generally not necessary before 4 months of age, in most cases they should be introduced no later than 6 months of age. By this time, infants need the additional calories that solid foods provide.[13,41,42] Also, it is appropriate at this time for the infant to be developing the skills that accompany solid food consumption.

Solid foods will displace some of the milk or formula in an infant's diet. Because both breast milk and infant formula are nutrient-dense foods, it is important that the solid foods offered are also nutrient dense. Parents must understand that solid foods are added specifically to meet the nutrient needs of the growing infant. The recommended diet for infants is 40% to 50% fat and 7% to 11% protein.[39,43] Both breast milk and infant formula meet these recommendations. The addition of solid foods will probably alter the macronutrient intake to some extent. Excessive intake of foods that are high in carbohydrate and low in both protein and fat, such as fruits and juices, can produce diets that are not ideal for infants.

Because the first solid foods for infants are always cereals, fruits, and vegetables, recommendations for introducing these foods are exactly the same for vegetarian infants as for those in omnivore households. The first solid food for infants is usually an iron-fortified cereal. Rice cereal is the best choice because it is hypoallergenic, and commercially prepared infant cereals are usually recommended. The cereal should be mixed with breast milk or formula to make it dilute for first feedings. Solid foods should always be fed from a spoon, not from a bottle. Even dilute cereal preparations should not be fed from the bottle. It is normal for infants to resist the unfamiliar spoon initially. If infants begin to choke or gag, however, this is an indication that they are not ready for solid foods.

Parents should offer one new food every 3 or 4 days, watching for signs of allergic reactions after the introduction of each new food. Iron-fortified barley or oat cereal is generally the next food to be introduced after rice cereal. Wheat and corn cereals can cause allergic reactions and should be delayed until the first birthday. First feedings will comprise just 1 or 2 tsp of cereal. Eventually, the infant can progress to two daily servings of cereal for a total of ⅓ to ½ cup of cereal per day.

Some parents may choose to prepare their own infant cereals. Oats, barley, or rice can be processed in a blender until they are finely ground and then cooked until they are smooth. Because these cereals are low in iron, however, breastfed infants should continue to receive an iron supplement, and bottle-fed infants should receive iron-fortified formula.

When infants are consuming ⅓ to ½ cup of cereal per day, mashed fruits and vegetables can be introduced. Again, it is important that parents introduce only one new food every 3 or 4 days so that any sources of allergies can be identified easily. Good choices for first fruits and vegetables are smooth applesauce, pureed canned peaches or pears (canned in their own juice, not in heavy syrup), strained potatoes, carrots, sweet potatoes, and green beans. Mashed banana and avocado are also good first foods for infants and can be easily prepared because they do not need to be cooked.

Most infants will begin to drink from a cup at about 7 to 8 months, and fruit juice can be introduced at that time. Apple juice is a good choice. Citrus juice should be avoided for the first year because it is potentially allergenic. At this point, infants are also ready to begin consuming some higher-protein foods.

First protein foods for vegetarian infants can be thoroughly cooked and pureed legumes or well-mashed tofu. Infants in lacto-ovo families can also have pureed cottage cheese, yogurt mixed with mashed fruit, or egg yolks. At this time, parents can introduce some of the stronger-tasting vegetables, such as kale, collards, or other greens. The flavors of these foods can be tempered by blending them with bland or sweet foods. Vegetables can be pureed with avocado, applesauce, tofu, or cottage cheese.

By 10 months, most infants can enjoy finger foods, such as tofu chunks, crackers, and bread. For infants who are teething, gnawing on frozen bagels can be soothing. By their first birthday, infants can have smooth nut and seed butters, such as almond or peanut butter or tahini.

Many parents prefer to use commercially prepared infant foods. Vegetarian parents should be encouraged to make their own baby foods, however, because commercial lines offer a limited variety of foods for vegetarian infants. Foods that will eventually play a significant role in the diets of vegetarian children (eg, legumes, tofu, and leafy green vegetables) should be introduced in infancy and are seldom available as commercial baby foods. Exhibit 9–1 offers guidelines for home preparation of infant foods.

Adequate calorie intake can be one concern in vegetarian infants. Parents can be counseled on ways to incorporate foods into infant diets that are particularly rich in calories and nutrients. Some ideas include legume spreads, mashed firm tofu (firm tofu tends to be higher in fat and calories than soft tofu), dried fruits processed in a blender with a few teaspoons of water or fruit juice to make a spread, mashed avocado, and nut and seed butters (after the first birthday).

COMPARISON OF SAMPLE MENU PLANS FOR 9-MONTH-OLD VEGAN AND OMNIVORE INFANTS

Vegan diets that follow the guidelines noted above provide roughly the equivalent nutrient intake of omnivore diets, as the sample meal plans for 9-month-old infants in Exhibit 9–2 indicate. The meal plans are for a vegan breastfed or soy formula–fed infant and a breastfed or cow's milk formula–fed nonvegetarian infant. These menu plans differ only in that the plant proteins in the vegan plan have been replaced with animal foods in the nonvegetarian plan. Table 9–3 compares the percentage of the recommended dietary allowances (RDAs) provided by each of these diets. In both cases, when infant formulas (either soymilk or cow's milk based) are used, the nutrient content meets or exceeds the RDAs for infants except for vitamin D. For breastfed infants, the nutrient content of the vegan and omnivore diets are adequate for most nutrients with the exception of vitamin B_6 and zinc. The levels of vitamins A, B_{12}, D, and C as well as thiamin, riboflavin, and niacin could be expected to vary depending on the mother's diet. In this

---

Exhibit 9–1 Home Preparation of Infant Foods

- Wash all fruits and vegetables thoroughly. If preparing beans, rinse dried beans under cold running water. Do not use canned vegetables or beans unless they are canned without added sodium.
- Remove skins, seeds, and stringy portions from fruits and vegetables.
- Cook the foods thoroughly until they are soft enough to puree.
- Puree foods in a blender, adding some cooking liquid to reach a smooth consistency.
- Press cooked legumes through a sieve to remove any skins.
- Home-prepared infant foods can be kept in the refrigerator for up to 2 days. They can also be prepared in large quantities and then frozen for later use. Freeze in ice cube trays and defrost only one serving at a time.

case, it is assumed that the mother of the vegan infant has a reliable source of vitamin B_{12} in her diet.

POTENTIAL CONCERNS IN INFANT FEEDING

Cow's Milk Formula and Diabetes

There has been much recent media attention to the link between consumption of cow's milk protein in early infancy and later development of insulin-dependent diabetes mellitus. For example, one study found that of the 142 diabetic children studied all exhibited blood levels of antibodies to cow's milk protein.[23] Levels of these antibodies were much lower in nondiabetic children. It is believed that the antibodies destroy the insulin-producing β cells of the pancreas.

Evidence shows that early exposure to cow's milk protein, either as unmodified cow's milk or in cow's milk infant formula, can raise the risk for diabetes in susceptible children.[23–26] Although this issue warrants further study, it is an additional reason to recommend breastfeeding for all infants.

Exhibit 9–2 Sample Diets for 9-Month-Old Vegan and Omnivore Infants

Meal	Vegan Infant*	Omnivore Infant†
Breakfast	1 tbsp mashed tofu, 2 tbsp iron-fortified cereal, 1 tbsp mashed banana, 1 cup infant soy formula or breast milk	1 tbsp egg yolk, 2 tbsp infant rice cereal, 1 tbsp mashed banana, 1 cup formula or breast milk
Midday	1 tbsp mashed potatoes, 1 tbsp mashed carrots, ¼ slice bread, 1 tbsp applesauce, 1 cup infant soy formula or breast milk	1 tbsp mashed potatoes, 1 tbsp applesauce, 1 tbsp mashed carrots, ¼ slice bread, 1 cup formula or breast milk
Evening	1 tbsp mashed pinto beans, ¼ slice bread, 1 tbsp strained pears, 1 tbsp prune spread, 1 cup infant soy formula or breast milk	1 tbsp strained chicken, 1/4 slice bread, 1 tbsp strained pears, 1 tbsp prune spread, 1 cup formula or breast milk
Bedtime	1 cup infant soy formula or breast milk	1 cup formula or breast milk

*Breastfed or soy formula fed.
†Breastfed or cow's milk formula fed.

Table 9–3 Percentage RDA Met by Vegan and Nonvegetarian Diets for 9-Month-Old Infants on Four Different Diets (Diets Described in Exhibit 9–2)

Nutrient	Vegan, Breastfed	Vegan, Soy Formula Fed	Omnivore, Breastfed	Omnivore, Cow's Milk Formula Fed
Kilocalories	99	94	102	97
Protein (g)	118	183	123	153
Iron (mg)	68	174	62	175
Calcium (mg)	73	116	72	99
Zinc (mg)	51	114	53	115
Vitamin A (µg)	260	221	283	246
α-Tocopherol (mg)	225	231	229	368
Thiamin (mg)	93	219	98	1,661
Riboflavin (mg)	115	236	125	1,965
Niacin (mg)	70	94	76	159
Pyridoxine (B_6) (mg)	51	86	54	100
Folate (µg)	252	195	228	352
Cobalamin (µg)	107	402	162	393
Vitamin C (mg)	150	193	150	174
Vitamin D (µg)	12	12	12	12
Vitamin K (µg)	209	973	209	524

Allergies

Between 4% and 6% of infants develop allergies to one or more foods.[44] Allergies to cow's milk protein are most common; it is estimated that 1% to 7% of infants are allergic to cow's milk protein.[45] Often, infants with cow's milk allergy are placed on infant soy formulas. There is some controversy about the advisability of doing so because many allergic infants will also develop allergies to soy formula.[46] Some pediatricians recommend switching infants directly to casein hydrolysates. The cost of these special formulas can be prohibitive for some families, however, and for some infants they may be unwarranted. Estimates are that between 15% and 50% of infants with cow's milk allergy will develop allergies to soy protein.[47–50] Therefore, soy formula can still be a viable option for many infants with milk allergy.

Infants who are allergic to cow's milk have a greater likelihood of developing allergies to other foods. In these high-risk infants, it is wise to delay introduction of potential problem foods until later in infancy, possibly as late as 12 months of age (Exhibit 9–3). Vegetarian foods that are most likely to cause allergic reactions include egg whites, nuts, peas, chocolate, citrus fruits, corn products, soy products, and wheat.[17]

Exhibit 9–3 Some Feeding Practices To Avoid in Infancy

- For the first year, avoid feeding infants whole, low-fat, or nonfat cow's milk; regular commercial soymilk; or goat's milk.
- Feed only breast milk, infant formula, or water in the infant's bottle. Diluted cereal preparations should not be fed in the bottle. Most infants are ready to drink from a cup when fruit juices are offered.
- Avoid foods that may cause adverse reactions, such as wheat, citrus, egg whites, and nut butters, before 1 year of age.
- Do not feed honey or corn syrup to infants younger than 1 year; both can cause botulism.[52,53]

Although breastfed infants appear to be less likely to develop food allergies, they can show adverse reactions to food components in the mother's diet that are passed into her milk. For example, cow's milk protein in the mother's diet can cause an allergic response in her infant.[51] Other foods that may cause discomfort include coffee, chocolate, cabbage and other gas-producing vegetables, onions, beans, and chili. Such problems occur in a minority of infants, however. Breastfeeding mothers need not modify their diets unless a specific problem arises.

MACROBIOTIC DIETS IN INFANCY

Several studies of macrobiotics in the United States and the Netherlands have revealed nutritional deficiencies in macrobiotic infants.[15,16] Nutrients of greatest concern are vitamin B_{12}, vitamin D, calcium, and iron. Energy levels have also been found to be too low in some macrobiotic infants.

The percentage of mothers who breastfeed is high among macrobiotics, and they tend to breastfeed for longer periods than the general population.[10] When macrobiotic infants are weaned, it is often onto a homemade grain-based milk that is low in protein, calories, iron, and calcium and devoid of vitamin B_{12} and vitamin D. These water-based cereal porridges can be the major component of the weanling's diet.[6] Tofu, legumes, and vegetables, including sea vegetables, may be added several months after weaning. Although some seeds, particularly sesame seeds, are used in the infant's diet, added fats are strongly discouraged among macrobiotics.

Potential problems with macrobiotic diets for infants center on the following:

- Tofu, legumes, vegetables, and sea vegetables may be the sole sources of calcium for weaned macrobiotic infants. Although these foods can provide adequate calcium for children and adults, they are consumed in amounts that are too small in the infant diet to meet calcium needs.

- A diet based solely on grains, vegetables, and legumes with no added fats appears to be too high in bulk to meet infant calorie needs.

- The use of fortified foods is often prohibited on macrobiotic diets.

- Although the macrobiotic diet is not always vegetarian (some macrobiotics use fish or fish oil), when the weaned infant is consuming only unfortified plant foods the diet contains no vitamin B_{12} or vitamin D.

Dietitians who counsel parents of macrobiotic infants may face some challenges in developing healthy infant diets that conform to macrobiotic guidelines. Many of these parents will be willing to make adjustments to the diets of their infants, however, especially if the nutrition counselor makes every possible effort to work within the guidelines of the macrobiotic principles. Also, proponents of macrobiotics actually follow many versions of the diet, so that it should not be assumed that all macrobiotic infants are being fed deficient diets. Many are well nourished. The following suggestions can help ensure safe macrobiotic diets for infants:

- It has recently been suggested that macrobiotic infants and children should receive milk in their diet.[15] Because dairy products have never been a part of macrobiotic diets, their adoption would represent a fundamental change in dietary philosophy that may not be acceptable to most macrobiotics. Soy products, however, such as tofu, miso, and soybeans, are included in macrobiotic meals; therefore, a fortified soy formula may be more acceptable.

- Sea vegetables should be limited in the diet of macrobiotic infants whose intake of vitamin B_{12} is low. Although these foods may contain some active B_{12}, they may also contain analogues that may interfere with the absorption of active vitamin B_{12}.[10] The amounts used in infant diets typically provide only negligible amounts of other nutrients, such as calcium.

- A source of dietary fat, such as margarine or vegetable oil added to other foods, should be included in the infant's diet.

- Fiber intake of infants should be reduced by sieving grains before cooking them or by using some refined grains.

- Frequent sun exposure should be encouraged to ensure adequate vitamin D synthesis.
- A vitamin B_{12} supplement should be provided.

FATTY ACIDS IN THE DIET OF VEGETARIAN INFANTS

The omega-3 fatty acids are thought to be especially important for development of the brain and central nervous system. In particular, docosahexaenoic acid (DHA) is found in large amounts in the retina and the brain membrane. Concern has been raised about the fact that the breast milk of vegetarian mothers is low in DHA because this fatty acid is not present in vegetarian diets. Infant formulas are also lacking in DHA. Although DHA can be synthesized from linolenic acid, this conversion appears to be reduced in infancy.[54] In one study, no differences in DHA status were seen between infants consuming a linolenic acid–free corn oil formula and those consuming a soy oil formula that did contain linolenic acid.[55]

Two studies have shown that breast milk of vegan mothers is much lower in DHA than milk from omnivores and lacto-ovo vegetarians.[56,57] Also, DHA content of red blood cells from breastfed infants of vegan mothers was lower than that of formula-fed infants or breastfed infants of omnivore mothers.[57] Other studies have found these levels to be similar.[58,59]

Despite reduced intake of DHA in vegan infants, their growth and development, as discussed earlier, appear to be comparable to those of omnivore infants. In one study, visual acuity was also found to be comparable between formula-fed infants and breastfed infants of omnivore mothers, although the formula did not contain any DHA and DHA blood levels were higher in the breastfed group.[59] Although it is possible that the breastfed infants in this study had higher DHA stores than vegetarian infants normally would, research suggests that infants born to vegetarian mothers have only slightly lower DHA levels than infants born to omnivore mothers.[59] It appears that fetal tissue is capable of synthesizing DHA.

Although the ability of infants to convert linolenic acid to DHA appears to be limited, and there are no apparent problems associated with low intakes of DHA, it may be prudent to recommend that vegan mothers of breastfed infants strive to include adequate amounts of linolenic acid in their diet until this issue is resolved.

CONCLUSION

Although infancy, particularly the period after weaning, can be a time of great nutritional vulnerability, it is relatively easy to provide nutritious vegetarian diets for these youngest family members. Parents can follow the feeding plan in Exhibit 9–2 and should be provided with the following general guidelines for feeding infants:

- Choose breast milk or a commercial infant formula for all milk feedings for the first year. Vegan infants who are not breastfed can receive soy infant formula.
- Use appropriate supplements as prescribed by the health care provider. These will include iron after 3 to 4 months for both breastfed and formula-fed infants and possibly vitamins D and B_{12} for breastfed vegan infants. Fluoride supplements are generally used also for breastfed infants and for bottle-fed infants when water is not fluoridated.
- Introduce iron-fortified cereal when the infant shows appropriate signs of readiness, usually between 4 and 6 months.
- Gradually offer additional solid foods, including pureed vegetables, fruits, beans, tofu, and cottage cheese. Nut butters can be introduced toward the end of the first year.

REFERENCES

1. Dwyer JT, Palombo R, Thorne H, Valadian I, Reed RB. Preschoolers on alternate life-style diets. *J Am Diet Assoc.* 1978;72:264–270.
2. O'Connell JM, Dibley MJ, Sierra J, Wallace B, Marks JS, Yip R. Growth of vegetarian children: The Farm study. *Pediatrics.* 1989;84:475–481.
3. Dwyer JT, Andrew EM, Valadian I, Reed RB. Size, obesity, and leanness in vegetarian preschool children. *J Am Diet Assoc.* 1980;77:434–439.
4. King JC, Stein T, Doyle M. Effect of vegetarianism on the zinc status of pregnant women. *Am J Clin Nutr.* 1981;34:1049–1055.
5. Dagnelie PC, van Staveren WA, van Klaveren JD, Burema J. Do children on macrobiotic diets show catch-up growth? *Eur J Clin Nutr.* 1988;42:1007–1016.
6. Dagnelie PC, van Staveren WA, Vergot FJVRA, et al. Nutritional status of infants aged 4 to 18 months on macrobiotic diets and matched omnivorous control infants: A population-based mixed-longitudinal study. II. Growth and psychomotor development. *Eur J Clin Nutr.* 1989;43:325–338.
7. Jacobs C, Dwyer JT. Vegetarian children: Appropriate and inappropriate diets. *Am J Clin Nutr.* 1988;48:811–818.
8. van Staveren WA, Dhuybetter JHM, Bons A, Zeelen M, Hautvast JGAJ. Food consumption and height/weight status of Dutch preschool children on alternative diets. *J Am Diet Assoc.* 1985;85:1579–1584.
9. Sanders TAB. Growth and development of British vegan children. *Am J Clin Nutr.* 1988;48:822–825.

10. Dagnelie PC, van Staveren WA, Verschuren SAJM, Hautvast JGAJ. Nutritional status of infants aged 4 to 18 months on macrobiotic diets and matched omnivorous control infants: A population-based mixed-longitudinal study. I. Weaning pattern, energy and nutrient intake. *Eur J Clin Nutr*. 1989;43:311–323.

11. Garza C. Infancy. In: Brown ML, ed. *Present Knowledge in Nutrition*. 6th ed. Washington, DC: International Life Sciences Institute–Nutrition Foundation; 1990:320–324.

12. Dwyer JT, Andrew EM, Berkey C, Valadian I, Reed RB. Growth in "new" vegetarian preschool children using the Jenss-Bayley curve fitting technique. *Am J Clin Nutr*. 1983;37:815–827.

13. Canadian Pediatric Society, Committee on Nutrition. Breast feeding. *Pediatrics*. 1978;62:591–660.

14. Committee on Nutrition, Academy of Pediatrics. Soy protein formulas: Recommendations for use in infant feeding. *Pediatrics*. 1983;72:359–363.

15. Dagnelie PC, van Staveren WA. Macrobiotic nutrition and child health: Results of a population-based, mixed-longitudinal cohort study in the Netherlands. *Am J Clin Nutr*. 1994;59(suppl):1187S–1196S.

16. Dagnelie PC, Vergot F, van Staveren WA, van den Berg H, Kingjan PG, Hautvast J. High prevalence of rickets in infants on macrobiotic diets. *Am J Clin Nutr*. 1990;51:202–208.

17. Groh-Wargo SL, Antonelli K. Normal nutrition during infancy. In: Queen PM, Lang CE, eds. *Handbook of Pediatric Nutrition*. Gaithersburg, Md: Aspen; 1993:107–144.

18. American Dietetic Association. Promotion of breastfeeding. *J Am Diet Assoc*. 1986;86:1580–1585.

19. Anderson GH. Human milk feeding. *Pediatr Clin North Am*. 1985;32:335–353.

20. Kovar MG, Serdula MG, Marks JS, et al. Review of the epidemiologic evidence for an association between infant feeding and infant health. *Pediatrics*. 1984;74:615–638.

21. Newton N, Newton M. Psychologic aspects of lactation. *N Engl J Med*. 1967;277:1179–1188.

22. Cunningham AS, Jelliffe DB, Jelliffe EFP. Breast-feeding and health in the 1980s: A global epidemiologic review. *J Pediatr*. 1991;118:659–666.

23. Gruskay FL. Comparisons of breast, cow, and soy feedings in the prevention of allergic disease. *Clin Pediatr*. 1982;21:486.

24. Karjalainen J, Martin JM, Knip M, et al. A bovine albumin peptide as a possible trigger of insulin-dependent diabetes mellitus. *N Engl J Med*. 1992;327:302–307.

25. Gerstein HC. Cow's milk exposure and type I diabetes mellitus. *Diabetes Care*. 1993;17:13–19.

26. Drash AL, Kramer AL, Swanson MS, Udall JN. Infant feeding practices and their possible relationship to the etiology of diabetes mellitus. *Pediatrics*. 1995;94:752–754.

27. Sanders TAB, Purves R. An anthropometric and dietary assessment of the nutritional status of vegan preschool children. *J Hum Nutr*. 1981;35:349–357.

28. Shull MW, Reed RB, Valadian I, Palombo R, Thorne H, Dwyer JT. Velocities of growth in vegetarian preschool children. *Pediatrics*. 1977;60:410–417.

29. Lubby AL, Cooperman JM, Donnfeld AM, et al. Observations on transfer of vitamin B_{12} from mother to fetus and newborn. *Am J Dis Child*. 1958;96:532–533.

30. Specker BL, Black A, Allen L, Morrow F. Vitamin B_{12}: Low milk concentrations are related to low serum concentrations in vegetarian women and to methylmalonic aciduria in their infants. *Am J Clin Nutr*. 1990;52:1073–1076.

31. Specker BL, Valanis B, Hertzberg V, et al. Sunshine exposure and serum 25-hydroxyvitamin D concentrations in exclusively breast-fed infants. *J Pediatr*. 1985;107:372–376.

32. Committee on Nutrition, American Academy of Pediatrics. Vitamin and mineral supplement needs in normal children in the United States. *Pediatrics*. 1980;66:1015–1021.

33. Greer FR, Searcy JE, Levin RS, et al. Bone mineral content and serum 25-hydroxyvitamin D concentrations in breast-fed infants with and without supplemental vitamin D: One year follow-up. *J Pediatr*. 1982;100:919–962.

34. Lawrence RA. *Breastfeeding—A Guide for the Medical Profession*. 3rd ed. St Louis, Mo: Mosby; 1989.

35. Pastel RA, Howanitz PJ, Oski FA. Iron sufficiency with prolonged exclusive breast-feeding in Peruvian infants. *Clin Pediatr*. 1981;20:625–626.

36. Fomon SJ, Filer LJ, Anderson TA, Ziegler EE. Recommendations for feeding normal infants. *Pediatrics*. 1979;63:52–59.

37. Owen GM, Garry PJ, Hooper EM, et al. Iron nutriture of infants exclusively breast-fed the first five months. *J Pediatr*. 1981;99:237–240.

38. Committee on Nutrition, American Academy of Pediatrics. Follow-up on weaning formulas. *Pediatrics*. 1989;83:1067.

39. Fomon S. *Infant Nutrition*. 2nd ed. Philadelphia, Pa: Saunders; 1974.

40. Ziegler EE. Milk and formulas for older infants. *J Pediatr*. 1990;117:S76–S79.

41. Ashworth A, Feachem RG. Interventions for the control of diarrhoeal disease among young children: Weaning and education. *Bull World Health Organization*. 1985;63:1115–1127.

42. Whitehead RG. Nutritional aspects of human lactation. *Lancet*. 1983;1:167–169.

43. Food and Nutrition Board, National Research Council, National Academy of Sciences. *Recommended Dietary Allowances*. 10th ed. Washington, DC: National Academy Press; 1989.

44. Sampson HA. Food hypersensitivity. In: Grant JA, ed. *Insights in Allergy*. St Louis, Mo: Mosby; 1986.

45. Olejer VL. Food hypersensitivities. In: Queen PM, Lang CE, eds. *Handbook of Pediatric Nutrition*. Gaithersburg, Md: Aspen; 1993:206–231.

46. Powell GK. Milk and soy induced enterocolitis of infancy: Clinical features and standardization of challenge. *J Pediatr*. 1978;93:553–560.

47. Gerrard JW, MacKenzie JWA, Goluboff N, Garson JZ, Maningas CS. Cow's milk allergy: Prevalence and manifestations in an unselected series of newborns. *Acta Paediatr Scand*. 1973;234(suppl):1–21.

48. Kjellman N-IM, Johansson SGO. Soy versus cow's milk in infants with a biparental history of atopic disease: Development of atopic disease and immunoglobulins from birth to 4 years of age. *Clin Allergy*. 1979;9:347–358.

49. Perkkio M, Savilahti E, Kuitunen P. Morphometric and immunohistochemical study of jejunal biopsies from children with intestinal soy allergy. *Eur J Pediatr*. 1981;137:63–69.

50. Brady MS, Rickard KA, Fitzgerald JF, Lemons JA. Specialized formulas and feedings for infants with malabsorption or formula intolerance. *J Am Diet Assoc*. 1986;86:191–200.

51. Kilshaw PJ, Cant AJ. Passage of maternal dater proteins into human breast milk. *Arch Allergy Appl Immunol*. 1984;75:8–15.

52. Centers for Disease Control and Prevention (CDC). *Infant Botulism: Botulism in the United States, 1899–1977. Handbook for Epidemiologists, Clinicians and Laboratory Workers*. Atlanta, Ga: CDC; 1979.

53. Kautter DA, Lilly T, Solomon HM, Lynt RK. *Clostridium botulinum* spores in infant foods: A survey. *J Food Prot.* 1982;45:1028.

54. Carlson SE, Rhodes PG, Ferguson MG. Docosahexaenoic acid status of preterm infants at birth and following feedings with human milk or formula. *Am J Clin Nutr.* 1986;44:798–804.

55. Ponder DS, Innis SM, Benson JD, Shegman JS. Docosahexaenoic acid status of term infants fed breast milk or infant formula containing soy oil or corn oil. *Pediatr Res.* 1992;32:683–688.

56. Sanders TAB, Ellis FR, Dickerson DJWT. Studies of vegans: The fatty acid composition of plasma choline phosphoglycerides, erythrocytes, adipose tissue, and breast milk, and some indicators of susceptibility to ischemic heart disease in vegans and omnivore controls. *Am J Clin Nutr.* 1978;31:805–813.

57. Sanders TAB, Reddy S. The influence of a vegetarian diet on the fatty acid composition of human milk and the essential fatty acid status of the infant. *J Pediatr.* 1992;120:871–877.

58. Specker BL, Wey HE, Miller D. Differences in fatty acid composition of human milk in vegetarian and nonvegetarian women: Long-term effect of diet. *J Pediatr Gastroenterol Nutr.* 1987;6:764–768.

59. Innis SM, Nelson CM, Rioux MF, King DJ. Development of visual acuity in relation to plasma and erythrocyte ω-6 and ω-3 fatty acids in healthy term gestation infants. *Am J Clin Nutr.* 1994;60:347–352.

CHAPTER 10

Preschool and School-Age Children

Feeding toddlers and preschoolers is a challenge to most parents, whether or not the family is vegetarian. Growth slows considerably toward the end of the first year, and with this slowed growth comes a decrease in appetite. Also, by age 2 most children are expressing the independence that is typical of preschoolers and that can manifest itself in picky eating habits. Many parents, both vegetarian and omnivore, face problematic eating behavior and are concerned about providing adequate nutrition for their children. National surveys have shown that several nutrients, including iron, zinc, calcium, and vitamins A and C, may be consumed in less than recommended amounts in the diets of omnivore American children.[1,2]

GROWTH OF VEGETARIAN CHILDREN

Growth of vegetarian children tends to vary depending on the type of vegetarian diet followed. Studies of Seventh-day Adventist children, who are mostly lacto-ovo vegetarians, show that growth rates equal or exceed those of nonvegetarians.[3–5] This is true even when the control group consists of children from southern California, who are taller and heavier than national standards.[6] When Adventist vegetarian children aged 7 to 18 years were compared with Adventist nonvegetarian children, the vegetarians were slightly taller.[4] One exception is seen in Seventh-day Adventist preadolescent girls, who tend to be slightly shorter than controls, a finding that may be linked to the fact that Adventist girls have a later onset of the adolescent growth spurt.[5] Later age of menarche has been observed in vegetarian girls.[7,8] There may be some health benefit to this because a later onset of menarche may reduce the risk of developing breast cancer.[9] According to the American Academy of Pediatrics, growth of vegan children is similar to that of omnivore children if menu planning is adequate.[10]

Growth of British vegan (nonmacrobiotic) toddlers and preschoolers has also been shown to be normal. In one study, vegans were lighter than but as tall as controls.[11] Similarly, a study of 404 vegan children aged 4 months to 10 years who lived on The Farm, a vegan community in western Tennessee, showed that although they were slightly shorter than controls at ages 1 through 3, they were comparable in height by age 10.[12] In another study of 48 children from The Farm, however, of 28 boys only 3 met or exceeded the 50th percentile for height, and 7 were below the 5th percentile.[13]

Poor growth in vegan children is observed primarily in macrobiotic populations.[14,15] Childhood feeding practices in macrobiotic families can be significantly different from those in other vegan families. Some macrobiotic diets may be too low in calories to support optimal growth because fats are often severely limited in these diets.[16] Smaller size in macrobiotic children has been attributed to inadequate calories,[13,15,17–21] calcium,[13,17,21,22] vitamin B_{12},[15,17,23,24] riboflavin,[22] and zinc.[24,25]

Most studies of growth of vegetarian children are relatively old and are based on relatively few cohorts. For example, for the studies of macrobiotic children noted above, the same group of Boston children were examined repeatedly, generating a fairly large body of literature on the growth of macrobiotics but all of it focusing on the same small group of children. Based on limited available data, it appears that lacto-ovo children exhibit growth similar to that of their nonvegetarian peers. Little information about the growth of nonmacrobiotic vegan children is available, although findings suggest that growth may be somewhat slower in younger children but that heights are similar to those of omnivores among older children.

Finally, although tall stature is generally perceived as more desirable and healthier, optimal health is not related to height. In fact, stature is tied to life style and dietary habits that may increase risk for a variety of diseases. For example, taller individuals appear to be at increased risk for both cancer[26] and hip fracture.[27] Therefore, perceptions of adequate growth in children who are following different diets may be biased somewhat by cultural ideas of what constitutes desirable growth.

DIETS OF VEGETARIAN CHILDREN

It is difficult to assess the dietary adequacy of vegetarianism in children. First, dietary intake varies considerably depending on the type of vegetarian diet followed. Second, much of the information that exists about vegan dietary intake is derived from studies of macrobiotic children. Macrobiotic diets can be much more restrictive than nonmacrobiotic vegan diets, and therefore nutritional profiles will be different. Finally, many of the studies of vegetarian children were conducted before vegetarian products fortified with calcium, vitamin D, and vitamin B_{12} were widely available. Also, better access to information about vegetarian diet serves to make it increasingly easy to plan healthy diets for vegetarian children.

Much attention has been focused on the question of whether vegetarian children have had healthy diets in the past. The more relevant question, however, is whether healthy diets can be planned for vegetarian children. The answer is that they can, and with ease. A brief review of findings on the intake of vegetarian children can help dietitians highlight appropriate foods in counseling sessions and focus on the particular areas of the diet that may deserve special attention.

PROTEIN

Average protein intake of vegetarian children (lacto-ovo, vegan, and macrobiotic) generally meets or exceeds recommendations,[13,15,21,24,28–30] although vegetarian children consume less protein than omnivore children.[29,30] Adequate energy intake is an important consideration in meeting protein needs; when diets are too low in calories, protein is catabolized for energy, raising total protein needs. Therefore, providing adequate calories is an important goal in diet planning for all children. Ways to ensure adequate calorie intake of vegetarian children are discussed later.

In comparison with adults, children have much higher protein needs on a body weight basis, and their essential amino acid requirements are higher. Their caloric intake relative to body weight is also high, however, so that the percentage of protein required in their diet is similar to that for adults. Although protein combining at meals is not necessary for adults, it may be helpful in meeting protein needs of infants and young children because of their somewhat higher need for essential amino acids. Because children eat frequently throughout the day, however, their meals are likely to be timed closely enough to provide the benefits of complementary amino acid profiles without conscious protein combining at each meal. Sample food combinations that will appeal to many vegetarian children are presented in Exhibit 10–1.

FAT

Fat intake among adult vegans averages about 30% of calories, which is lower than the intake among the general population and comes closer to meeting dietary guidelines than omnivore diets. Vegetarian children also

Exhibit 10–1 Examples of Meals and Snacks That Offer Children Complementary Proteins

- Rice pudding made with soymilk
- Bagel or bread spread with almond butter, sunflower butter, or tahini
- Hummus in pita bread
- Bean burrito with pinto beans in a flour tortilla
- Textured soy protein taco with corn tortilla
- Soup with barley and diced tofu
- Soup with macaroni and beans

consume a diet that is lower in fat than that of omnivore children.[22,31] As long as calories are adequate, relatively low-fat diets support growth in children. In a study of 3- to 4-year-old nonvegetarian children, there were no differences in growth between those whose fat intake averaged 27% of calories and those whose fat intake averaged more than 38% of calories.[32] Similarly, no differences in growth according to fat intake were noted among children in an Australian retrospective study.[33] Children ($N = 140$) were divided into three categories according to the percentage of calories derived from fat (less than 30%, 30.0% to 34.9%, and greater than 34.9%) and were followed up to 15 years of age.

There has been much legitimate concern about fat in the diets of American children. Many children consume diets that are too high in fat and have blood cholesterol levels that are too high.[34] Eating habits formed in childhood may influence adult eating behavior and therefore may theoretically affect risk for chronic disease. The Pediatric Panel of the National Cholesterol Education Program recommends that all children older than 2 years consume a diet that derives 30% of calories or less from fat and no more than 10% of calories from saturated fat.[34] It is clear that vegetarian children have the edge here because they consume diets that are lower in total fat[22,31] and cholesterol[24] and have lower blood cholesterol levels than nonvegetarian American children.[24,35]

With the emphasis on low-fat diets, however, there has been a trend, particularly in some popular publications, toward recommending very low–fat diets (10% to 15% of calories) for all children older than 2 years. These diets sometimes eliminate all high-fat foods (eg, nuts and seeds) and added fats and oils, and they greatly limit or eliminate soy products, which tend to be higher in fat.

Although it is not clear that such diets are harmful to children, there is no indication that they are any healthier than vegetarian diets that derive 20% to 25% of calories from fat. In addition, the inclusion of small amounts of nuts, seeds, and soy products can make it easier for vegan children to meet nutrient needs. Because toddlers and preschoolers can have difficulty meeting calorie needs, especially on vegetarian diets, which tend to be higher in bulk, the judicious use of added fats can support adequate energy intake in these children. On the other hand, parents of all children, including vegetarian children, should understand that the more flexible guidelines for fat in the diets of children do not allow for a free-for-all with fatty foods.

It is generally recommended that fat not be restricted in the diets of children younger than 2 years. After this age, it is wise to limit foods that are high in saturated fat and to use food high in total fat only in moderate amounts. Children in lacto-ovo families should consume primarily only low-fat dairy products, and the use of these products should be moderate. In all families, it is wise to limit the use of processed foods, snack foods, and baked goods, all of which can be high in fat and sodium and sometimes offer negligible nutrients. Although calories are an important concern for the young vegetarian child, so is nutrient density.

CALCIUM

Limited data indicate the calcium intake of lacto-ovo vegetarian children exceeds the recommended dietary allowance (RDA).[31] This is to be expected because, in many cases, dairy products replace meat in lacto-ovo vegetarian diets. The calcium content of adult vegan diets is lower than that of both lacto-ovo vegetarian and nonvegetarian diets (see Appendix G), and limited data indicate that the calcium content of diets of vegan children is lower than recommended levels.[17,36] Calcium intake of some macrobiotic children has been shown to be quite low.

Adequate calcium is especially important during childhood. Although factors common to vegan diets, such as a lower protein intake, may decrease calcium needs, the precise calcium needs of vegetarian children are unknown. In many cultures, particularly those with a high incidence of lactose intolerance, dairy products are not commonly used, and calcium intakes are much lower than in Western countries with no apparent ill effect. Genetics may be an important factor, however, and life style differences between Western vegetarian children and children in developing countries may also contribute to different calcium needs.

Although Western vegan children may need less calcium than nonvegetarian children, there are no data available upon which to base a vegan RDA for calcium for children. Until such information is available, it is prudent to recommend that all vegan children consume the RDA for calcium.

As discussed in Chapter 4, many plant foods are rich in calcium. The calcium needs of small children can be met by using plant foods that are naturally high in calcium. For example, a 2-year-old with a good appetite might consume the following amounts of foods in 1 day:

- ¼ cup of grains
- two slices of bread
- ½ cup of vegetables
- ½ cup of legumes
- 3 cups of soymilk
- 2 tbsp of nuts/seeds
- ½ cup of fruit
- 1 tbsp of blackstrap molasses

When calcium-rich foods in each of these groups are consumed, it is possible to meet the RDA for calcium without the use of fortified foods. Table 10–1 illustrates food choices for the groups listed above that would produce a diet that meets the calcium RDA.

Appetite and calorie needs vary greatly among preschoolers, however, and many children may eat less than the amounts noted in Table 10–1. Also, children who are picky eaters may not always be willing to consume many foods that are calcium rich. Therefore, most guidelines for feeding vegan children recommend regular use of a calcium-fortified soymilk.[37,38] If children dislike soymilk or are allergic to it, calcium fortified rice milk is an

---

Table 10–1 Food Choices That Meet the RDA for Calcium

Food	Calcium Content (mg)
¼ cup cooked rice	5
One slice bread	15
½ English muffin	46
¼ cup cooked broccoli	45
¼ cup cooked collards	89
¼ cup tofu	60
¼ cup baked beans	32
2 tbsp almond butter	86
3 cups soymilk	252
1 tbsp blackstrap molasses	187
½ orange	23
Total	840

Source: Data from *Bowes & Church's Food Value of Portions Commonly Used.* 16th ed., by J. Pennington, Lippincott-Raven, 1994, and package information.

alternative. It has a sweeter taste that may appeal to many children. Soymilk is more nutrient rich overall, however, and is a better first choice. Ways to incorporate milk into a child's diet are discussed later in this chapter. Calcium-fortified orange juice is also a good choice for children, although juices should be used in moderation in children's diets. Even with the use of fortified foods, it is important to emphasize foods that are naturally rich in calcium in the diets of all children.

The addition of even small amounts of foods that are rich in calcium can significantly increase calcium intake. Although many children may refuse sea vegetables, some may tolerate small amounts of these mineral-rich foods in a broth or wrapped around a child-sized nori roll. Adding blackstrap molasses to recipes can also boost calcium intake considerably.

VITAMIN D

Children can make adequate vitamin D with sun exposure. For light-skinned children in sunny climates, exposing the hands and face to the sun two or three times a week for about 20 to 30 minutes each is enough to provide adequate vitamin D, so that a dietary source of this nutrient may not be required for all children.[39] In fact, in most instances, for active children and adults it is casual everyday exposure to sunlight that provides them with their vitamin D requirement.[40]

Nevertheless, a regular source of dietary vitamin D is recommended for children who are otherwise at risk for vitamin D deficiency. This would include dark-skinned children or those who live in northern urban areas. Furthermore, because sun exposure may be erratic, consumption of a dietary source of vitamin D is prudent for all children.

Although fish oil and egg yolk can provide some natural vitamin D, this nutrient is poorly supplied by foods; fortification is nearly always depended upon to provide adequate vitamin D in the diets of children and adults. In the United States, milk is the most commonly recognized fortified food. Lacto-ovo vegetarian children will generally have no problem meeting vitamin D needs if they consume cow's milk. By law, vitamin D-fortified cow's milk must provide 10 µg of vitamin D per quart. Recently, there has been some concern about the wide variation in vitamin D content of cow's milk, with some samples containing potentially toxic levels of the vitamin (see Chapter 6).

Rickets due to vitamin D deficiency has been seen in some macrobiotic children.[41–44] A number of vegan products are vitamin D fortified, however, including some brands of soymilk or rice milk and many commercial cereals (see Exhibit 7–1 for examples of cereals that are fortified with vitamin D).

VITAMIN B$_{12}$

Because dairy products are rich in vitamin B$_{12}$, lacto-ovo vegetarians generally get enough of this nutrient, although their intake is lower than that of omnivores. Vegan diets are theoretically devoid of this nutrient unless fortified foods are used, however. Although there are few diet-related instances of vitamin B$_{12}$ deficiency, in some macrobiotic children vitamin B$_{12}$ deficiency has been seen when fortified foods were not used.[45,46] Fortunately, a variety of B$_{12}$-fortified products are available, including some brands of soymilk, meat analogues, and breakfast cereals.

IRON

Iron deficiency anemia is the most common childhood nutritional problem and is most likely to occur between the ages of 18 and 24 months. The iron density of vegetarian diets is generally higher (see Appendix H) than nonvegetarian diets. This appears also to be the case for the iron intake of vegetarian children, particularly vegan children.[17,36] Iron deficiency is no more likely to occur in vegetarian children, but all parents need to give attention to including iron-rich foods in their children's diets since iron bioavailability is lower in vegetarian diets.

Excessive consumption of milk and other dairy products can raise the risk for iron deficiency because milk is devoid of iron and, in the diets of young children, can displace iron-rich foods in the diet. It can also inhibit iron absorption[47-49] and cause iron loss through intestinal bleeding.[50,51] Because young children have fairly high iron needs and eat relatively small quantities of food, it is important to stress the inclusion of iron-dense foods in the diet.

Many plant foods are high in iron, but because the iron from plant foods is less well absorbed than that from meat, it is important to maximize the absorption of iron in the diets of children. It can be helpful to include some iron-fortified or iron-enriched refined foods in children's meals. Fortified cereals and enriched bread, rice, and pasta are good choices. Vitamin C greatly enhances the absorption of nonheme iron in the diet;[52,53] it is important to help parents plan meals for toddlers that include both an iron-rich food and a vitamin C–rich food at the same time. Good meal combinations include pasta with tomato sauce, cereal with orange juice, fruit salad with dried fruits added, and soymilk and strawberry shake. Some vegetables, such as spinach, broccoli, and other greens, are rich in both iron and vitamin C.

ZINC

There is little available information about the zinc content of the diets of vegetarian children. Although many plant foods are rich in zinc, bioavailability is lower on a vegetarian diet. Both fiber and phytate may inhibit zinc absorption. Serving more refined foods can reduce the zinc content of the diet, however, because much of the zinc is lost from a food when it is processed.

GUIDELINES FOR MEAL PLANNING FOR VEGETARIAN CHILDREN

Children can follow the same menu-planning guidelines as adults. Their diets should emphasize a wide variety of grains, legumes, vegetables, fruits, nuts, and seeds. Foods emphasized for children will be somewhat different than for adults, however, and serving sizes are, of course, much smaller. Although not a dietary necessity, vegetarian children will meet nutrient needs most easily if some type of milk (vegetable or cow's) is consumed. Milk can be a fortified soymilk or other vegetable milk (eg, Vegelicious) or low-fat cow's milk (or whole cow's milk before the age of 2 years). These milks can provide significant amounts of calcium and vitamin D in the diet. The food guides included in this chapter all recommend three servings a day of some type of milk for children. Of course, breast milk is also an option, and some children may consume breast milk well into their second year.

As noted earlier, children can meet vitamin D needs via sun exposure under optimal conditions, and calcium needs can be met using a variety of plant foods that are naturally rich in this nutrient. Even so, children, particularly toddlers and preschoolers, tend to consume small quantities of vegetables and legumes. Also, sun exposure can vary depending on climate. Therefore, it may be somewhat difficult to meet these needs without the use of fortified products.

Nuts and seeds may also play an important role in children's diets. Because these foods are high in fat, they are considered optional for adults, but for children they provide an easy way to boost calorie intake and intake of minerals such as zinc and manganese. For this reason, it is advisable that vegetarian children, particularly vegans, include a daily serving of nuts or seeds in their diet.

The use of supplemental foods can also add significantly to a child's nutrient intake. Good choices are a tablespoon each day of nutritional yeast (Red Star brand T6635 is reliably rich in vitamin B_{12}) and blackstrap molasses. Ideas for including these foods in the diets of children include the following:

- **Blackstrap molasses**

  Add to baked beans

  Use in muffin, cake, or cookie batter

  Mix into milkshakes

  Add to bean or vegetable stews

  Mix with peanut butter or other nut butters and spread thinly on sandwiches

- **Nutritional yeast**

  Mix into baked beans or other bean dishes

  Mix into white sauce to create a cheeselike sauce to use over vegetables or macaroni

  Sprinkle over popcorn (for older children)

  Add to veggie burgers or loaves

  Add to scrambled tofu

It is important that parents of vegan children identify a regular source of vitamin B_{12} to be included in the diet. This might be a fortified soymilk (although many brands of soymilk are not fortified with B_{12}, so that parents should be careful to read labels), nutritional yeast, fortified breakfast cereals, fortified meat analogues, or a vitamin supplement. Parents of macrobiotic children in particular should understand that sea vegetables and soy products such as tempeh and miso are not reliable sources of vitamin B_{12}.

The meal-planning guidelines presented in Appendix 10–A use the food guide presented in Chapter 7. For ages 1 to 6 years, total amounts of food rather than number of servings in the vegetable, fruit, legume, nuts, and milk groups is presented for ease of use. A number of other food guides have been developed for vegetarian children. Meal-planning guidelines based on these food guides are also presented in Appendix 10–A.

MILK IN THE DIETS OF VEGETARIAN CHILDREN

Milk can be a favorite food of children, vegetarian or otherwise. As noted above, milk can play an important nutritional role in children's diets. The type of milk chosen—breast milk, cow's milk, soymilk, or other vegetable milks such as rice milk or Vegelicious—will depend upon the child's diet (vegan children will consume soy or rice milk) and age (breast milk is not commonly consumed beyond 2 years of age, and its consumption is actually quite uncommon in the United States beyond the first birthday).

Where consumption of cow's milk is excessive, iron deficiency can be one outcome because cow's milk contains virtually no iron and because calcium and milk both inhibit iron absorption, although the long-term effects of high calcium intakes on iron status are less certain. Therefore, cow's milk should be limited in the diets of young children to no more than 3 cups per day. Although soymilk contains some iron, it is not well absorbed, and overconsumption of this food can displace other nutrient-rich foods in the diet.

Recently, there have been reports in the literature of an increased risk of diabetes among susceptible children when cow's milk is consumed (see Chapter 2 for more detail on this subject). Initial reports linked consumption of cow's milk, either as unmodified milk or as cow's milk infant formula, during the first year of life to elevated risk for diabetes.[54] More recently, however, it has been shown that cow's milk consumption throughout childhood is associated with development of juvenile onset diabetes.[55]

Whether these findings justify limiting or even eliminating cow's milk in children's diets remains an issue of debate. It is clear, however, that no one food group should be depended upon to provide a particular nutrient. It is important that dietitians instruct all clients in choosing calcium-rich foods from all the food groups.

COUNSELING PARENTS OF VEGETARIAN CHILDREN

The food intake of children can seem fairly erratic because their appetite tends to follow their rate of growth. Appetite is generally good in infancy, when a child is growing quickly, but by the preschool years both growth and appetite slow, and children begin to form strong food and eating preferences. Disinterest in food is generally evident in most toddlers and preschoolers.

General guidelines for encouraging good eating habits in a young child combine a respect for the child's independence with a healthy dose of parental control. It is believed that allowing the child to make food decisions in an environment that includes a wide variety of nutritious foods will eventually lead to a wider acceptance of healthful foods.

Introducing New Foods

Familiarity is an important dimension of food preference for toddlers and preschoolers.[56] Therefore, acceptance of a new food may be a multistep process for young children. They may need to see the food on their plate several times before they are willing to try it. It is particularly important for parents of vegetarian children to understand this. Foods that are emphasized in vegetarian diets may not be typical fare for the average young child, and vegetarian children are unlikely to see these foods in preschool or at friends' homes. If a particular food is refused on the first offer, it is sometimes assumed by the parent that it is a food the child will not eat. Frequent offerings of the item may eventually lead to acceptance, however.

The attitude with which parents present foods is also important. Children learn which foods are acceptable and which are not in part by observing adult reactions to foods. Therefore, it is imperative that children see parents enjoying a wide range of healthy vegetarian foods.

When parents are introducing new foods to a preschooler, it may help to include one well-liked food in a meal and to offer the new food in a tiny amount. Food preferences can be erratic at this age, however; a food that is a favorite one week may be refused the next week. Similarly, children may suddenly begin to eat a food that they previously disliked.

Getting Children To Eat Vegetables and Legumes

Most children enjoy a varied selection of grains, fruits, juices, and nuts. Many, however, will reject a variety of vegetables and legumes. These foods can be important contributors of nutrients in the diets of vegetarian children and should be introduced early and regularly. Some tips for introducing more of these foods into the diets of children include the following:

- Make foods as easy to eat as possible. Young children like finger foods, which may include chunks of braised tofu or strips of steamed vegetables.
- Make mealtimes fun by incorporating raw vegetables into salads in the shapes of animals and other familiar objects.
- Vary the ways in which foods are served. Raw vegetables may be more acceptable than cooked ones. Offer these vegetables with dips. A child who rejects chunks of tofu may enjoy it pureed into a cheese sauce with macaroni. Researchers at Southern Illinois University found that tofu incorporated into familiar dishes was well accepted by preschoolers.[57]
- Involve children in food preparation to increase their interest in a new meal. Family gardens can be one way to pique a child's interest in vegetables.
- Dilute the taste of strongly flavored vegetables, such as kale, collards, or other greens, by blending them with bland-tasting foods, such as tofu, avocado, or ricotta cheese.
- Some vegetables can be incorporated in small amounts into well-liked dishes. Greens can be finely shredded and mixed into soups or spa-

ghetti sauce. Finely chopped vegetables can be added to nut or bean loaves or burgers. Shredded carrots and zucchini can be added to muffin or quick bread batters.

Getting Children To Drink Milk

The following suggestions are for any type of milk (soy, nonsoy vegetable milks, or cow's milk):

- Use milk in shakes with frozen or fresh fruit.
- Cook hot cereals with milk.
- Use milk in cream soups.
- Add milk to the batter of baked goods.

Meeting Calorie Needs

A first step in helping children meet calorie needs is providing an atmosphere that fosters good eating habits at mealtime. Children should be rested, and mealtime should be pleasant with no distractions, such as toys or television.

If appetite is poor in a toddler or preschooler, it can be made worse by a plate that is overloaded with food. Parents should serve small portions and let the child ask for more. Appetite will vary from day to day in the same child and will be different among different children within the same age group. Children need to judge when they are full and should not be forced to finish everything on their plate.

Because children have considerable calorie and nutrient needs and their stomach capacity is small, a pattern of three meals per day will not be sufficient for the average child. Snacks are an important means of meeting nutrient needs. Research indicates that children who eat more than six times per day are more likely to have higher intakes of calories, calcium, and vitamin C than average, whereas those who eat less than four times a day have lower than average intakes of iron and protein.[58] Good snack ideas for vegetarian children include the following:

- muffins
- fruit-flavored milkshakes using cow's or vegetable milk
- vegetable soup with crackers
- crackers spread thinly with nut butter
- trail mix (for older children)
- oatmeal cookies or graham crackers with juice

- frozen bananas
- frozen juice bars
- dried fruits
- yogurt with fruit

The high fiber content of vegetarian meals can fill a child up quickly. Where calorie needs are not easily being met, parents may wish to limit the use of high-fiber foods in their child's diet. Good choices for nutritious refined grains are hot cereals such as farina or Cream of Rice, many ready-to-eat cereals, muffins made with 1/2 white flour and 1/2 whole wheat flour, applesauce, fruit juice, and white rice. Parents can also peel fruits such as apples to make them easier to eat.

High-calorie foods can also play a role in the diets of vegetarian children. Good choices include legume spreads, nut butters, tofu and nut butter spreads, avocado as a sandwich spread or in small chunks, soymilk shakes with fruits, and dried fruit spreads. Small amounts of added fats, such as mayonnaise (eggless mayonnaise is available for vegans) on sandwiches, a small amount of margarine on vegetables, or foods sauteed in oil, can also help boost a child's calorie intake.

VEGETARIAN DIETS FOR SCHOOL-AGE CHILDREN

Growth during the school years is slow and steady and appetite will reflect this to some degree. Food-related problems, such as food jags, have usually played themselves out by this time, although strong food preferences (and dislikes) can persist.

The overall eating behavior of children is bound to change when they enter school. For one thing, snacks will be less frequent, so that well-balanced meals become more important than ever. If children are left to get themselves ready for school in the morning, there may be a tendency to skip breakfast. After-school activities may interfere with after-school snacks and perhaps even with family mealtime. Many children may also participate in the school's lunch program, which may offer few options for vegetarian children.

Some children may exhibit discomfort with their vegetarian diet. Peer pressure is an important influence in this age group. Also, children may be exposed to nutrition education lessons in school that are at variance with the family's eating practices. The child may learn for the first time that vegetarianism is an "alternative" dietary choice. Among older school-age children, however, vegetarian diet is increasingly viewed as attractive, so that many vegetarian children will continue to be comfortable with this choice. Where children are not comfortable with being different, parents can pack lunches that appear more "mainstream" if they are acceptable to the child. For example, sandwiches can be made using soy cheese or meat analogues. Soymilk can be saved for snacks and at-home meals, and juice can be packed in bag lunches.

The decision to let a child experiment with foods that are not a part of the family's chosen diet is strictly a family decision that is based on philosophical concerns and needs to be assessed in reference to the family's own values. Where children are resistant to the family's vegetarian diet, the outcome will be different among families, and there is no right or wrong resolution to the issue.

SCHOOL LUNCH

The National School Lunch Program (NSLP) was started in the 1940s to provide low-cost, nutritious meals to hungry children. Today, it serves more than 25 million students daily and is a critically important means of ensuring adequate nutrient intake among low-income children. Schools that participate in the NSLP must serve meals that provide a third of the RDA for protein and several other nutrients. In an effort to keep costs low, school lunch programs depend on millions of dollars' worth of donated foods from the US Department of Agriculture (USDA) each year. These foods, which include eggs, cheese, butter, ground pork, ground beef, and milk, represent 20% to 30% of the food served in school cafeterias.[59]

Although the NSLP is successful in providing nutrient-rich meals, it has been criticized for providing meals that are too high in fat, saturated fat, and cholesterol. School lunches provide 37% fat and 15% saturated fat. Children who eat school lunches have higher-fat diets than children who do not.[59]

Few (if any) lunch offerings in most schools are vegetarian. Some vegetarian foods are not allowable items in the school lunch program. For example, tofu cannot be served as a meat substitute despite the fact that the protein quality of tofu is equal to that of animal foods and that the American Dietetic Association has recommended the inclusion of this food in school lunches.[60] Particularly in school districts with a high percentage of Asian students, tofu would be a popular item.

Also, meals must include specific servings from food groups. A more useful way to plan meals is to rate them on their total nutrient content. Presently, the USDA is testing a program that would allow schools to do this. Changes such as these would allow the introduction of more vegetarian meals into schools. Consumer demand will be the biggest determinant of whether this happens, however.

BAG LUNCH

Although studies show that lunches brought from home are lower in nutrient content than the school lunch menus, they actually may provide a better option for most school children, particularly for vegetarian children.[61] Parents can plan lunches around a child's food preferences, so that there is more likelihood that all the meal will be consumed. Parents have much greater control over the amount of fat in the diet. For children in vegetarian families, there is the opportunity for much greater variety in these meals, and for vegan children lunches brought from home are the only viable option in most school systems.

The following suggestions for bag lunches will appeal to many children:

- **Sandwiches**
  Hummus spread with sliced tomatoes and lettuce
  Almond or peanut butter with shredded carrots
  Peanut butter blended with pureed tofu, ricotta cheese, or dried fruits
  "Missing egg salad" (egg salad with chopped tofu in place of the eggs and vegan mayonnaise)
  Avocado blended with chopped or shredded raw vegetables
  Peanut butter mixed with crushed pineapple and raisins
  "No tuna salad" (chopped chickpeas flavored with kelp powder and lemon in place of tuna)
  Submarine sandwich with cheese (soy or dairy), lettuce, tomatoes, and other sliced vegetables
  Cheese with sliced apples
- **Lunch box stuffers**
  Fresh fruit
  Raw carrots, celery, or zucchini rounds or strips
  Trail mix
  Dried fruit
  Rice cakes
- **Beverages**
  Individual containers of soy, rice, or almond milk
  Juice

- **Treats**

Oatmeal cookies

Homemade small fruit pies

Graham crackers

When perishable items are packed in a lunch box, an ice pack should be used. A small container of frozen juice can also be used and should keep foods cold but defrost by lunchtime.

REFERENCES

1. Nutrition Monitoring Division, Human Nutrition Information Service. Nationwide food consumption survey—Continuing survey of food intake by individuals—1985. *Nutr Today.* 1986;21:18–22.
2. Nutrition Monitoring Division, Human Nutrition Information Service. Nationwide food consumption survey—Continuing survey of food intake by individuals—1986. *Nutr Today.* 1987;22:36–39.
3. Sabaté J, Linsted KD, Harris RD, Johnston PK. Anthropometric parameters of schoolchildren with different life-styles. *Am J Dis Child.* 1990;144:1159–1163.
4. Sabaté J, Linsted KD, Harris RD, Sanchez A. Attained height of lacto-ovo vegetarian children and adolescents. *Eur J Clin Nutr.* 1991;45:51–58.
5. Sabaté J, Llorca C, Sanchez A. Lower height of lacto-ovovegetarian girls at preadolescence: An indicator of physical maturation today? *J Am Diet Assoc.* 1992;92:1263–1264.
6. Hamill PVV, Drizd TA, Johnson CL, Reed RB, Roche AF, Moore WM. Physical growth: National Center for Health Statistics percentiles. *Am J Clin Nutr.* 1979;32:607–629.
7. Kissinger DG, Sanchez A. The association of dietary factors with the age of menarche. *Nutr Res.* 1987;7:471–479.
8. Sanchez A, Kissinger DG, Phillips RJ. A hypothesis on the etiologic role of diet on age of menarche. *Med Hypotheses.* 1981;7:139–145.
9. De Waard F, Trichopoulos D. A unifying concept of the aetiology of breast cancer. *Int J Cancer.* 1988;41:666–669.
10. American Academy of Pediatrics, Committee on Nutrition. Nutritional aspects of vegetarian diets. In: Committee on Nutrition, *Paediatric Nutrition Handbook,* 3rd ed. Elk Grove Village, Ill: American Academy of Pediatrics; 1993:302–313.
11. Sanders TAB. Growth and development of British vegan children. *Am J Clin Nutr.* 1988;48:822–825.
12. O'Connell JM, Dibley MJ, Sierra J, Wallace B, Marks JS, Yip R. Growth of vegetarian children: The Farm study. *Pediatrics.* 1989;84:475–481.
13. Fulton JR, Hutton CW, Stitt KR. Preschool vegetarian children. *J Am Diet Assoc.* 1980;76:360–365.
14. Dagnelie PC, van Staveren WA, Vergote FJVRA, et al. Nutritional status of infants aged 4 to 18 months on macrobiotic diets and matched omnivorous control infants: A population-based mixed-longitudinal study. II. Growth and psychomotor development. *Eur J Clin Nutr.* 1989;43:325–338.

15. Dwyer JT, Andrew EM, Berkey C, Valadian I, Reed RB. Growth in "new" vegetarian pre-school children using the Jenss-Bayley curve fitting technique. *Am J Clin Nutr.* 1983;37:815–827.

16. Kushi M, Kushi A. *Macrobiotic Child Care and Family Health.* Tokyo, Japan: Japan Publications; 1986.

17. Sanders TAB, Purves R. An anthropometric and dietary assessment of the nutritional status of vegan preschool children. *J Hum Nutr.* 1981;35:349–357.

18. Shull MW, Reed RB, Valadian I, Palombo R, Thorne H, Dwyer JT. Velocities of growth in vegetarian preschool children. *Pediatrics.* 1977;60:410–417.

19. Shull M, Valadian I, Reed RB, Palomobo R, Thorne H, Dwyer J. Seasonal variations in preschool vegetarian children's growth velocities. *Am J Clin Nutr.* 1978;31:1–11.

20. Dwyer JT, Andrew EM, Valadian I, Reed RB. Size, obesity, and leanness in vegetarian preschool children. *J Am Diet Assoc.* 1980;77:434–439.

21. Brown PT, Bergan JG. The dietary status of "new" vegetarians. *J Am Diet Assoc.* 1975;67:455–459.

22. van Staveren WA, Dhuyvetter JHM, Bons A, Zeelen M, Hautvast JGAG. Food consumption and height/weight status of Dutch preschool children on alternative diets. *J Am Diet Assoc.* 1985;85:1579–1584.

23. Dagnelie PC, van Staveren WA, Vergote FJVRA, Dingjan PG, van den Berg H, Hautvast JGAG. Increased risk of vitamin B12 and iron deficiency in infants on macrobiotic diets. *Am J Clin Nutr.* 1989;50:818–824.

24. Dwyer JT, Dietz WH Jr, Andrews EM, Suskind RM. Nutritional status of vegetarian children. *Am J Clin Nutr.* 1982;35:204–216.

25. Kramer LB, Osis D, Coffey J, Spencer H. Mineral and trace element content of vegetarian diets. *J Am Coll Nutr.* 1984;3:3–11.

26. Albanes D, Taylor PR. International differences in body height and weight and their relationship to cancer incidence. *Nutr Cancer.* 1990;14:69–77.

27. Hemenway D, Azruel DR, Rimm EB, Feskanich D, Willett WC. Risk factors for hip fracture in US men aged 40 through 75 years. *Am J Public Health.* 1994;84:1843–1845.

28. Dwyer JT, Miller LC, Arduino NL, et al. Mental age and IQ of predominantly vegetarian children. *J Am Diet Assoc.* 1980;76:143–147.

29. van Staveren WA, Dhuyvetter JHM, Bons A, Zeelen M, Hautvast JGAJ. Food consumption and height/weight status of Dutch preschool children on alternative diets. *J Am Diet Assoc.* 1985;85:1579–1584.

30. Dagnelie PC, van Staveren WA, Verschuren SAJM, Hautvast JGAJ. Nutritional status of infants aged 4 to 18 months on macrobiotic diets and matched omnivorous control infants: A population-based mixed longitudinal study. I. Weaning pattern, energy and nutrient intake. *Eur J Clin Nutr.* 1989;43:311–323.

31. Tayter M, Stanek KL. Anthropometric and dietary assessment of omnivore and lacto-ovo-vegetarian children. *J Am Diet Assoc.* 1989;89:1661–1663.

32. Nicklas TA, Webber LS, Koschak ML, Berenson GS. Nutrient adequacy of low fat intakes for children: The Bogalusa Heart Study. *Pediatrics.* 1992;89:221–228.

33. Boulton TJC, Magarey AM. Effects of differences in dietary fat on growth, energy and nutrient intake from infancy to eight years of age. *Acta Paediatr.* 1995;84:148–150.

34. National Cholesterol Education Program. Highlights of the report of the Expert Panel on Blood Cholesterol Levels in Children and Adolescents. *Pediatrics.* 1992;89:495–500.

35. Ruys J, Hickie JB. Serum cholesterol and triglyceride levels in Australian adolescent vegetarians. *Br Med J*. 1976;2:87.

36. Sanders TAB, Manning J. The growth and development of vegan children. *J Hum Nutr Diet*. 1992;5:11–21.

37. Haddad EH. Development of a vegetarian food guide. *Am J Clin Nutr*. 1995;59(suppl).

38. Mangels AR. Nutrition Section. In: Wasserman D, *Simply Vegan*. Baltimore, Md: Vegetarian Resource Group; 1995:191.

39. Specker BL, Valanis B, Hertzberg V, et al. Sunshine exposure and serum 25-hydroxyvitamin D concentrations in exclusively breast-fed infants. *J Pediatr*. 1985;107:372–376.

40. Holick MF. Importance of an adequate source of vitamin D for calcium metabolism. Presented at the National Institutes of Health Consensus Development Conference on Optimal Calcium Intake; June 6–8, 1994; Bethesda, Md.

41. Jacabs C, Dwyer JT. Vegetarian children: Appropriate and inappropriate diets. *Am J Clin Nutr*. 1988;48:811–818.

42. Dagnelie PC, Vergote FJRVA, van Staveren WA, van den Berg H, Dingjan PG, Hautvast JGAJ. High prevalence of rickets in infants on macrobiotic diets. *Am J Clin Nutr*. 1990;51:202–208.

43. Salmon P, Rees JRP, Flanagan M, O'Moore R. Hypocalcaemia in a mother and rickets in an infant associated with a Zen macrobiotic diet. *Isr J Med Sci*. 1981;150:192–193.

44. Dwyer JT, Dietz WH Jr, Hass G, Suskind R. Risk of nutritional rickets among vegetarian children. *Am J Dis Child*. 1979;133:134–140.

45. Higginbottom MC, Sweetman L, Nyhan WL. A syndrome of methylmalonic aciduria, homocysteinuria, megoblastic anemia and neurologic abnormalities of a vitamin B12-deficient breast-fed infant of a strict vegetarian. *Am J Med*. 1970;48:390–397.

46. Specker BL, Black A, Allen L, Morrow F. Vitamin B12: Low milk concentrations are related to low serum concentrations in vegetarian women and to methylmalonic aciduria in their infants. *Am J Clin Nutr*. 1990;52:1073–1076.

47. Gleerup A, Rossander-Hultén L, Gramatkovski E, Hallberg L. Iron absorption from the whole diet: Comparison of the effect of two different distributions of daily calcium intake. *Am J Clin Nutr*. 1995;61:97–104.

48. Hallberg L, Rossander-Hultén L, Brune M, Gleerup A. Calcium and iron absorption; Mechanism of action and nutritional importance. *Eur J Clin Nutr*. 1992;46:317–327.

49. Hallberg L, Brune M, Erlandsson M, Sandberg A-S, Rossander-Hultén L. Calcium: Effect of different amounts on nonheme- and heme-iron absorption in humans. *Am J Clin Nutr*. 1991;53:112–119.

50. Ziegler EE, Foman SJ, Nelson SE, et al. Cow milk feeding in infancy: Further observations on blood loss from the gastrointestinal tract. *J Pediatr*. 1990;16:11–18.

51. Woodruff CW, Clark JL. The role of fresh cow's milk in iron deficiency. *Am J Dis Child*. 1972;124:18–23.

52. Monsen ER, Balintfy JL. Calculating dietary iron bioavailability: Refinement and computerization. *J Am Diet Assoc*. 1982;80:307–311.

53. Cook JD, Monsen ER. Vitamin C, the common cold, and iron absorption in man. *Am J Clin Nutr*. 1977;30:225–241.

54. Gerstein HC. Cow's milk exposure and type I diabetes mellitus. *Diabetes Care*. 1994;17:13–19.

55. Fava D, Leslie RDG, Pozzilli P. Relationship between dairy product consumption and incidence of IDDM in childhood in Italy. *Diabetes Care.* 1994;17:1488–1490.

56. Hammer LD. The development of eating behavior in childhood. *Pediatr Clin North Am.* 1992;39:379–394.

57. Ashraf H-R, Schoeppel C, Nelson JA. Use of tofu in preschool meals. *J Am Diet Assoc.* 1990;90:1114–1116.

58. Eppright ES. The North Central Regional Study of diets of preschool children III. Frequency of eating. *J Home Econ.* 1970;62:407.

59. US Department of Agriculture, Food and Nutrition Service. *Dietary Status of School Children.*

60. ADA comments on proposed rule for meat alternates used in child nutrition programs. *J Am Diet Assoc.* 1986;86:530–531.

61. Ho CS, Gould RA, Jensen LN, et al. Evaluation of the nutrient content of school, sack and vending lunch of junior high students. *Sch Food Serv Res Rev.* 1991;15:85.

62. Truesdell DD, Acosta PB. Feeding the vegan infant and child. *J Am Diet Assoc.* 1985;85:837–840.

63. Vyhmeister IB, Register UD, Sonnenberg LM. Safe vegetarian diets for children. *Pediatr Clin N Amer.* 1977;24:203–210.

Meal-Planning Guidelines for Children

Food Group	1–4 Years	5–6 Years	7–12 Years
Grains	Four servings	Six servings	Seven servings
Vegetables			
Leafy green	2–4 tbsp	¼ cup	One serving
Other	¼–½ cup	¼–½ cup	Three servings
Fruits	¾–1½ cups	1–2 cups	Three servings
Legumes	¼–½ cup	½–1 cup	Two servings
Nuts and seeds	1–2 tbsp	1–2 tbsp	One serving
Soymilk, cow's milk, First Alternative or Vegelicious, breast milk	3 cups	3 cups	3 cups
Fats	3 tsp	4 tsp	5 tsp
Red Star nutritional yeast T6635, blackstrap molasses	Use these foods frequently to flavor dishes		

OTHER FOOD GUIDES

Haddad Food Guide*

	Number of Servings		
Food Group	1–4 Years	5–6 Years	7–12 Years
Breads, grains, cereals	Three–four	Four–five	Five–six
Legumes, plant proteins	One half	One	One
Vegetables	One–two	Two–three	Two–three
Fruits	Two–three	Two–three	Three–four
Nut butter or nuts	One quarter	One half	One
Milk, yogurt, cheese, fortified soymilk	Two–three	Two–three	Two–three
Eggs (optional)	One half	One half	One half
Margarine and oils	Two	Three–four	Four
Sugar	Three	Three–six	Six

*Based on Reference 37.

Mangels Food Guide*

Food Group	1–4 Years	5–6 Years	7–12 Years
Bread	Three slices	Four slices	Four–five slices
Cereals and grains	½ cup	1 cup	1 cup
Nuts, nut butter, legumes, tofu	3 tbsp–1 cup	3 tbsp–1 cup	3 tbsp–1½ cups
Fats	3 tsp	4 tsp	5 tsp
Fruits			
Citrus	½–1 cup	½–1 cup	½–1 cup
Other	¼–¾ cup	½–1 cup	1–1½ cups
Vegetables			
Leafy green or yellow	2–3 tbsp	¼–⅓ cup	½–1 cup
Other	¼–⅓ cup	¼–⅓ cup	1–1½ cups
Soymilk	3 cups	3 cups	3–4 cups
Nutritional yeast	1 tbsp	1 tbsp	1 tbsp
Blackstrap molasses	1 tbsp	1 tbsp	1 tbsp

*Based on Reference 38 and adapted from references 62, 63.

CHAPTER 11

Vegetarian Diets for Adolescents

Vegetarian adolescents represent a rapidly growing segment of the vegetarian population. Teens are often attracted to both animal rights and environmental arguments for a meatless diet. Although some teens grow up in vegetarian households, an increasing number who live in omnivore households are choosing a vegetarian diet. As a result, teens' diets may be a subject of great concern to parents, and some adolescents may not have the support of parents in planning vegetarian meals.

Few data are available on the eating habits of vegetarian teenagers (Appendixes L, M, N, and O). Omnivore teenagers tend to have diets that are too high in fat and sugar and low in fiber and complex carbohydrates.[1] Obesity is a significant problem among American teenagers.[2] Teens' diets also are often too low in folate, calcium, iron, vitamin C, and magnesium.[3] Because adult vegetarians typically consume less fat and more fiber than adult omnivores and have diets that are high in vitamin B_6 and folate (and calcium for lacto-ovo vegetarians), it is reasonable to speculate that vegetarian teenagers will enjoy the same advantages. For example, a recent study found that female vegetarian adolescents consume 40% more fiber and 20% more vitamin C than omnivore adolescents;[4] these data are consistent with other studies of adolescents (Appendixes L and M). Nutrition is often a low priority for all teens, however, and problematic eating habits can be typical of teenagers no matter what type of diet they choose.

GROWTH OF VEGETARIAN ADOLESCENTS

Growth is faster during the growth spurt of adolescence than at any other time in life, with the exception of infancy. Fifty percent of adult weight and 20% of adult height are acquired during puberty.[5] During the 2 to 3 years of fastest adolescent growth, a boy can add 10 inches to his height. Nearly half the skeleton is formed during the adolescent years as well. Growth is erratic during this period, however. The actual growth spurt lasts only 1½ to 2 years. For girls, it generally occurs between the ages of 10 and 13, and the fastest growth is seen in the year preceding menarche. For boys, the growth spurt occurs later, generally between the ages of 12 and 15 years. During this time, nutrient needs can be twice as high as at other times of adolescence.[6] Boys grow faster and for a longer period of time than girls, and they also gain more muscle tissue, whereas girls deposit more fat. As a result, boys require more iron, zinc, and protein. They also are likely to need more calcium, although this is not reflected in the recommended dietary allowances (RDAs)[7] (Table 11–1).

Although nutrient needs can be high during some periods in adolescence, appetite tends to follow growth, so that teens eat more when they are growing fastest. Also, calorie needs are quite high compared with nutrient needs, so that appropriate nutrient density of diets can actually be lower in adolescence than in adulthood.

There are limited data available on the growth of vegetarian adolescents, although studies suggest there is little difference between vegetarians and omnivores.[4,8–10] In a study of 1,800 lacto-ovo vegetarians between the ages of 7 and 18 years, vegetarians were slightly taller than omnivores; among Adventists, vegetarians were taller than nonvegetarians.[11] The exception was

Table 11–1 Daily Increments in Body Content Due to Growth in Adolescence

Nutrient	Average for Ages 10–20 Years (mg)	During Peak of Growth Spurt (mg)
Calcium (mg)		
Male	210	400
Female	110	240
Iron (mg)		
Male	0.57	1.1
Female	0.23	0.9
Nitrogen (mg)		
Male	320	610 (3.8 g protein)
Female	160	360 (2.2 g protein)
Zinc (mg)		
Male	0.27	0.50
Female	0.18	0.31

Source: Forbes GB, Nutritional requirements in adolescence. In: Suskind RM, ed: *Textbook of Pediatric Nutrition.* Raven Press: New York; 1981.

11- and 12-year-old girls, who were slightly shorter than their omnivore peers. This probably reflects the fact that vegetarian girls have a later menarche than omnivore girls[12,13] and is consistent with the observation that girls in countries that consume plant-based diets also have a later onset of menstruation.[14,15] Later menarche has not been associated with any health risks and in fact may reduce risk for breast cancer later in life.[16,17]

NUTRIENT NEEDS OF VEGETARIAN ADOLESCENTS

There are few studies on the nutrient needs of adolescents; consequently, the RDAs for adolescents are based on scant data. The RDAs are stated for three different age groups for adolescents, but growth varies considerably among individuals within the same age group. Some teens may experience their growth spurt at age 13, whereas for others it may not occur until several years later. Therefore, the age divisions in the RDAs may not reflect the actual growth pattern of the individual adolescent.

Individual needs can be better calculated based on the adolescent's height. Dividing the total RDA of a nutrient by the reference individual's height provides the amount of the nutrient needed per centimeter of height and can be used to determine an individual's specific needs. For example, the protein RDA for a 12-year-old boy is 45 g, and the height of the reference individual for this age is 157 cm (62 inches); this gives 0.29 g of protein per centimeter (45 g ÷ 157 cm = 0.29 g/cm). Therefore, for a boy who is 145 cm tall, the specific protein RDA would be 42 g (0.29 g/cm × 145 cm = 42 g), but for a boy who is 175 cm tall it would be 51 g.

Calorie Needs

Teenagers have high calorie needs. On a body weight basis, they require about 50% more calories than adults. Energy needs will actually vary considerably among teenagers, however, and in the same teen over time depending on the growth rate at any given age and the level of physical activity. Some teens who are involved in athletics may have exceptionally high calorie needs. This represents an advantage because it encourages greater food consumption among teenagers and increases the likelihood of meeting nutrient needs. For proper growth and development, it is important that teenagers meet those calorie needs. At the same time, it is important to recognize that American teens tend to have diets that are too high in fat, and a significant percentage of these teenagers are overweight. On the other hand, very low-fat diets can jeopardize calorie intake, especially during the growth spurt. Limited data suggest little difference in caloric intake between vegetarian and omnivore adolescents (Appendix L).

Protein

Protein should provide about 7% to 8 % of calories in a teenager's diet (45 to 59 g/day). This amount of protein actually represents a slightly smaller percentage of calories than is the case for adults. Vegetarian adults easily meet protein needs; even vegans consume between 10% and 12% of their calories in the form of protein. Consequently, it is extremely likely that vegetarian teens will meet their protein needs because, relatively speaking, they actually need less protein than adults. Limited data suggest protein intake to be above requirements and similar to nonvegetarians (Appendix I). There is no need to emphasize protein in the diet when counseling vegetarian adolescents.

Calcium

The RDA for calcium for teenagers is 1,200 mg/day. Some experts believe that calcium needs are higher, as high as 1,500 mg/day.[18] Other countries, however, including some Western countries, set much lower recommendations. For example, calcium recommendations for adolescents in the United Kingdom are just 700 mg/day.[19] Calcium needs will probably vary considerably throughout the teenage years according to the rate of growth.

Omnivore teenagers, particularly girls, often do not meet the calcium RDA.[3] Adult lacto-ovo vegetarian intake of calcium is equal to or higher than omnivore intake. Nevertheless, limited data indicate lacto-ovo vegetarian adolescents do not meet the RDA for calcium (Appendix O). Vegan calcium intake is considerably lower than lacto-ovo vegetarians and omnivores. Vegans consume less total protein and no animal protein and perhaps somewhat less sodium; these factors may help compensate for their lower calcium intake. Worldwide, populations that consume less calcium than Western populations frequently experience a lower rate of hip fracture.[20] Nevertheless, there are many genetic and life style factors that affect bone health and hip fracture, so that extrapolation from one culture to another must be done cautiously. Furthermore, there are no studies on the bone health of life-long vegans residing in Western countries.

For those reasons, it is prudent for vegetarian teenagers to strive to meet the calcium RDA. Calcium-rich foods that are likely to appeal to teenagers include calcium-fortified orange juice, almond butter, tahini, figs, calcium-fortified soymilk, calcium-set tofu, textured soy protein, soynuts, English muffins, and corn tortillas. Beans and dark leafy green vegetables can also boost calcium intake considerably but may not be well liked by all teens. The use of some type of calcium-rich milk may be advisable for most teenagers. This can include fortified soymilk, fortified rice milk, Vegelicious, or cow's milk. Nondairy fortified vegetable milks can be good choices because cow's milk is devoid of iron. Regardless of the type of milk chosen, it is wise to encourage all teenagers to explore a variety of calcium-rich foods rather than depend on one food group to provide this nutrient.

Teens should also be encouraged to avoid full-fat dairy products. When cow's milk is chosen, skim or 1% should be used. Cheese and ice cream can provide calcium, but they do so at the risk of an increased intake of saturated fat and cholesterol and should be used on a limited basis unless they are reduced-fat versions.

Iron

Iron deficiency anemia is the most common nutritional deficiency in the world and in American adolescents.[21,22] Teenage girls in particular, because of their lower calorie intake and their greater iron needs, require a particularly iron-dense diet. Vegetarian diets, particularly vegan diets, are often higher in iron than omnivore diets, although nonheme iron is more poorly absorbed. In a study of US adolescents, lacto-ovo vegetarians consumed more iron than omnivores (11.4 mg vs 9.5 mg).[10] But a study of Canadian female adolescents found iron intake was similar between lacto-ovo vegetarians and omnivores, and twice as many vegetarians as omnivores had ferritin levels indicative of depleted iron stores. Fewer vegetarians, however, had two or more abnormal indices of iron status.[4] Excessive use of dairy products can be a disadvantage because dairy foods are devoid of iron, and both calcium and milk are potent inhibitors of iron absorption.[23] Although the long-term effects of calcium and iron status have yet to be determined, adolescents should be counseled to use milk in moderation and to include iron-rich foods in their diets. Excellent sources of iron that will appeal to many teenagers include bran flakes, instant oatmeal, bread, nuts, nut butters, potatoes, and dried fruits.

Vitamin B12

The RDA for vitamin B12 is 50% higher for adolescents than for children. These recommendations can easily be met by lacto-ovo vegetarians who consume 2 cups of cow's milk or the equivalent. Vegans need to use fortified foods or supplements.

Zinc

Zinc is needed for growth and sexual maturation in adolescence. Both protein and phosphorus may raise zinc requirements.[24] Consequently, vegetarians, particularly vegans, may need less zinc. Zinc is absorbed somewhat less well from vegetarian diets than from omnivore diets, however, so that it is important that all teenagers get enough of this nutrient.[25] In Canadian female adolescents, zinc intake was about 15% lower among vegetarians than omnivores.[4] However, in a small study of British adolescents, vegetarian zinc intake was higher (9.3 mg vs 7.6 mg) than that of omnivores.[26] Dairy products can significantly contribute to the zinc intake of lacto-ovo vegetarians. Good plant sources of zinc for teenagers include whole grains, legumes, and nuts.

MEAL-PLANNING GUIDELINES FOR VEGETARIAN ADOLESCENTS

Adolescents can follow meal-planning guidelines that are similar to those for adults and can use the same serving sizes, but they will often require more servings from most of the food groups. As is true for adults, there are many different food patterns that can offer adequate nutrition. As with children, adolescents in Western countries may find it easiest to meet nutrient needs if the use of a nutrient-rich milk, either a vegetable milk or cow's milk, is continued. Three servings per day are recommended in the food guide shown in Table 11–2. If teens prefer not to use milks at all or do not consume the recommended number of servings, however, they can still meet nutrient needs by choosing other calcium-rich foods.

As for adults, the number of servings in each of the food groups represents the minimum, and in some cases teens who are not at a rapid stage of growth may actually require less food than this. Boys and those who are at a period of rapid growth or who are physically active may require more than the number of servings represented in Table 11–2, however.

Dietitians may be called upon to counsel vegetarian teenagers or families with vegetarian teenagers in planning appropriate menus. Special care may

---

Table 11–2 Food Guide for Vegetarian Adolescents

Food Group	Number of Servings Per Day
Grains, breads, cereals	10
Legumes, nuts, seeds, milks	
Legumes	2
Nuts/seeds	1
Fortified soymilk, fortified rice milk, Vegelicious, cow's milk	3
Vegetables	
Leafy green	1–2
Other	3
Fruit	4
Fats	4

be required in discussing food habits with teenagers because these clients can interpret criticism of food habits as personal criticism. Also, food choices can be a point of intense conflict in families, especially where teenagers choose a diet that is different from that of the rest of the family. It is important to elicit support for, and interest in, the teen's diet from the parents. Many nonvegetarian parents will agree to allow a teenager to choose vegetarianism but may be reluctant to participate actively in menu planning and food preparation to support this dietary choice. Wherever possible, dietitians should encourage parents to become active participants in the teen's efforts to consume a vegetarian diet. Some adolescents may experience difficulty in planning appropriate vegetarian diets if parents do not willingly cooperate by purchasing "special" foods such as soymilk, beans, vegetarian burgers, and so forth. Good nutrition is not a high priority with most teenagers, so that they may need some supervision from parents in planning menus. Sincere interest in and acceptance of the vegetarian eating plan will encourage teens to accept some menu-planning guidance from parents.

Introducing more vegetarian meals that the whole family enjoys, such as spaghetti with tomato sauce or bean burritos, can be a unifying approach to mealtime, especially in a family where the teen's dietary change has disrupted family mealtimes. So can using more meals that can be served with and without meat. Spaghetti can be served meatless to the vegetarian teen and with meat to the rest of the family. Mealtime can include a variety of ingredients for tacos, and individuals can make their own according to their preferences. Stir fries can be made with meat added at the last minute after a portion for the vegetarian teen has been removed.

If parents are especially resistant to the idea of serving more vegetarian options at mealtimes, then the dietitian may need to work with the teenager to plan meals that the teenager can prepare himself or herself. Also, many vegetarian teens who have been raised in omnivore households will not be familiar with many foods that can be important staples in vegetarian diets, such as whole grains, leafy green vegetables, soymilk, nut butters, legumes, and tofu. The dietitian may need to work with both the teenager and the parents to identify stores in the community that sell these foods and to explore ways to introduce these foods into the teen's diet.

In planning menus for adolescents, it is important to consider that teens are likely to have different eating styles compared with those of adults and children. Teenagers consume many of their calories as snacks and consume many meals away from home. Some teenagers may begin to skip breakfast because of lack of time or because they are not hungry in the morning. Often meals will be purchased out, but portable meals and snacks can make it easier for vegetarian adolescents to have constant access to nutritious food choices. Parents can improve the chances that teenagers will make appropriate meal choices by stocking the kitchen with foods that can serve as quick snacks, portable meals, and even breakfasts that can be consumed en route to school. Exhibit 11–1 lists some ideas for portable snacks and meals.

EATING DISORDERS

Because vegetarianism is somewhat common among adolescents who have anorexia nervosa or bulimia, there has been some concern that vegetarianism is in some way linked to causation of these eating disorders. In fact, eating disorders have a much more complex etiology and are not causally linked in any way to the teenager's desire to eat a meatless diet.

The spectrum of physical symptoms that characterize eating disorders ranges from obesity to anorexia nervosa. Eating disorders are associated with a failure to accomplish the developmental tasks of adolescence. Some developmental problems associated with eating disorders in adolescents include the following:[27]

- inability to experience bodily sensations originating within themselves as normal
- unrealistic perceptions of body size
- preoccupation with weight and food, reflecting dependence on social opinion and judgment
- unrealistic expectations for themselves
- failure to develop autonomy

Anorexia nervosa is most common in adolescents compared with other age groups because it is closely tied to body image distortion and adolescents are most likely to experience body image problems. Characterized by

---

Exhibit 11–1 Ideas for Quick and Portable Snacks and Meals for Teenagers

- Dried fruits
- Trail mix
- Popcorn
- Rice cakes
- Yogurt
- Leftover pizza or frozen pizza slices
- Milkshakes
- Hummus in pita bread
- Muffin and juice
- Bagel with peanut butter
- Peanut butter and banana sandwich
- Almond butter on crackers
- Instant soup

self-starvation, it affects about 4% of girls and young women between the ages of 13 and 18 years.[28] Approximately 5% of those with this disease die.[28]

Adolescents with anorexia nervosa can show all the physical symptoms of advanced starvation, including muscle wasting, dry skin, hirsutism, alopecia, postural hypotension, and inability to regulate body temperature. Loss of menstruation is thought to have some psychologic component because amenorrhea sets in before body fat loss is sufficient to explain it.[29]

Bulimia nervosa is a bingeing and purging syndrome that affects about 8% of girls and young women between the ages of 13 and 24 years.[28] Body weight in bulimics tends to be closer to normal than in anorexia nervosa, and distortions in body image and weight loss goals may be less severe.

Vegetarian diet is somewhat more common among patients with eating disorders, particularly those with anorexia.[30] This dietary choice may represent one way of controlling calorie intake. It may also be a result of advanced anorexia. People with symptoms of wasting disease often lose the taste for meat.[30,31] As stated earlier, there is no causal relationship between vegetarianism and a propensity toward eating disorders. Eating disorders are multifaceted and complex. In the past, vegetarianism was often prohibited for patients recovering form eating disorders. Current recommendations are to adjust the diet of these patients to allow them to follow a vegetarian diet if desired.[29]

REFERENCES

1. Carruth BR. Adolescence. In: Brown ML, et al, eds. *Present Knowledge in Nutrition*. 6th ed. Washington, DC: International Life Sciences Institute; 1990.

2. Dietz WH. Obesity in infants, children and adolescents in the United States. I. Identification, natural history, and after effects. *Nutr Res*. 1983;3:43–50.

3. Human Nutrition Information Service (HNIS), US Department of Agriculture. *Nationwide Food Consumption Survey, 1977–1978. Nutrient Intake: Individuals in 48 States, Year 1977–1978*. (HNIS report 1-2). Washington, DC: Government Printing Office; 1985.

4. Donovan UM, Gibson RS. Iron and zinc status of young women aged 14–19 years consuming vegetarian and omnivorous diets. *J Am Coll Nutr*. 1995;14:463–472.

5. Tanner JM. *Fetus into Man: Physical Growth from Conception to Maturity*. Cambridge, Mass: Harvard University Press; 1978.

6. Forbes GB. Nutritional requirements in adolescence. In: Suskind RM, ed. *Textbook of Pediatric Nutrition*. New York, NY: Raven Press; 1981:381–392.

7. Mahan KL, Rosebrough RH. Nutritional requirements and nutritional status assessment in adolescence. In: Mahan KL, Rees JM, eds. *Nutrition in Adolescence*. St Louis, Mo: Times Mirror/Mosby; 1984:40–76.

8. Hardinge MG, Stare FJ. Nutritional studies in vegetarians. 1. Nutritional, physical, and laboratory studies. *J Clin Nutr*. 1954;2:73–82.

9. Cooper R, Allen A, Goldberg R, et al. Seventh-day Adventist adolescents—life-style patterns and cardiovascular risk factors. *West J Med*. 1984;140:471–477.

10. Persky VW, Chatterton RT, Van Horn LV, Grant MD, Langenberg P, Marvin J. Hormone levels in vegetarian and nonvegetarian teenage girls: Potential implications for breast cancer risk. *Cancer Res.* 1992;50:578–583.

11. Sabate J, Linsted KD, Harris RD, Sanchez A. Attained height of lacto-ovo vegetarian children and adolescents. *Eur J Clin Nutr.* 1991;45:51–58.

12. Sanchez A, Kissinger DG, Phillips RL. A hypothesis on the etiological role of diet on age of menarche. *Med Hypothesis.* 1981;7:1339–1345.

13. Kissinger DG, Sanchez A. The association of dietary factors with the age of menarche. *Nutr Res.* 1987;7:471–479.

14. Kagawa Y. Impact of westernization on the nutrition of Japanese: Changes in physique, cancer, longevity and centenarians. *Prev Med.* 1978;7:205–217.

15. Lin W-S, Chen ACN, Su JZX, et al. The menarcheal age of Chinese girls. *Ann Hum Biol.* 1992;19:503–512.

16. De Waard F, Trichopoulos D. A unifying concept of the etiology of breast cancer. *Int J Cancer.* 1988;41:666–669.

17. Peeters PHM, Verbeek ALM, Krol A, Matthyssen MMM, de Waard F. Age of menarche and breast cancer risk in nulliparous women. *Breast Cancer Res Treat.* 1994;33:55–61.

18. Rowe PM. New US recommendations on calcium intake. *Lancet.* 1994;343:1559–1560.

19. Shils ME, Olson JA, Shike M. *Modern Nutrition in Health and Disease,* 8th ed. Philadelphia: Lea & Febiger; 1994: A–23.

20. Abelow BJ, Holford TR, Insogna KL. Cross-cultural association between dietary animal protein and hip fracture: A hypothesis. *Calcif Tissue Int.* 1992;50:14–18.

21. DeMaeyer EM, Adiels-Tegman M. The prevalence of anemia in the world. *World Health Stat Q.* 1985;38:302–316.

22. Life Sciences Research Office. *Assessment of Iron Nutritional Status of the United States Population Based on Data Collected in the Second NHANES Survey, 1976–1980.* Bethesda, Md: Federation of American Societies for Experimental Biology; 1984.

23. Hallberg L, Rossander-Hultén, Brune M, Gleerup A. Calcium and iron absorption: Mechanism of action and nutritional importance. *Eur J Clin Nutr.* 1991;46:317–327.

24. Sandstead HH. Availability of zinc and its requirement in human subjects. In: Prasad AS, ed. *Clinical, Biochemical, and Nutritional Aspects of Trace Elements.* New York, NY: Liss; 1982:83–101.

25. Hunt JR, Matthys LA, Lykken GI. Reduced zinc absorption from a lacto-ovo vegetarian diet. *Am J Clin Nutr.* 1995;61:908.

26. Treuherz J. Possible inter-relationship between zinc and dietary fibre in a group of lacto-ovo vegetarian adolescents. *J Plant Foods.* 1982;4:89–95.

27. Rees JML. Eating disorders. In: Mahan LK, Rees JM, eds. *Nutrition in Adolescence.* St Louis, Mo: Times Mirror/Mosby; 1984:104–137.

28. Johnson C, Connors M. *The Etiology and Treatment of Bulimia Nervosa.* New York, NY: Basic Books; 1987.

29. Huse DM, Lucas AR. Dietary patterns in anorexia nervosa. *Am J Clin Nutr.* 1984;40:251–254.

30. Rock CL, Yager J. Nutrition and eating disorders: A primer for clinicians. *Int J Eating Dis.* 1987;6:267–280.

31. De Wys WD. Taste and feeding behavior in patients with cancer. In: Winick M, ed. *Nutrition and Cancer.* New York, NY: Wiley; 1977.

CHAPTER 12

Vegetarian Diets for Older People

A 1992 poll found that 55% of vegetarians were over age 40.[1] Further age breakdowns are unavailable, so that it is not known how many vegetarians are over the age of 65. There is reason to believe, however, that the number of older vegetarians is on the rise. First, in the United States the older segment of the population is growing more rapidly than any other age group. By the 21st century, it is expected that 20% of the population, or about 60 million people, will be 65 or older.[2] Also, the number of vegetarians is growing, and those who choose a meatless diet appear to make this a long-term choice.[1] As a result, dietitians need to be prepared to address the concerns of older vegetarians. Diet is an issue of importance for all older Americans because there is evidence of significant changes in nutrient needs and that are not always met.

DIETARY STATUS OF OLDER VEGETARIANS

There are few studies of older vegetarians. The available data indicate, however, that nutrient intake of older vegetarians is at least as good as, if not better than, that of older nonvegetarians (Appendix R). In a study of Dutch vegetarians, for example, aged 65 to 99 years, intakes of fiber, carbohydrate, fat, and protein were closer to recommendations than intakes of nonvegetarians. Intake of zinc was somewhat low, however, and although iron intake was adequate there was a higher incidence of poor iron status among the vegetarians.[3] In another study, elderly Canadian Seventh-day Adventist women had lower protein and energy intakes but higher copper, selenium, and magnesium intakes than nonvegetarians.[4] Adventist women with an average age of 71 years consumed less cholesterol and saturated fat and more carbohydrate, fiber, magnesium, vitamin A, vitamin E, thiamin, pantothenic acid, copper, folate, and manganese than nonvegetarians. The nonvegetarians also had diets that were low in vitamins B6 and E. Both groups had low intakes of vitamin D and zinc.[5] Two other studies of older Adventist vegetarian women also indicate intake to be equal to or superior to that of nonvegetarians.[6,7]

Although studies indicate that most older vegetarians have dietary intakes that are comparable to those of omnivores, dietary adequacy of all older people is an issue of concern. One problem in assessing adequacy is that nutrient needs of older people are not fully defined. The full impact of the physiologic changes of aging on nutrient needs is not well understood. The extent to which nutrient needs may differ between older vegetarians and older omnivores is also not clear. There are several potential problems with the recommended dietary allowances (RDAs) for this age group:

- The most recent (10th) edition of the RDAs groups all people over the age of 50 together for the purpose of establishing nutrient recommendations. Previous editions established separate recommendations for those over the age of 75. It is probable that nutrient needs are considerably different between people in their 50s and those in their 70s and 80s.

- The most recent RDAs were published in 1989, at a time when there were few data on the nutrient needs of older persons. Therefore, nutrient recommendations are often extrapolated from studies of requirements of younger adults. Since 1989, considerably more information has been amassed.

- Both chronic disease and the use of multiple prescription drugs (polypharmacy), both of which are more common in the elderly, can affect nutrient needs.

Consequently, there is some debate about how well the RDAs reflect the actual nutrient needs of older Americans. In the discussion of nutrient intake and needs of older vegetarians that follows, both the RDAs and some more recent studies that affect our understanding of these needs are considered.

NUTRIENT NEEDS OF OLDER VEGETARIANS

Calories

As people age, muscle mass decreases and percentage body fat increases in response to both hormonal changes and decreased physical activity. These changes can be significant. Men and women in their late 60s may have 26 (11.8 kg) and 11 (5 kg) fewer pounds of muscle tissue, respectively, than they did at age 25.[8] These changes result in decreased calorie needs.

According to the RDAs, energy needs decrease by 600 and 300 calories after the age of 51 for men and women, respectively. Clearly, the reduction in calorie needs is gradual; it may be more pronounced in people older than 75. Most of the reduction is due to reduced metabolic rate, although a small amount is also due to decreased physical activity.

The RDAs for energy are 2,300 kcal for older men and 1,900 kcal for older women. Even with lower energy requirements, however, there is some concern that older people do not meet those needs. One US survey revealed that older men and women consumed an average of only 1,800 and 1,300 kcal/day, respectively.[9] Also, the RDAs for energy represent average needs and do not include a margin of safety. Older editions of the RDAs indicated, however, that after the age of 75 calorie needs may be as low as 2,050 kcal/day for men and 1,600 kcal/day for women. Thus meeting caloric needs may be less of a problem for those in their 70s and 80s, for whom energy needs may actually be quite low.

Decreased calorie intake is not a problem as long as ideal body weight is maintained, but it does make it more difficult to meet nutrient needs. Some older people may have energy intakes so low that appropriate nutrient densities are difficult to achieve.[10,11] Caloric intake of elderly vegetarians appears to be slightly lower than that of nonvegetarians, but the data vary considerably (Appendix P).

Protein

The lower muscle mass of older people may reduce their protein needs somewhat. Protein is used less efficiently with aging, however, and the low calorie intake of older people may also increase protein needs. The net effect may be an increased protein requirement for older people. Some research has suggested that needs may be as high as 1.00 to 1.25 g per kilogram body weight, although the RDA (0.8 g/kg) is not increased for older people.[12]

Given their possible increased protein needs, older Americans may be consuming too little protein. In a study of 1,000 people older than 60, protein intake was 0.86 and 0.81 g/kg for men and women, respectively.[13] Vegetarians, including older vegetarians, consume diets that are lower in protein than omnivore diets (Appendix P). With the reduction in caloric intake with aging, it becomes especially important that older vegetarians consume protein-dense foods, such as legumes and soy products.

Nevertheless, vegetarians may have an advantage by consuming less protein and a greater proportion of plant protein. Excess protein may exacerbate the decline in kidney function that is often seen in aging (see Chapter 2). Replacing animal protein with plant protein may help preserve kidney function. Additionally, lower protein diets may decrease the loss of calcium from bones, as discussed in Chapter 4. This may be particularly important for the elderly, since the kidney's ability to excrete acid (which occurs as a result of increased protein intake) may deteriorate with age.[14] Therefore, older vegetarians who consume lower amounts but adequate protein and derive most of that protein from plant foods may have a distinct health advantage.

Calcium

Bone loss begins at around age 40 and increases with advancing age. Women are at much greater risk for osteoporosis because they start out with less bone and lose bone mass more quickly, particularly in the years after menopause. Women between the ages of 20 and 29 have about 76% the bone matter of men; by their 70s this decreases to about 60%.[15]

Calcium needs probably increase with aging because absorption becomes less efficient.[16,17] Absorption efficiency may decrease by as much as 25% by age 60 compared with age 40. Some studies have shown that a high intake of calcium can help maintain bone calcium content.[17,19] Calcium intake in these studies was typically greater than 1,500 mg/day, however, an amount that is likely to be achievable only through supplementation.

Given the effect of high protein intake on calcium loss, it is likely that older vegetarians need less calcium than omnivores. Until more is understood about these needs, however, dietitians should work with older patients to ensure that they come close to meeting the RDA for calcium, which is 800 mg, or utilize foods that are especially rich in well-absorbed calcium to ensure that biologic needs are met (see Chapter 4).

The incidence of lactose intolerance increases with age;[19] consequently, many older people are unable to drink milk without experiencing some discomfort,[20] although small quantities of milk can be tolerated.[21] Also, a recent study found that, among individuals who described themselves as lactose intolerant, most did not experience symptoms in response to milk consumption when measured objectively.[22] If milk has represented an important part of the diet in the past, it may be difficult for the older person to identify alternative sources of calcium. Lactase-fortified milk can be one option. Many older people may also enjoy calcium-fortified soymilk and rice milks. Dietitians can help older clients identify a wide variety of calcium-rich foods, including calcium-rich vegetables, beans, and nuts.

Vitamin D

Vitamin D synthesis is decreased in the elderly. Also, older people who are homebound or institutionalized may be at increased risk for vitamin D deficiency because they have less sun exposure.[23] In a study of homebound and institutionalized patients aged 68 to 96 years, mean dietary vitamin D was twice the RDA, but 7 of 22 patients had low circulating vitamin D levels.[24,25] Also, those living in northern regions are more likely to experience vitamin D deficiency. In older people living in Great Britain who experienced hip fractures, as many as 30% to 40% were vitamin D deficient.[26]

Older people may be at increased risk for vitamin D deficiency for the following reasons (see Exhibit 12–1):

- less sun exposure due to decreased mobility
- decreased vitamin D synthesis compared with younger people (the efficiency of synthesis in older people is the same, but the absolute concentration of substrate for vitamin D synthesis is lower;[27] as a result, young adults make two to three times more vitamin D in their skin than older adults[28,29])
- impaired renal synthesis of 1,25-dihydroxyvitamin D, possibly due to a decreased renal mass and/or an impaired response to parathyroid hormone[30]
- increased vitamin D requirements due to medications commonly used by the elderly[31]
- vitamin D intake is typically lower compared with younger people[32]

Exhibit 12–1 Checklist for Diagnosing Vitamin D Deficiency in the Elderly

Diet Consumption of <2 to 3 8-oz glasses of fortified milk/day, or daily use of other vitamin D fortified products?	**Yes** or **No**
Endogenous synthesis Hands and face exposed for <20 minutes/day, 3 times per week? Renal or hepatic insufficiency?	**Yes** or **No** **Yes** or **No**
Absorption Malabsorption due to laxative abuse or cholestyramine?	**Yes** or **No**
Nutrient-drug interactions Interference from anticonvulsant?	**Yes** or **No**
If response is yes to any of the above questions, consider vitamin D supplementation.	

Source: Adapted from Ryan C, Eleazer P, Egbert J. Vitamin D in the elderly. An overlooked nutrient. *Nutrition Today.* 1995;30:228–233. Used with permission.

As a result of these factors, vitamin D requirements of the elderly may be twice as high as for younger adults, although the RDA for vitamin D for older people remains at 5 μg. In lieu of adequate sun exposure, fortified foods or vitamin D supplements are the only reliable means of ensuring adequate vitamin D status. The only foods that naturally provide this vitamin are eggs and some fatty fish. In the United States, fortified milk is an important source of vitamin D. As noted above, however, many older people do not drink cow's milk. Other good sources of this nutrient include fortified soymilk and rice milks and fortified breakfast cereals.

Vitamin B$_{12}$

Older people, regardless of dietary habits, may be at risk for vitamin B$_{12}$ deficiency. A study of 500 older people found that 40% had low B$_{12}$ levels compared with 18% of younger subjects.[33] Several instances of either extremely low levels of vitamin B$_{12}$ or outright B$_{12}$ deficiency have been seen in older vegans.[34–40]

There is evidence that some of the symptoms often attributed to aging might actually be caused by marginal vitamin B$_{12}$ deficiency. These include depression, restlessness, irritability, mood swings, panic disorders, phobic disorders, impotence, confusion, disorientation, memory loss, concentration difficulties, dementia, chronic fatigue, apathy, insomnia, and even psychotic episodes.[41–45]

It is also worthwhile noting that among the elderly, serum levels of vitamin B$_{12}$ have been shown to underestimate the true prevalence of vitamin B$_{12}$ deficiency.[46] Furthermore, lower vitamin B$_{12}$ levels have been associated with increased serum homocysteine, which is thought to be a risk factor for vascular disease among both the young and the elderly.[47] A high incidence of atrophic gastritis, which interferes with vitamin B$_{12}$ absorption, is seen in aging and may be one reason for low serum B$_{12}$ levels. Atrophic gastritis may occur in as much as 50% of the population older than 60.[48] This condition also leads to increases in levels of bacteria in the intestines that may compete for vitamin B$_{12}$,[49,50] although these bacteria may also synthesize vitamin B$_{12}$.[51]

Vitamin B$_{12}$ needs of the elderly may be higher than those of younger adults, although again this is not reflected in the RDAs.[52] Therefore, identifying regular sources of vitamin B$_{12}$ in the diets of older vegetarians is prudent. Because of malabsorption problems, however, it is not clear that increasing B$_{12}$ intake among older people will actually increase blood levels.[53–55] Increasing B$_{12}$ intake may compensate for mildly impaired B$_{12}$ absorption, however. If absorption is poor, it may be necessary to use injections of vitamin B$_{12}$.

Both eggs and dairy products provide significant amounts of vitamin B_{12} for lacto-ovo vegetarians. As noted in Chapter 6, however, it is effectively absent in plant foods. Therefore, vegans must use fortified foods (nutritional yeast, fortified breakfast cereals, fortified soymilk, and meat analogues) or supplements.

Riboflavin

Because riboflavin requirements are linked to caloric intake, the RDA for riboflavin decreases slightly in the elderly as a result of their decreased calorie needs. There is good evidence now, however, that older people may actually need just as much riboflavin as younger adults.[56] Older vegetarians, however, might require somewhat less riboflavin (about 5% to 10% less) than older omnivores because, in a metabolic feeding study, subjects consuming a high-carbohydrate, low-fat (20% fat) diet required less dietary riboflavin to achieve normal riboflavin status than subjects consuming a high-fat diet (30% fat).[56] This may be because a high-carbohydrate diet leads to greater riboflavin synthesis by the intestinal bacteria, some of which is absorbed.[56] This finding would seem to apply to younger individuals consuming low-fat, high-carbohydrate diets as well.

MEAL PLANNING FOR OLDER PEOPLE

Much attention is given in dietetics to the challenges of meeting nutritional needs of growth phases: infancy, childhood, adolescence, and pregnancy and lactation. Often the challenge of meeting nutrient needs in aging is overlooked. Indeed, nutritionists have only begun to define those needs. It is increasingly evident, however, that nutritional needs of older people demand the attention of dietitians. This is a stage where energy needs begin to decrease while nutrient needs remain the same or may even increase. It is clear that changes in dietary habits are warranted and that special attention should be given to nutrient-dense foods. In addition, there are certain challenges to meeting dietary needs of older people. A variety of physical, social, and psychologic conditions that may accompany aging can affect food choices; also, life-long dietary habits can be difficult to change. Food habits of people in their 70s and 80s may require special attention because some research indicates that those aged 60 to 70 years make more healthful food choices than those aged 75 to 85 years.[57]

Dietitians need to work closely with older clients to develop strategies for meeting dietary requirements in the face of many complicating factors whether the client is vegetarian or not. Older vegetarians can follow the same meal-planning guidelines for younger vegetarian adults outlined in Chapter 7. By avoiding the use of "empty calorie" foods, it should be possible to achieve adequate nutrient intake within an appropriate caloric allowance. It is especially important to include daily servings of foods that are fortified with vitamins D and B_{12}. A medical assessment of vitamin B_{12} status can be used to ascertain whether B_{12} supplements and/or B_{12} injections are warranted. Older people should also be encouraged to include plenty of fluids in their diets to help prevent constipation and dehydration.

Factors That Affect Food Choices

In helping older people make food choices, it is important to evaluate a variety of factors that may affect those choices.

Decreased Appetite

Taste acuity diminishes with aging. At age 70, people have only 30% of the taste buds they had as young adults.[58] Loss of smell can also occur, which can make it more difficult to distinguish weak tastes. When foods taste bland, appetite can be poor. There may be a tendency to oversalt foods to make them more flavorful. Dietitians can help clients choose flavorful foods that are low in sodium. A number of salt-free herb blends are available. Lemon juice, herb-flavored vinegars, and other condiments can help perk up food flavors. Spicy dishes may also appeal to some older people. In formulating recommendations, however, it is necessary to realize that many older Seventh-day Adventists avoid pepper and sometimes vinegar as well.

Many older people may show an increased desire for sweets. In younger people intensely sweet foods are perceived as unpleasant, but with aging this response to sweet foods diminishes, and sweet flavors are more acceptable.[59] Dietitians can take advantage of this by encouraging consumption of sweet foods that offer good nutrition. Some examples are chopped dried fruits mixed into hot cereals, fruit smoothies or fruit-flavored milkshakes, blackstrap molasses added to bean dishes, baked fruits, and fruit-oat crisps.

Anorexia can also be a side effect of drugs. Poor appetite can be exacerbated by loneliness and isolation. Feelings of loneliness have been found to be inversely related to caloric intake.[60]

Decreased Mobility and Dexterity

For many older people, cooking may present some difficulties. In one study, approximately 4% and 17% of noninstitutionalized Americans older than 65 and 85, respectively, reported that they could not prepare their own meals because of a health or physical problem.[61] More than 30% of homebound older persons reported difficulties in preparing meals.[62]

Using some convenience foods and foods that are easily prepared can help older people with limited cooking ability choose healthy meals. Although many of these are high in fat and sodium, they can be used occasionally provided that most of the dietary choices are whole foods that are low in fat and sodium. Vegetarian meals and snacks that take little preparation include the following:

- pasta with prepared sauce
- canned soup with crackers (choose low-sodium soups where possible)
- textured vegetable protein with canned Sloppy Joe sauce
- frozen vegetarian burgers
- vegetarian baked beans
- peanut butter sandwich
- instant soup (many are lower in sodium than canned soups)
- bagel with fruit spread or nut butter
- cereal with milk
- instant hot cereal with fresh, canned, or dried fruit
- frozen pizza
- cottage cheese and fruit
- prepared bean tacos
- homemade bean tacos using canned refried beans
- instant flavored rice mixes tossed with cooked frozen vegetables
- three-bean salad
- baked potatoes
- tofu marinated in barbecue sauce and baked in the oven

Many convenience foods that are healthy and easy to prepare and can round out meals are available, such as instant mashed potatoes, canned low-sodium vegetables, frozen vegetables, and canned and instant soups. Frozen entrees with reduced fat and sodium are also available, although these tend to be expensive. Also, many packaged items, particularly those wrapped tightly in cellophane, can be difficult to open for older people with poor hand strength and coordination. All these factors need to be considered in helping older people make food choices that include easy-to-prepare items.

Appliances that make preparation easier include microwave ovens, food processors, and Crock-Pots. Many older people may need to be taught to use these, however. Also, older people with poor eyesight may not be able to read preparation directions on packages, so that unfamiliar cooking techniques may require some help.

Finally, the dietitian may be able to help clients identify community resources for seniors. Meals on Wheels offers meals to those who are homebound, and many community centers offer meals to seniors at congregate sites. In most cases, there are no vegetarian options. Exhibit 12–2 lists fed-

Exhibit 12–2 Possible Substitutions in the Title III-C Meal Pattern That Would Produce Meals Suitable for Vegetarians

---

Substitutions for 1 ounce cooked meat:
 1 egg
 1 ounce cheddar cheese
 ½ cup cooked dried beans, peas, or lentils
 ¼ cup cottage cheese
Example of combination that meets the standard of 3 ounces of meat or equivalent:
 Cheese enchilada (1 ounce cheddar cheese and 1 cup refried beans)

---

eral guidelines that offer suggestions for menu substitutions. These could meet the needs of vegetarians and also could result in meals that are more likely to appeal to minority populations, who tend to use these services less often.[63] It may also be possible to arrange for special meals where resources allow. In more populated areas, some Seventh-day Adventist churches may be involved in providing low-cost vegetarian meals to seniors. Cafeterias in Seventh-day Adventist hospitals also offer inexpensive vegetarian meals.

Problems with Chewing

Many older people have problems chewing tough or hard foods. A dental referral may be advised to make sure that dentures are properly fitted. A healthy diet can also easily be planned around foods that are soft and easy to chew. Some suggestions for foods that are easy to eat include the following:

- Refined grains, such as white bread and rolls, couscous, and white rice, can be easier to chew than their whole grain counterparts. Although adequate fiber is an important concern in the diets of older people, vegetarians are likely to be consuming much more fiber than their nonvegetarian peers. As long as some whole, fiber-rich foods are emphasized in the diet, the moderate use of refined foods is certainly acceptable in the diets of vegetarians.
- Many fiber-rich foods can be easy to eat. These include baked potatoes (fiber rich even without the skin), sweet potatoes, oatmeal, multigrain hot cereals, cooked vegetables (especially softer vegetables such as zucchini, winter squash, and eggplant), and stewed or baked fruits.
- Tofu is easy to chew and can be used in a variety of ways, including cubes of tofu in soups, creamed tofu pureed with vegetables and served as a cream soup or sauce over rice, and crumbled tofu mixed with mayonnaise as a sandwich filling.

- Textured soy protein, particularly the granular form, has a texture similar to that of ground beef and makes an easy-to-prepare meat substitute.
- Cream of vegetable soups or soups with pasta and well-cooked vegetables are popular with many older people.
- Beans can be cooked to a tender stage to make them easy to chew and digest.
- Nut butters on soft bread provide a nutrient- and calorie-rich meal or snack.

Cost Constraints

Limited income is a common constraint for senior citizens and may affect food purchases. Dietitians can help seniors plan low-cost meals that are nutritious. This can be particularly difficult in view of some of the other potential restrictions discussed above. For example, seniors who are cooking for themselves only and/or have trouble preparing meals are likely to gravitate toward convenience foods, which tend to be expensive. Some con-

Exhibit 12–3 2-Day Menu for Older Vegetarians

Meal	Day 1	Day 2
Breakfast	¾ cup quick oatmeal with ½ cup fortified soymilk and ½ sliced banana, 1 cup calcium-fortified orange juice	1 cup bran flakes with ½ cup fortified soymilk; one slice toast; coffee, tea, or herbal tea
Snack	½ cup canned peaches, 1 oatbran muffin, 1 cup herb tea	Fruit smoothie with ½ cup calcium-fortified orange juice, 1/2 banana, ¼ cup strawberries
Lunch	Sloppy Joes (½ cup textured soy protein with ½ cup Manwich sauce), one whole wheat hamburger bun, ½ cup cooked squash, 1 cup water	1 cup spaghetti with 1 cup spaghetti sauce, 1 cup steamed broccoli, 1 cup juice
Snack	One slice toast with 2 tbsp almond butter	Four saltines with 2 tbsp almond butter
Dinner	One small baked potato, ½ cup vegetarian baked beans, 1 cup steamed frozen or fresh kale, one slice bread, 1 cup decaffeinated coffee	1 cup canned or instant lentil soup, four crackers, 1 cup steamed frozen or fresh asparagus, sliced tomatoes, ½ cup canned fruit cocktail, 1 cup water

venience foods are inexpensive, however, and some low-cost foods are relatively easy to prepare. The following are some examples:

- macaroni and cheese mix from a box
- canned beans (more expensive than dried beans, but still a relatively inexpensive source of excellent nutrition)
- baked potatoes
- peanut butter
- quick (not instant) oatmeal
- textured soy protein
- frozen greens
- supplemental food items such as blackstrap molasses, nutritional yeast, and wheat germ (used in small quantities and excellent nutritional values for the money; adding just a tablespoon of these items to various dishes every day can boost the nutrient intake of seniors considerably)

Where seniors are unable to meet their living expenses, the dietitian needs to be able to make referrals to the appropriate social agencies to arrange for financial help. Local food banks and charitable institutions can also offer assistance.

Sample Menus for Older Vegetarians

When one is planning meals for seniors, there may be many factors to take into consideration. Important goals include helping clients choose foods that are nutrient rich and are enjoyed, that fit well within the senior's budget, and that consider any constraints in meal preparation ability and eating ability. The menus shown in Exhibit 12–3 follow the meal-planning guide in Chapter 7 and utilize foods that are likely to meet the needs of seniors.

REFERENCES

1. *The American Vegetarian: Coming of Age in the 90s* (a study of the vegetarian marketplace conducted for *Vegetarian Times* by Yankelovich, Skelly, and White/Clancy, Shulman, Inc). Oak Park, Ill; 1992.

2. Kane RL, Kane RA. Long-term care: Can our society meet the needs of the elderly? *Annu Rev Public Health*. 1980;1:227–253.

3. Brants HAM, Lowik MRH, Westenbrink S, Hulshof KFAM, Kistemaker C. Adequacy of a vegetarian diet at old age (Dutch Nutrition Surveillance System). *J Am Coll Nutr*. 1990;9:292–302.

4. Gibson RS, Anderson BM, Sabry JH. The trace metal status of a group of postmenopausal vegetarians. *J Am Diet Assoc.* 1983;82:246–250.

5. Nieman DC, Underwood BC, Sherman KM, et al. Dietary status of Seventh-Day Adventist vegetarian and non-vegetarian elderly women. *J Am Diet Assoc.* 1989;89:1763–1769.

6. Hunt IF, Murphy NJ, Henderson C. Food and nutrient intake of Seventh-Day Adventist women. *Am J Clin Nutr.* 1988;48:850–851.

7. Marsh AG, Christiansen DK, Sanchez TV, Mickelsen O, Chaffee FL. Nutrient similarities and differences of older lacto-ovo-vegetarian and omnivorous women. *Nutr Rep Int.* 1989;39:19–24.

8. Forbes GB, Reina JC. Adults' lean body mass declines with age: Some longitudinal observations. *Metabolism.* 1970;19:653–663.

9. Carroll MD, Abraham S, Dresser CM. *Dietary Intake Source Data: United States, 1976–1980* (Vital and Health Statistics series 11, no. 231). Hyattsville, Md: National Center for Health Statistics, Public Health Service, US Department of Health and Human Services; 1983. Dept of Health and Human Services publication (PHS) 83–1681.

10. Kohns MB. A rational diet for the elderly. *Am J Clin Nutr.* 1982;36:735–736.

11. Shannon B, Smicklas-Wright H. Nutrition education in relation to the needs of the elderly. *J Nutr Educ.* 1979;11:85–89.

12. Campbell WW, Crim MC, Dallal GE, Young VR, Evans WJ. Increased protein requirements in elderly people: New data and retrospective reassessments. *Am J Clin Nutr.* 1994;60:501–509.

13. Hartz SC, Russel RM, Rosenberg IH. Nutrition in the elderly: The Boston Nutritional Status Survey. London, England: Smith-Gordon; 1992.

14. Adler S, Lindeman RD, Yiengst MJ, Beard ES. The effect of acute acid loading on the urinary excretion of acid by the aging human kidney. *J Lab Clin Med.* 1968;72:278–282.

15. Widdowson EM. Physiological processes of aging: Are there special nutritional requirements for elderly people? Do McCay's findings apply to humans? *Am J Clin Nutr.* 1992;55:1246–1249.

16. Heaney RP, Gallagher JC, Johnston CC, Neer R, Parfitt AM, Whedon GD. Calcium nutrition and bone health in the elderly. *Am J Clin Nutr.* 1982;36:986–1013.

17. Weaver CM. Age related calcium requirements due to changes in absorption and utilization. *J Nutr.* 1994;124:1418s–1425s.

18. Heaney RP, Recker RR, Saville PD. Menopausal changes in calcium balance. *J Lab Clin Med.* 1978;92:953–963.

19. Welsh JD, Russel LC, Walker AW Jr. *Gerontology.* 1974;75:847–855.

20. Debongnie JC, Newcomer AD, Mcgill DB, Phillips FS. Absorption of nutrients in lactase deficiency. *Dig Dis Sci.* 1979;24:225–231.

21. Johnson AO, Semenya JG, Buchowski MS, Enwonwu CO, Scrimshaw NS. Adaptation of lactose maldigesters to continued milk intakes. *Am J Clin Nutr.* 1993;58:879–881.

22. Suarez FL, Saviano DA, Levitt MD. A comparison of symptoms after the consumption of milk or lactose-hydrolyzed milk by people with self-reported severe lactose intolerance. *N Engl J Med.* 1995;333:1–4.

23. Morris HA, Morrison GW, Burr M, et al. Vitamin D and femoral neck fractures in elderly South Australian women. *Med J Aust.* 1984;140:519–521.

24. Aksnes I, Rodland O, Aarskog D. Serum levels of vitamin D_3 and 25-hydroxyvitamin D_3 in elderly and young adults. *Bone Miner.* 1988;3:351–357.

25. Gloth FM, Tobin JD, Sherman SS, Hollis BW. Is the recommended daily allowance for vitamin D too low for homebound elderly? *J Am Geriatr Soc.* 1991;39:137–141.

26. Aron JE, Gallagher JC, Anderson J, et al. Frequency of osteomalacia and osteoporosis in fractures of the proximal femur. *Lancet.* 1974;1:229–233.

27. MacLaughlin J, Holick MF. Aging decreases the capacity of human skin to produce vitamin D₃. *J Clin Invest.* 1985;76:1536–1538.

28. Norman AW. *Vitamin D: The Calcium Homeostatic Steroid Hormone.* New York, NY: Academic Press; 1979.

29. Raist LG, Johannesson A. Pathogenesis, prevention, and therapy of osteoporosis. *J Med.* 1984;15:267–278.

30. Tsai KS, Health H III, Kumar R, Riggs BL. Impaired vitamin D metabolism with aging in women: Possible role in pathogenesis of senile osteoporosis. *J Clin Invest.* 1984;73:1668–1672.

31. Roe DA. *Drug-Induced Nutritional Deficiencies.* Westport, Conn: AVI; 1986.

32. Abraham S, Johnson C. *Dietary intake findings, United States 1976–1980.* Hyattsville, Md: National Center for Health Statistics, US Department of Human Services; 1982.

33. Lindenbaum J, Rosenberg IH, Wilson PWF, Stabler SP, Allen RH. Prevalence of cobalamin deficiency in the Framingham elderly population. *Am J Clin Nutr.* 1994;60:2–11.

34. Murphy MF. Vitamin B₁₂ deficiency due to a low-cholesterol diet in a vegetarian. *Ann Intern Med.* 1981;94:57–58.

35. Wokes F, Badenoch J, Sinclair HM. Human dietary deficiency of vitamin B₁₂. *Voeding.* 1955;16:590–602.

36. Wokes F. Anaemia and vitamin B₁₂ dietary deficiency. *Proc Nutr Soc.* 1956;15:134–141.

37. Harrison RJ, Booth CC, Mollin DL. Vitamin-B₁₂ deficiency due to defective diet. *Lancet.* 1956;1:727–728.

38. Connor PM, Pirola RC. Nutritional vitamin B₁₂ deficiency. *Med J Aust.* 1963;2:451–453.

39. Winawer SJ, Strieiff RR, Zamcheck N. Gastric and hematological abnormalities in a vegan with nutritional vitamin B₁₂ deficiency: Effect of oral vitamin B₁₂. *Gastroenterology.* 1967;3:130–135.

40. Carmel R. Nutritional vitamin B₁₂ deficiency. Possible contributory role of subtle vitamin B₁₂ malabsorption. *Ann Intern Med.* 1978;88:647–649.

41. Dommisse J. Subtle vitamin-B₁₂ deficiency and psychiatry: A largely unnoticed but devastating relationship? *Med Hypotheses.* 1991;34:131–140.

42. Fine EJ, Soria ED. Myths about vitamin B₁₂ deficiency. *South Med J.* 1991;84:1475–1481.

43. Hector M, Burton JR. What are the psychiatric manifestations of vitmain B₁₂ deficiency? *J Am Geriatr Soc.* 1988;36:1105–1112.

44. Karnaze DS, Carmel R. Low serum cobalamin levels in primary degenerative dementia. *Arch Intern Med.* 1987;147:429–431.

45. Unrecognized cobalamin-responsive neuropsychiatric disorders. *Nutr Rev.* 1989;47:208–210.

46. Joosten E, van den Berg A, Riezler R, et al. Metabolic evidence that deficiencies of vitamin B₁₂ (cobalamin), folate, and vitamin B₆ occur commonly in elderly people. *Am J Clin Nutr.* 1993;58:468–476.

47. Malinow MR, Kang SS, Taylor LM, et al. Prevalence of hyperhomocyst(e)inemia in patients with peripheral arterial occlusive disease. *Circulation.* 1989;79:1180–1188.

48. Krasinski SD, Russel RM, Samloff M, et al. Fundic atrophic gastritis in an elderly population. Effect on hemoglobin and several serum nutritional indicators. *J Am Geriatr Soc.* 1986;34:800–806.

49. Suter PM, Golner BB, Goldin BR, Morrow FD, Russel RM. Reversal of protein-bound vitamin B12 malabsorption with antibiotics in atrophic gastritis. *Gastroenterology.* 1991;101: 1039–1045.

50. Nilsson-Ehle H, Landahl S, Lindstedt G, et al. Low serum cobalamin levels in a population study of 70- and 75-year-old subjects. Gastrointestinal causes and hematological effects. *Dig Dis Sci.* 1989;34:716–723.

51. Herbert V. Vitamin B12: Plant sources, requirements, and assay. *Am J Clin Nutr.* 1988;48:852–858.

52. Russel RM, Suter PM. Vitamin requirements of elderly people: An update. *Am J Clin Nutr.* 1993;58:4–14.

53. Allen LH, Casterline J. Vitamin B12 deficiency in elderly individuals: Diagnosis and requirements. *Am J Clin Nutr.* 1994;60:12–14.

54. Herbert V. Vitamin B12 and elderly people. *Am J Clin Nutr.* 1994;59:1093–1094.

55. Russel RM. Vitamin B12 and elderly people. Reply to V Herbert. *Am J Clin Nutr.* 1994;59:1094–1095.

56. Boisvert WA, Russell RM. Riboflavin requirement of healthy elderly humans and its relationship to macronutrient composition of the diet. *J Nutr.* 1993;123:915–925.

57. Fischer CA, Crokett SJ, Heller KE, Skauge LH. Nutrition knowledge, attitudes, and practices of older and younger elderly in rural areas. *J Am Diet Assoc.* 1991;91:1398–1401.

58. Schiffman SS, Moss J, Erickson RP. Thresholds of food odors in the elderly. *Exp Aging Res.* 1976;2:389–398.

59. Kamath SK. Taste acuity and aging. *Am J Clin Nutr.* 1982;36:766–775.

60. Walker D, Beauchene RE. The relationship of loneliness, social isolation, and physical health to dietary adequacy of independently living elderly. *J Am Diet Assoc.* 1991;91:300–304.

61. US Department of Health and Human Services (DHHS), Public Health Service, Centers for Disease Control and Prevention. *Physical Functioning of the Aged—United States, 1984.* Hyattsville, Md: DHHS; 1989. DHHS publication (PHS) 89–1595.

62. Smicklas-Wright H. Aging. In: Brown ML, ed. *Present Knowledge in Nutrition.* 6th ed. Washington, DC: Nutrition Foundation, International Life Sciences Institute; 1990:333–340.

63. O'Shaughnessy C. *Older Americans Act Nutrition Program: CBS Report for Congress.* Washington, DC: Congressional Research Service; 1990.

Practical Applications for Counseling Vegetarians

CHAPTER 13

Counseling Vegetarian Clients

Dietitians may be called upon frequently to counsel clients who follow a vegetarian diet. Often these will be clients who are referred for a specific clinical condition and who happen to be vegetarians. Sometimes, healthy clients may seek assistance in planning well-balanced vegetarian diets, especially if they are new vegetarians. In some cases, health care providers may refer a client with a problem believed to be related to poor dietary choices.

When one is counseling vegetarian clients, the same guidelines used in other counseling situations are helpful. The dietitian needs to pay particular attention to dietary concerns as expressed by the vegetarian client, however. It is important to listen to the client's definition of his or her vegetarian diet because it may differ from one's own definition. For example, many vegans avoid honey, and some will not consume white sugar (processing of white sugar can involve the use of animal bones). Although some health-motivated vegans may willingly consume foods that have small amounts of animal products in the ingredient list, most ethically motivated vegans will choose to avoid foods that contain even small amounts of animal-derived ingredients, such as whey, casein, or egg whites. Many of these ingredients are used extensively in processed foods, baked goods, cereals, and so forth.

Some vegans also avoid commercially fortified products because of the concern that vitamins added to the product might be derived from animals. Seventh-day Adventist vegetarians may avoid acidic foods, such as vinegar, and foods flavored with hot peppers. Some vegetarians may opt for a low-fat eating plan. Dietitians need to be prepared to help plan diets within the confines of whatever guidelines the client chooses to adopt.

Some clients may choose diets that are somewhat unfamiliar to many dietitians, such as a macrobiotic eating plan. Although these diets can be planned to meet nutrient needs, dietitians who have not worked with macrobiotic clients before may need to become more familiar with macrobiotic philosophy, dietary guidelines, and frequently consumed foods.

Dietitians will also need to be familiar with the preparation, use, and nutrient content of foods that are frequently used in vegetarian diets. With a growing selection of commercial vegetarian products available, it is not possible to be completely knowledgeable about all products on the market, but a working knowledge of a variety of whole grains, beans, soy products, and meat analogues is essential. It is also important to know about sources of these foods in the community because new vegetarians may not know where to find many specialty items. Chapter 16 provides some basic techniques for using and preparing vegetarian foods (see the Glossary of vegetarian foods).

DIETARY ASSESSMENT

Counseling protocol will always involve some assessment of the client's initial dietary or nutritional status. Assessment may be limited to a review of the current eating habits but is more likely to involve some additional elements, such as a medical history review, anthropometric measurements, clinical observations, and review of laboratory data. Any or all of these techniques can be used to assess the nutritional status or needs of vegetarian clients. A medical history review is especially important to ascertain special dietary needs. Along with biochemical assessment, it can also be used to ascertain any long-term problems of malnutrition. In children, ongoing anthropometric measurements are especially useful in this regard.

Some studies have shown slightly reduced rates of growth in young vegetarian children.[1-3] Breastfed infants grow more slowly than formula-fed infants, however.[4] Because breastfeeding is more common among vegetarians and may be of longer duration in vegetarian families, vegetarian infants and toddlers may be slightly lighter than their peers.[5] Nevertheless, vegetarian children whose diets are well balanced are generally within normal ranges for growth. Therefore, their growth can be assessed using the National Center for Health Statistics reference data.

Although laboratory measures are among the most objective means of establishing nutritional status, they are affected by many factors. For example, anemia may not be present in vegetarians despite an inadequate intake of vitamin B_{12} levels because of their higher folate intake. In older clients, a low vitamin B_{12} status may reflect not inadequate intake but rather poor absorption due to atrophic gastritis.[6] Similarly, reduced serum zinc levels might actually be the result of reduced levels of albumin (to which zinc is bound) brought about by illness.[7] Although biochemical assessment is a useful and direct means of ascertaining nutritional status, in vegetarian clients, as in all clients, it must be carried out in conjunction with other medical and dietary evaluations before appropriate conclusions can be drawn.

Methods of dietary assessment often require some adjustment for vegetarian clients. In particular, food frequency questionnaires may not include some foods or categories of foods that are a regular part of the client's diet and are important sources of certain nutrients. For example, some individuals may consume all their vitamin B12 in the form of nutritional yeast added to dishes, or they may consume much of their calcium from fortified soymilk. Both these foods are likely to be absent from food frequency questionnaires. As a result, it is possible to draw erroneous conclusions about the adequacy of an individual's diet based on the use of standard food frequency questionnaires. A food diary that includes both weekdays and weekend days before the counseling session is a much better means of establishing usual intake and dietary adequacy.

COUNSELING CLIENTS TO PLAN MENUS BASED ON VEGETARIAN FOOD GUIDES

Some clients may experience difficulty in meeting the minimum number of servings for each of the food groups. There may be an expressed dislike of foods in certain groups, particularly vegetables and legumes. Clients may feel that amounts of some foods are excessive. Food models can help clients better visualize serving sizes. Also, clients need to be assured that, although variety is an important component of planning healthy meals, eight servings of grains do not necessarily mean eight servings of *different* grains each day. Larger servings of one food can count toward several servings from a particular food group.

When counseling new vegetarians or vegetarians who experience problems in meeting nutrient needs, dietitians should be prepared to help the client choose foods that are well liked and practical and that fit into the client's budget. There are a variety of approaches for increasing food choices from each of the food groups.

Grains

One of the easiest ways to increase consumption from this group is to increase the number of servings of bread, a food that requires no preparation and is portable and generally well liked. Clients should be encouraged to choose whole grain bread as often as possible, although refined bread can also play a role in the diet. Clients should be encouraged to make all meals grain based. That is, grains should become "center of the plate" choices, a concept that is important for planning healthy menus in both vegetarian and omnivore diets. Exploring ethnic cuisine can help clients introduce more grains into meals. Table 13–1 offers some suggestions for using ethnic dishes as a means of introducing more grains into the diet.

If clients are not willing to spend time on preparation or have limited time, grains can be prepared in simple but appealing ways by cooking them in vegetable broth or by using apple juice for part of the cooking liquid and by tossing the grains with herbs, chopped dried fruits, or nuts.

Breakfasts provide a good opportunity for clients to consume more grains as well because staples of this meal include cereals, breads, muffins, pancakes, and French toast. The use of whole grain cereals should be encouraged where possible. Ready-to-eat cereals that are fortified with vitamins B_{12} and D can be good choices for vegans if they are acceptable. Clients should try to build breakfasts around whole grain breads, bagels, low-fat muffins, hot cereals, and whole grain ready-to-eat cereals. Lunch ideas that make good use of whole grains include sandwiches, cold pasta or rice salads, and soups with pasta, rice, or barley. Snacks can also be grain based. Good snack ideas include popcorn, bread, muffins, graham crackers, oatmeal cookies, bagels, and pretzels.

Table 13–1 Introducing Grains into Meals Using Ethnic Menus

Ethnic Cuisine	Grains Used	Menu Ideas
Italian	Polenta, wheat (pasta)	Spaghetti or other pasta with tomato sauce, pasta primavera, polenta with sauteed vegetables
Latin American	Rice, corn (tortillas)	Tacos, burritos, beans with rice, enchiladas
Asian	Rice (noodles), millet	Stir-fried rice with vegetables, millet with steamed vegetables, soups with ramen noodles, lo mein noodles with steamed vegetables
Mediterranean	Couscous, rice	Salads with couscous, chickpeas, vegetables; rice pilaf; rice salads
African	Rice, corn (cornmeal), millet	Rice with sauteed vegetables flavored with spicy peanut sauce, millet with sauteed vegetables, baked cornmeal with vegetables
Indian	Rice, wheat (flat breads)	Samosas, curried vegetables or beans over rice

Vegetables

Vegetables should be emphasized in all diets. Many clients will express difficulty in including three to five servings of these foods in their diet each day. The green leafy vegetables, such as kale, collards, and mustard, turnip, and dandelion greens, are especially valuable in providing a wide variety of nutrients (particularly calcium). These foods are uncommon in many American households, however, and clients may need some ideas for their preparation.

To boost vegetable intake with fairly simple preparation, clients can consume a serving of raw vegetables each day (eg, raw carrot sticks) and include at least one salad per day in their menus. When dark green leafy vegetables are purchased as tender young greens, they can be consumed raw in salads. Vegetables can be flavored with salad dressing, nonfat salad dressing, flavored mustards, herb vinegars, or Parmesan cheese. If clients do not care for the strong taste of some of the green leafy vegetables, these flavors can be tempered with more bland ingredients by blending them with a cream sauce made with soymilk or cow's milk. They can also be torn into small pieces and added to tomato-based dishes, stews, or vegetable soups. Exploring ethnic cuisines that make frequent use of these vegetables is useful also. Collards are common in African cooking and are often served as spicy dishes that will appeal to many clients.

Sea vegetables are exceptionally rich in many minerals and make a good addition to any type of diet. For the most part, however, they are common only in Asian diets. Sea vegetables are generally served as an ingredient in soups or stir fries rather than as a vegetable side dish. Recipes for vegetarian sushi using nori can be found in many vegetarian or Asian cookbooks.

Legumes

Many Americans have limited exposure to legumes beyond occasional servings of baked beans. These foods are important components of many world cuisines, however, and can play an important role in the diets of vegetarians. Canned beans are a good choice for those who have limited time to prepare these long-cooking foods, although a pressure cooker can greatly speed their preparation. Chapter 16 includes instructions for cooking beans to reduce gas production. Where flatulence and discomfort persist, clients can be encouraged to make greater use of legumes that are less gas producing, such as lentils or split peas. Also, gradual introduction of small amounts of legumes often leads to better tolerance. Finally, over-the-counter products such as Beano can be used to aid in digestion of the sugars in beans that cause gas.

New vegetarians in particular may find it a challenge to introduce more legumes into their diet. Familiar dishes such as chili, baked beans, and lentil soup can provide good starting points for introducing more legumes into family meals. Beans can also be added to salads and vegetable soups. Gradual exploration of ethnic dishes, such as dal (a curried lentil dish), hummus, and pasta fagioli, can provide clients with new ideas for eating more beans.

Clients should be encouraged to explore more creative ways to use beans in meals. For example, well-cooked beans can be pureed with olive oil and herbs to create sandwich spreads. The addition of a small amount of olive oil can turn these into a dip or paté. Beans mixed with salsa and blended to a chunky consistency can also serve as a dip.

Soyfoods are included in the legume food group and provide an easy way for clients to add versatility to meals and to consume more legumes. Chapter 16 includes suggestions for using tofu and textured soy protein in meals. Other soyfoods include soymilk, tempeh, and meat analogues made from soy.

Fruits

Fruits are generally well liked, so that introducing more fruits into the diet is generally not a problem. Fruit juice is especially popular with young children and can often displace other nutritious foods. Where possible, all vegetarians should be encouraged to make more use of whole fruits rather than fruit juice. Stewed or cooked, mashed fruits can be an excellent option for older people or young children who have problems chewing.

Milks

In the United States, cow's milk and dairy products have long held an important role in diet planning. Experience with eating habits among healthy populations in other parts of the world, however, indicates that cow's milk is a dietary option rather than an essential. Nutritious and satisfying diets are easily planned without the use of cow's milk.

Vegans and macrobiotics do not use any dairy products. Many lacto-ovo vegetarians choose to use milk substitutes rather than cow's milk some of the time. Dietitians who counsel vegetarians, regardless of the type of vegetarian diet, need to be familiar with nondairy sources of calcium and products that are available as milk substitutes. It is faulty nutrition guidance to advise consumers to meet total needs for a nutrient from one food group. Rather, clients should always be encouraged to explore a wide variety of foods that provide calcium.

Many clients choose to include vegetable milks in their diet, such as soymilk, rice milk, or almond milk. These foods can be used in most of the same ways that cow's milk is used in meals and food preparation. For example, they can be served over cereal, consumed as a beverage, and used in place of cow's milk in baked goods, cream soups, or sauces. Soymilk is a particularly high-protein food; rice and almond milk are fairly low in protein. A number of soymilks and rice milks are fortified with calcium, vitamin D, and/or vitamin B_{12}. These foods can be especially valuable in the diets of children, who may have picky eating habits and may experience difficulty meeting nutrient needs.

VEGETARIAN DIETS AS DIETARY THERAPY

Because the vegetarian eating pattern tends to be lower in total fat, saturated fat, cholesterol, total protein, and animal protein and higher in complex carbohydrates and fiber, it has been used with some success in the management of a number of clinical conditions, including diabetes, and hypercholesterolemia. It has also been used for weight control.

Recent popular literature has led to increased interest in vegetarian diets as a means of producing weight loss or reducing blood cholesterol. Therefore, dietitians are likely to encounter omnivore clients who wish to adopt a vegetarian eating plan specifically to lose weight or to improve heart disease risk. These clients present a special challenge to dietitians because they may not be familiar with vegetarian foods and guidelines for planning vegetarian menus; they may also need instruction to identify high-fat vegetarian foods.

Cardiovascular Disease

Vegetarian diets may be a successful means of reducing risk for cardiovascular disease for the following reasons:

- Whole plant foods, with the exception of nuts and seeds, are generally lower in fat than animal foods (Table 13–2).
- Whole plant foods tend to be low in saturated fat compared with animal foods.
- Plant foods contain no cholesterol.
- Plant foods contain fiber; soluble fiber has been shown to reduce blood cholesterol levels.[8]
- Plant foods are rich in antioxidants, which may help inhibit low-density lipoprotein cholesterol oxidation and thus lower heart disease risk.[9]

Table 13–2 Fat in Selected Plant and Animal Foods

Food/Serving Size	Total Calories	Total Fat	Percentage Fat
Baked potato, one	220	0.2	<1
Black beans, ½ cup	120	0.3	2
Pasta, ½ cup	100	0.45	4
Brown rice, ½ cup	108	0.9	7.5
Banana, one medium	105	0.6	5
Broccoli, ½ cup	22	0.3	12
Whole wheat bread, one slice	61	1.1	16
Broiled chicken breast (no skin), one half	142	3.1	20
Broiled perch, 4 oz	132	1.3	8
Low-fat milk, 1 cup	121	4.7	34
Whole milk, 1 cup	150	8.2	49
Sirloin steak, 3.5 oz	245	13.9	51
Egg, one large	77	5.3	61
Cheddar cheese, 1 oz	114	9.4	74

Source: Data from *Bowes & Church's Food Value of Portions Commonly Used.* 16th ed., by J. Pennington, Lippincott-Raven, 1994.

- Diets based on plant foods are higher in folate, which in turn can help to lower serum levels of homocysteine, an independent risk factor for heart disease (see Chapter 2).
- Plant-based diets are associated with lower blood pressure, and a lower incidence of hypertension.
- Plant-based diets are less calorically dense, which may decrease risk of obesity.

Because of a combination of factors, vegetarian diets may offer some advantage over more traditional approaches to lowering blood cholesterol, such as the American Heart Association's Step One Diet, which is fairly high in fat (30%) and makes liberal use of both meat and dairy foods.

Ornish et al[10] showed that a low-fat vegetarian diet, combined with a comprehensive plan that included exercise and stress management, successfully lowered cholesterol and perhaps affected other factors, to the extent that atherosclerosis was reversed. Previous studies demonstrating the regression of atherosclerosis involved drug therapy.[11] Standard approaches to management of hypercholesterolemia, such as the Step One Diet advocated by the National Cholesterol Education Program and the American Heart Association, are successful only in slowing the process of atherosclerosis, not in stopping or reversing it. The study by Ornish et al, however, utilized a

10% fat, nearly vegan diet, which is considerably different from the way the average Western vegetarian eats.

Average blood cholesterol levels are lower in both lacto-ovo vegetarians and vegans than in the general US population, and heart disease rates are lower among vegetarians as well.[12,13] Lacto-ovo vegetarians typically consume a diet that is between 30% and 36% fat, however, and vegan diets contain 30% fat on average (see Appendix A). Thus typical diets of vegetarians are not lower in total fat than what is recommended by most government agencies. Vegetarians, especially vegans, have the added overall benefits of lower intakes of saturated fat and cholesterol and higher fiber and antioxidant consumption. Nevertheless, it is probable that in patients who are at elevated risk for heart disease some adjustments to standard vegetarian eating practices to reduce overall fat intake may be beneficial. In lacto-ovo vegetarian diets in particular, it may be necessary to provide guidance on avoiding saturated fats from dairy foods and eggs.

Weight Control

Vegetarian diets have also been used with some success in producing weight loss. Plant-based eating plans are less calorically dense than omnivore diets. The best approach to weight control remains elusive, however, and studies show that short-term success is common but that one third to two thirds of the weight loss is regained within 1 year and almost all is regained within 5 years.[14] Current research has focused on low-fat diets as a promising approach to weight management. Advantages of low-fat diets include the following:

- Low-fat diets tend to be lower in calories. Although individuals can increase their calorie intake by eating more food to compensate for the lower caloric density of low-fat foods, several studies show that at least in the short term this often does not occur.[15-17] In one study of 24 women who consumed diets ranging from 15% to 50% fat, those who ate low-fat diets ate slightly more food but did not consume as many calories as those eating the high-fat plans.[16] In a similar study at Cornell University, subjects who consumed a 20% to 25% fat diet did not eat as many calories as those whose diet was 35% to 40% fat.[18] Vegetarian diets are also higher in fiber; fiber decreases caloric density, promotes satiety and fullness, and has been shown to be effective in weight loss.[19-23]

- Fat metabolism is more efficient than the metabolism of either carbohydrate or protein, so that calories from fat are more available. In a Stanford study there was no relationship between total number of calories consumed by male subjects and total body fat, but there was a relationship between total fat consumed and body fat.[24]

- Some research suggests that carbohydrate calories are not readily converted into fat, at least not to the extent that fat calories are.[25]
- Results from studies in which diets with different energy expenditures were fed to men indicate that consuming calories in the form of protein and carbohydrate reduces subsequent energy intake, whereas fat calories do not have this effect.[26] On a mixed diet, excess energy in the form of fat tends to promote fat storage.[27]
- Some data indicate vegetarians have a higher basal metabolic rate than nonvegetarians (see Chapter 2).

The lower fat content of vegetarian diets presents a clear advantage in weight management on a population basis. In general, vegetarians tend to be leaner than nonvegetarians (Appendix A). On an individual basis, however, usual vegetarian practices may not be adequate to produce weight loss in those clients who have experienced long-term weight control problems. That is, changing from an omnivore food pattern to a vegetarian food pattern is not necessarily enough to produce weight loss. Most clients will need additional guidance on reducing the fat content of their vegetarian plan. In addition, despite the overall leanness of the vegetarian population, individual vegetarians may be overweight and may require guidance in reducing the fat content in their diet.

A variety of approaches have been used to help vegetarians lose weight:

- Clients who seek structured guidelines for meal planning can utilize the exchange lists for meal planning presented in Chapter 14. Exchange list diets can be planned based on an appropriate caloric intake and on a fat intake that is conducive to weight loss (such as 15% to 20% of calories from fat).
- An increasingly popular approach to managing fat intake involves counting grams of fat consumed each day. An upper limit is set to reflect what would typically be a 15% to 20% fat diet based on a recommended caloric intake for the client.
- Some practitioners advocate free consumption of certain foods with other foods being greatly restricted in the diet. For example, the client would be allowed unrestricted consumption of legumes (except for soybeans and peanuts), whole grains, vegetables, and fruits. Soyfoods, nonfat dairy products, and nonfat commercial products (crackers, soups, fat-free ice cream, etc) might be limited to a particular number of servings each day, and foods that are very limited in the diet might include meat, chicken, fish, avocados, olives, nuts, seeds, full-fat or

low-fat dairy foods, added sugars, and alcohol. Many clients prefer these types of guidelines, which require no calculations or meal-planning guidelines.

Bear in mind, however, that the greater availability of low-fat and nonfat products has not been associated with a decrease in obesity; in fact, the opposite is true. It has been proposed that the greater use of these products leads to overconsumption of calories, which, in turn, promotes weight gain.[28]

REDUCING FAT IN VEGETARIAN DIETS

As noted above, vegetarian diets can be used successfully both to manage hypercholesterolemia and to reduce weight, but many clients will require instruction on reducing fat intake in vegetarian diets. The guidelines presented in Table 13–3 can be used to help clients make appropriate choices

Table 13–3 Low-Fat and High-Fat Food Choices in Vegetarian Food Groups

Food Group	Lower-Fat	Higher-Fat
Grains	Whole and refined grains (eg, white or brown rice, barley, quinoa, kamut, wheat berries, bulgur, couscous), regular hot breakfast cereals, some dry cereals, breads (pita, bagels, English muffins), corn tortillas (fat content varies)	Some dry cereals with added fat, baked goods prepared with fat (eg, muffins, biscuits, pastries), pancakes, waffles, breads with added fat, flour tortillas, crackers
Legumes	Most cooked dried beans, textured vegetable protein, low-fat tofu	Soybeans, soynuts, tempeh, regular tofu, some meat analogues
Nuts and seeds		All nuts, seeds, nut and seed butters
Milks	Nonfat cow's milk, nonfat cow's milk yogurt, low-fat or nonfat soymilk, rice milks, Vegelicious	Low-fat and whole cow's milk, regular soymilk
Vegetables	All raw or steamed vegetables	Olives, avocado, vegetables prepared with added fat or sauces
Fruits	All fruit and fruit juices	
Fats	Fat-free margarine, low-fat or nonfat salad dressings	All other fats (oil, margarine, butter, mayonnaise, regular salad dressing)
Other foods	Fruit ices, sorbets, pretzels, fat-free chips, popcorn	Cheese, eggs, ice cream, most baked goods, microwave popcorn, most snack foods

within each food group. Exhibit 13–1 gives some general guidelines for reducing fat in vegetarian meals. Exhibit 13–2 lists vegetarian foods that are high in fat and may need to be limited in the diet, and Exhibit 13–3 lists some low-fat snack foods that may appeal to vegetarian clients who are watchful of their fat intake.

REDUCING FOOD COSTS ON VEGETARIAN DIETS

Vegetarian diets at their most basic should represent a low-cost way of cooking. Grains and beans, the foundation of vegetarian meals, are among the least expensive foods, especially when prepared from scratch. As the vegetarian population has grown, however, hundreds of new products have become available to meet demands. Many of these, such as fortified soymilk and nutritional yeast, make it even easier to plan well-balanced meals. Meat analogues introduce more opportunities for variety in vegetarian meal plans, and a number of convenience products, such as instant soups, grain mixes, and prepared dinners, serve to make meal preparation faster and easier for vegetarians. Nevertheless, because demand for such foods remains small compared with the demand for foods that fit into more traditional Western diets, these foods are largely viewed as specialty items, and their prices are

---

Exhibit 13–1 Guidelines for Reducing Fat in Vegetarian Meals

- Reduce use of fatty spreads, such as butter, margarine, and peanut butter, by using the following:
  bean spreads made from cooked beans pureed with chopped onions and celery, herbs, and lemon juice or salsa
  fruit spreads made by pureeing dried fruits with a small amount of water or fruit juice
  low-fat tofu blended with herbs and lemon juice to make a dip or sandwich spread
- Reduce the fat in homemade baked goods by reducing the oil or margarine in a recipe by 25% or more, or replace some of the fat in a baked product with mashed bananas, blended tofu, or pureed prunes. Because fat intensifies flavors, it may be necessary to increase amounts of vanilla extract or spices in low-fat baked goods.
- Use nonfat salad dressings.
- Sauté onions and other vegetables in recipes in sherry, dry wine, vegetable broth, tomato juice, or apple juice instead of oil.
- Flavor dishes with nonfat flavor enhancers, such as sun-dried tomatoes, fresh ginger, freshly squeezed lemon or lime juice, and fresh herbs.
- Use low-fat tofu in place of regular tofu in recipes.
- Blend low-fat tofu to add to dishes that call for cream, or thicken soups or sauces with blended vegetables, legumes, or mashed potatoes.

Exhibit 13–2 Popular Vegetarian Items That Are Relatively High in Fat on a Caloric Basis

• Falafel	• Regular soymilk
• Tofu ice cream	• Tofu
• Some meat analogues and veggieburgers (low-fat or nonfat versions are increasingly available)	• Commercially prepared cookies and cakes
• Soy cheese	• Oils
• Hummus	• Avocado
• Nut butters	• Olives
• Tahini	• Coconut
	• French fries
	• Snack chips

high even compared with meat, the most costly item on most American grocery lists. Frequent use of such products can make vegetarian diet costs prohibitive for some. It is somewhat of an irony that the diet that mimics the eating patterns of many poorer populations throughout the world has to some extent been transformed into a pattern based on expensive, often hard to find, specialty items.

For families that need to keep food costs low, it is helpful to dispel some of the myths of meal planning. One of these is that diets must contain a wide variety of foods to be healthy. Although it is important to choose foods from different food groups throughout the day, healthy diets can be planned using relatively few types of food. Throughout the world, most populations derive most of their calories from a fairly limited selection of food items. The following suggestions can help families plan healthy vegetarian meals at minimal cost.

- *Gardening.* Fresh produce is one of the most costly items on both omnivore and vegetarian shopping lists. Small gardens can yield con-

Exhibit 13–3 Low-Fat Vegetarian Snacks

• Baked potatoes	• Bagels
• Steamed vegetables	• Nonfat crackers
• Salad with nonfat dressing	• Rice cakes
• Fresh fruit salad	• Popcorn
• Ready-to-eat cereals	• Soft pretzels with mustard
• Whole grain breads	• Baked fruit dusted with cinnamon

siderable savings during the growing season, and preserving foods from a large garden can contribute to savings throughout the year. Where space or time constraints make full-scale gardening difficult, clients can be encouraged to grow small vegetables in containers on balconies or patios.

- *Compare costs of frozen and fresh vegetables.* Consumers often believe that vegetables purchased fresh are more nutritious than frozen vegetables. Studies of nutrient content show that this is not true, however.[29] Especially when vegetables are out of season, frozen vegetables can offer a less expensive option. Fresh vegetables and fruits are often a good buy when they are locally grown and in season.

- *Use dry beans rather than canned beans.* Dry beans offer a twofold to threefold savings over canned varieties, although they do require much more cooking time. Clients can plan schedules to speed up cooking time by putting beans to soak each night for the next night's dinner, cooking beans in large batches and freezing leftovers, and using either a pressure cooker or a Crock-Pot (slow cooker).

- *Shop at ethnic grocery stores.* Many items that are exotic specialties in traditional supermarkets are actually basic essentials in the diets of some populations. Therefore, tofu and sea vegetables, both fairly expensive items in most stores, often sell for 50% to 75% less in Asian markets. These stores are easier to find in urban areas and are more common in some parts of the country than others.

- *Use refined grains.* Although whole foods are often the most nutritious, vegetarian diets that are largely based on whole foods and are rich in fiber can make some use of refined products without sacrificing overall dietary quality. White rice typically is less expensive than brown rice, and pasta made from refined grains is less expensive than whole wheat pasta.

- *Comparison shop among different types of foods.* Many vegans make wide use of dark green leafy vegetables to help meet calcium needs. Many of the less popular but easily grown vegetables, such as collards and kale, are far less expensive than broccoli and are actually richer in calcium.

- *Choose foods that offer the most nutritional value for the money.* Vegetarians may make wide use of a variety of foods that are nutrient dense but are also expensive, such as soymilk, tofu, calcium-fortified orange juice, quinoa, and almond butter. Although these foods can make it easy to meet nutrient needs, none is a dietary necessity. Clients can be encouraged to focus on foods that are nutrient rich and inexpensive, such as dried beans, oatmeal, peanut butter, rice, potatoes, fresh or frozen greens, and textured vegetable protein. Of course, more expensive items in vegetarian diets (eg, whole grain bread, tofu, and soymilk) can all be made from scratch if clients have the time and inclination to do so. The acceptability of this suggestion will vary among clients and will depend on a variety of factors.

REFERENCES

1. Fulton JR, Hutton CW, Stitt KR. Preschool vegetarian children. *J Am Diet Assoc.* 1980;76:360–365.

2. Dwyer JT, Andrew EM, Berkey C, Valadian I, Reed RB. Growth in "new" vegetarian pre-school children using the Jenss-Bayley curve fitting technique. *Am J Clin Nutr.* 1983;37: 815–827.

3. Dwyer JT, Palombo R, Thorne H, Valadian I, Reed RB. Preschoolers on alternate life-style diets. *J Am Diet Assoc.* 1978;72:264–270.

4. Garza C, Frongillo E, Dewey KG. Implications of growth patterns of breast-fed infants for growth references. *Acta Paediatr.* 1994;402(suppl):4–10.

5. Shull MW, Reed RB, Valadian I, Palombo R, Thorne H, Dwyer JT. Velocities of growth in vegetarian preschool children. *Pediatrics.* 1977;60:410–417.

6. Krasinski SD, Russel RM, Samloff M, et al. Fundic atrophic gastritis in an elderly population. Effect on hemoglobin and several serum nutritional indicators. *J Am Geriatr Soc.* 1986;34:800–806.

7. McMahon MM, Bistrian BR. The physiology of nutritional assessment and therapy in pro-tein-calorie malnutrition. *Dis Mon.* 1990;36:373–417.

8. Glore SR, Van Treeck DV, Knehans AW, Guild M. Soluble fiber and serum lipids: A litera-ture review. *J Am Diet Assoc.* 1994;94:425–436.

9. Steinberg D, Witztum JL. Lipoproteins and atherogenesis. *J Am Diet Assoc.* 1990;264:3047–3052.

10. Ornish D, Brown SE, Scherwitz LW, et al. Can lifestyle changes reverse coronary heart disease? *Lancet.* 1990;336:129–133.

11. Loscalzo J. Regression of coronary atherosclerosis. *N Engl J Med.* 1990;323:1337–1339.

12. Phillips RL, Lemon FR, Beeson L, Kuzma JW. Coronary heart disease mortality among Seventh-Day Adventists with differing dietary habits: A preliminary report. *Am J Clin Nutr.* 1978;31:S191–S198.

13. Snowdon DA, Phillips RL, Fraser GE. Meat consumption and fatal ischemic heart disease. *Prev Med.* 1984;13:490–500.

14. NIH Technology Assessment Conference Panel. Methods for voluntary weight loss and control. *Ann Intern Med.* 1992;116:942–949.

15. Pi-Sunyer F. Effect of the composition of the diet on energy intake. *Nutr Rev.* 1990;48:94–105.

16. Lissner L, Levitsky DA, Strupp BJ, Kalkwarf HJ, Roe DA. Dietary fat and the regulation of energy intake in human subjects. *Am J Clin Nutr.* 1987;46:886–892.

17. Kendall A, Levitsky DA, Strupp BJ, Lissner L. Weight loss and a low-fat diet: Consequences of the imprecision of the contribution of food intake in humans. *Am J Clin Nutr.* 1991;53:1123–1129.

18. Duncan KH, Bacon JA, Weinser RL. The effects of high and low energy density diets on satiety, energy intake, and eating time of obese and nonobese subjects. *Am J Clin Nutr.* 1983;37:763–767.

19. Rigaud D, Ryttig KR, Angel LA, Apfelbaum M. Overweight treated with energy restriction and a dietary fibre supplement: A 6-month randomized, double-blind, placebo-controlled trial. *Int J Obesity.* 1990;14:763–769.

20. Ophir O, Peresecenschi GP, Gilad J, Blum M, Aviram A. Low blood pressure in vegetarians: The possible role of potassium. *Am J Clin Nutr.* 1983;37:755–762.

21. Astrup A, Vrist E, Quaade F. Dietary fibre added to very low calorie diet reduces hunger and alleviates constipation. *Int J Obesity.* 1990;14:105–112.

22. Rigaud D, Ryttig KR, Leeds AR, Bard D, Apfelbaum M. Effects of a moderate dietary fibre supplement on hunger rating, energy input and faecal energy output in young, healthy volunteers. *Int J Obesity.* 1987;11(suppl 1):73–78.

23. Haber GB, Heaton KW, Murphy D, Burroughs LF. Depletion and disruption of dietary fibre. Effects on satiety, plasma-glucose, and serum-insulin. *Lancet.* 1977;2:679–682.

24. Dreon DM, Frey-Hewlett B, Ellsworth N, et al. Dietary fat:carbohydrate ratio and obesity in middle-aged men. *Am J Clin Nutr.* 1988;47:995–1000.

25. Flatt JP. Dietary fat, carbohydrate balance, and weight maintenance: Effects of exercise. *Am J Clin Nutr.* 1987;45:296–306.

26. Stubbs RJ, Harbron G, Murgatroyd PR, Prentice AM. Covert manipulation of dietary fat and energy density: Effect on substrate flux and food intake in men eating ad libitum. *Am J Clin Nutr.* 1995;62:316–329.

27. Abbot WGH, Howard BV, Christin L, et al. Short-term energy balance: Relationship with protein, carbohydrate and fat balances. *Am J Physiol.* 1988;255:E332–E337.

28. Alfred JB. Too much of a good thing? *J Am Diet Assoc.* 1995;95:417–418.

29. Fennema O. Effects of freeze preservation on nutrients. In: Karmas E, Harris RS, eds. *Nutritional Evaluation of Food Processing.* 3rd ed. New York, NY: AVI; 1988:3–5.

CHAPTER 14

Diabetes

The incidence of diabetes varies considerably throughout the world. Diabetes is nearly nonexistent in some cultures, whereas in others nearly 50% of the population has the disease.[1] Some estimates are that as many as one third of all diabetics in the world live in the United States, where between 5% and 10% of the population has been diagnosed with this disease.[2]

Although hereditary factors greatly influence the risk of developing diabetes, life style is also thought to play a significant role. For example, within a given ethnic population, rural dwellers are far less likely to have diabetes than urban dwellers.[3] Migration studies reveal that westernization of diet and life style is associated with an increased incidence of diabetes. The rate of diabetes is higher among Japanese who move to Hawaii or California than among those who live in Japan and is higher among Yemenites who move to Israel than among those who live in Yemen.[4] International comparisons generally show that the prevalence of diabetes correlates positively with serum cholesterol levels and with intake of fat, animal fat, protein, animal protein, and sugar; it correlates negatively with intakes of carbohydrate and vegetable fat.[5,6]

The first person to describe diabetes was a Hindu physician who noted 3,000 years ago that the disease occurred in people who were "gluttonous and obese."[2] Today, it is well recognized that obesity dramatically elevates the risk for non–insulin-dependent diabetes mellitus (NIDDM). In fact, the only factor consistently linked to the prevalence of NIDDM is body weight.[4] Duration of obesity also correlates with risk; the younger the age of onset of obesity, the greater the risk for diabetes.[7] Abdominal fat is much more closely related to diabetes risk than hip and thigh fat.[4,8] More than 90% of the diabetics in the United States have NIDDM.[2] In the past 50 years, the number of people diagnosed with NIDDM has risen by a factor of 5 to 10.

Insulin-dependent diabetes mellitus (IDDM) is the most common chronic disease of American children. More than 13,000 new cases are diagnosed each year, and more than 300,000 Americans have this disease.[9] The incidence of IDDM has increased since the 1960s, and in the latter half of the 1980s the increase in incidence of IDDM among young children was of almost epidemic proportion. It was especially prevalent in boys and nonwhite children.[10]

The cause of IDDM is unknown, but there are a number of suspected etiologic factors. Viral infections can cause diabetes by attacking the pancreatic cells that produce insulin.[11,12] Milk consumption during infancy, particularly before 3 months of age[13,14] but also during childhood, has been linked to risk for diabetes.[15] Intolerance to milk protein may lead to production of antibodies that can destroy insulin-producing pancreatic cells.

DIET THERAPY FOR DIABETES

The beneficial effect of caloric restriction in the treatment of diabetes has been known for decades. During both World Wars, when food was scarce and fat intake was low, death from diabetes-related complications was reduced by approximately half.[16] Because it was recognized several centuries ago that diabetics excreted sugar in their urine, early recommendations for diabetics were to restrict carbohydrates, especially simple sugars. In contrast, the more recent understanding of diabetes is that diets high in complex carbohydrates are associated with lower risk for the disease. In populations consuming high–complex carbohydrate diets, diabetes is often quite rare; for example, in a study of 1,381 inhabitants of various villages in West Africa, whose diet was more than 80% carbohydrate, not a single person was found to have diabetes.[17]

The goals of diet therapy in diabetes include the following:

- to meet nutrient needs
- to prevent postprandial hyperglycemia
- to prevent periods of hypoglycemia in patients receiving insulin by timing meals appropriately
- to achieve and maintain ideal weight
- to prevent or delay development of diabetic complications (cardiovascular, renal, neurologic, and retinal disorders)

In planning diabetic diets, particular attention is given to the distribution of fat, carbohydrate, and protein. Both fiber and simple sugars are also usually addressed in the planning of these diets.

Fat

Total fat, saturated fat, and cholesterol are all restricted on diabetic diets. There are three reasons for this. First, a primary goal of diet therapy for diabetics is to lower blood cholesterol levels. Diabetics are at greater risk for complications related to atherosclerosis. Insulin-dependent diabetics are eight times more likely to have coronary artery disease than their age- and sex-matched peers.[18] Second, achieving and maintaining ideal weight are particularly important for non–insulin-dependent diabetics. Low-fat diets should help in this regard. Third, low-fat diets may help in the control of blood glucose levels. In a study at the Pritikin Longevity Center, diabetics followed a 10% fat diet containing just small amounts of animal products in conjunction with an exercise program for 4 weeks. Of the 18 patients who were on exogenous insulin therapy, 13 were able to discontinue its use, and of the 31 patients using oral hypoglycemic agents, 24 were able to stop.[19,20]

The type of fat in the diet may have some bearing on control of blood glucose. Some research has shown that diets high in monounsaturated fatty acids may specifically help in the control of diabetes, and monounsaturated fats are effective in helping reduce blood cholesterol levels when they replace saturated fat.[21–24]

The American Diabetes Association recommends that less than 30% of calories come from fat and less than 10% of calories come from saturated fat. Diabetics may benefit by a further reduction in fat intake, however. To improve glucose tolerance control, promote weight loss, and lower blood cholesterol levels, an upper limit of 20% fat may be advisable.

Carbohydrate

High-carbohydrate diets aid in the control of diabetes.[19,20,22,25] This was first demonstrated more 60 years ago by Himsworth,[16] but only recently have relatively high-carbohydrate diets been officially recommended. In fact, between 1921 and 1986 recommendations for the carbohydrate content of diabetic diets increased from 20% to about 60%.[26] The consumption of low-fat, high-starch, high-fiber diets has been shown to increase insulin receptors on monocytes in insulin-dependent diabetics[27] and to increase peripheral insulin sensitivity in both young and old individuals and in normal and diabetic subjects.[28,29]

The American Diabetes Association recommends that diabetic diets include between 55% and 60% of calories from carbohydrate. The average American consumes a diet that is approximately 50% carbohydrate. In contrast, vegetarians typically consume diets that are 50% to 65% carbohydrate.

There may be some advantage to diabetics in consuming a diet that is higher than 60% carbohydrate in order to decrease fat intake further.

Fiber

Low-fat, high-fiber diets help reduce blood glucose more effectively than diets that are low in fat but not rich in fiber.[19,22] Soluble fiber in particular may aid in control of blood glucose levels. Insoluble fiber is less effective. The American Diabetes Association recommends 20 to 35 g of fiber per day, which is far in excess of the 12–15 g/day that is consumed on average by Americans.

Protein

The American Diabetes Association recommends that diabetics consume diets that are 10% to 20% protein. It is best to aim for the low end of that recommendation, however, because protein can adversely affect kidney function, and diabetics are prone to diabetic nephropathy.[30] The type of protein may also affect kidney function. When individuals with IDDM were placed on a vegetarian diet, kidney function, as assessed by glomerular filtration rate (GFR) and renal plasma flow (RPF), was favorably affected when compared to consuming a nonvegetarian diet containing similar amounts of protein.[31] Consistent with these findings, a vegetarian diet in which soy protein provided nearly all of the protein was shown to favorably affect kidney function in nephrotic patients as assessed by GFR and RPF.[32] The vegetarian diet in this study did, however, contain less overall protein. Thus, in addition to the advantage of vegetarian diets containing less overall protein, there are at least interesting preliminary data indicating the consumption of diets containing a higher proportion of plant protein may be particularly advantageous for individuals with diabetes.

Sugar

Sugar and other caloric sweeteners were once considered taboo for diabetics. There is no evidence that they raise blood glucose more than other types of carbohydrates, however, when included as part of a total meal and a balanced, healthy diet. Consequently, according to the most recent American Diabetes Association guidelines, it is not necessary for diabetics to avoid sweeteners completely.[27]

Exercise

The importance of exercise should be stressed for all diabetics. In addition to helping with weight loss, exercise may also increase insulin sensitivity and the number of insulin receptors.[33–36] The Nurse's Health Study found that physical activity was associated with a decreased risk of developing NIDDM in women.[37]

VEGETARIANS AND DIABETES

Not surprising, there is some evidence that vegetarians have lower rates of diabetes than the general population.[38] Vegetarians are often leaner than omnivores and have lower fat and higher fiber intakes (Appendix A) than the general population. In comparison with omnivores, their diet comes closer to the eating pattern that reduces risk for diabetes and is closer to the guidelines for controlling diabetes.

Rates of diabetes among Seventh-day Adventists are less than half the rates seen in the general population. Also, Seventh-day Adventist vegetarians have lower rates of diabetes than nonvegetarian Seventh-day Adventists.[38] In a large prospective study involving more than 25,000 Adventists, the prevalence of diagnosed diabetes was 1.9 and 1.4 times higher for nonvegetarian men and women, respectively.[38] In men, as meat consumption increased, diabetes incidence also increased. Relative risk in men consuming no meat and those consuming meat 1 to 2 days per week, 3 to 5 days per week, and 6 days or more per week was 1.0, 1.3, 1.5, and 2.4, respectively. Among women, only those consuming meat 6 days or more per week were at increased risk for diabetes.

In addition to affecting overall risk of developing diabetes, vegetarianism may also have therapeutic effects in diabetic patients. Meat consumption is positively related to blood glucose levels, and saturated fat intake may increase insulin secretion and possibly lead to insulin insensitivity.[39,40] In a 25-day inpatient program, when researchers placed patients with diabetic neuropathy on a low-fat vegetarian diet regimen that included regular exercise, 17 of the 21 patients experienced a remission of pain in less than 2.5 weeks. This was accompanied by a drop in average fasting blood sugar from 169 to 121 mg/dL. Six of the subjects were also able to discontinue either insulin or oral hypoglycemic medication.[41]

THE DIABETIC EXCHANGE LISTS

The term *diabetic diet* is no longer used in planning diets for people with this disease. According to the American Diabetes Association, diets should be planned according to individual needs. Diets that meet the general goals of diet therapy for diabetics are appropriate. This can be achieved in a variety of ways. The diabetic exchange lists that were once used for all diabetic patients are now considered unnecessary for many. The exchange lists are useful where strict calorie control and macronutrient distribution are important, however. The exchange lists allow dietitians to plan diets with their clients that will ensure nutritional adequacy and the desired distribution of macronutrients.

For most vegetarian diabetes patients, the exchange lists need to be modified to meet their needs better. Many foods that are common in the diets of some vegetarians, such as tempeh, soymilk, and sea vegetables, are not included in the standard exchange lists. The exchange lists for vegetarians given in Appendix 14-A may be helpful in developing diets for vegetarian diabetics.

Some vegetarians may prefer not to use foods from the milk exchange list in their diet. In some cases, low-fat soymilk can be used as a milk exchange. As long as diets are planned according to the goals set forth by the patient, the dietitian, and the physician, however, there is no reason why the milk exchange list cannot be omitted. As long as nutrient balance is achieved, the diet is low in fat, and blood glucose levels are controlled, adjustments in the way the exchange lists are used are perfectly reasonable. Where clients choose not to include dairy alternatives such as fortified soymilk in their diet, it is important to identify calcium-rich foods from the other exchange lists. Also, for vegan clients regular use of vitamin B_{12}–fortified foods or a vitamin B_{12} supplement must be stressed.

REFERENCES

1. Davidson JK, DiGirolamo M. Non–insulin-dependent diabetes mellitus. In: Davidson JK, ed. *Clinical Diabetes Mellitus, a Problem Oriented Approach*. 2nd ed. New York, NY: Thieme Medical; 1991:11–34.

2. Hazlett BE. Historical perspective: The discovery of insulin. In: Davidson JK, ed. *Clinical Diabetes Mellitus, a Problem Oriented Approach*. 2nd ed. New York, NY: Thieme Medical; 1991:2–10.

3. King H, Rewers M. Diabetes in adults is now a Third World problem. *Bull World Health Organ*. 1991;69:643–648.

4. West KM. *Epidemiology of Diabetes and Its Vascular Lesions*. New York, NY: Elsevier/North-Holland; 1978.

5. West KM, Kalbfleisch JM. Influence of nutritional factors on prevalence of diabetes. *Diabetes*. 1971;20:99–108.

6. West KM, Kalbfleisch JM. Glucose tolerance, nutrition, and diabetes in Uruguay, Venezuela, Malaya, and East Pakistan. *Diabetes*. 1966;15:9–18.

7. Everhart JE, Petitt DJ, Bennett PH, Knowler WC. Duration of obesity increases the incidence of NIDDM. *Diabetes*. 1992;41:235–240.

8. Björntorp P. Abdominal obesity and the development of non–insulin-dependent diabetes mellitus. *Diabetes Metab Rev*. 1988;4:615–622.

9. Libman I, Songer T, LaPorte R. How many people in the US have IDDM? *Diabetes Care.* 1993;16:841–842.

10. Dokheel TM. An epidemic of childhood diabetes in the United States. Evidence from Allegheny County, Pennsylvania. *Diabetes Care.* 1993;16:1606–1611.

11. Yoon JW, Ray U. Perspectives on the role of viruses in insulin-dependent diabetes. *Diabetes Care.* 1985;8:39–44.

12. Yoon JW, Austin M, Onodera T, Notkins AL. Isolation of a virus from the pancreas of a child with diabetic ketoacidosis. *N Engl J Med.* 1979;300:1173–1179.

13. Gerstein HC. Cow's milk exposure and type I diabetes mellitus. *Diabetes Care.* 1993;17: 13–19.

14. Dahl-Jørgensen K, Joner G, Hanssen KF. Relationship between cow's milk consumption and incidence of IDDM in childhood. *Diabetes Care.* 1991;14:1081–1083.

15. Fava D, Leslie RDG, Pozzilli P. Relationship between dairy product consumption and incidence of IDDM in childhood in Italy. *Diabetes Care.* 1994;17:1488–1490.

16. Himsworth HP. Diet in the etiology of human diabetes. *Proc R Soc Med.* 1949;42:323:9–12.

17. Teuscher T, Rosman JH, Baillod P, Teuscher A. Absence of diabetes in a rural West African population with a high carbohydrate/cassava diet. *Lancet.* 1987;1:765–768.

18. Dorman LS, Laporte RE, Kuller LH, et al. The Pittsburgh insulin-dependent diabetes mellitus (IDDM) morbidity and mortality study; mortality results. *Diabetes.* 1984;33:271–276.

19. Barnard RJ, Massey MR, Cherny S, O'Brien LT, Pritkin N. Longterm use of high–complex-carbohydrate high-fiber diet and exercise in the treatment of NIDDM patients. *Diabetes Care.* 1983;6:268–273.

20. Barnard RJ, Lattimore L, Holly RG, Cherny S, Pritkin N. Response of non–insulin-dependent diabetic patients to an intensive program of diet and exercise. *Diabetes Care.* 1982;5:370–374.

21. Lerman-Garber I, Ichazo-Cerro S, Zamora-Gonzalez J, Carddoso-Saldana G, Posada-Romero C. Effect of a high-monounsaturated fat diet enriched with avocado in NIDDM patients. *Diabetes Care.* 1993;17:311–315.

22. Garg A, Bantle JP, Henry RR, et al. Effects of varying carbohydrate content of diet in patients with non–insulin-dependent diabetes mellitus. *JAMA.* 1994;271:1421–1428.

23. Rivellese AA, Auletta P, Marotta G, et al. Long term metabolic effects of two dietary methods of treating hyperlipidaemia. *Br Med J.* 1994;308:227–331.

24. Gustafsson I-B, Vessby B, Nydahl M. Effects of lipid-lowering diets enriched with monounsaturated and polyunsaturated fatty acids on serum lipoprotein composition in patients with hyperlipoproteinaemia. *Atherosclerosis.* 1992;96:109–118.

25. Simpson HCR, Lousley S, Geekie M, et al. A high carbohydrate leguminous fibre diet improves all aspects of diabetes control. *Lancet.* 1981;1:1–5.

26. Anderson JW, Herman RH, Zakim D. Effect of high glucose and high sucrose diets on glucose tolerance of normal men. *Am J Clin Nutr.* 1973;26:600–607.

27. Executive Committee of the American Diabetes Association. Nutrition recommendations and principles for people with diabetes mellitus. *J Am Diet Assoc.* 1994;94:504–506.

28. Anderson JW, Zeigler JA, Deakins DA, et al. Metabolic effects of high-carbohydrate, high-fiber diets for insulin-dependent diabetes in individuals. *Am J Clin Nutr.* 1991;54:936–943.

29. Hjollund E, Pedersen O, Richelsen B, Beck-Nielsen H, Sorensen NS. Increased insulin binding to adipocytes and monocytes and increased insulin sensitivity of glucose transport

and metabolism in adipocytes from non–insulin dependent diabetics after a low fat/high starch/high fiber diet. *Metabolism*. 1983;32:1067–1075.

30. Brenner BM, Meyer TW, Hostetter TH. Dietary protein intake and the progressive nature of kidney disease: The role of hemodynamically medicated glomerular injury in the pathogenesis of progressive glomerular sclerosis in aging, renal ablation, and intrinsic renal disease. *N Engl J Med*. 1982;307:652–659.

31. Kontessis P, Bossinakou I, Sarika L, et al. Renal, metabolic, and hormonal responses to proteins of different origin in normotensive, nonproteinuric type I diabetic patients. *Diabetes Care*. 1995;18:1233–1240.

32. D'amico G, Gentile M, Manna G, et al. Effect of vegetarian soy diet on hyperlipidaemia in nephrotic syndrome. *Lancet*. 1992;335:1131–1134.

33. Koivisto VA, Soman V, Conrad P, Hendler R, Nadel E, Felig P. Insulin binding to monocytes in trained athletes. *J Clin Invest*. 1979;64:1011–1015.

34. Saltin B, Lindgrade F, Houston M, Horlin R, Nygard E, Gad P. Physical training and glucose tolerance in middle-aged men with chemical diabetes. *Diabetes*. 1979;28(suppl 1):30–32.

35. Björntorp P, Jounge KD, Sjostrom L, Sullivan L. The effect of physical training on insulin production in obesity. *Metabolism*. 1970;19:631–638.

36. Le Blanc J, Nadeau A, Boulay M, Rousseau-Migneron S. Effects of physical training and adiposity on glucose metabolism and ^{25}I-insulin binding. *J Appl Physiol*. 1979;46:235–239.

37. Manson JE, Rimm EB, Stampfer MJ, et al. Physical activity and incidence of non–insulin-dependent diabetes mellitus. *Lancet*. 1991;33:744–748.

38. Snowdon DA, Phillips RL. Does a vegetarian diet reduce the occurrence of diabetes? *Am J Public Health*. 1985;75:507–512.

39. Gear JS, Mann JI, Thorogood M, Carter R, Jeffs R. Biochemical and haematological variables in vegetarians. *Br Med J*. 1980;1:1414–1415.

40. Collier G, O'Dea K. The effect of coingestion of fat on the glucose, insulin, and gastric inhibitory polypeptide responses to carbohydrate and protein. *Am J Clin Nutr*. 1983;37:941–944.

41. Crane MG, Sample C. Regression of diabetic neuropathy on total vegetarian (vegan) diet. *J Nutr Med*. 1995;4:431–439.

Exchange Lists for Meal Planning

STARCHY FOODS

A starch exchange provides approximately 15 g of carbohydrate, 3 g of protein, a trace of fat, and 80 calories.

Breads

½ bagel
½ hamburger bun
½ English muffin
½ 6-inch pita

1 6-inch chapati (Indian bread)
1 6-inch poori (Indian bread)
1 dinner roll
1 slice whole grain bread
1 6-inch corn or flour tortilla

Cereals/Grains

⅓ cup bran cereal
½ cup bran, corn, or other flakes
½ cup shredded wheat
1 shredded wheat biscuit
3 tbsps Grapenuts
1½ cups puffed rice or wheat
½ cup cooked cereal (oatmeal, 7-grain, oat
    bran, bear mush, farina, Wheatena, etc)
½ cup cooked grits
⅓ cup cooked rice (white or brown)
½ cup cooked bulgur

⅓ cup cooked couscous
⅓ cup cooked millet
⅓ cup cooked quinoa
½ cup cooked pasta
¾ cup mung bean (cellophane) noodles
⅓ cup polenta
⅓ cup cooked wheat berries
3 cups air-popped popcorn
3 tbsp wheat germ
5 tbsp bran

Starchy Vegetables

½ cup corn
1 6-inch corn on the cob
½ cup lima beans
⅔ cup parsnips
½ cup green peas
½ cup plantain
1 3-oz potato
½ cup mashed potatoes
1 cup winter squash
⅓ cup sweet potatoes or yams
¼ cup chestnuts

Dried Beans

½ cup vegetarian baked beans, cooked
   beans, peas, or lentils*
3 tbsp miso

Crackers/Cookies

4 Rye Krisps
3 graham crackers
5 oblong melba toasts
2 rice cakes
¾-oz matzo
8 animal crackers
2 thin bread sticks
2 Fig Newtons
3 ginger snaps
2 oatmeal cookies
6 vanilla wafers

Other†

¼ cup bread dressing
1 2½-inch biscuit
1 2-inch square corn bread
¼ cup granola
1 4-inch pancake
2 4-inch crisp taco shells
½ cup chow mein noodles

*Count as 1 exchange of starch plus 1 exchange of protein.
†Count each as 1 exchange of starch plus 1 exchange of fat.

VEGETABLES

An exchange provides approximately 5 g of carbohydrate, 2 g of protein, no fat, and 25 calories. One exchange of vegetables is equal to ½ cup of cooked or 1 cup of raw vegetables (any of the following). Note that starchy vegetables such as potatoes and winter squash are included on the starchy foods exchange list.

Alfalfa sprouts	Eggplant	Radicchio
Artichoke	Greens (kale, collards,	Rutabaga
Asparagus	mustard, turnip greens,	Sauerkraut
Bamboo shoots	beet, Swiss chard)	Sea vegetables
Beans (green, wax,	Jicama	Spinach
Italian)	Kohlrabi	Summer squash and
Beets	Leeks	zucchini
Bok choy	Mushrooms	Tomatoes
Brussels sprouts	Okra	Tomato or vegetable
Cabbage	Onions	juice
Carrots	Pea pods	Turnips
Cauliflower	Pepper	Water chestnuts

FRUITS AND JUICES

One exchange of fruit provides approximately 15 g of carbohydrate, no protein or fat, and about 60 calories.

Fresh Fruits

1 apple
½ cup unsweetened applesauce
4 apricots
½ banana
¾ cup blackberries
¾ cup blueberries
1 cup cantaloupe chunks
12 cherries
½ grapefruit
15 grapes
⅛ honeydew melon or 1 cup honeydew cubes
1 kiwifruit

½ mango
1 nectarine
1 orange
1 cup papaya or ½ papaya
1 peach
1 pear
¾ cup pineapple
2 plums
1 cup raspberries
1¼ cup strawberries
2 tangerines
1¼ cup watermelon cubes

Dried Fruits

7 apricot halves
2½ dates
1½ figs
3 prunes
2 tbsp raisins

Juices

½ cup apple juice or cider
⅓ cup cranberry juice cocktail
⅓ cup grape juice
½ cup grapefruit juice
½ cup orange juice
½ cup pineapple juice
⅓ cup prune juice

PROTEIN FOODS

One protein exchange provides 7 g of protein and 3 g of fat.

½ cup tofu
1 tofu hot dog
¼ cup tempeh
1 oz seitan
¼ cup roasted soynuts
¼ cup prepared textured soy protein
2 tbsp Parmesan cheese
3 egg whites
1 whole egg
¼ cup egg substitute

Count as 1 protein exchange plus 1 starch exchange:

½ cup cooked dried beans

Count as 1 protein exchange plus 1 fat exchange:

1 oz soy cheese
1 oz dairy cheese
1 veggieburger

Count as 1 protein exchange plus 2 fat exchanges:

2 tbsp peanut butter, tahini, almond butter, or other nut or seed butter
2 tbsp nuts
1 tbsp seeds

MILKS

One milk exchange provides approximately 12 g of carbohydrate, 8 g of protein, between 0 and 2 g of fat, and about 90 calories.

1 cup "light" soymilk
1 cup Vegelicious
1 cup Rice Dream
1 cup skimmed cow's milk
1 cup buttermilk
½ cup skimmed milk cottage cheese
¾ cup nonfat plain yogurt

Count as 1 milk exchange plus 1 fat exchange:

1 cup 2% cow's milk

Count as 1 milk exchange plus 2 fat exchanges:

1 cup whole cow's milk

Count as 1 milk exchange plus 1 fat exchange:

1 cup regular soymilk

Count as 1 milk exchange plus 1 fruit exchange:

¾ cup fruit-flavored, nonfat yogurt

FATS

One fat exchange provides approximately 5 g of fat and about 45 calories.

⅛ avocado
1 tsp mayonnaise
1 tbsp reduced-calorie mayonnaise
1½ tbsp tofu mayonnaise (Nayonnaise)
1 tsp vegetable oil
10 small or 5 large olives
2 tsp mayonnaise type salad dressing
2 tbsp low-fat salad dressing
1 tsp margarine

1 tsp butter
1 tbsp reduced-calorie margarine
1 tbsp cream cheese
1 tbsp tofu cream cheese
2 tbsp sour cream
2 tbsp shredded coconut
1 tbsp coconut cream
1 tbsp coconut milk

CHAPTER **15**

Vegetarian Diets for Athletes

The benefits of exercise have been expounded for centuries. The earliest records of organized exercise as a formal means of health promotion are from the ancient Chinese, written in approximately 2500 BC. Hua To, a legend in Chinese surgery, encouraged exercises modeled on the movements of animals, principally the tiger. These formed the basis for the Chinese martial art Kung Fu.[1] Hippocrates also promoted the benefits of exercise and is quoted as saying "To keep well, avoid too much food, too little toil."[2]

Despite recommendations by health professionals, however, knowledge of the importance of exercise has had little impact on the behavior of many Americans. On the whole, most Americans lead sedentary lives; in fact, daily energy expenditure has decreased by 200 kcal since 1965.[3] Reportedly, less than 20% of adults and 37% of adolescents in the United States exercise regularly.[4]

According to some research, vegetarians exercise more than their non-vegetarian counterparts.[5] Also, Seventh-day Adventist men exercise more than non-Adventists.[6] Most of the data do not support these findings, however, and it seems that vegetarians are not more likely to be physically active than nonvegetarians.[7–10]

Vegetarian or nearly vegetarian diets are a popular choice with some elite athletes (Exhibit 15–1). A recent report found that most top triathletes were on high-carbohydrate, nearly vegetarian diets and that these diets were viewed by athletes as most supportive of vigorous training schedules.[11] Similarly, results of a recent survey of female runners who had competed nationally revealed that 40% did not eat red meat for health reasons.[12] According to Whorton,[13] a number of prominent athletes consumed vegetarian diets even a century ago:

Exhibit 15–1 Well-Known Vegetarian Athletes

Surya Bonaly, French Olympic figure skater
Andreas Cahling, champion body builder
Chris Campbell, Olympic medalist in wrestling
Desmond Howard, Heisman trophy winner and professional football player
Billy Jean King, tennis champion
Bill Manetti, powerlifting champion
Martina Navratilova, tennis champion
Paavo Nurmi, long distance runner with 20 world records
Bill Pearl, four time Mr. Universe
Dave Scott, six-time Ironman winner

- Will Brown, who switched to a vegetarian diet for health reasons, went on to thrash all records for the 3,218-km bicycle race in the 1890s.
- Vegetarian cyclist Margarita Gast established a women's record for the 1,606-km race near the turn of the century.
- In the 1893 walking race from Berlin to Vienna, the first two competitors to cover the 599-km course were vegetarians.
- Near the turn of the century, 11 of 14 finishers of the 100-km race in Germany were vegetarian.
- In 1912, a vegetarian was the first man to complete a marathon in less than 2 hours and 30 minutes.

VEGETARIAN DIETS AND ATHLETIC PERFORMANCE

A few early investigations of vegetarian diet and athletic performance have been published. One was a Yale study, published in 1906, that involved vegetarian and nonvegetarian athletes and a group of health professionals employed by the Battle Creek Sanitarium. Three simple tests were used to measure endurance: holding the arms horizontally as long as possible, deep knee bending, and leg raising with the subject lying on his back.[14] Omnivore athletes were able to hold their arms for only half as long as the vegetarian athletes. Only 3 of 9 "flesh eaters" did 325 or more knee bends compared with 17 of 21 vegetarians. In fact, in one test, even the sedentary vegetarian health professionals greatly outperformed nonvegetarian athletes. In 1907, another Yale study found that over a 5-month period, when athletes switched from an omnivore diet to a mainly lacto-ovo vegetarian one, their strength increased and their fatigue decreased.[15]

More recent studies, however, show little difference between vegetarian and nonvegetarian athletes. An Israeli study published in 1986 used a battery of tests to compare vegetarian (31 lacto-ovo vegetarians, 13 lacto vegetarians, and 5 vegans) with nonvegetarian athletes matched for age, sex, body size, and type of athletic activity. No significant differences were found between groups for a variety of physical fitness, anthropometric, and metabolic variables, including aerobic and anaerobic capacity, hand grip and back strength, hemoglobin, total serum protein, and pulmonary function.[16]

These results agree with those of Raben et al,[17] who found that in male endurance athletes no significant differences in physical performance existed when subjects were fed either a lacto-ovo vegetarian diet or a mixed diet containing meat for 6 weeks. Of course, the short duration of this study may have prevented any potential dietary effects on athletic performances from manifesting.

Two studies have examined the effects of vegetarian diet on physical fitness and physiologic factors that underlie the capacity for exercise not in athletes but in sedentary individuals. In one study, subjects included 23 individuals who had consumed a vegan diet supplemented with vitamin B_{12} for between 3 and 23 years (average 11.9 years), 66 omnivore homemakers with a similar social background as the vegans, and 20 omnivore office workers with a comparable level of customary activity.[18] Essentially, no differences were noted in any of the parameters examined, which included forced expiratory volume, forced vital capacity, cycle ergometer, and measures of muscle and skinfold thickness. Similarly, Nieman et al[7] found no differences between elderly vegetarian and nonvegetarian women in a variety of metabolic and electrocardiographic parameters during graded maximal treadmill testing except for a lower resting heart rate in the vegetarians.[7] The vegetarians did, however, have lower low-density lipoprotein cholesterol and a lower BMI.

Immune function may be a particularly important consideration related to physical activity because athletes in heavy training may be more susceptible to infections than sedentary individuals.[19] In a short-term study (6 weeks), immune function in subjects who had consumed a meat-rich diet (69% animal protein sources) was similar to that after consumption of a lacto-ovo vegetarian diet (82% vegetable protein sources).[20] These findings conflict somewhat with the results of a German study that found that, in comparison with omnivore men, vegetarian men had much higher blood levels of natural killer cells, which can destroy tumor cells and viruses.[21] Because low-fat diets have been shown to increase natural killer cell activity,[22] results of these two studies may reflect the different fat content of the diets to some extent. In the short-term study in which natural killer cell activity was no higher among vegetarians, fat intake of both groups was similar. It is also possible that subjects need to follow a vegetarian diet for longer than 6 weeks to produce changes in immune function.

Vegetarian diets more closely resemble dietary recommendations for athletes than omnivore diets. There is considerable debate over the nutrient needs of athletes, however. The slight increase in nutrient needs of casual exercisers can be met easily when such individuals increase their food intake to compensate for the increased energy expenditure.

NUTRITION NEEDS OF ATHLETES

The discussion that follows centers on the needs of competitive or elite athletes, including those who engage in endurance training (running, cycling, swimming, race walking, etc.) at least 1 hour or more five times per week or who are following rigorous strength-training programs.

Protein

The emphasis on protein for athletic performance has a long history, culminating in the traditional steak dinner that was until recently the standard pregame meal of competitive athletes. For example, ancient Greek athletes were heavy meat eaters.[23] The preeminent 19th century physiologic chemist von Liebig proposed that the energy for all muscular movement was produced by the oxidation of protein.[24] The customary diets of heavy laborers and athletes were found to be high in protein, and this was accepted by nutritionists as a physical necessity. The biochemist Atwater found that crew members of the Yale and Harvard rowing teams consumed 150 to 170 g of protein per day, two thirds of which was from animal sources.[25] By the 1860s, scientists knew that the major fuels for exercising muscle were fatty acids and carbohydrates. Today, it is recognized that protein supplies only 5% to 15% of the fuel or energy used during endurance training.[26,27]

Nevertheless, protein was favored well into the 20th century. Many athletes still consume high-protein diets in an effort to increase muscle mass. Two recent surveys found that athletes (football players and triathletes) consume more protein than the typical nonathlete and about 2.5 times more than the recommended dietary allowance (RDA) for protein,[28,29] although there is a wide variation in intake among athletes.[30]

In setting the RDA for protein, the National Research Council does not make an allowance for work or training.[31] It is believed that the margin of safety included in the protein RDA precludes any need to recommend increased protein intake for athletes. This conflicts with more recent research and with the position of the American and Canadian Dietetic Associations, which recommend that athletes consume 1.5 g of protein per kilogram body weight, essentially twice the RDA of 0.8 g/kg.[32] The higher value is thought to be the amount of protein that allows for maximum protein deposition provided that energy intake is adequate.[33-35]

In both endurance and strength athletes, the theoretical basis for the increased need for dietary protein results from an increase in the oxidation (catabolism) of amino acids, which occurs as muscles are being exercised. Increased protein needs for actual lean tissue deposition are small because muscles are three-quarters water. On the basis of only increased muscle mass, adding half a pound (227 g, only 56 g of which is protein) of lean tissue per week (an amount unlikely to be achieved by most individuals) would require an additional 8 g of protein per day assuming 100% efficiency of protein utilization.

Not all experts agree with the positions of the American and Canadian Dietetic Associations, however. For example, in a review on this subject, Millward and colleagues,[36] from the Nutritional Metabolism Research Group at the University of Surrey in England, concluded that there were insufficient data to justify recommendations for athletes to increase protein intake. Young,[37] from the Massachusetts Institute of Technology, suggests that between 1.0 and 1.5 g of protein per body weight is needed to support the needs of all athletes. Other estimates, however, are even higher than those stated in the positions of the Canadian Dietetic Association and the American Dietetic Association.[38]

Energy intake is a crucial factor in meeting the protein needs of athletes. It is also important for athletes to maintain adequate glycogen stores because, when exercising for long periods of time (such as an hour), athletes with low glycogen stores metabolize twice as much protein as those with high stores primarily because protein will be used for gluconeogenesis.[39]

Vegetarians can easily meet the increased protein needs of endurance exercise even if those needs are twice the RDA. A 175-lb (80-kg) male lacto-ovo vegetarian athlete has a dietary protein requirement of 120 g/day assuming a requirement of 1.5 g/kg. This 80-kg man would consume approximately 3,700 kcal/day (2,900 kcal/day to meet normal, nonexercising needs and an additional 800 kcal/day for exercise). Assuming that this subject consumes a 12.5% protein diet (on a caloric basis), his protein intake would be 116 g/day, which is nearly equal to his protein needs. Because vegan diets are generally lower in protein (about 11%), the same athlete consuming a vegan diet might ingest only 102 g of protein, somewhat less than requirements. Therefore, vegan athletes would need to give some attention to consuming high-protein foods, such as soy products or other legumes (see Chapter 3 for a discussion of protein needs and vegetarian diets).

Meeting protein needs may be somewhat more difficult for vegetarian strength athletes, whose calorie, and therefore, protein intake is lower. For example, an 80-kg weight lifter who consumes 3,500 kcal/day would consume 109 g of protein on a lacto-ovo vegetarian diet and 96 g on a vegan diet. For these athletes, some dietary adjustment to include more protein-rich foods, such as legumes and soy products, might be advised. Elite weight lifters, however, for whom the increased protein requirements are primarily intended, often train for more than 1 hour per day, so that their caloric expenditure and protein intake may be much greater than presented here, and therefore less adjustment would be required. Exhibit 15–2 illustrates a sample menu plan that can meet the needs of a vegan strength athlete.

Protein increases urinary calcium excretion.[40-44] Athletes consuming twice the RDA for protein could theoretically be at increased risk for osteoporosis. Exercise strongly promotes bone health; consequently, the overall effect of increased exercise and the protein needed to support it is still likely to be beneficial. Calcium loss may be a problem in female athletes who are amenorrheic. However, these women produce less estrogen, which will have an adverse effect on bone health. For amenorrheic female athletes, and perhaps also to some extent for male athletes, limiting protein-induced calcium excretion may be important.

As discussed in Chapter 3, legume proteins (because of their lower sulfur amino acid content), are thought to cause less urinary calcium excretion in comparison with animal protein.[45,46] Plant-based diets overall may also cause

Exhibit 15–2 Sample Menu for Vegan Weight Lifter (3,450 kcal, 14% Protein, 16% Fat, 70% Carbohydrate)

Breakfast	Lunch	Dinner	Snacks throughout the Day
½ cup bran flakes, 1 cup soymilk, 1 banana, 3 slices toast with 3 tsp margarine	2 tofu salad sandwiches, one apple, carrot sticks, tossed salad with 2 tbsp dressing, two oatmeal cookies, 1 cup soymilk	3 cups pasta, 1 cup spaghetti sauce with ½ cup textured vegetable protein, ½ cup steamed broccoli, one roll with 1 tsp margarine, 1½ cups rice pudding made with soymilk	½ cup orange juice, one pear, five gingersnap cookies, bagel with 2 tbsp almond butter, ½ cup soynuts, one low-fat bran muffin

less calcium excretion. Therefore, vegetarian athletes who increase their intake of protein by consuming more soy and bean products will probably
have an advantage over those who increase their protein intake by consuming more flesh foods. It is therefore prudent to suggest that even
nonvegetarian female athletes consume more plant sources of protein.

Excessive protein intake can also raise the risk for kidney stones. In a
large prospective study involving 45,000 men aged 40 to 75 years, Curhan et
al[47] found that animal protein intake (≥77 g/d vs ≤50 g/d) increased risk of
kidney stones by 30%. The kidney itself may also be adversely affected by
high protein intakes. High-protein diets may increase kidney disease risk,
particularly in susceptible individuals.[48] Some work suggests that soy protein, and perhaps plant protein in general, may have advantages over animal
protein in this regard.[49] Consequently, there are several reasons for both
vegetarian and nonvegetarian athletes to meet increased protein needs by
consuming more protein-rich plant foods.

Iron

The iron needs of athletes have been the subject of much discussion. Iron is
essential in the transport and delivery of oxygen to the mitochondria of the
working cell through the proteins hemoglobin and myoglobin. Athletes are
well aware of the key role of hemoglobin. Blood doping has been a common
practice among athletes.[50] About 2 months before competition, the athlete has
2 U (2 pints) of blood withdrawn. The red cells are separated from the plasma
and stored, and about 1 week before competition they are added back to the
donor athlete. Through this increase in the number of red blood cells, more
oxygen is available to be used for energy production. Blood doping is effective, but it was also banned by the International Olympic Committee.[51,52]

Iron deficiency anemia can adversely affect physical performance, particularly aerobic performance.[53] The number of athletes with true anemia is
around 10%, although the percentage is believed to be higher among endurance athletes.[54,55] Also, in general, both male and female athletes have lower
hemoglobin levels and poorer iron status than the sedentary population.[56,57]
Nevertheless, it is still not clear to what extent, if any, these generally lower
levels among athletes affect performance,[58] although some evidence does
indicate that the poor iron status of athletes, even in the absence of anemia,
can impair performance.[56,59] Studies have shown that long-distance runners
consuming vegetarian or semivegetarian diets have lower iron stores than
runners consuming an omnivore diet.[60,61]

The lower hemoglobin level of athletes has been referred to as sports
anemia. This is somewhat of a misnomer in that the lower hemoglobin

levels are due to an exercise-induced increase in blood volume that dilutes the concentration of red blood cells. This has led some investigators to suggest, perhaps erroneously, that iron intakes of athletes should be increased.[53] Also, increased perspiration increases iron loss somewhat. For example, one study found that when subjects were placed in a dry sauna until body temperatures reached the same temperature that endurance athletes experience during training on a medium sunny day, they lost 1.3 L of sweat per hour containing about 0.5 mg of iron.[62] Not all studies support this finding, but because iron is poorly absorbed any increased loss could increase dietary iron needs significantly.

There is also a phenomenon called footstrike hemolysis, which refers to an increased destruction of red blood cells (hemodialysis). This was initially thought to be due entirely to the force created by exercises such as running, but even swimmers have been shown to experience this effect.[63-65] There may be other factors associated with physical activity that increase iron loss as well, such as increased gastrointestinal blood loss.[66-68]

In the absence of research indicating that routine iron supplementation improves athletic performance, supplementation is not advised. High levels of stored iron have been associated with increased risk for heart disease and cancer.[69,70] Clearly, if anemia is present, then iron supplements or dietary modifications are needed. It is recommended that all athletes, but particularly vegetarian athletes because of their lower iron stores, have their iron status monitored. One of the most important factors determining iron status of athletes is the adequacy of iron reserves.[53] Measures of iron status should include hemoglobin, hematocrit, and serum ferritin levels. Female athletes are at an even greater risk for iron deficiency than males as a result of blood loss from menstruation.

Carbohydrate

The energy source for exercising muscle is determined by the duration and intensity of exercise and the fitness level of the athlete. The ability to exercise at high intensity is related to the preexercise level of muscle glycogen. Muscle glycogen is used specifically for the purpose of supplying a quick source of energy for the muscle because the glucose derived from glycogen cannot be released into the bloodstream for use by peripheral tissues.

Exercise of high intensity and short duration (70% or more of aerobic capacity, such as sprinting) relies primarly on anaerobic glycolysis for the production of energy. Although this is often said to be due to oxygen insufficiency, more current thinking suggests this is not the cause. Consequently, only glucose derived primarily from the breakdown of muscle glycogen can be used as fuel. When metabolized anaerobically, muscle glycogen provides energy at a rate that is almost 20 times faster than when glucose is metabolized aerobically.

Exercise of low to moderate intensity (up to 60% of aerobic capacity) can be fueled almost entirely through aerobic metabolism. Hormonal changes that occur with exercise promote the release of fatty acids from adipose tissue into the bloodstream, where they can be delivered to muscle tissue and used for energy. Also, training, particularly endurance training, promotes storage of fat within muscle that serves as a more immediate source of fuel. About half the energy for low- to moderate-intensity exercise comes from fat, and about half comes from glycogen and blood glucose. A small percentage is supplied by protein. Fat cannot sustain metabolic rates during exercise much above 50% of $\dot{V}_{O_2}$ max.[71] As the duration of an exercise increases, and consequently as the intensity decreases, the percentage of energy derived from fat increases to as high as 70%.[72,73]

Recommendations are for athletes to consume between 60% and 70% of their calories in the form of carbohydrate. The upper range is intended for those athletes who train to exhaustion on successive days or who compete in prolonged endurance events.[32] It may be that, regardless of total energy intake, the consumption of between 500 and 800 g of carbohydrate (2,000 to 3,200 calories) is necessary for maximizing glycogen stores for greater endurance.[74,75] Muscle exhaustion during prolonged, hard exercise is tied to low muscle glycogen levels as is fatigue during repeated bouts of high intensity exercise such as sprints.[76]

Glycogen stores in athletes can be twice as high as in sedentary individuals.[77] After a strenuous workout, when glycogen stores are depleted, a high carbohydrate diet will replete these stores, whereas a low-carbohydrate, high-fat diet will not.[75,78] The carbohydrate intake of typical nonvegetarian athletes (around 50%) is generally too low for optimal athletic performance.[30] In fact, many omnivore athletes are unwilling to eat the recommended level of carbohydrate, perhaps because of concerns about including enough protein in their diet.[79] Vegetarians, particularly vegans, consume more of their calories in the form of carbohydrate, and thus their diet is actually better suited for maximizing glycogen stores.

Calories

Individuals engaged in different physical training programs have varied but increased energy needs, ranging from 2,000 to 6,000 kcal/day or more. The caloric density of vegetarian diets, particularly of vegan diets, tends to be low because of their low fat and high fiber content. Tactics for increasing calorie intake include eating more frequent meals, eating planned snacks, using some refined carbohydrates and adding concentrated sources of energy such as dried fruit, avocados, nuts, and seeds. Exhibit 15–3 illustrates an example of a vegan diet that provides 5,500 calories.

Water

Muscular activity produces heat, which is partially dissipated through the production of sweat. Dehydration not only adversely affects both endurance and strength performance but, if prolonged, can have serious consequences, such as heat exhaustion and life-threatening heat stroke.[79,80] Also, every unit of stored glycogen carries with it three units of water, thus adding to the need for adequate hydration. Furthermore, increased protein intake requires additional water for proper excretion of urea.

Some individuals lose up to 8 lb of sweat per hour during strenuous activity. For every pound lost, 16 oz of water should be consumed. One note of caution: Vigorous exercise can delay the thirst mechanism, so that it is important not to rely on thirst alone as the indicator of fluid status. Athletes, especially those in hot climates, should consume water at regular intervals.

Other Nutrients

Several extensive reviews have been written on the micronutrient needs of athletes.[81,82] The following is a brief discussion of those needs.

Exhibit 15–3 Sample Menu for Vegan Diet Providing 5,500 kcal (13% Protein, 17% Fat, 70% Carbohydrate)

Breakfast	Lunch	Dinner	Snacks throughout the Day
2 cups oatmeal, 1 cup soymilk, four slices toast, 4 tsp margarine, one banana	Two hummus sandwiches, 1½ cups potato salad, tossed salad with 2 tbsp dressing, carrot sticks, one apple, four oatmeal cookies	1 cup black beans, 3 cups rice, two rolls with 2 tsp margarine, 1 cup corn, 1 cup broccoli, ½ cup strawberries	Two bagels with fruit spread, ½ cup bean soup, pasta salad (2 cups pasta with 1 cup steamed vegetables), four slices bread, one orange, one peach, carrot sticks

Thiamin (Vitamin B₁)

Thiamin is used in the metabolism of all three macronutrients: fat, carbohydrate, and protein. The main effects of thiamin deficiency, however, are disturbances in carbohydrate metabolism. Increased carbohydrate intake and exercise can increase thiamin needs. The RDAs of 1.5 and 1.1 mg for adult men and women, respectively, are based on the assumption that thiamin requirements are 0.5 mg per 1,000 kcal. As long as reasonable food choices are made, the increased caloric intake required to compensate for the increased energy expenditure in athletes will be adequate to meet thiamin needs. Because thiamin is widely available in grains and other plant foods, vegetarians should have no difficulty meeting needs.

Riboflavin (Vitamin B₂)

Riboflavin also plays a role in energy production. Consequently, the RDAs of 1.7 and 1.3 mg for adult men and women, respectively, are based on a requirement of 0.6 mg of riboflavin per 1,000 kcal. Although the National Research Council states that the current RDA is adequate for athletes, several studies have shown that riboflavin needs are directly increased as a result of exercise.[83,84] If athletes do need slightly more riboflavin than sedentary individuals, their increased energy intake should be enough to provide this amount on both vegetarian and omnivore diets.

Niacin

Niacin, as part of the coenzyme nicotinamide adenine dinucleotide (NAD), is used to produce adenosine triphosphate (ATP) from the glycolysis of glucose (anaerobic metabolism). There is, however, little or no evidence to suggest that niacin supplementation will increase athletic performance. Also, the amino acid tryptophan is converted into niacin. On average, plant proteins contain about 1% tryptophan, so that an increased intake of 50 or 60 g of protein by athletes is equivalent to about 50 to 60 mg of tryptophan or 8 to 10 niacin equivalents, which is about 50% of the US RDA.[85] Similarly, the extra food consumed to meet caloric needs will also directly provide some niacin.

Pyridoxine (Vitamin B₆)

Pyridoxine functions as a coenzyme for as many as 60 enzymes that help regulate nitrogen metabolism; it is also involved in hemoglobin and myoglobin formation. Vitamin B₆ requirements increase with increased protein consumption.[86,87] Because the RDAs of 2.0 and 1.6 mg for adult men and women, respectively, are based on a protein intake that is twice the RDA, it should cover the needs of athletes with elevated protein requirements, although this does not allow for any margin of safety. Vitamin B6 is normally found in plentiful amounts in high-protein foods, so that its intake generally increases as protein intake increases. Research indicates that supplementation of vitamin B6 does not enhance athletic performance.[88] Also, plant foods tend to have a better ratio of protein to vitamin B6 than animal foods, thus vegetarian athletes will not have problems meeting requirements.

Cyanocobalamin (Vitamin B12)

Because red blood cells may be destroyed at a faster rate in athletes and vitamin B12 is needed for their synthesis, it is often thought that vitamin B12 needs are increased with vigorous exercise. Injections of vitamin B12 are sometimes used by athletes because of the belief that oxygen delivery will be increased and thus endurance enhanced.[88] Studies have failed to demonstrate any beneficial effects of vitamin B12 supplementation on athletic performance in the absence of outright vitamin B12 deficiency, however.[89,90] Nevertheless, vegan athletes, just as vegan sedentary individuals, need to take vitamin B12 supplements and/or B12 fortified foods.

Pantothenic Acid, Folate, and Biotin

Relatively little work has been conducted on these vitamins in relation to physical performance. Pantothenic acid is widely distributed among plant foods, so that adequate intake is easily achieved. It is involved in the metabolism of fatty acids for energy, and some work suggests a possible relationship between pantothenic acid and exercise, but no firm conclusions can be drawn at this time. Folate is involved in DNA synthesis and red blood cell production, and at least one study has shown that folate needs are increased with an increased production of red blood cells.[91] Consequently, because in athletes red blood cells may be destroyed at a faster rate than in sedentary people, folate needs of athletes may be increased somewhat. Also, iron status and folate are related; low iron status can impair folate utilization, and visa versa.[92] Vegetarians consume substantially more folate than nonvegetarians. Finally, biotin is involved in gluconeogenesis and theoretically could be involved in athletic endurance, but this hypothesis has not been studied.

Vitamin C

Vitamin C is a potent antioxidant. Vitamin C supplementation is popular among athletes,[93] and one study reported that work conducted under high temperatures (in this study, mine workers were examined) increased vitamin C needs significantly.[94] Thus athletes exercising in hot climates may also need more vitamin C. Inadequate vitamin C intakes have been shown to have an adverse effect on the working capacity of athletes,[95] but vitamin C supplementation in athletes with adequate vitamin C intake has not improved athletic performance.[96] Vegetarians consume about 50% more vitamin C than nonvegetarians.

Vitamin E

It has been theorized that vitamin E supplementation may help keep red blood cells intact during exercise by preventing oxidation of cell membrane phospholipids. Vitamin E deficiency increases red blood cell destruction because it leaves red blood cells more fragile and more easily damaged.[97] A recent study of athletes found that running on a treadmill decreased tissue levels of vitamin E by 30%, and when subjects exercised at high altitudes (above 5,000 ft) vitamin E supplementation in excess of the RDA improved performance.[98] Supplementation in athletes with adequate stores of vitamin E has not been found to improve performance, however.[99] Vegetarian vitamin E intake is higher than omnivorous intake.

Zinc

Several reports have indicated that strenuous exercise and increased perspiration increase zinc requirements and that many athletes ingest inadequate amounts of zinc.[100,101] For example, one survey of competitive triathletes found that 60% had zinc intakes below the RDA.[102] Some endurance athletes have low resting blood levels of zinc, whereas others have normal levels. Zinc red blood cell levels have been found to be unrelated to $\dot{V}_{O_2}$ max, however. Also, there are few (if any) data suggesting that zinc supplementation in healthy individuals improves performance.

Creatine

Most of the creatine in the body is found in skeletal muscle where it exists both as free creatine and as creatine phosphate. Creatine phosphate serves as a storage form of energy, ATP is produced during the conversion of creatine phosphate to creatine. Creatine is synthesized extramuscularly in a two-step process involving the kidey and liver, but dietary intake can lead to an increase in the body pool of creatine, including the amount in skeletal muscle. For this reason, some athletes consider increasing creatine intake.

Creatine is found primarily in meats; consequently, creatine intake by vegetarians is extremely low. One study reported that serum levels of creatine were about 40% lower in both male and female vegetarians compared with the general population.[103] Also, the authors of this study estimated that both the body creatine content and the endogenous synthesis rate of creatine by vegetarians was lower than the general population. Whether the lower creatine levels of vegetarians affect athletic performance is yet to be determined. Vegetarian athletes, however, need not consume meat to increase their intake of creatine, since creatine supplements are available.

RISK OF AMENORRHEA IN FEMALE VEGETARIANS AND FEMALE VEGETARIAN ATHLETES

Exercise promotes the acquisition of bone and may compensate for relatively low intakes of calcium. A substantial number of women athletes undergoing intense training stop menstruating, however.[104] This type of menstrual abnormality is due to hypothalamic dysfunction and results in low circulating levels of estrogen.[105] Because estrogen promotes bone health, the withdrawal of estrogen at any age increases bone loss.[106] It was previously thought that exercise would completely compensate for the negative effects of amenorrhea on bone health.[107] It has now been clearly established, however, that athletes with amenorrhea have deficits in vertebral bone mass as well as in other regions, including appendicular weightbearing bones, compared with eumenorrheic athletes or sedentary controls.[108–113]

Amenorrhea may have adverse consequences in teenage girls in particular because this is the period during which bone development reaches a peak. According to one report, young women who have missed 50% of their menstrual periods are likely to reach the age of 20 with reduced peak bone mass, putting them at greater risk for the development of osteoporosis.[114] This may have particular relevance for vegetarians.

Vegetarians have been reported to have lower blood levels of estrogen and higher levels of sex hormone–binding globulin, which would effectively lower the amount of biologically active estrogen in the circulation.[115–119] Also, prolactin levels are lower in vegetarians, which may also affect the menstrual cycle.[120] These effects may be due to the high fiber and low fat intake of vegetarians.[120–123] Menstrual cycle disturbances have been observed in both sedentary and active vegetarian women.

Researchers at the College of Obstetrics and Gynecology, College of Medicine, Pennsylvania State University studied diet and menstrual cycle and found that only 4.9% of nonvegetarian women experienced menstrual irregularities (3 to 10 menses per year), whereas about five times that many vegetarians (26.5%) experienced irregularities.[124] Regularity was associated with protein and cholesterol consumption, irregularity with fiber consumption. Consistent with these findings are results showing that seven of nine healthy women who adopted a vegetarian diet became anovulatory, whereas none of the nonvegetarian women experienced any irregularities.[120] The results of this study should be viewed cautiously, however, since subjects consumed only about 800 kcal/d and lost approximately 1 kg/week during the length of the study.

In a study of nearly 500 women athletes, it was observed that a high percentage were amenorrheic (runners, 25.7%; swimmers, 12.3%; cyclists, 12.1%) compared with an average of about 2.0% expected for age-matched nonathletes.[125] In a closer look at the data, a comparison between 11 amenorrheic and 15 regularly menstruating runners revealed that 82% (9) of the amenorrheic athletes were vegetarians, whereas only 13% (2) of the nonamenorrheic athletes were vegetarians.[126] Subjects were considered vegetarian if they consumed less than 200 g (7 oz) of meat per week. The only other major dietary difference between the two groups was fat intake. Women with regular menstruation consumed 98 g/day, whereas amenorrhoeic women consumed only 68 g/day. No differences were reported in body fat between the two groups.

Similar findings were reported by researchers at the Melpomene Institute for Women's Health Research in St Paul, Minnesota.[127] Women studied were engaged in physical activity vigorous enough to work up a sweat at least twice a week. Of the 45 vegetarians in the group, 14 (31%) had secondary amenorrhea (less than three menstrual cycles during the previous year), 6 (14%) of the 44 women who described their diet as high in carbohydrate and low in fat were amenorrheic, but only 3 (4%) of the 84 women who consumed a nonvegetarian, more typical Western diet were classified as amenorrheic. Other studies have also reported a higher incidence of amenorrhea or irregular cycles among vegetarian compared with nonvegetarian athletes[12,128] and sedentary individuals.[10] In addition, the adoption of a mixed diet by sedentary amenorrheic women consuming a vegetarian (composed largely of raw foods) or semi-vegetarian diet resulted in ovulation, but this was likely due to a decrease in the high serum carotene levels in the vegetarians, rather than any specific effect of animal products.[129,130]

In contrast to the above data, however, several studies involving both athletes and nonathletes suggest that vegetarianism and amenorrhea are unrelated. For example, although 12 of the 36 cyclists participating in the 1982 Coors Classic bicycle race who were amenorrheic consumed a vegetarian or semivegetarian diet, 20 of the 24 women with regular menstruation also consumed a vegetarian diet or a modified vegetarian diet.[127] Similarly, an Israeli study of athletes found no differences in menstrual cycle patterns between vegetarians and nonvegetarians.[58]

In two studies involving nonathletes, no differences were noted in mean menstrual days per year or menstrual cycle interval between lacto-ovo vegetarian (mean age, 28.9 years) and omnivorous (mean age, 31.0) women[131] and no differences between lacto-ovo vegetarian adolescents (mean age, 16.2 years) and omnivorous adolescents (mean age, 16.7 years) was observed in the percentage of girls with ovulatory cycle.[132] Finally, Barr et al[133] specifically examined the relationship between vegetarianism and menstrual cycle patterns in 23 vegetarians and 22 nonvegetarian sedentary individuals.

Exhibit 15–4 Food Guide for Young Female Athletes (2,000 Calories, 13% Protein, 25% Fat, 62% Carbohydrate, 1,600 mg Calcium)

11 servings grains
1 serving legumes
2 servings nuts/seeds
2 servings green leafy vegetables
2 servings other vegetables
4 servings fruit
3 servings milk (calcium-fortified soymilk, Vegelicious, or 2% cow's milk)
4 servings fat

In this 6-month prospective study, vegetarians actually had a higher proportion of normal ovulatory cycles than nonvegetarians (76.7% versus 61.9%).

Clearly, data on vegetarian diet and menstrual cycle patterns are conflicting. In addition, results are difficult to compare because studies differ significantly in experimental design, including such factors as study duration and subject inclusion criteria. Dietary factors that have been hypothesized to affect menstrual cycle patterns and typically differ between vegetarians and nonvegetarians are fiber, fat, and meat intake.[128,134–136] Some work has suggested that high blood carotene levels may increase the risk of irregular menstrual cycles,[129,130] and, as noted in Chapter 6, vegetarians have higher carotene levels than nonvegetarians. Also, there are phytoestrogens in plant foods (such as isoflavones in soy and lignans in unrefined cereals[137,138]) that may affect menstrual cycle length,[139] although no evidence indicates that the consumption of these substances leads to amenorrhea. The etiology of amenorrhea among athletes is undoubtedly multifactorial; vegetarian diet may be one factor that increases risk, but this has not been clearly established because of the many confounding variables in studies reporting such effects. Diets that include higher levels of fat and high levels of calcium may be advised for female vegetarian athletes. Exhibit 15–4 offers guidelines for menu planning to achieve these goals.

REFERENCES

1. Lyons AS, Petrucelli RJ. *Medicine: An Illustrated History*. New York, NY: Abradale; 1978.
2. Robinson RS. *Sources for the History of Greek Athletes*. Cincinnati, Ohio: RS Robinson; 1955.
3. Grilo CM. Physical activity and obesity. *Biomed Pharmacother*. 1994;48:127–136.

4. Serdula M, Collins ME, Williamson DF, Anda RF, Pamuk ER, Byers TE. Weight control practices in US adolescents and adults: Youth risk behavior survey and behavioral risk facts surveillance system. *Ann Intern Med.* 1993;119:667–671.

5. Slattery ML, Jacobs R Jr, Hilner JE, et al. Meat consumption and its associations with other diet and health factors in young adults: The CARDIA study. *Am J Clin Nutr.* 1991;54:930–935.

6. Fraser GE, Dysinger W, Best C, Chan R. IHD risk factors in middle aged Seventh-Day Adventist men and their neighbors. *Am J Epidemiol.* 1987;126:638–646.

7. Nieman DC, Sherman KM, Arabatzis K, et al. Hematological, anthropometric, and metabolic comparisons between vegetarians and nonvegetarian elderly women. *Int J Sports Med.* 1989;10:243–250.

8. McKenzie J. Profile on vegans. *Plant Foods Hum Nutr.* 1971;2:79–88.

9. Shickle D, Lewis PA, Charny M, Farrow S. Differences in health, knowledge and attitudes between vegetarians and meat eaters in a random population sample. *R Soc Med.* 1989;82:18–20.

10. Lloyd T, Schaeffer JM, Walker MA, Demers LM. Urinary hormonal concentrations and spinal bone densities of premenopausal vegetarian and nonvegetarian women. *Am J Clin Nutr.* 1991;54:1005–1010.

11. Holly RG, Barnard RJ, Rosenthal M, Applegate E, Pritikin E. Triathlete characterization and response to prolonged strenuous competition. *Med Sci Sports Exerc.* 1986;18:123–127.

12. Clark N, Nelson M, Evans W. Nutrition education for elite female runners. *Physician Sportsmed.* 1988;16:274.

13. Whorton JC. *Crusaders for Fitness.* Princeton, NJ: Princton University Press; 1982.

14. Fisher I. The influence of flesh eating on endurance. *Yale Med J.* 1907;8:205–221.

15. Chittenden RH. *The Nutrition of Man.* London, England: Heinemann; 1907.

16. Hanne N, Dlin R, Rostein A. Physical fitness, anthropometric and metabolic parameters in vegetarian athletes. *J Sports Med.* 1986;26:180–185.

17. Raben A, Kiens B, Richter EA, et al. Serum sex hormones and endurance performance after a lacto-ovo vegetarian and mixed diet. *Med Sci Sports Exerc.* 1992;24:1290–1297.

18. Cotes JE, Dabbs JM, Hall AM, et al. Possible effect of a vegan diet upon lung function and the cardiorespiratory response to submaximal exercise in healthy women. *J Physiol.* 1970;209:30P–32P.

19. Fitzgerald L. Exercise and the immune system. *Immunol Today.* 1988;9:337–339.

20. Richter EA, Kiens B, Raben A, Tvede N, Pedersen BK. Immune parameters in male athletes after a lacto-ovo vegetarian diet and a mixed Western diet. *Med Sci Sports Exerc.* 1991;23:517–521.

21. Malter M, Schriever G, Eilber U. Natural killer cells, vitamins, and other blood components of vegetarian and omnivorous men. *Nutr Cancer.* 1989;12:271–278.

22. Barone J, Herbert JR, Reddy MM. Dietary fat and natural-killer-cell activity. *Am J Clin Nutr.* 1989;50:861–867.

23. Ryan AJ. Anabolic steroids are fool's gold. *Fed Proc.* 1981;40:2683–2688.

24. von Liebig J. *Animal Chemistry.* Cambridge, 1842.

25. Atwater WO, Bryant AP. *Dietary Studies of University Boat Crews* (Office of Experimental Stations bulletin 25). Washington, DC: US Department of Agriculture; 1900.

26. Lemon PWR, Nagle FJ. Effects of exercise on protein and amino acid metabolism. *Med Sci Sports Exerc.* 1981;13:141–149.

27. Dohm GL, Williams RT, Kasperek GJ, van Rij AM. Increased excretion of urea and *N*-methylhistidine by rats and humans after a bout of exercise. *J Appl Physiol.* 1982;52:27–33.

28. Short SH, Short WR. Four year study of university athletes' dietary intake. *J Am Diet Assoc.* 1983;82:632–645.

29. Burke LM, Read RSD. Diet patterns of elite Australian male triathletes. *Physician Sportsmed.* 1987;15:140–155.

30. Brotherhood JR. Nutrition and sports performance. *Sports Med.* 1984;1:350–389.

31. National Research Council. *Recommended Dietary Allowances.* 10th ed. Washgton, DC: National Academy Press; 1989.

32. Plomden MS, Benardot D. Position of the American Dietetic Association and the Canadian Dietetic Association for physical fitness and athletic performance. *J Am Diet Assoc.* 1993;93:691–696.

33. Paul GL. Dietary protein requirements for physically active individuals. *Sports Med.* 1987;8:154–176.

34. Butterfield G, Cady C, Moynihan S. Effect of increasing intake on nitrogen balance in recreational weight lifters. *Med Sci Sports Exerc.* 1992;24:S-71. Abstract.

35. Lemon PWR. Protein and exercise: Update 1987. *Med Sci Sports Exerc.* 1987;19:S179–S190.

36. Millward J, Bowtell JL, Pacy P, Rennie MJ. Physical activity, protein metabolism and protein requirements. *Proc Nutr Soc.* 1994;53:223–240.

37. Young VR. Protein and amino acid metabolism in relation to physical exercise. In: Winick M, *Nutrition and Exercise.* New York, NY: Wiley; 1986:9–32.

38. Colgan M. *Optimum Sports Nutrition.* Ronkonkoma, NY: Advanced Research Press; 1993.

39. Lemon PWR, Mullin JP. Effect of initial muscle glycogen levels on protein catabolism during exercise. *J Appl Physiol.* 1980;48:624–629.

40. Anand CR, Linkswiler HM. Effect of protein intake on calcium balance of young men given 500 mg calcium daily. *J Nutr.* 1974;104:695–700.

41. Margen S, Chu J-Y, Kaufman NA, Calloway DH. Studies in calcium metabolism I. The calciuretic effect of dietary protein. *Am J Clin Nutr.* 1974;27:584–589.

42. Linkswiler HM, Zemel MB, Hegsted M, Schuette S. Protein-induced hypercalciuria. *Fed Proc.* 1981;40:2429–2433.

43. Hegsted M, Schuette SA, Zemel MB, Linkswiler HM. Urinary calcium and calcium balance in young men as affected by level of protein and phosphorus intake. *J Nutr.* 1981;111:553–562.

44. Kerstetter JE, Allen LH. Dietary protein increases urinary calcium. *J Nutr.* 1990;120:134–136.

45. Breslau NA, Brinkley L, Hill KD, Pak CYC. Relationship of animal protein–rich diet to kidney stone formation and calcium metabolism. *J Clin Endocrinol Metab.* 1988;66:140–146.

46. Gonick HC, Goldberg G, Mulcare D. Reexamination of the acid-ash content of several diets. *Am J Clin Nutr.* 1968;21:898–903.

47. Curhan GC, Willet WC, Rimm EB, Stampfer MJ. A prospective study of dietary calcium and other nutrients and the risk of symptomatic kidney stones. *N Engl J Med.* 1993;328:833–838.

48. Brenner BM, Meyer TW, Hostetter TH. Dietary protein intake and the progressive nature of kidney disease: The role of hemodynamically mediated glomerular injury in the pathogenesis of progressive glomerular sclerosis in aging, renal ablation, and intrinsic renal disease. *N Engl J Med.* 1982;307:652–659.

49. Kontessis P, Jones S, Dodds R, et al. Renal, metabolic and hormonal responses to ingestion of animal and vegetable proteins. *Kidney Int.* 1990;38:136–144.

50. Higden H. Blood doping among endurance athletes; rationalizations, results, and ramifications. *Am Med News.* September 27, 1985:37.

51. Williams MH, Wesseldine S, Somma T. The effect of induced erythrocythemia upon 5-mile treadmill time. *Med Sci Sports Exerc.* 1981;13:169–175.

52. Brien AJ, Simon TL. The effects of red blood cell infusion on 10 km race time. *JAMA.* 1987;257:2761–2765.

53. Sherman AR, Krammer B. Iron, nutrition and exercise. In: Wolinsky I, Hickson JF, eds. *Nutrition in Exercise and Sport.* Boca Raton, Fla: CRC; 1989:291–300.

54. Clement D, Asmundson R. Nutritional intake and hematological parameters in endurance runners. *Physician Sportsmed.* 1982;10:37–43.

55. Magnusson B, Hallberg L, Rossander L, et al. Iron metabolism and "sports anemia." I. A study of several iron parameters in elite runners with differences in iron status. *Acta Med Scand.* 1984;216:149–155.

56. Pate R. Sports anemia: A review of the current research literature. *Physician Sportsmed.* 1983;11:115–126.

57. Expert Scientific Working Group. Summary of a report on assessment of the iron nutritional status of the United States population. *Am J Clin Nutr.* 1985;42:1318–1330.

58. Magnusson B, Hallberg L, Rossander L, et al. Iron metabolism and "sports anemia." II. A hematological comparison of elite runners and control subjects. *Acta Med Scand.* 1984;216:157–164.

59. Colgan M, Fielder S, Colgan LA. Micronutrient status of endurance athletes affects hematology and performance. *J Appl Nutr.* 1991;43:17–30.

60. Seiler D, Nagel D, Franz H, Hellstern P, Leitzmann C, Jung K. Effects of long-distance running on iron metabolism and hematological parameters. *Int J Sports Med.* 1989;10:357–362.

61. Snyder AC, Dvorak LL, Roepke JB. Influence of dietary iron source on measurement of iron status among female runners. *Med Sci Sports Exerc.* 1989;21:7–10.

62. Vellar OD. Studies on sweat loss of nutrients. *Scand J Clin Lab Invest.* 1968;21:157–167.

63. Williamson MR. Anemia in runners and other athletes. *Physician Sportsmed.* 1981;9:73–78.

64. Ehn L, Carlmark B, Hoglund S. Iron status in athletes involved in intense physical activity. *Med Sci Sports Exerc.* 1980;12:61–70.

65. Siegel A, Hennekens C, Solomon S, et al. Exercise-related hematuria. Findings in a group of marathon runners. *JAMA.* 1979;241:391–392.

66. Fisher RL, McMahon LF Jr, Ryan MJ, et al. Gastrointestinal bleeding in competitive runners. *Dig Dis Sci.* 1986;31:1226.

67. Puhl JL, Runyan WS. Hematological variations during aerobic training of college women. *Res Q Exerc Sport.* 1980;51:533–541.

68. Jenkins RR. Free radical chemistry: Relationship to exercise. *Sports Med.* 1988;5:156–170.

69. Beard JL. Are we at risk for heart disease because of normal iron status? *Nutr Rev.* 1993;51:112–115.

70. Weinberg ED. Roles of iron in neoplasia. *Biol Trace Elem Res.* 1992;34:123–140.

71. Gollnick PD. Metabolism of substances; energy substrate metabolism during exercise and as modified by training. *Fed Proc.* 1985;44:353–357.

72. Astrand PO, Rodahl K. *Textbook of Work Physiology.* New York, NY: McGraw-Hill; 1977.

73. McArdle WD, Katch FL, Katch VL. *Exercise Physiology: Energy, Nutrition and Human Performance.* Philadelphia, Pa: Lea & Febiger; 1981.

74. Zachwieja J. Influence of muscle glycogen depletion of the rate of resynthesis. *Med Sci Sports Exerc.* 1991;23:44–48.

75. Costil DL, Sherman WM, Fink WJ, Maresh C, Witten M, Miller JM. The role of dietary carbohydrate in muscle glycogen resynthesis after strenous running. *Am J Clin Nutr.* 1981;34:1831–1836.

76. Sherman WM, Costill DL. The marathon: Dietary manipulation to optimize performance. *Am J Sports Med.* 1984;12:44–51.

77. Coyle EF, Coggan AR. Effectiveness of carbohydrate feeding in delaying fatigue during prolonged exercise. *Sports Med.* 1984;1:446–458.

78. Costill DL, Miller JM. Nutrition for endurance sports: Carbohydrate and fluid balance. *Int J Sports Med.* 1980;1:2–14.

79. Costill DL. Carbohydrate nutrition before, during, and after exercise. *Fed Proc.* 1985;44:364–368.

80. Aldman V, Karoven M. Weight reduction by sweating in wrestlers and its effects on physical fitness. *J Sports Med Phys Fit.* 1962;7:58.

81. Clarkson PM. Vitamins and trace minerals. In: Lamb DR, Williams R, eds. *Perspectives in Exercise Science and Sports Medicine.* Carmel, Ind: Benchmark; 1991;2.

82. Williams MH. Vitamins, iron and calcium supplementation: Effect on human physical performance. In: Haskell W, Scala J, Whittan J, eds. *Nutrition and Athletic Performance.* Palo Alto, Calif: Bull; 1982.

83. Belko AZ, Meredith MP, Kalwarf HJ, et al. Effects of exercise on riboflavin requirements: Biological validation in weight reducing women. *Am J Clin Nutr.* 1985;41:270–277.

84. Belko AZ, Obarzanek E, Roach R, et al. Effects of aerobic exercise and weight loss on riboflavin requirements of moderately obese, marginally deficient young women. *Am J Clin Nutr.* 1984;40:553–561.

85. Horwitt MK, Harper AE, Henderson LM. Niacin–tryptophan relationships for evaluating niacin equivalents. *Am J Clin Nutr.* 1981;34:423–427.

86. Schultz TD, Leklem JE. Urinary 4-pyridoxic acid, urinary vitamin B_6 and plasma pyridoxal phosphate as measures of vitamin B_6 status and dietary intake of adults. In: Leklem JE, Reynolds RD, eds. *Methods in Vitamin B_6 Nutrition: Analysis and Status Assessment.* New York, NY: Plenum: 297–320.

87. Miller LT, Linkswiler HM. Effect of protein intake on the development of abnormal tryptophan metabolism by men during vitamin B_6 depletion. *J Nutr.* 1967;93:53–59.

88. Williams MH. Vitamin and mineral supplements to athletes: Do they help? *Clin Sports Med.* 1984;3:623–627.

89. Than T-M, May M-W, Khin-Sann-Aung, Mya-Tu M. The effect of vitamin B12 on physical performance capacity. *Br J Nutr.* 1978;40:269–273.

90. Montoye HJ, Spata P, Pinckney V, Barron L. Effects of vitamin B12 supplementation on physical fitness and growth of young boys. *J Appl Physiol.* 1955;7:589–592.

91. Rodriguez MS. A conspectus of research on folacin requirements of man. *J Nutr.* 1981;108:1983–2130.

92. Milne DB, Johnson LK, Mahalko MS, Sandstead HH. Folate status of adult males living in a metabolic unit: Possible relationships with iron nutriture. *Am J Clin Nutr.* 1983;37:768–773.

93. Gerster H. The role of vitamin C in athletic performance. *J Am Coll Nutr.* 1989;8:636–643.

94. Visagie ME, DuPlessies JP, Laubscher NF. Effects of vitamin C supplementation on black mineworkers. *S Afr Med J.* 1975;49:889–892.

95. Buzina R, Sobuticanec K. Vitamin C and physical working capacity in adolescents. *Int J Vitam Nutr Res.* 1985;27(suppl):157–166.

96. Keren G. The effect of high dosage vitamin C intake on aerobic and anaerobic capacity. *J Sports Med Phys Fit.* 1980;20:145–148.

97. Leonard PJ, Losowsky MS. Relationship between plasma vitamin E level and peroxide hemolysis test in human subjects. *Am J Clin Nutr.* 1967;20:795–802.

98. Bowles DK, et al. Effects of acute submaximal exercise on skeletal muscle vitamin E. *Free Radical Res Commun.* 1991;14:139–143.

99. Shephard RJ, Campbell R, Pimm P, Stuart D, Wright GR. Vitamin E, exercise, and the recovery from physical activity. *Eur J Appl Physiol.* 1974;33:119–126.

100. Couzy F, Lafargue P, Guezennec CY. Zinc metabolism in the athlete: Influence of training, nutrition, and other factors. *Int J Sports Med.* 1990;11:263–266.

101. Baer MT, King JC. Tissue zinc levels and zinc excretion during experimental zinc depletion in young men. *Am J Clin Nutr.* 1984;39:556–570.

102. Worme JD. Dietary patterns, gastrointestinal complaints and nutrition knowledge of recreational triathletes. *Am J Clin Nutr.* 1990;51:690–697.

103. Delanghe J, De Slypere J-P, De Buyzere M, et al. Normal reference values for creatine, creatinine, and carnitine are lower in vegetarians. *Clin Chem.* 1989;35:1802–1803.

104. Jones KP, Ravnkar VA, Tulchinsky D, Schiff I. Comparison of bone density in amenorrheic women due to athletics, weight loss, and premature menopause. *Obstet Gynecol.* 1985;66:5–8.

105. Boyden TW. Prolactin responses, menstrual cycles and body composition of women runners. *J Clin Endocrinol Metab.* 1982;54:711–713.

106. Christiannsen C, Christiannsen MS, McNair P, Hagen C, Stocklund E, Transbol I. Prevention of early postmenopausal bone loss: Controlled 2-year study in 315 normal females. *Eur J Clin Invest.* 1980;10:273–279.

107. Lutter JM. Mixed message about osteoporosis in female athletes. *Physician Sportsmed.* 1983;11:154–165.

108. Cann CEM, Martin C, Genant HK, Jaffe R. Decreased spinal mineral content in amenorrheic women. *JAMA.* 1984;251:626–629.

109. Drinkwater BL, Nilson K, Chesnut III CH, Bremner WJ, Shainholtz S, Southworth MB. Bone mineral content of amennorrheic and eumenorrheic athletes. *N Engl J Med.* 1984;311:277–281.

110. Lindberg J, Fears W, Hunt M, Powell M, Boll D, Wade C. Exercise induced amenorrhea and bone density. *Ann Intern Med.* 1984;101:647–648.

111. Marcus R, Cann C, Madvig P, et al. Menstrual function and bone mass in elite women distance runners. Endocrine and metabolic features. *Ann Intern Med.* 1985;102:158–163.

112. Nelson ME, Fisher EC, Catsos PD, Meredith CN, Turksoy RN, Evans WJ. Diet and bone status in amenorrheic runners. *Am J Clin Nutr.* 1986;43:910–916.

113. Myburgh KH, Bachrach LK, Lewis B, Kent K, Marcus R. Low bone mineral density at axial and appendicular sites in amenorrheic athletes. *Med Sci Sports Exerc.* 1993;25:1197–1202.

114. Lloyd T, Myers C, Buchman JR, Demers LM. Collegiate women athletes with irregular menses during adolescence have decreased bone density. *Obstet Gynecol.* 1988;72:639–642.

115. Goldin BR, Adlercreutz H, Gorbach SL, et al. Estrogen excretion patterns and plasma levels in vegetarian and omnivorous women. *N Engl J Med*. 1982;307:1542–1547.

116. Barbosa JC, Shultz TD, Filley SJ, Nieman DC. The relationship among adiposity, diet, and hormone concentrations in vegetarian and nonvegetarian postmenopausal women. *Am J Clin Nutr*. 1990;51:798–803.

117. Musey PI, Collins DC, Bradlow HL, Gould KG, Preedy JRK. Effect of diet on oxidation of 17β-estradiol in vivo. *J Clin Endocrinol Metab*. 1987;65:792–795.

118. Longscope C, Gorbach S, Goldin B, et al. The effect of a low fat diet on estrogen metabolism. *J Clin Endocrinol Metab*. 1987;64:1246–1250.

119. Armstrong BK, Brown JB, Clark HT, et al. Diet and reproductive hormones: A study of vegetarian and nonvegetarian postmenopausal women. *J Natl Cancer Inst*. 1981;67:761–767.

120. Pirke KM, Schweiger U, Laessle R, Dickhaut B, Schweiger M, Waechtler M. Dieting influences the menstrual cycle: Vegetarian versus nonvegetarian diet. *Fertil Steril*. 1986;46:1083–1088.

121. Rose DP, Boyar AP, Cohen C, Strong LE. Effect of a low-fat diet on hormone levels in women with cystic breast disease. I. Serum steroids and gonadotropins. *J Natl Cancer Inst*. 1987;78:623–626.

122. Prentice RL, Thompson D, Clifford C, Gorbach S, Goldin B, Byar D. Dietary fat reduction and plasma estradiol concentration in healthy postmenopausal women. *J Natl Cancer Inst*. 1990;82:129–134.

123. Rose DP, Goldman M, Connolly JM, Strong LE. High-fiber diet reduces serum estrogen concentrations in premenopausal women. *Am J Clin Nutr*. 1991;54:520–525.

124. Pedersen AB, Bartholomew MJ, Dolence LA, Aljadir LP, Netteburg KL, Lloyd T. Menstrual differences due to vegetarian and nonvegetarian diets. *Am J Clin Nutr*. 1991;53:879–885.

125. Sanborn CF, Martin BJ, Wagner WW. Is athletic amenorrhea specific to runners? *Am J Obstet Gynecol*. 1982;143:859–861.

126. Brooks SM, Sanborn CF, Albrecht BH, Wagner WW Jr. Diet in athletic amenorrhoea. *Lancet*. 1984;1:559–560.

127. Slavin J, Lutter J, Cushman S. Amenorrhoea in vegetarian athletes. *Lancet*. 1984;1:1974–1975.

128. Kaiserauer S, Snyder AC, Sleeper M, Zierath J. Nutritional, physiological, and menstrual status of distance runners. *Med Sci Sports Exerc*. 1989;21:120–125.

129. Martin-Du Pan RC, Hermann W, Chardon F. Hypercaratinemia, amenorrhea and vegetarian diet. *J Gynaecol Obstet Biol Reprod*. 1990;19:290–294.

130. Kemmann E, Pasquale SA, Skaf R. Amenorrhea associated with carotenemia. *JAMA*. 1983;249:926–928.

131. Worthington-Roberts BS, Breskin MW, Monsen ER. Iron status of premenopausal women in a university community and its relationship to habitual dietary sources of protein. *Am J Clin Nutr*. 1988;47:275–279.

132. Persky VW, Chatterton RT, Van Horn LV, et al. Hormone levels in vegetarian and nonvegetarian teenage girls: Potential implications for breast cancer risk. *Cancer Res*. 1992;50:578–583.

133. Barr SI, Janelle KC, Prior JC. Vegetarian vs nonvegetarian diets, dietary restraint, and subclinical ovulatory disturbances: Prospective 6-mo study. *Am J Clin Nutr*. 1994;60:887–894.

134. Nelson ME, Fisher EC, Catsos PD, Meredith CN, Turksoy RN, Evans WJ. Diet and bone status in amenorrheic runners. *Am J Clin Nutr*. 1986;43:910–916.

135. Myerson M, Gutin B, Warren MP, et al. Resting metabolic rate and energy balance in amenorrheic and eumenorrheic runners. *Med Sci Sports Exerc.* 1987;19:546–556.

136. Deuster PA, Kyle SB, Moser PB, Vigersky RA, Singh A, Schoomaker EB. Nutritional survey of highly trained women runners. *Am J Clin Nutr.* 1986;44:954–962.

137. Price KR, Fenwick GR. Naturally occurring oestrogens in foods—A review. *Food Addit Contam.* 1985;2:73–106.

138. Folman Y, Pope GS. Effect of norethisterone acetate, dimethylstilbestrol, genistein and coumestrol on uptake of [³H]oestradiol by uterus, vagina, and skeletal muscle of immature mice. *J Endocrinol.* 1969;44:213–218.

139. Cassidy A, Bingham S, Setchell KDR. Biological effects of a diet of soy protein rich in isoflavones on the menstrual cycle of premenopausal women. *Am J Clin Nutr.* 1994;60:333–340.

CHAPTER 16

Vegetarian Food Preparation

Vegetarian diets often include foods that are unfamiliar to many Americans. Clients may have questions about the preparation and use of these products. There are many excellent cookbooks (see Resources section at the end of the book) that can be recommended to vegetarian clients who request recipe suggestions or who wish to hone their cooking skills. In counseling vegetarians, however, it is helpful for the dietitian to have a basic understanding of food preparation. This is especially true for dietitians who offer community presentations on vegetarian diets.

PREPARING GRAINS

The technique for cooking grains is generally the same for most grains, although the amounts of water used and the cooking times vary (Tables 16–1 and 16–2):

1. Rinse the grain thoroughly.
2. Pretoast the grain. This step is optional, although in many cases it helps grains cook more evenly and enhances flavor. To toast grains, heat a large, heavy skillet, add the rinsed grain, and stir until the water has evaporated. Continue stirring until the grain begins to pop.
3. Measure liquid into a heavy pot with a tight-fitting lid, and bring the water to a boil. Grain can be cooked in water, vegetable broth, or, for a sweeter flavor, in a mixture of water and apple juice. Grain will not cook well in tomato sauce, so add any tomato products after cooking is completed.
4. Add the grain, return to a boil, then lower heat to simmer. Cover and cook until all the water is absorbed.
5. Most grains will cook best if salt is added after cooking is completed.

PREPARING BEANS

Soaking Methods

The first step in preparing dried beans is to rinse them thoroughly. Then, to reduce cooking time greatly, most beans (except lentils and split peas) should be soaked for several hours. Small beans require only about 4 hours soaking time; large beans should be soaked for 8 hours or overnight. Use any of the following soaking methods.

Soaking Method 1

1. Place the beans in a large bowl or pot, and add 2 cups of fresh cold water for each cup of dried beans.
2. Place in the refrigerator, and allow to soak for 4 to 8 hours.
3. Drain the beans thoroughly.

Soaking Method 2

Clients who experience gas when consuming beans may wish to try this soaking technique:

1. Place the rinsed beans in a large pot with 3 cups of water for each cup of dried beans. Bring to a boil, and boil for 2 minutes. Drain the beans.
2. Add fresh water, again using 3 cups of water for each cup of beans. Let soak for 6 hours or longer in the refrigerator.
3. Drain the beans thoroughly.

Table 16–1 Cooking Times for Grains (Amounts Are for 1 Cup Dry, Uncooked Grain)

Grain	Cups (Liquid)	Cooking Time	Yield (Cups)
Amaranth	2½	20–25 minutes	3
Barley (hulled)	3	1½ hours	3½–4
Barley (pearl)	3	50 minutes	3½
Bulgur	2	20 minutes	3
Couscous	2	5 minutes	3
Kamut	3	2 hours	2¾
Millet	2	25 minutes	3
Quinoa	2	15 minutes	3
Spelt	3	2 hours	3
Triticale	3	2 hours	2½
Wheat berries	3	2 hours	3

Table 16–2 Grain Cooking Times for Pressure Cookers (Instructions Are for 1 Cup Dried, Uncooked Grain)

Grain	Cups (Liquid)	Cooking Time (Minutes) under High Pressure	Yield (Cups)
Amaranth	1¾	4	2
Barley (hulled)	3	40	3½
Barley (pearl)	3	18	3½
Buckwheat	1¾	3	2
Bulgur	1½	6	3
Kamut	3	40–45	2½
Millet	2–2½	12	3½
Spelt	3	40–45	2½
Triticale	3	35–45	2
Wheat berries	3	35–45	2

Soaking Method 3: The Quick-Soak Method

1. Cover the beans with water, and bring to a boil.
2. Remove from heat, cover, and let stand at room temperature for 1 hour.

Cooking Dried Beans

Soaked beans should be drained and then cooked in fresh water. Place the beans in a large, heavy pot with 3 cups of water for each cup of soaked beans or 4 cups of water for each cup of unsoaked beans. Bring the water to a boil. Reduce the heat, cover, and simmer until the beans are tender. Table 16–3 gives approximate cooking times for different varieties of beans.

Because beans take such a long time to cook, a pressure cooker is an excellent way to prepare them. Follow these steps for pressure cooking beans.

1. Use 3 cups of water for each cup of soaked beans or 4 cups of water for each cup of unsoaked beans.
2. If using a jiggle-top pressure cooker, add 1 tbsp of oil for each cup of dried beans.
3. Lock the lid into place, and bring to high pressure.
4. Cook at high pressure for the time indicated in Table 16–4.
5. Release the pressure quickly, according to the directions for the cooker.

Table 16–3 Cooking Times for Beans (Yields Are for 1 Cup of Dried, Uncooked Beans)

Beans	Cooking Time (Hours)		Yield (Cups)
	Soaked	Unsoaked	
Anasazi	2	2½–3	2
Adzuki	1–1½	2–3	2
Black	1½–2	2–3	2
Black-eyed peas	½	1	2
Cannellini	1–1½	2	2
Chickpeas	2	3½–4	2½
Cranberry	2	2–3	2½
Great northern	1–1½	2–3	2¼
Kidney	1½–2	2–3	2
Lentils*		½–¾	2
Lima	¾–1	1½	2
Navy	1½–2	2½–3	2
Pinto	1½–2	2–3	2
Soybeans	2–3	3–4	2½
Split peas*		¾	2

*No need to soak before cooking.

6. Test the beans, and return to high pressure for a few minutes if they are not quite done.

USING TOFU

Tofu is still an unfamiliar food to many Westerners. Its versatility and ease of use make it a staple in many vegetarian kitchens, however. Tofu has been a staple in Chinese cooking since around 200 BC and is still used every day in most households throughout much of Asia. It is made fresh daily in small tofu shops and sold by street vendors.

Two distinctive features make tofu an especially versatile food. First, it is relatively bland. It does not compete with other flavors and contributes no strong flavors of its own to a dish. Second, it is a spongy, porous food that absorbs flavors and sauces well. Therefore, tofu works well in a wide variety of dishes, from spicy chili to banana cream pie.

Tofu is made from soymilk, the liquid expressed from soaked soybeans. A curdling agent is added to the tofu, usually a salt such as calcium sulfate, which causes large curds to form. The curds are pressed into a solid block of tofu.

Tofu is a nutritious product. When it is made with a calcium salt, it is an excellent source of calcium. In addition, like all soy products, tofu is rich in high-quality protein. It is also a good source of several minerals and vita-

Table 16–4 Cooking Times for Beans in a Pressure Cooker (Instructions Are for 1 Cup of Dried, Uncooked Beans)

	Cooking Time (Minutes) under High Pressure		
Beans	*Soaked*	*Unsoaked*	*Yield (Cups)*
Adzuki	5–9	14–20	2
Anasazi	4–7	20–22	2
Black	9–11	20–25	2
Black-eyed peas*		9–11	2
Cannellini	9–12	22–25	2
Chickpeas	10–12	30–40	2½
Cranberry	9–12	30–35	2¼
Great northern	8–12	25–30	2¼
Kidney	10–12	20–25	2
Lentils*		7–10	2
Lima	5–7	12–15	2½
Navy	6–8	15–25	2
Pinto	4–6	22–25	2¼
Soybeans	9–12	25–35	2¼
Split peas*		8–10	2

*No need to soak before cooking.

mins. Although tofu tends to be fairly high in total fat, it is low in saturated fat and is often lower in fat than the meat and dairy products it replaces in recipes. Reduced-fat tofu is also available. Firm tofu tends to be higher in fat than soft tofu.

There are a variety of types of tofu on the market. Firm tofu works well for stir-fried dishes, for grilling, in salads, or for scrambled tofu. Soft tofu is a much more delicate product with a higher water content. It can be blended to produce a creamy product for sauces, dressings, fruit shakes, cream pies, dips, cheese type fillings for pasta, and salad dressings. Silken tofu is a soft, custardy product. It is more delicate than the other two kinds of tofu and is especially appropriate for shakes and desserts. In addition to regular firm, soft, and silken tofu, there are a number of baked and flavored tofu products available.

Tofu can be frozen for up to 5 months. Once defrosted, it has a spongy, chewy texture that is pleasant grilled and in stews or baked in a sauce.

Tofu is available in water tubs, vacuum packs, or aseptic brick packages. It is usually found in the produce section of the supermarket, although it can also be found in the dairy case. Bulk tofu is often available in food cooperatives or in Asian markets. Unless it is aseptically packaged, tofu should be kept cold. Once the package is opened, the tofu should be rinsed, covered with fresh water (which should be changed daily), and used within a week.

The following ideas can help vegetarian clients introduce tofu into their meals:

- Marinate tofu chunks in tamari or any sauce, and add them to soups and stews.
- Mash tofu with cottage cheese and fresh herbs to make a dip or a sandwich spread.
- Make tofu burgers: mash tofu with bread crumbs, chopped onions, celery, and seasonings. Form into patties and fry or bake.
- Defrost frozen tofu, marinate it in barbecue sauce, and cook it on the grill. Serve it in rolls with sliced tomatoes and onions.
- Sauté crumbled firm tofu with chopped onion, and add a package of taco seasoning and tomato sauce to create a filling for tacos.
- Blend dried onion soup mix into soft or silken tofu to make an onion dip.
- Blend soft tofu with fresh lemon juice, salt, and fresh herbs for a baked potato topping.
- Blend soft tofu with melted chocolate chips to make a pie filling or a pudding type dessert.
- Replace all or part of the cream in creamed soups with blended silken tofu.
- Replace all or part of the cooked egg in egg salad with diced tofu.
- Use blended soft tofu instead of ricotta cheese in stuffed shells or lasagna.
- Use blended soft tofu in creamy ranch or Thousand Island dressing in place of mayonnaise.

USING TEXTURED VEGETABLE PROTEIN

TVP, which stands for Texured Vegetable Protein, is actually a brand name; the generic name for this product is *texured soy protein*. *TVP* is the commonly used term, however, and TVP is often sold in bulk in natural food stores under this name. TVP is made from soy flour and is low in fat and rich in protein, fiber, calcium, iron, and zinc.

TVP is available as a dried, granular product. When boiling water is added to it, it takes on a tender, chewy consistency similar to that of ground beef. TVP is also sold in chunks and is sometimes available as a product flavored to taste like beef or chicken. Flavored TVP chunks can be used in stir-fried dishes, soups, stews, and curries. Most TVP sold in grocery stores or natural foods stores is the unflavored, granular variety, however. Both unflavored and flavored TVP is also sold by mail.

To use TVP, pour ⅞ cup of boiling water over 1 cup of dry TVP. Let it sit for a few minutes. Chunk style TVP requires 1 full cup of water for each cup of TVP and may need to be simmered or cooked in a microwave oven to rehydrate fully.

Studies show that TVP tastes best in dishes that are flavored with tomato sauce. It works well as a replacement for the ground beef in chili, tacos, spaghetti sauce, stuffed peppers, stuffed cabbage, and Sloppy Joes. Rehydrate the TVP, and use it to replace an equal amount of ground beef in those dishes.

USING EGG SUBSTITUTES

Eggs have two important functions in recipes. First, because the protein in eggs coagulates upon heating, eggs help thicken mixtures and hold them together. For example, most meatloaf recipes contain eggs to bind the rest of the ingredients together. Second, eggs help leaven baked goods, making them lighter and fuller. Eggs also add some moisture to these baked goods.

For vegans or others who prefer to cook without eggs, there are a number of ingredients that can take on these roles in most dishes.

Baked Goods

In baked goods, eggs leaven and add some moisture. The following can be used in place of eggs in baking.

- *Flax seed.* Grind 3 level tbsp of flax seed in a blender for several minutes to produce a fine powder. Then add ½ cup of cold water, and blend until the mixture is frothy and viscous and has a texture similar to that of well-beaten whole eggs. This mixture is the equivalent of about two large eggs and can be added to batter whenever eggs are called for. It can also be refrigerated for several days.

- *Soy flour.* Soy flour has properties not found in other flours that help it serve some egglike functions in baked goods. For each egg in a recipe, substitute 1 heaping tbsp of soy flour and 1 tbsp of water.

- *Mashed fruits.* The addition of mashed banana, applesauce, or pureed prunes can replace the moisture of an egg and make a product somewhat tender. Use ¼ cup of mashed banana, applesauce, or pureed prunes to replace one egg. This will change the flavor of the product and will result in a slightly heavier baked good. When using fruit to replace the egg in baked goods, try adding an extra ½ tsp of baking powder for each egg omitted from the recipe.

In some products that do not require a great deal of leavening and call for only one egg (eg, pancakes), it is usually acceptable to leave the egg out. Two or three additional tablespoons of liquid should be added to the batter. The following mixture can replace one egg in the batter of other kinds of baked goods: 2 tbsp white flour, ½ tbsp vegetable oil, 2 tbsp water, and ½ tsp baking powder. Finally, commercial egg replacer is also available. This is a powdered mixture of potato starch, tapioca flour, and leavening agents.

Binding

The following substitutions will bind recipes together like an egg:

- tomato paste (thin just a bit with water, but not too much or it will lose its capacity to hold the recipe together)
- tahini mixed with tomato paste
- blended tofu (blended with or without white flour)
- thickened white cream sauce made from flour, margarine, and soymilk
- mashed potatoes
- mashed banana
- flour, matzo meal, or quick oats (use these sparingly because they can give burgers or loaves a heavy, dense quality)
- moistened bread crumbs

COOKING WITH SWEETENERS

Many vegans choose to avoid white sugar because animal products are involved in its processing; most also avoid honey. Many other sweeteners can be substituted for sugar in recipes, but substituting sweeteners can sometimes change the end result of the product. Also, when sugar is replaced with a liquid sweetener, other liquids in the recipe must be reduced. The following can substitute for 1 cup of refined white sugar.

- ⅔ cup fructose
- ¾ cup maple syrup (reduce the liquid in the recipe by 3 to 4 tbsp)
- 1¼ cup molasses (reduce the liquid in the recipe by 6 tbsp; use molasses for only half the sugar in a recipe)
- 1 cup Sucanat (see Glossary at the end of the book)
- 1 cup barley malt (reduce the liquid in the recipe by ½ cup)
- 1 cup brown rice syrup (reduce the liquid in the recipe by ½ cup)

Glossary of Vegetarian Foods

Adzuki beans: a small brownish bean used frequently in Japan and often served mixed in with brown rice or other grains. Popular in macrobiotic cooking.

Agar: sometimes called agar-agar; a sea vegetable that can be used in place of gelatin. Sold in flakes or bars and is taste free. Add 2 tbsp agar flakes to 2 cups of simmering water. Continue to simmer until the flakes are dissolved, then allow to gel for 35 minutes in the refrigerator or for 1 hour at room temperature.

Alaria: a sea vegetable similar to Japanese wakame; it is harvested off the coast of Maine. Used frequently in soups. Remove the midrib before cooking to speed cooking time.

Almond butter: a spreadable paste made from ground, toasted almonds. Refrigerate for up to 4 months.

Almond milk: milk made from almonds and sometimes flavored. Sold in aseptic packages.

Amaranth: an ancient grain used by the Aztecs. It has a taste that is faintly reminiscent of corn. The seeds are yellowish brown and tiny; cooked amaranth tends to be soupy rather than fluffy, and it is often mixed with other grains. Can also be used to thicken soups.

Anasazi beans: maroon and white speckled beans that are native to the American southwest and are good in Mexican and Southwestern dishes. Can be used interchangeably with pinto beans. Considered an heirloom bean.

Arame: a precooked, mildly flavored sea vegetable. The large leaves are usually sliced and dried into thin black strands that can be crumbled into soups and stews. Requires little cooking time.

Barley: an ancient grain with a chewy quality and mild taste. Barley is available as either hulled barley (the whole grain, also called Scotch barley) or pearled barley (which has the bran removed). It is frequently used in soups and stews or sauteed with onions and mushrooms.

Barley malt syrup: a liquid sweetener extracted from sprouted, roasted barley. It is only about 50% as sweet as sugar.

Bear mush: a whole wheat version of Cream of Wheat cereal.

Black-eyed peas (cowpeas): brought to the United States by African slaves and somewhat important to cuisine of the southern United States, they are used in salads and often flavored with hot peppers. Because they are quick cooking, they do not require presoaking.

Black turtle beans: natives of the Carribean and Central and South America, these beans are important to the cuisine of those areas. They are used frequently in black bean soup and chili and are sold as canned refried black beans.

Blue corn: a purple-blue–hued corn. Blue cornmeal is increasingly available in natural foods stores. It has a finer texture and more delicate flavor than regular cornmeal. It is often used to make tortillas.

Bragg liquid amino acids: a salty, unfermented condiment similar to, and used like, soy sauce.

Brewer's yeast: a byproduct of beer making, it is rich in many vitamins and minerals; usually used in supplement form.

Brown beans: also called Swedish brown beans, they are used in baked beans.

Brown rice cream: cracked brown rice that cooks up into a creamy rice cereal.

Buckwheat: toasted buckwheat is a Russian grain called kasha; it has a decidedly strong, earthy flavor that works best when mixed with other, mellower grains. Untoasted buckwheat is milder in flavor. All types of buckwheat cook quickly.

Buckwheat flour: a dark, strong-tasting flour made from toasted buckwheat and traditionally used to make Japanese soba noodles and Russian blini (pancakes).

Bulgur (bulghur): whole wheat that has been precooked and dried. It is common in Middle Eastern cuisine and is used to make the popular salad tabouli.

Cannellini beans: small white beans used frequently in Italian cooking, especially to make the popular Italian soup pasta fagioli. When thoroughly cooked, they have a creamy consistency and can be blended with lemon, garlic, and herbs to produce paté or sandwich spreads.

Carob (St John's bread): a mildly sweet powder made by grinding the pods of the tropical carob tree. The flavor is somewhat comparable to that of cocoa. Carob is often used as a chocolate substitute.

Chickpeas: called garbanzo beans in Mexican cooking and cecis in Italian cooking. Popular in vegetarian cooking, especially to produce the Middle Eastern sandwich spread called hummus. Also used frequently in Indian curries.

Cornmeal: ground, dried corn. It is used most frequently to make cornbread or muffins or to make polenta, a corn-based Italian porridge. It can also be added to home-baked breads.

Couscous: a quick-cooking grain made from steamed, dried wheat and used extensively in North Africa. Available as both refined and whole wheat products.

Cowpeas: *see* black-eyed peas

Cranberry beans: brownish beans with red spots. These are traditional in New England style baked beans.

Dulse: a red-colored sea vegetable that does not require cooking and is added to soups and stews.

Egg replacer: commercial, egg-free, powdered egg replacer for use in baked products.

Falafel: Middle Eastern chickpea croquettes flavored with spices, deep fried, and served in pita bread, usually with a sauce of tahini.

Fava beans: large brown beans that are a staple in Middle Eastern and Mediterranean cooking. The tough skins must be removed before eating.

Flax seeds: tiny brown seeds that are sometimes added to cereals. Ground flax seeds can be used as an egg replacer. They are prone to rancidity and must be stored in the freezer.

Garbanzo beans: *see* chickpeas

Grain coffee: caffeine-free coffee substitute made from a variety of grains.

Greens: a wide range of dark green leafy vegetables that are important in the diets of vegans because most are rich in calcium. They include collards, dandelion greens, kale, mustard greens, and turnip greens.

Hijiki: a black-colored sea vegetable that looks like strands of angel hair pasta. Should be soaked for several minutes before cooking to reduce saltiness. Often added to soups, stews, and vegetables.

Hoison sauce: a sweet, salty, and spicy Chinese condiment used in many types of Asian dishes.

Hummus (hummous): a Middle Eastern dip or sandwich spread made from pureed chickpeas, tahini, garlic, lemon, and parsley. Traditionally served in pita bread or as a dip with pita wedges.

Great northern beans: large white beans with a mild flavor, used in baked beans or bean soups.

Job's tears: an Asian grain resembling barley that can be added to soups or stews.

Kasha: *see* buckwheat

Kamut: an ancient Egyptian wheat berry with a chewy consistency and a rich taste.

Kelp: a sea vegetable usually sold in powdered form to add a salty, briny taste to vegetables or grains.

Kidney beans: available as either a red or white bean. The red variety is traditional in chili.

Kombu: a sea vegetable that grows as long, flat strips. Often added to beans while they are cooking to improve digestibility.

Lentils: one of the oldest foods known to humankind, lentils are used frequently in the cuisines of India and Middle Eastern and Mediterranean countries. Brown-colored lentils are most commonly available, but yellow and orange types are also sold.

Lima beans: used as a fresh green bean or a dried tan-colored bean. Dried, they are sometimes called butter beans. Available as large or baby limas; used in soups and stews.

Mayonnaise: eggless varieties made from tofu are available.

Millet: a tiny, round, yellowish grain widely used in Asia and Africa. It is often served as a simple grain dish tossed with chopped onions and herbs.

Miso: fermented soybean paste with a salty, earthy flavor. An essential condiment in Japanese cooking, it is used to make miso soup and to flavor sauces, stews, grains, and bean dishes.

Miso soup: a soup made from a broth flavored with miso and any of a wide variety of vegetables. Chunks of tofu and sea vegetables are commonly used.

Mochi: cooked sweet rice that has been pounded into flat sheets, which have a sticky consistency. Mochi puffs up when baked or cooked in an ungreased skillet and can be added to soups or eaten as a snack.

Mung beans: tiny green beans used in soups and purees.

Navy beans (pea beans): small, roundish, tan-colored beans frequently used in soups or baked beans. Most commercial canned baked beans use navy beans.

Nori: a sea vegetable sold in flat, dried sheets and often used to make sushi or nori rolls.

Nutritional yeast: an inactive yeast grown on a nutrient-rich culture to produce a condiment that is rich in vitamins and minerals. Red Star brand T6635 is reliably rich in vitamin B_{12}.

Oat flour: flour made from rolled oats. Use small amounts to add flavor to baked goods.

Pea beans: *see* navy beans

Pinto beans: pale beige or pinkish beans with dark brown speckles. A southwestern staple used in chili and spicy bean stews or to make refried beans.

Polenta: cornmeal porridge popular in Italian cooking.

Portabello mushrooms: sometimes called the steak of vegetarians, these large mushrooms are sliced and grilled or sauteed in olive oil with herbs.

Quinoa: called the Mother Grain by the Incans, this grain was a staple in the diet of that civilization. Quinoa is coated with saponin and must be thoroughly rinsed before it is cooked.

Ramen noodles: thin, curly noodles used in Chinese soups.

Rice: comes in three basic varieties. Long grain rice is fluffy when cooked and is excellent for pilafs. Medium grain rice is moist and tender right after cooking but becomes sticky as it cools. Short grain rice is higher in starch and tends to stick together when cooked; it is the traditional rice used in Chinese and Japanese cooking. Within these categories, there are many types of rice.

- *brown rice:* the whole rice kernel (with just the outer hull removed). It is available as long, medium, or short grain and has a nutty flavor and a chewy texture.
- *white rice:* polished or milled rice. The bran and germ are both removed, so that this rice is slightly more tender than brown rice and cooks more quickly. In the United States it is nearly always enriched with B vitamins and iron.
- *arborio rice:* a high-starch, short grain rice used to make risotto, a northern Italian dish that is especially rich and creamy. Other types of rice that can be used to make risotto are vialone, nano, and canaroli, but these are much more difficult to find. In a pinch, any short grain white rice (often sold as pearled rice) can be used to make risotto, especially when it is made in the pressure cooker.
- *basmati rice:* an aromatic, long grain rice imported from India and Pakistan. It is available as both a brown and a white rice.
- *japonica rice:* a Japanese rice that tends to stick together when cooked. It is a good choice for Asian dishes.
- *jasmine rice:* a long grain, aromatic rice imported from Thailand. Try this rice in cold salads because it stays fluffy even after it has cooled.
- *wild rice:* actually not a rice at all. Wild rice belongs to a completely different family of grasses that grow wild in the lakes of upper Michigan and Wisconsin. It is traditionally harvested by hand and is fairly costly, but 1 cup of wild rice expands to produce 4 cups of cooked grain.

Rice milk: a rice-based beverage with a somewhat sweet taste. Used to replace cow's milk in the diet.

Seitan: sometimes called wheat meat and made from gluten (wheat protein). It is baked and can be used in a variety of dishes as a meat substitute.

Seven-grain cereal: a combination of seven grains (grains used vary) prepared as a hot cereal.

Shiitake mushrooms: sold in fresh or dried form and used frequently in Asian cooking.

Soba noodles: Japanese noodles made from buckwheat.

Soybeans: a high-protein, high-fat bean used to make a variety of products that are of great importance in the cuisine of Asian cooking. Products made from soybeans include tofu, tempeh, tamari (soy sauce), miso, and soymilk. The whole bean can be used in stews and soups. Green immature soybeans are consumed in Asia as a vegetable but are generally not available in the United States.

Soy cheese: an imitation cheese made from soybeans. It is generally not vegan because most brands contain casein.

Soy flour: flour made from soybeans; can be full fat or defatted.

Soymilk: the rich liquid expressed from soaked soybeans. It is sold in powdered form or as a liquid in aseptic containers and is often flavored, sweetened, defatted, or fortified. Used in the same ways that dairy milk is used.

Soynuts: roasted, soaked soybeans used for snacks or in salads.

Soy yogurt: a nondairy yogurt made from soybeans.

Split peas: available as green or yellow beans. When well cooked, they develop a creamy consistency and are used to make soup or sauces to use over grains. A staple in Indian cooking.

Sucanat: a sweetener made from evaporated and granulated sugar cane juice. Can be used to replace sugar in equal amounts.

Swedish brown beans: *see* brown beans

Tabouli: a Middle Eastern salad made with bulgur and flavored with lemon and mint.

Tahini: made from pureed sesame seeds to produce a product that is slightly more liquid than peanut butter. A popular ingredient in Middle Eastern cooking.

Take Care: fortified soy protein beverage sold in powdered form.

Tamari: soy sauce made in the traditional Asian way, which requires long periods of fermentation and aging. It has a much richer taste than commercial, American soy sauce.

Tempeh: a traditional Indonesian product made from fermented soybeans pressed into a solid cake. It can be marinated and grilled, baked in sauces, or used to make sandwich spreads.

Textured Vegetable Protein (TVP): a brand name for textured soy protein, made from soy flour. Available as either granules or chunks and sometimes flavored to taste like meat. Used in place of ground beef in dishes such as chili and tacos or in stews and soups.

Tofu: a mild-tasting porous product made by curdling soymilk and pressing the curds into a solid block.

Tofu hotdogs: hot dogs made from tofu.

Tofu ice cream: nondairy frozen dessert similar to ice cream and made from tofu.

Udon noodles: flat whole wheat noodles used in Asian cuisine.

Umeboshi plum paste: a pickled plum paste with a salty flavor used in marinades.

Vegelicious: a substitute for cow's milk made from potatoes and soy protein and sold in powdered form.

Vegetarian Worcestershire sauce: Worcestershire sauce made without anchovies; many commercial low-sodium brands are vegetarian.

Veggieburgers: vegetarian burgers made from a wide variety of products. Available as frozen, ready-made burgers, as powdered mixes to be rehydrated and cooked, or from home recipes.

Wakame: a sea vegetable with a tough midrib that should be removed before cooking. Often sliced into soups, especially miso soup.

Wasabi: a hot Japanese radish available in powdered or paste form. Used to make sushi.

Wheat germ: the nutrient-rich germ of the wheat kernel, often added to baked goods or cereals.

Wheat berries: the whole kernel of wheat. Ground wheat berries produce whole wheat flour. Whole wheat berries have a chewy quality and are often mixed in with other grains.

Whole wheat pasta: pasta made from whole wheat.

Resources on Vegetarian Diet

VEGETARIAN RESOURCES FOR DIETITIANS

Organizations That Provide Information about Vegetarian Diet

Vegetarian Nutrition Dietetic Practice Group of the American Dietetic
  Association
  216 West Jackson Boulevard
  Chicago IL 60606-6995
  (312) 899-0040

Seventh-day Adventist Dietetic Association
  PO Box 75
  Loma Linda CA 92354
  (714) 793-8918

Vegetarian Resource Group
  PO Box 1463
  Baltimore MD 21203
  (410) 366-8343

Printed Materials on Vegetarian Diet

Diet Manual Including a Vegetarian Meal Plan
  Available from the Seventh-day Adventist Dietetic Association, PO Box
  75, Loma Linda CA 92354.

Vegetarian Journal's Foodservice Update
  Quarterly newsletter for dietitians and food service directors that
  includes tips and recipes for introducing vegetarian meals into food
  service settings. Available from the Vegetarian Resource Group, PO Box
  1463, Baltimore MD 21203, (410) 366-8343.

Vegetarian Quantity Food Recipes

Twenty-eight recipes with nutritional analyses; quantities given for 25 and 50 people. This book also includes a listing of companies that produce vegetarian food items in institutional sizes. Available from the Vegetarian Resource Group, PO Box 1463, Baltimore MD 21203, (410) 366-8343.

The Gold Plan

Twelve vegan recipes that serve 48 people each. The Gold Plan is a comprehensive plan to promote nutrition education in a cafeteria setting; it includes a variety of materials for distribution to patrons, including copies of the recipes formulated to serve six to eight people. Available from the Physicians Committee for Responsible Medicine, 5100 Wisconsin Avenue NW, Washington DC 20016, (202) 686-2210.

The Vegetarian Food Pyramid

Available from the Health Connection, 55 West Oak Ridge Drive, Hagerstown MD 21740, (800) 548-8700. Single copies are $1.50 each or $2.00 for a laminated copy. Posters are $5.95 each plus $3.50 postage. Bulk prices are available.

The New Four Food Groups Poster

Vegan food guide available from the Physicians Committee for Responsible Medicine, 5100 Wisconsin Avenue NW, Washington DC 20016, (202) 686-2210.

RESOURCES FOR VEGETARIAN CLIENTS

National Organizations That Provide Vegetarian Information

The Vegetarian Resource Group
PO Box 1463
Baltimore MD 21203
(410) 366-8343

North American Vegetarian Society
PO Box 72
Dolgeville NY 13329
(518) 568-7970

American Vegan Society
501 Old Harding Highway
Malaga NJ 08328
(609) 694-2887

Physicians Committee for Responsible Medicine
PO Box 6322
Washington DC 20015
(202) 686-2210

Vegetarian Education Network (VE-Net)
  PO Box 3347
  West Chester PA 19381
  (Promotes vegetarian perspective in schools and supports young vegetarians)

Vegetarian Nutrition Dietetic Practice Group
  c/o The American Dietetic Association
  216 West Jackson Boulevard, Suite 800
  Chicago IL 60606-6995

Cookbooks

There are many cookbooks on the market aimed at vegetarian cooks, including ones that specialize in certain types of vegetarian cuisine. The following lists can help clients identify some of the most popular and available choices.

General Vegetarian Cooking

- *The New Laurel's Kitchen,* by Laurel Robertson, Carol Flinders, and Brian Ruppenthal (Berkeley, CA: Ten Speed Press, 1986). This is the updated, lower-fat version of the original vegetarian classic published in 1976. It is a selection of both lacto-ovo vegetarian and vegan recipes and includes information about vegetarian cookery and nutrition.

- *Simply Vegan,* by Debra Wasserman and Reed Mangels, PhD, RD (Baltimore, MD: Vegetarian Resource Group, 1991). This is a collection of vegan recipes with an emphasis on ease of preparation and low-fat dishes. Includes a nutrition section written by Mangels. A good choice for new vegans.

- *Recipes from an Ecological Kitchen,* by Lorna Sass (New York, NY: Morrow, 1992). All recipes are vegan. This book includes an extensive glossary of foods and information about basic preparation of a wide variety of grains and beans. Cooking with a pressure cooker is emphasized, but standard stove-top instructions are included for all recipes. This cookbook is also available in soft cover under the title *Lorna Sass' Complete Vegetarian Kitchen* (New York, NY: Hearst Books, 1995).

- *The Farm Vegetarian Cookbook,* edited by Louise Hagler (Summertown, TN: Book Publishing, 1978). This book celebrates the cuisine of the best known vegetarian community in the United States: The Farm in Summertown, Tennessee. These are homestyle vegan recipes with an emphasis on soy products. The book includes instructions for making soymilk, tofu, tempeh, and other products.

- *American Wholefoods Cuisine,* by Nikki Goldbeck and David Goldbeck (New York, NY: New American Library, 1983). This is a huge collection of recipes—more than 1,200 of them—that covers the whole spectrum of basic vegetarian cooking. Although it is lacto-ovo vegetarian, many recipes are free of animal products.

- *Moosewood Restaurant Cooks at Home,* by the Moosewood Collective (New York, NY: Simon & Schuster, 1994). From the renowned restaurant in Ithaca, New York, this collection of recipes emphasizes ease of preparation. The recipes are interesting and appealing. This is a lacto-ovo vegetarian cookbook, but there are many vegan choices (some fish recipes as well).

- *The Complete Vegetarian Cuisine,* by Rose Elliot (New York, NY: Pantheon, 1988). A lacto-ovo vegetarian cookbook that includes attractive color photographs and descriptions of the foods used in vegetarian cooking. The recipes tend to be somewhat high in fat. This book is recommended for special occasion cooking.

- *The Compassionate Cook,* by People for the Ethical Treatment of Animals (PETA; New York, NY: Warner, 1993). A collection of vegan recipes, all easy to prepare. Some are contributed by a few of PETA's better known supporters, including Linda McCartney and Rue McClanahan.

- *The Complete Whole Grains Cookbook,* by Carol Gelles (New York, NY: Fine, 1989). Extensive information about whole grains and their preparation. Most recipes are vegan.

- *The Savory Way,* by Deborah Madison (New York, NY: Bantam, 1990). Slightly more complicated recipes for sophisticated vegetarian cuisine.

Seventh-day Adventist Cookbooks

The Seventh-day Adventist Church has been producing vegetarian cookbooks for many decades. These are valuable guides to a type of family style cooking that contains no animal products and has been perfected over many years of homestyle cooking and community cooking demonstrations. A few of these books have become classics. The following are the most popular.

- *Country Life,* edited by Diana J. Fleming (Sunfield, MI: Family Health, 1990). A collection of recipes from the Country Life chain of Seventh-day Adventist–run restaurants, including those in France, Korea, and Japan. Recipes are vegan and easy to prepare.

- *Ten Talents,* by Frank J. Hurd and Rosalie Hurd (Chisholm, MN: 1968). This pioneering vegan cookbook boasts more than 750 recipes and has sold more than 250,000 copies since its original publication in 1968. This is the classic Seventh-day Adventist cookbook.

Specialty Cookbooks

- *Aveline Kushi's Introducing Macrobiotic Cooking,* by Aveline Kushi and Wendy Esko (New York, NY: Japan Publications, 1987). Recipes for a macrobiotic diet for those who are new to this way of eating, written by two of the best known macrobiotic cooks.

- *Great Vegetarian Cooking under Pressure,* by Lorna Sass (New York, NY: Morrow, 1994). Vegan recipes for the pressure cooker.

- *The Low Fat Jewish Vegetarian Cookbook,* by Debra Wasserman (Baltimore, MD: The Vegetarian Resource Group, 1994). This book celebrates a cultural cooking tradition that ranges from the most basic homestyle dishes to truly festive offerings. It offers low-fat, vegan versions of traditional favorites.

- *The Uncheese Cookbook,* by Joanne Stepaniak (Summertown, TN: Book Publishing, 1994). Cheeselike dishes based on beans, nuts, and various condiments. All recipes are vegan.

- *The Book of Tofu,* by William Shurtleff and Akiko Aoyagi (New York, NY: Ballantine, 1988). Extensive information about the history, culture, preparation, and use of tofu by two of the world's experts on the topic.

- *The Art of Indian Vegetarian Cooking,* by Yamuna Devi (New York, NY: Dutton, 1987). A true classic of Indian cooking, this book is the first vegetarian cookbook ever to win the Cordon Bleu's cherished Cookbook of the Year award. It contains more than 500 recipes and volumes of information about Indian cooking. Some recipes use dairy products.

- *World of the East Vegetarian Cooking,* by Madhur Jaffrey (New York, NY: Knopf, 1981). A wonderful selection of more than 400 recipes from the kitchens of India, Bali, Japan, China, and Middle Eastern countries. Many recipes are vegan. This is a perfect introduction to vegetarian cooking from other cultures.

Low-Fat Cooking and Eating

- *Simple, Low-Fat and Vegetarian,* by Suzanne Havala, MS, RD, with recipes by Mary Clifford, RD (Baltimore, MD: Vegetarian Resource Group, 1994). A guide to simple changes that will cut the fat from vegetarian diets in a variety of settings: in restaurants, amusement parks, cruise ships, and so forth or at the movies.

- *The No-Cholesterol (No Kidding!) Cookbook,* by Mary Carroll, with Hal Straus (Emmaus, PA: Rodale, 1991). Mary Carroll created the recipes used by Dr Dean Ornish in his study on reversing heart disease. This is an excellent collection of low-fat, no-cholesterol, vegan recipes for both beginner and seasoned cooks.

- *Eat More, Weigh Less,* by Dean Ornish, MD (New York, NY: Harper Collins, 1993). This is actually a cookbook preceded by a short discussion of diet and weight control. All recipes are vegetarian (some nonfat dairy is used) and were developed by some of the world's best chefs. Many tend to be a bit time consuming and will appeal most to those who enjoy cooking.

Books Providing General Vegetarian Nutrition Information

- *Eating for the Health of It,* by Winston Craig, PhD, RD (Eau Claire, MI: Golden Harvest, 1993). Sound, reliable vegetarian nutrition information written by a nutrition professor at Andrews University, a Seventh-day Adventist university. It presents a good overview of nutrition issues and practical advice on meeting nutrient needs on a plant-based diet.

- *Simply Vegan,* by Debra Wasserman and Reed Mangels, PhD, RD (Baltimore, MD: Vegetarian Resource Group, 1991). This book is listed above with recommended cookbooks, but the nutrition section, written by vegetarian nutritionist Mangels, deserves a separate mention. This is a brief overview of nutrition issues that are especially relevant to vegans. New vegetarians will find the information especially useful.

- *Food for Life,* by Neal Barnard, MD (New York, NY: Harmony, 1993). Presents evidence for a vegan diet as the optimal eating plan that will dramatically decrease risk for cancer, heart disease, and other chronic, life-threatening conditions. A 21-day menu plan and recipes by vegetarian cook Jennifer Raymond make this a comprehensive guide for adults who want practical advice on how to change their diet.

- *Vegan Nutrition: Pure and Simple,* by Michael Klaper, MD (Umatillo, FL: Gentle World, 1987). An easy-to-read guide to planning healthy vegan diets. It includes guidelines for meal planning, sample menus, recipes, and information about nutrients and vegetarian foods.

- *Vegan Nutrition: A Survey of Research,* by Gil Langley, PhD (Oxford, England: Vegan Society, 1988). A comprehensive survey of the scientific research supporting the safety of vegan diets for all age groups.

Books on the Rationale for Vegetarian Diet

- *Compassion: The Ultimate Ethic: An Exploration of Veganism* by Victoria Moran (Malaga, NJ: American Vegan Society, 1991). Describes vegan philosophy, diet, and life style. This book also explores the historical background of vegetarianism and veganism in daily life.

- *Animal Factories,* by Jim Mason and Peter Singer (New York, NY: Crown, 1980). An in-depth look at the mass production of animals for food and how this affects the lives of consumers, farmers, and the animals themselves.
- *Diet for a Small Planet,* by Frances Moore Lappé (New York, NY: Bantam, 1982). The 10th anniversary edition of this classic book corrects some misinformation about protein combining in the original edition. Lappé explores the relationship between food production and the use of the earth's resources in this important work.
- *A Vegetarian Sourcebook,* by Keith Akers (Denver, CO: Vegetarian Press, 1989). This book makes the argument for vegetarian diet from health, ethical, and environmental perspectives and includes an interesting discussion of vegetarianism in the context of the world's major religions.

Materials Especially for Young People

- *A Teen's Guide to Going Vegetarian,* by Judy Krizmanic (New York, NY: Viking Children's Books, 1994). Written specifically for teens, this book explores the reasons for choosing a vegetarian diet and then sets young people on the right track toward planning healthy vegetarian diets.
- *Good Food Today, Great Kids Tomorrow,* by Jay Gordon, MD, with Antonia Barnes Boyle (Studio City, CA: Michael Wiese Productions, 1994). Gordon is a sort of pediatrician to the stars, and his patients include the offspring of many Hollywood celebrities. In this book, he gives sound nutrition advice that favors a vegan eating plan and is presented in a pleasant question-and-answer format. The book includes a series of transition menus (including recipes) that include small amounts of nonfat dairy foods; they are especially valuable to families who are working toward a vegan diet in a more gradual fashion. Despite the use of some dairy, some of these menus need to be supplemented with additional calcium-rich foods.
- *How on Earth!,* a periodical published four times a year on vegetarianism, ecology, and animal rights. It is written by and for teenagers. Available from *How on Earth!,* PO Box 3347, West Chester, PA 19381.

Vegetarian Restaurant Guide

- *Vegetarian Journal's Guide to Natural Foods Restaurants in the US and Canada,* by the Vegetarian Resource Group (Garden City Park, NY: Avery, 1993).

Vegetarian Magazines

Vegetarian Gourmet
  PO Box 7641
  Riverton NJ 08077-7641
  Quarterly

Vegetarian Journal
  PO Box 1463
  Baltimore MD 21203
  Bimonthly

Vegetarian Times
  PO Box 446
  Mount Morris IL 61054
  Monthly

Veggie Life
  PO Box 57159
  Boulder CO 80323
  Quarterly

Vegetarian Voice
  PO Box 72
  Dolgeville NY 13329

ON-LINE SERVICES

Each of the on-line services (American Online, Prodigy, CompuServe, etc) offers bulletin boards especially for people with an interest in vegetarian diet. The following are other Internet services for vegetarians.

Mailing Lists

- Veglife: To subscribe, address mail to listserv@vtvm1.bitnet. Your message should read "sub veglife<your first and last name> set veglife digest".

- Veggie: To subscribe, address mail to veggie-request@maths.bath.ac.uk. Your message should contain a brief request to subscribe to the mailing list.

- Vegan-l: To subscribe, address mail to listserv@templevm.bitnet. Your message should read "sub vegan-l <your first and last name> set vegan-l digest".

- Veg-Cook: To subscribe, address mail to listserv@netcom.com. Your message should read "SUBSCRIBE veg-cook".

Internet Newsgroups

- rec.food.veg
- rec.food.veg.cooking
- alt.food.fat-free

World Wide Web

- The Vegetarian Page (http://catless.ncl.ac.uk/Vegetarian): This home page includes a comprehensive list of vegetarian restaurants and organizations around the world as well as links to recipe sites and other vegetarian resources on the Internet.
- Vegetarian Recipes (http://www-sc.ucssc.indiana.edu/cgi-bin/recipes/): A searchable database of more than 800 vegetarian recipes.

MAIL-ORDER VEGETARIAN FOODS

The Mail Order Catalog
  PO Box 180
  Summertown TN 38483
  (800) 695-2241
  Nutritional yeast, gluten, tempeh starter, TVP, other food products, and many, many vegetarian books

Harvest Direct
  PO Box 4514
  Decatur IL 62525-4514
  (800) 835-2867
  Many flavors of TVP, burger mixes, pasta and sauces, soymilk, and cookbooks

Dixie Diner's Club
  PO Box 55549
  Houston TX 77255-5549
  (713) 688-4993
  Flavored TVP products, condiments, and kitchen gadgets; emphasis on low-fat cookery

Appendixes

APPENDIX A

Fiber, Cholesterol, and Macronutrient Intakes of Adult Vegetarians and Nonvegetarians

(Ref)/ year	Group/ Gender(N)	Country	Age (years)	SDA/ NSDA[2]	Kcal[3]	Protein[4] (%)	Fat[4] (%)	CHO[4] (%)	Sat fat[5] (g or %)	PUFA or LA[6]	PUFA: Sat fat[7]	Chol (mg)	Fiber[8]
(1) 1954	LOV M (15)	United States	55	NSDA	3020	13.0	32.1		33.4 g	14.8	0.44	333	16.3
	VEG M (14)		51		3260	10.2	35.9		21.3 g	19.0	0.89		23.9
	NV M (15)		57		3720	13.4	42.5		67.4 g	16.3	0.24	914	10.7
	LOV F (15)		58		2451	13.4	33.9		32.4 g	10.5	0.33	350	12.6
	VEG F (11)		49		2400	10.2	36.3		28.3 g	22.2	0.78		20.7
	NV F (15)		57		2690	14.0	41.6		46.8 g	11.2	0.24	612	8.4
(2) 1963	LOV F (26)	Australia	19	NSDA	1980	10.7	31.8						6.4
	NV F (25)		20		2115	12.2	40.8						4.0
(3) 1968	LOV M/F (206)	United States	15–74	SDA		14.6	32.8		11.1%	5.5%		193	5.7
	NV M/F (106)		15–74	SDA		16.3	37.4		14.1%	5.5%		361	3.8
(4) 1978	VEG M/F (23)	United States	27	NSDA	2233	17.0	32.0	51.0			1.9		
	NV M/F (39)		27		2264	16.0	42.0	41.0			0.44	424	
(5) 1978	LOV F (42)	United States	57	SDA	1600	16.3	32.2	54.8	13.7 g			185	5.9
	NV F (36)		59	NSDA	1579	17.0	35.7	48.9	21.5 g			307	3.9
(6) 1980	LOV M/F (57)	United States	18–40	NSDA	2270	12.2	34.5	51.5					8.9
	LV M/F (14)		18–40		1830	12.2	30.5	59.0					10.8
	VEG M/F (8)		18–40		1665	8.2	28.6	69.9					16.1
	NV F (41)		18–40		2072	16.2	40.0	41.7					4.5
(7) 1980	LOV M (7)	Netherlands	20–26	NI	2833	13.1	34.0	49.7		25.8	0.30	272	48.1
	NV M (7)		18–25		2619	14.2	38.5	44.6		16.6	0.18	279	33.1
(8) 1980	LOV M (15)	United States	28	NSDA	2624	13.7	34.0	54.7				298	
	NV M (25)		27		2684	16.7	40.2	41.1				453	
	LOV F (13)		26		2174	14.5	38.5	51.0				241	
	NV F (24)		26		1859	16.4	38.7	40.5				287	

(Ref)/year	Group[1]/Gender(N)	Country	Age (years)	SDA/NSDA[2]	Kcal[3]	Protein[4] (%)	Fat[4] (%)	CHO[4] (%)	Sat fat[5] (g or %)	PUFA or LA[6]	PUFA: Sat fat[7]	Chol (mg)	Fiber[8]
(9) 1980	LOV F (49)	Canada	53	SDA	1630	14.2							30.9
(10) 1981	LOV M (11)	Great Britain	28–80	NSDA	2015	13.1	39.3	49.4					36.7
	NV M (18)		28–80		2300	14.3	40.1	46.5					24.5
	LOV F (14)		28–80		1737	12.9	42.4	48.5					30.1
	NV F (28)		28–80		1656	15.4	41.1	44.3					19.5
(11) 1981	LOV F (5)	United States	22	NI	1329	15.3	34.5	51.8	17.0 g			340	6.2
(12) 1982	LOV F (101)	United States	57	NI	1565	15.2	32.3	56.8	13.2 g			157	6.3
	NV F (107)		62		1573	17.4	36.5	47.6	22.1 g			319	4.0
(13) 1982	LOV F (10)	United States	27	NI	1649	13.3	30.6		17.0 g				28.0
	NV F (10)		25		1572	15.8	40.1		27.0 g				12.0
(14) 1982	VEG M (8)	United States	30	NSDA	2910	16.0	43.0	42.0			2.5		
	VEG F (8)		29		2451	14.0	41.0	46.0			2.7		
(15) 1983	LOV M (36)	United States	31	NSDA	2532	13.0	36.6	47.7	37.0	23.0	0.66	340	7.1
	NV M (18)		31		2836	14.0	39.4	42.3	46.0	20.0	0.45	482	4.6
(16) 1983	LOV M/F (75)	United States	NI	SDA		13.5	36.1						
(17) 1983	LOV M (47)	Australia	33	SDA	2610	14.1	34.4	54.1	33.7 g	25.1 g	0.83	191	44.3
	NV M (59)		34	NSDA	2767	14.9	41.3	46.4	50.3 g	18.4 g	0.41	398	24.3
	LOV F (51)		34	SDA	2036	14.2	36.8	51.3	29.2 g	19.0 g	0.77	208	32.6
	NV F (54)		33	NSDA	2007	15.8	41.3	44.6	35.4 g	14.2 g	0.46	308	19.7
(18) 1983	LOV F (14)	United States	33	SDA	1865	13.5	30.9	58.6	16.0 g	12.8	.80	136	
	NV F (9)		36	NSDA	1711	14.7	41.0	44.7	22.6 g	10.6	.47	322	
(19) 1983	LOV M (20)	United States	36	SDA	2324	12.7	28.7	60.9	18.8 g	15.4 g	.81	186	
	NV M (17)		44	NSDA	2652	14.6	39.4	46.8	37.2 g	15.0 g	.40	404	
	LOV F (31)		46	SDA	1776	13.5	30.4	58.6	14.8 g	11.8 g	.80	168	
	NV F (36)		44	NSDA	1754	14.1	40.0	44.7	22.9 g	11.2 g	48.9	284	

(Ref)/year	Group/Gender/(N)	Country	Age (years)	SDA/NSDA[2]	Kcal[3]	Protein[4] (%)	Fat[4] (%)	CHO[4] (%)	Sat fat[5] (g or %)	PUFA or LA[6]	PUFA: Sat fat[7]	Chol (mg)	Fiber[8]
(20) 1983	LOV F (36)	Canada	69	SDA	1615	14.5							33.2
	NV F (30)		60	NSDA	1727	15.6							20.2
(21) 1984	LOV M (25)	United States	39–65	SDA	2128	13.2	27.5	62.4					
	VEG M (9)		39–65	SDA	2259	11.7	25.9	67.1					
	NV M (25)		39–65	NSDA	2335	17.5	37.8	42.3					
	LOV F (25)		39–65	SDA	1615	12.9	34.6	55.2					
	VEG F (9)		39–65	SDA	1497	12.9	22.8	68.7					
	NV F (25)		39–65	NSDA	1821	14.7	40.0	43.1					
(22) 1984	VEG M (10)	Great Britain	NI	NSDA	2548	11.0	35.3	53.8					48.0
	NV M (12)				2524	13.3	40.3	43.3					22.0
	VEG F (12)				2214	12.5	33.7	55.8					38.0
	NV F (12)				1976	14.6	38.3	45.7					18.0
(23) 1985	LOV M/F (17)	Great Britain	34	NSDA	2290	11.5	38.5	48.6					37.0
	VEG M/F (17)		31		2381	10.2	33.6	56.3					47.0
	NV M/F (17)		35		2313	14.5	40.9	44.3					23.0
(24) 1985	LOV M (12)	United States	57	SDA	2667	14.1	34.1	54.0	31.0	17.0		197	37.0
	NV M (8)		56	NSDA	2617	12.7	39.9	38.7	32.0	17.0		438	20.0
(25) 1985	LV M/F (9)	Great Britain	37	NSDA	NI	14.1	38.5	45.1				296	49.0
	VEG M/F (10)		35		NI	11.4	32.6	54.5					40.0
	NV M/F (10)		39		NI	14.0	41.0	38.5				375	22.0
(26) 1986	LOV M (14)	South Africa	29	SDA/	2717	11.4	36.6	49.7	13.4	7.7	0.72	292	38.6
	NV M (10)		29	NSDA	3167	14.1	37.5	41.7	13.1	7.9	0.63	467	22.4
	LOV F (19)		27	SDA/	1916	12.1	38.0	48.5	14.9	8.0	0.58	191	25.6
	NV F (12)		27	NSDA	1890	14.6	38.3	41.0	13.8	8.1	0.60	272	17.3
(27) 1986	LOV M (60)	Israel	55	NSDA	3290	12.1	30.3	57.2					74.4
	NV M (53)		50		2896	16.7	31.0	50.8					42.4
	LOV F (32)		51		2544	11.6	29.6	58.6					58.5
	NV F (60)		52		2389	18.8	32.8	47.4					33.6

(Ref)/ year	Group[1]/ Gender(N)	Country	Age (years)	SDA/ NSDA[2]	Kcal[3]	Protein[4] (%)	Fat[4] (%)	CHO[4] (%)	Sat fat[5] (g or %)	PUFA or LA[6]	PUFA: Sat fat[7]	Chol (mg)	Fiber[8]
(28) 1986	LOV M (14)	Canada	28	NSDA	2401	11.8	37.1	53.5	31.0			245	35
	NV M (14)		21		2809	14.1	38.4	46.7	30.0			368	21
	LOV F (22)		26		1760	14.5	37.3	54.8	21.0			206	25
	NV F (18)		22		2097	15.3	37.8	46.5	29.0			249	19
(29) 1986	VEG M (8)	Great Britain	18–40	NSDA	2429	11.1	40.7	47.0					46
	NV M (8)		18–40		2381	13.3	39.6	41.4					21
	VEG F (10)		18–40		2071	11.2	34.3	52.4					25
	NV F (10)		18–40		2333	14.9	37.8	43.1					19
(30) 1987	VEG M (11)	Great Britain	32	NSDA	2643	11.0	40.7	47.0			1.18		50
	NV M (11)		31		2381	15.4	39.6	41.4			0.35		22
	VEG F (11)		28		1881	11.6	34.3	52.4			1.15		39
	NV F (11)		24		1833	15.1	37.8	43.1			0.45		27
(31) 1988	LOV F (88)	United States	73	SDA	1533	14.2	32.9	56.4				167	5.6
	NV F (278)		79	NSDA	1633	17.1	48.5	46.1				305	4.2
(32) 1988	LOV F (20)	United States	31	NSDA	1814	14.2	31.8	54.9					
	NV F (16)		29		1788	17.0	39.3	44.1					
(33) 1988	LOV M (14)	United States	34	SDA/	2444	12.8	33.6	54.6					7.0
	NV M (13)		35	NSDA	2329	13.9	35.6	48.2					3.9
	LOV F (15)		34	SDA/	1742	12.4	33.1	54.4					5.9
	NV F (16)		34	NSDA	1656	14.3	37.2	47.2					3.5
(34) 1989	LV/LOV F (11)	Finland	36	NSDA	1820	12.8	33.5	52.3	33.4	10.3			22.9
	NV F (12)		32		1910	15.0	38.4	43.8	43.2	9.3			17.4
(35) 1989	LOV (9)	United States	58	SDA	1452	13.3	29.3	59.0	16.5 g	12.4		142	27.0
	NV (10)		56	NSDA	1799	16.6	36.9	45.4	28.0 g	14.3		350	16.8
(36) 1989	LOV M (15)	Canada	29	NI	2700	12.6	29.7	58.4	27.0	19.0		296	38.0
	NV M (14)		27		2620	16.6	36.8	48.4	43.0	12.0		524	14.0
(37) 1989	LOV F (144)	United States	67	SDA	1474	14.1	30.8	58.6	15.0			155	20.0
	NV F (146)		66	NSAA	1563	16.2	34.9	49.1	20.6			243	16.0

(Ref)/year	Group[1]/Gender(N)	Country	Age (years)	SDA/NSDA[2]	Kcal[3]	Protein[4] (%)	Fat[4] (%)	CHO[4] (%)	Sat fat[5] (g or %)	PUFA or LA[6]	PUFA: Sat fat[7]	Chol (mg)	Fiber[8]
(38) 1989	LOV F (10)	United	67	NI	1612	13.9	36.0				0.75	194	5.2
	NV F (10)	States	65		1641	16.6	42.0				0.48	294	4.7
(39) 1989	B-LOV M/F (51)	United	55	SDA	2406	11.1	28.0	50.0					10.8
	B-NV M/F (49)	States	56	SDA	2504	15.5	36.9	51.4					10.2
	W LOV M/F (163)		52	SDA	2340	13.7	31.7	60.0					13.2
	W-NV (89)		53	SDA	2225	14.5	36.0	53.6					9.6
(40) 1989	LOV M (11)	France	37	NSDA	2100	12.0	33.9	53.1			1.00	296	
	NV M (33)		40		2600	14.8	37.7	39.2			0.40	497	
	LOV F (26)		35		1700	12.0	36.0	51.8			0.90	188	
	NV F (36)		49		1800	16.2	41.5	39.8			0.40	373	
(41) 1990	LOV F (23)	United	72	SDA	1452	12.9	31.7	60.0	12.1%	9.2%	0.845	89	21.5
	NV F (14)	States	71	SDA	1363	16.2	35.9	50.2	16.5%	7.9%	0.506	183	13.0
(42) 1990	LOV F (12)	United	76	SDA	1425	13.2	31.6	60.6	10.0	7.0		72.0	24.0
	NV F (12)	States	72	SDA	1334	16.2	36.4	49.8	17.0	7.0		181	13.0
(43) 1990	LOV M (18)	Netherlands	83	NSDA	1960	12.2	37.2	50.8	15.0	8.5	0.57	200	33.7
	NV M		elderly		2412	13.6	40.8	41.8	17.3	6.8	0.39	356	27.4
	LOV F (26)		81		1667	13.1	37.3	49.8	15.8	8.3	0.53	216	28.7
	NV F		elderly		1879	14.9	40.1	43.2	17.2	6.5	0.38	294	23.7
(44) 1990	LOV M (15)	Netherlands	82	NSDA	2014	11.7	39.3	49.5					33.0
	NV M (225)		72		2414	13.6	41.0	41.6					27.0
	LOV F (17)		82		1681	12.8	39.1	48.1					28.0
	NV F (216)		72		1874	14.9	40.3	42.7					23.0
(45) 1990	LOV F (8)	United	27	NSDA	1814	14.7	27.9	62.8			0.60		11.6
	NV F (8)	States	23		2542	14.3	35.4	49.9			0.50		4.7
(46) 1990	LOV M (20)	United	26	SDA	2489	12.7	33.3	56.4	23	10		184	34.0
	VEG M (15)	States	30	SDA	2915	10.7	30.6	65.2	15	22			50.0
	NV M (18)		26	SDA	2061	14.8	34.9	51.6	23	7		195	16.0

(Ref)/year	Group[1]/Gender/(N)	Country	Age (years)	SDA/NSDA[2]	Kcal[3]	Protein[4] (%)	Fat[4] (%)	CHO[4] (%)	Sat fat[5] (g or %)	PUFA or LA[6]	PUFA: Sat fat[7]	Chol (mg)	Fiber[8]
(47) 1990	LOV F (18)	Great Britain	30	NSDA	1826	11.9	35.1	48.0				104	29.3
	NV F (22)		34		1779	15.8	40.3	40.3				199	16.6
(48) 1990	LOV M (26)	Great Britain	41	NSDA	2619	12.2	36.4	47.7	35.2%		0.73	267	41.8
	VEG M (26)		41		2571	11.3	33.5	52.5	17.7%		1.85		55.3
	NV M (26)		41		2548	14.6	38.1	43.0	37.4%		0.56	306	35.0
	LOV F (26)		45		1952	12.4	39.6	46.4	31.0%		0.63	201	31.3
	VEG F (26)		44		1905	12.2	36.2	51.4	15.7%		1.77		42.7
	NV F (26)		44		1952	15.5	38.7	43.2	30.8%		0.49	266	26.8
(49) 1991	LOV F (23)	United States	35	NSDA	1939	12.8	33.9	56.5	21.0 g	15.0 g		106	24.0
	NV F (36)		36		1835	16.6	35.8	48.6	24.0 g	11.0 g		261	14.0
(50) 1991	LOV F (34)	United States	36	SDA/	1819	13.9	33.2	58.1	16.0	13.0		133	26.0
	NV F (41)		29	SDA/	1700	17.6	32.3	51.3	19.0	9.0		198	15.0
(51) 1991	LOV M/F (79)	United States	18–30	NSDA	2800	13.7	34.0	53.8			0.66		10.7
	NV M/F (4821)		18–30		2980	14.9	37.6	45.9			0.50		6.0
(52) 1992	LOV F (28)	United States	63	SDA/	1652	15.2	30.5	58.7	16.5 g	10.1 g		98	10.3
	NV F (28)		63	SDA/	1657	18.5	33.6	48.1	19.1 g	10.9 g		214	7.6
(53) 1992	LOV F (20)	Scotland	NI	NI	1690	13.0	34.8	53.9					
	NV F (13)		NI		2143	13.0	37.1	52.0					
(54) 1993	LOV M (16)	Great Britain	21–40	NSDA	2238	11.8	37.4	50.0	32.6	19.2	0.71	275	34.0
	VEG M (18)		21–40		2190	11.9	34.9	52.8	18.0	28.6	1.79		44.0
	NV M (386)		NI		2452	14.2	38.2	44.4	42.5	14.5	0.36	396	26.0
	LOV F (36)		21–40		1826	12.3	38.0	48.4	25.1	18.5	0.94	155	33.0
	VEG F (20)		21–40		1750	10.7	34.5	55.5	15.7	22.4	1.47		36.0
	NV F (377)		NI		1733	15.2	39.5	45.5	31.9	10.4	2.96	296	20.0
(55) 1993	LV M/F (14)	Finland	44	NSDA	2029								31.0
	VEG M/F (10)		42		1927								41.0
	NV M/F (12)		33		1778								16.0

(Ref)/year	Group[1]/Gender(N)	Country	Age (years)	SDA/NSDA[2]	Kcal[3]	Protein[4] (%)	Fat[4] (%)	CHO[4] (%)	Sat fat[5] (g or %)	PUFA or LA[6]	PUFA: Sat fat[7]	Chol (mg)	Fiber[8]
(56) 1993	B-LOV M (23)	United States	69	SDA	1900	14.0	30.8	59.8	13.5 g	**15.0 g**	.90	84.0	
	B-NV M (29)		65	SDA	2487	14.5	37.1	52.3	25.5 g	**24.7 g**	.97	303	
	W-LOV M (83)		67	SDA	2336	13.6	30.8	61.1	17.8 g	**19.4 g**	1.09	137	
	W-NV M (43)		65	SDA	2078	14.1	33.8	56.8	20.1 g	**18.3 g**	.91	183	
(57) 1993	LV M (23)	Taiwan	23	NSDA	2071	11.8	25.1	62.8	9.0	30.0	3.40	9.0	5.6
	NV M (20)		21		2119	14.7	33.2	52.9	18.5	25.9	1.30	434	5.8
	LV F (32)		25		1881	12.4	29.5	57.5	10.0	31.8	3.30	14.0	4.9
	NV F (39)		20		1500	16.0	37.2	47.5	14.9	19.2	1.30	408	6.5
(58) 1994	LOV M/F (50)	New Zealand	26–30	NSDA	2272	12.3	35.4		32.3 g	19.2			34.4
	VEG F (5)		26–30		1842	12.0	29.6		14.0 g	19.7			36.0
	NV M/F (50)		26–30		2608	12.8	34.4		41.5 g	14.8			28.2
(59) 1994	LV/VEG M (17)	United States	25	NI	3005	13.3	26.1	59.8					
	NV M (40)		24		2906	14.6	34.4	52.4					
(60) 1994	LOV (8 M, 4 F)	Finland	36	NI	2298	12.1	31.8	56.5	34.8 g	18.0 g	0.69	303	
	NV M (14)		50		2507	15.9	40.8	40.8	54.7 g	15.6 g	0.28	803	
(61) 1994	LOV M/F (64)	United States	47	SDA	2272	12.8	30.0	59.7	16.3	19.5	1.20	110	36.0
	NV M/F (44)		47	SDA	2603	14.7	31.6	56.6	24.9	20.7	0.83	248	33.8
(62) 1995	LV F (15)	Canada	26	NI	2024	11.3	33.6	57.0	23.8 g	16.1 g	0.70	152	24.7
	VEG F (8)		29		1923	10.8	30.1	62.3	15.1 g	17.3 g	1.36		35.0
	NV F (22)		28		2086	14.8	32.4	54.5	25.2 g	14.6 g	0.64	231	22.4
(63) 1995	VEG (25)	United States	36	NI		12	26	62					42.5
	NV (20)		33			16	33	50					17.6

Notes: [1]Abbreviations: LV, lactovegetarian; LOV, lacto-ovo vegetarian; VEG, vegan; and NV, nonvegetarian; NI, not indicated; SDA, Seventh-day Adventist; SDA/NSDA, Seventh-day Adventist/non-Seventh-day Adventist; CHO, carbohydrates; Sat fat, saturated fat; PUFA, polyunsaturated fat; LA, linoleic acid; Chol, cholesterol; B, Black; W, White.

[2]SDA indicates the vegetarians were specifically identified as Seventh-day Adventists whereas NSDA indicates the vegetarians were not exclusively SDAs although some SDAs may have been included in the vegetarian group. NI indicates the process by which subjects were recruited for the study was not indicated or the extent to which SDAs comprised the vegetarian groups was not possible to determine by the information provided.

[3]When energy intake was listed as kilojoules, a factor of 4.2 was used to convert kilojoules into kilocalories.

[4]Values for protein, fat, and carbohydrate are the percentage of calories contributed by each nutrient. The percentage of calories contributed by protein, fat, and carbohydrate was determined by multiplying the number of grams consumed per day, by 4, 9, and 4 calories per gram respectively, and then dividing the calories provided by each macronutrient by the total number of calories listed in the reference. In some cases, this led to differences between the calculated percentage of calories contributed by each nutrient and the percentage listed in the reference and often resulted in the total percent not equalling 100. In cases where only the percentage of calories for each nutrient was listed and not grams, those percentages were used.

[5]Values for saturated fat are in grams unless indicated by (%), which represents the percentage of total calories provided by saturated fat.

[6]Values for PUFA and LA or in grams unless indicated by (%), which represents the percentage of total calories provided by PUFA or LA.

[7]PUFA::Sat fat ratios represent values as listed in the reference, or were determined by dividing the number of grams of PUFA or linoleic acid by the number of grams of saturated fat.

[8]No cholesterol values were listed for vegans since theoretically vegans do not consume cholesterol, although in some studies small amounts of milligrams were reportedly consumed.

[9]Values for fiber are listed as either dietary fiber (g) or crude fiber (g) (references 2, 3, 5, 6, 11, 12, 15, 31, 33, 38, 39, 42, 45, 51, 52, 57). Typically, one gram of crude fiber represents between 3 and 4 grams of dietary fiber.

ANNOTATED REFERENCES

1. Hardinge MG, Stare FJ. Nutritional studies of vegetarians. 1. Nutritional, physical, and laboratory studies. *J Clin Nutr.* 1954;2:73–82. Hardinge MG, Stare FJ. Nutritional studies of vegetarians. Dietary and serum levels of cholesterol. *J Clin Nutr.* 1954;2:83–88.

2. Hitchcock NE, English RM. A comparison of food consumption in lacto-ovo-vegetarians and non-vegetarians. *Food Nutr Notes Rev.* 1963;20:141–146.

3. West RO, Hayes OB. Diet and serum cholesterol levels. *Am J Clin Nutr.* 1968;21:853–862. *Note:* NV consisted of individuals considered to be moderate meat consumers.

4. Burslem J, Schonfeld G, Howald MA, Weidman SW, Miller JP. Plasma apoprotein and lipoprotein lipid levels in vegetarians. *Metabolism.* 1978;27:711–719.

5. Mason RL, Kunkel ME, Ann Davis T, Beauchene RE. Nutrient intakes of vegetarian and nonvgetarian women. *Tenn Farm Home Science.* 1978;1:18–20.

6. Freeland-Graves JH, Bodzy PW, Eppright MA. Zinc status of vegetarians. *J Am Diet Assoc.* 1980;77:655–661.

7. Huijbregtys AWM, Van Schaik A, Van Berge-Henegouwen GP, Van Der Werf SDJ. Serum lipids, biliary composition, and bile acid metabolism in vegetarians as compared to normal controls. *Eur J Clin Invest.* 1980;10:443–449.

8. Taber LAL, Cook RA. Dietary and anthropometric assessment of adult omnivores, fish-eaters, and lacto-ovo-vegetarians. *J Am Diet Assoc.* 1980;76:21–29.

9. Anderson BM, Gibson RS, Sabry JH. The iron and zinc status of long-term vegetarian women. *Am J Clin Nutr.* 1981;34:1042–1048.

10. Burr ML, Bates CJ, Fehily AM, Leger AS ST. Plasma cholesterol and blood pressure in vegetarians. *J Human Nutr.* 1981;35:437–441.

11. King JC, Stein JC, Doyle M. Effect of vegetarianism on the zinc status of pregnant women. *Am J Clin Nutr.* 1981;34:1049–1055.

12. Beauchene RE, Kunkel ME, Bredderman SH, Mason RL. Nutrient intake and physical measurements of aging vegetarian and nonvegetarian women. *J Am Coll Nutr.* 1982;1:131.

13. Goldin BR, Adlercreutz H, Gorbach SL, et al. Estrogen excretion patterns and plasma levels in vegetarian and omnivorous women. *N Engl J Med.* 1982;307:1542–1547.

14. Lock DR, Varhol A, Grimes S, Patsch W, Schonfeld G. Apolipoprotein E levels in vegetarians. *Metabol.* 1982;31:917–921.

15. Liebman M, Bazzarre TL. Plasma lipids of vegetarian and nonvegetarian males: effects of egg consumption. *Am J Clin Nutr.* 1983;38:612–619.

16. Phillips RL, Snowdon DA, Brin BN. Cancer in Vegetarians. In: Wynder EL, Leveille GA, Weisburger GA, Livingston GE, eds. *Environmental Aspects of Cancer.* The Role of Macro and Micro Components of Foods. Food and Nutrition Press, Inc; 1983.

17. Rouse IL, Armstrong BK, Beilin LJ. The relationship of blood pressure to diet and lifestyle in two religious populations. *J Hypertension.* 1983;1:65–71.

18. Shultz TD, Leklem JE. Nutrient intake and hormonal status of premenopausal vegetarian Seventh-day Adventists and premenopausal nonvegetarians. *Nutr Cancer.* 1983;4:247–259.

19. Shultz TD, Leklem JE. Dietary status of Seventh-Day Adventists and nonvegetarians. *J Am Diet Assoc.* 1983;83:27–33.

20. Gibson RS, Anderson BM, Sabry JH. The trace metal status of a group of post-menopausal vegetarians. *J Am Diet Assoc.* 1983;82:246–250. *Note:* Eight of the 36 LOV were vegans.

21. Calkins BM, Whittaker DJ, Nair PP, Rider AA, Turjman N. Diet, nutrition intake, and metabolism in populations at high and low risk for colon cancer. *Am J Clin Nutr.* 1984;40:896–905.

22. Roshanai F, Sanders TAB. Assessment of fatty acid intakes in vegans and omnivores. *Human Nutr: Applied Nutr.* 1984;38A:345–354. *Note:* The intake (g) of saturated fat, linoleic acid and linolenic acid for 10 vegetarians and their controls was 18, 26, and 1.5 for vegetarians and 31, 10 and 1.0 for the nonvegetarian controls. Subject ages were not provided, but vegetarians were age and sex matched with omnivores.

23. Davies GJ, Crowder M, Dickerson JWT. Dietary fibre intakes of individuals with different eating patterns. *Human Nutr: Appl Nutr.* 1985;39A:139–148.

24. Howie BJ, Schultz TD. Dietary and hormonal interrelationships among vegetarian Seventh-Day Adventists and nonvegetarian men. *Am J Clin Nutr.* 1985;42:127–134.

25. Lockie AH, Carlson E, Kipps M, Thomson J. Comparison of four types of diet using clinical, laboratory, and psychological studies. *J Royal Coll Gen Prac.* 1985;35:333–336.

26. Faber M, Gouws E, Benadé AJS, Labadarios D. Anthropometric measurements, dietary intake and biochemical data of South African lacto-ovovegetarians. *S Afr Med J.* 1986;69:733–738.

27. Levin N, Rattan J, Gilat T. Energy intake and body weight in ovo-lacto vegetarians. *J Clin Gastroenterol.* 1986;8:451–453.

28. Locong A. Nutritional status and dietary intake of a selected sample of young adult vegetarians. *Can Diet Assoc J.* 1986;47:101–106.

29. Rana SK, Sanders TAB. Taurine concentrations in the diet, plasma, urine and breast milk of vegans compared with omnivores. *Br J Nutr.* 1986;56:17–27.

30. Sanders TAB, Key TJA. Blood pressure, plasma renin activity and aldosterone concentrations in vegans and omnivores. *Human Nutr: Appl: Nutr.* 1987;41A:204–211.

31. Tylavsky FA, Anderson JJB. Dietary factors in bone health of elderly lactoovovegetarian and omnivorous women. *Am J Clin Nutr.* 1988;48:842–849.

32. Worthington-Roberts BS, Breskin MW, Monsen ER. Iron status of premenopausal women in a university community and its relationship to habitual dietary sources of protein. *Am J Clin Nutr.* 1988;47:275–279.

33. Kelsay JL, Frazier CW, Prather E, Canary JJ, Clark WM, Powell AS. Impact of variation in carbohydrate intake on mineral utilization by vegetarians. *Am J Clin Nutr.* 1988;48:875–879.

34. Adlercreutz H, Fotsis T, Hockerstedt K, et al. Diet and urinary estrogen profile in premenopausal omnivorous and vegetarian women and in premenopausal women with breast cancer. *J Steroid Biochem.* 19889;34:527–530.

35. Adlercreutz H, Hamalainen E, Gorbach SL, Goldin BR, Woods MN, Dwyer JT. Diet and plasma androgens in postmenopausal vegetarian and omnivorous women and postmenopausal women with breast cancer. *Am J Clin Nutr.* 1989;49:433–442.

36. Bélanger A, Locong A, Noel C, et al. Influence of diet on plasma steroid and sex plasma binding globulin levels in adult men. *J Steroid Biochem.* 1989;32:829–833.

37. Hunt I-F, Murphy NJ, Henderson C, et al. Bone mineral content in postmenopausal women: comparison of omnivores and vegetarians. *Am J Clin Nutr.* 1989;50:517–523.

38. Marsh AG, Christensen DK, Sanchez TV, Mickelsen O, Chaffee FL. Nutrient similarities and differences of older lacto-ovo-vegetarian and omnivorous women. *Nutr Rep Int.* 1989;39:19–24.

39. Melby CL, Goldflies DG, Hyner GC, Lyle RM. Relation between vegetarian/nonvegetarian diets and blood pressure in black and white adults. *Am J Publ Health.* 1989;79:1283–1288.

40. Millet P, Guilland JC, Fuchs F, Klepping J. Nutrient intake and vitamin status of healthy French vegetarians and nonvegetarians. *Am J Clin Nutr.* 1989;50:718–722.

41. Nieman DC, Underwood BC, Sherman KM, et al. Dietary status of Seventh-Day Adventist vegetarian and nonvegetarian elderly women. *J Am Diet Assoc.* 1989;89:1763–1769.

42. Barbosa JC, Shultz TD, Filley SJ, Nieman DC. The relationship among adiposity, diet and hormone concentrations in vegetarian and nonvegetarian postmenopausal women. *Am J Clin Nutr.* 1990;51:798–803.

43. Brants HAM, Löwik MRH, Westenbrink S, Hulshof KFAM, Kistemaker C. Adequacy of a vegetarian diet at old age (Dutch Nutrition Surveillance System). *J Am College Nutr.* 1990;9:292–302. *Note:* Values for NV from a separate nationwide survey.

44. Löwik MRH, Schrijver J, van den Berg H, Hulshof KFAM, Wedel M, Ockhuizen T. Effect of dietary fiber on the vitamin B6 status among vegetarian and nonvegetarian elderly (Dutch Nutrition Surveillance System). *J Am College Nutr.* 1990;9:241–249.

45. Oberlin P, Melby CL, Poehlman ET. Resting energy expenditure in young vegetarian and nonvegetarian women. *Nutr Res.* 1990;10:39–49.

46. Pusateri DJ, Roth WT, Ross JK, Schultz TD. Dietary and hormonal evaluation of men at different risks for prostate cancer: plasma and fecal hormone-nutrient interrelationships. *Am J Clin Nutr.* 1990;51:371–377.

47. Reddy S, Sanders TAB. Haematological studies on premenopausal Indian and Caucasian vegetarians compared with Caucasian omnivores. *Br J Nutr.* 1990;64:331–338.

48. Thorogood M, Roe L, McPherson K, Mann J. Dietary intake and plasma lipid levels: lessons from a study of the diet of health conscious groups. *Br Med J.* 1990;300:1297–1301.

49. Lloyd T, Schaeffer JM, Walker MA, Demers L. Urinary hormonal concentrations and spinal bone densities of premenopausal vegetarian and nonvegetarian women. *Am J Clin Nutr.* 1991;54:1005–1010.

50. Pederson AB, Bartholomew MJ, Dolence LA, Aljadir LP, Netteburg KL, Lloyd T. Menstrual differences due to vegetarian and nonvegetarian diets. *Am J Clin Nutr.* 1991;53:879–885.

51. Slattery ML, Jacobs DR, Hilner JE Jr, et al. Meat consumption and its association with other diet and health factors in young adults: the CARDIA study. *Am J Clin Nutr.* 1991;54:930–935.

52. Tesar R, Notelovitz M, Shim E, Kauwell G, Brown J. Axial and peripheral bone density and nutrient intakes of postmenopausal vegetarian and omnivorous women. *Am J Clin Nutr.* 1992;56:699–704.

53. Ball D, Robertson JD, Maughan RJ. Acid-based status of pre-menopausal vegetarian and omnivorous women. *Proc Nutr Soc.* 1992;51:32A (abstr).

54. Draper A, Lewis J, Malhotra N, Wheeler E. The energy and nutrient intakes of different types of vegetarian: a case for supplements. *Br J Nutr.* 1993;69:3–19. *Note:* Approximately 70% and 75% of the vegetarians and nonvegetarians were between 21 and 40 years of age. NV data taken from a separate nationwide survey.

55. Lamberg-Allardt C, Kärkkäinen M, Seppänen R, Biström H. Low serum 25-hydroxyvitamin D concentrations and secondary hyperparathyroidism in middle-aged white strict vegetarians. *Am J Clin Nutr.* 1993;58:684–689.

56. Melby CL, Goldflies DG, Toohey ML. Blood pressure differences in older black and white long-term vegetarians and nonvegetarians. *J Am Coll Nutr.* 1993;12:262–269. *Note:* Subjects in this study may consist of a subset of older individuals included in reference 39.

57. Pan W-H, Chin C-J, Sheu C-T, Lee M-H. Hemostatic factors and blood lipids in young Buddhist vegetarians and omnivores. *Am J Clin Nutr.* 1993;58:354–359. *Note:* The vegetar-

ian diet was described as including no flesh foods, and although milk was allowed, large amounts of milk were reportedly not consumed. No mention was made regarding egg use but the cholesterol intake indicates eggs were not consumed.

58. Alexander D, Ball MJ, Mann J. Nutrient intake and haematological status of vegetarians and age-sex matched omnivores. *Eur J Clin Nutr.* 1994;48:538–546. *Note:* Of the 50 LOV, 5 were vegans. Data for vegans are also reported separately.

59. Toth MJ, Poehlman ET. Sympathetic nervous system activity and resting metabolism rate in vegetarians. *Metabolism.* 1994;43:621–625.

60. Vuoristo M, Miettinen TA. Absorption, metabolism, and serum concentrations of cholesterol in vegetarians: effects of cholesterol feedings. *Am J Clin Nutr.* 1994;59:1325–1331.

61. Melby CL, Toohey M, Cebrick J. Blood pressure and blood lipids among vegetarian, semivegetarian, and nonvegetarian African Americans. *Am J Clin Nutr.* 1994;59:103–109. *Note:* All subjects were black; of the initial 66 vegetarians, 16 were vegans, and 50 were lactoovo vegetarians, there were 46 women and 20 men. Of the nonvegetarians, 34 were women and 11 men.

62. Janelle KC, Barr SI. Nutrient intakes and eating behavior scores of vegetarian and nonvegetarian women. *J Am Diet Assoc.* 1995;95:180–189. *Note:* Eleven of the 15 vegetarians ate eggs.

63. Berk LS, Hubbard RW, Haddad E, et al. Basal fasting cytokine levels in vegans and omnivores. *Am J Clin Nutr.* 1995;61:904 (abstr 74).

APPENDIX B

Lipid Levels in Adult Vegetarians and Nonvegetarians

(REF)/year	Group[1]/Gender (N)	Age (years)[2]	Serum TC[3]	Serum LDL[3]	Serum HDL[3]	Serum TC:HDL[4]	Serum TAG[3]
(1) 1954	LOV M (15)	55	243				
	VEG M (14)	51	206				
	NV M (15)	57	288				
	LOV F (15)	58	269				
	VEG F (11)	49	206				
	NV F (15)	57	295				
(2) 1966	VEG M/F (249)	13–87	159				62.0
	NV M/F (157)	NI	180				73.0
(3) 1970	VEG M (12)	22–80	181				
	NV M (12)	NI	240				
	VEG M (14)	18–68	NDR				
	NV M (14)	NI	NDR				
(4) 1975	LV/LOV (115)	16–62	126	73.0	43	2.93	59.0
	NV (115)	16–62	184	118	49	3.76	86.0
(5) 1978	LOV M/F (20)	39	175				80.0
	NV M/F (39)	37	229				102
(6) 1978	VEG M (17)	20–30	125	79.0	37	3.38	
	NV M (28)	20–30	184	118	48	3.83	
	VEG M (8)	30–40	137	78	37	3.70	
	NV M (7)	30–40	196	130	48	4.08	
	VEG F (24)	20–30	133	81.0	43	3.09	
	NV F (32)	20–30	174	114	50	3.48	
	VEG G (7)	30–40	147	94.0	43	3.42	
	NV F (11)	30–40	193	128	50	3.86	

(REF)/year	Group[1]/Gender (N)	Age (years)[2]	Serum TC[3]	Serum LDL[3]	Serum HDL[3]	Serum TC:HDL[4]	Serum TAG[3]
(7) 1979	LOV M/F (8)	21–66	6.30				1.19
	NV M/F (8)	21–66	6.70				1.51
	VEG M/F (22)	21–66	4.10				0.95
	NV M/F (22)	21–66	6.10				1.35
(8) 1979	LOV M (45)	18–35	4.25		1.04	4.09	
	NV M (48)	18–35	5.28		1.19	4.44	
	LOV F (52)	18–35	4.42		1.17	3.78	
	NV F (22)	18–35	5.26		1.42	3.70	
(9) 1979	LOV M/F (104)	NI	6.00				
	NV M/F (104)		6.60				
(10) 1980	LOV/VEG M (25)	40	4.70				1.20
	NV M (211)	50	6.00				1.68
	LOV/VEG F (25)	44	5.20				0.92
	NV F (71)	52	6.70				1.22
(11) 1980	LOV M (7)	20–26	4.31	2.64	1.34	3.22	1.06
	NV M (7)	18–25	4.84	2.87	1.52	3.18	1.20
(12) 1980	LOV M/F (91)	30–69	5.50		1.70		1.20
	NV M/F (264)	30–69	6.50		1.70		1.40
(13) 1981	LOV M (8)	40	4.70	1.14			
	NV M (50)	44	5.87	1.09			
	LOV M (21)	69	5.49	1.27			
	NV M (32)	69	5.65	1.20			
	LOV F (28)	43	5.41	1.40			
	NV F (85)	45	5.90	1.41			
	LOV F (28)	68	5.93	1.45			
	NV F (48)	68	6.52	1.47			
(14) 1981	LOV F (46)	67	6.80		1.61	4.22	1.70
	NV F (47)	66	7.20		1.54	4.68	1.60

(REF)/year	Group[1]/Gender (N)	Age (years)[2]	Serum TC[3]	Serum LDL[3]	Serum HDL[3]	Serum TC:HDL[4]	Serum TAG[3]
(15) 1982	LOV M (56)	34	4.7		1.40	3.36	0.45
	NV M (52)	35	5.5		1.20	4.58	0.38
(16) 1982	VEG M (8)	30	135	85.0	42.0	3.21	57.0
	NV M (10)	33	185	NI	NI	NI	154
	VEG F (28)	29	137	77.0	49.0	2.80	53.0
	NV F (26)	31	178	NI	NI	NI	82.0
(17) 1983	VEG M (86)	61	167				
	NV M (86)	61	193				
	VEG F (353)	60	173				
	NV F (353)	60	201				
(18) 1983	LOV M (36)	31	183	117	43.0	4.26	79.0
	NV M (18)	31	195	126	45.0	4.33	98.0
(19) 1984	LOV M (12)	52	177		37.1	4.77	166
	VEG M (9)	55	136		32.8	4.15	154
	NV M (13)	51	220		53.5	4.11	128
	LOV F (9)	51	205		56.0	3.66	120
	VEG F (13)	60	163		40.3	4.04	193
	NV F (13)	52	211		56.3	3.75	76
(20) 1984	VEG M (11)	NI	3.57	1.91	1.33	3.33	0.72
	NV M (12)	NI	4.62	3.01	1.32	3.50	0.64
	VEG F (12)	NI	3.74	2.02	1.45	2.58	0.60
	NV F (12)	NI	4.03	2.21	1.49	2.70	0.73
(21) 1980	LOV M/F (15)	20–47	150	100	45.0	3.33	95.0
	NV M/F (10)	20–47	170	114	46.0	3.70	103
	VEG M/F (10)	20–47	135	89.0	36.0	3.75	103
	NV M/F (15)	20–47	177	117	55.0	3.22	79
(22) 1986	LOV M (14)	29	185		53.0	3.49	153
	NV M (10)	27	180		53.0	3.40	162
	LOV F (12)	29	191		66.0	2.89	139
	NV F (19)	27	193		71.0	2.72	132

(REF)/year	Group¹/Gender (N)	Age (years)²	Serum TC³	Serum LDL³	Serum HDL³	Serum TC:HDL⁴	Serum TAG³
(23) 1987	VEG M (11)	21	4.40				
	NV M (11)	22	5.30				
	VEG F (11)	21	4.60				
	NV F (11)	21	4.90				
(24) 1987	LOV M/F (1550)	37–39	4.88	2.74	1.50	3.25	
	VEG M/F (114)	36–37	4.29	2.28	1.49	2.88	
	NV M/F (1198)	40–41	5.31	3.17	1.49	3.56	
(25) 1989	LOV F (23)	72	5.62	3.34	1.62	3.47	1.43
	NV F (13)	71	6.46	4.08	1.76	3.67	1.33
(26) 1989	LOV M/F (17)	37	5.26		1.18	4.46	1.07
	NV M/F (11)	31	5.66		1.32	4.29	0.92
(27) 1990	LOV M (26)	41	5.30	3.14	1.57	3.38	
	VEG M (26)	41	5.00	2.89	1.56	3.21	
	NV M (26)	41	5.90	3.52	1.56	3.78	
	LOV F (26)	45	5.38	3.19	1.68	3.20	
	VEG F (26)	44	4.84	2.72	1.62	2.99	
	NV F (26)	44	5.95	3.79	1.73	3.44	
(28) 1990	LV M/F (25)	29	189				81.0
	NV M/F (100)	28	192				80;0
(29) 1991	LOV M/F (79)	18–30	4.09	2.38	1.40	2.92	6.20
	NV M/F (4821)	18–30	4.58	2.83	1.37	3.34	7.22
(30) 1992	LOV M (18)	20–35	121				
	NV M (18)	20–35	206				
	LOV M (10)	36–50	122				
	NV M (10)	36–50	207				
	LOV F (34)	20–35	136				
	NV F (34)	20–35	183				
	LOV F (17)	36–50	143				
	NV F (17)	36–50	196				

(REF)/year	Group[1]/Gender (N)	Age (years)[2]	Serum TC[3]	Serum LDL[3]	Serum HDL[3]	Serum TC:HDL[4]	Serum TAG[3]
(31) 1992	VEG M (10)	32	3.52	1.85	1.31	2.69	0.76
	NV M (10)	33	4.77	3.14	1.34	3.56	0.65
	VEG F (10)	32	3.74	2.02	1.45	2.58	0.60
	NV F (10)	32	4.21	2.34	1.53	2.75	0.76
(32) 1992	LOV F (18)	30	4.44	2.25	1.83	2.43	0.80
	NV F (22)	34	5.19	3.19	1.66	3.13	0.98
(33) 1993	VEG M (23)	23	3.52				0.57
	NV M (20)	21	4.16				0.62
	VEG F (32)	25	3.50				0.77
	NV F (38)	20	4.43				0.75
(34) 1994	LV/LOV M (31)	19–30	4.34	2.61	1.30	3.34	0.94
	NV M (24)	19–30	5.39	3.41	1.33	4.05	1.44
	LV/LOV F (28)	19–30	4.11	2.39	1.32	3.11	0.89
	NV F (26)	19–30	5.26	3.30	1.36	3.87	1.32
(35) 1994	LOV M/F (12)	36	4.50	2.76	1.35	3.33	0.91
	NV M (14)	50	6.14	4.38	1.47	4.18	1.42
(36) 1994	LOV M/F (64)	47	4.70	3.10	1.20	3.92	1.10
	NV M/F (44)	48	5.40	3.60	1.30	4.15	1.50

Notes: [1]Abbreviations: LV, lactovegetarian; LOV, lacto-ovo vegetarian; VEG, vegan; and NV, nonvegetarian; NI, not indicated and NDR, no difference reported between vegetarians and nonvegetarians although no data were reported. Only one type of vegetarian was listed in cases where a small percentage of the vegetarians in that group may have been of a different type.

[2]In some cases, only data on age was specifically provided for vegetarians, but generally it was similar to or matched with vegetarians. In addition, vegetarians were often matched for BMI and generally only healthy subjects were eligible for recruitment.

[3]Values for TC, total cholesterol; LDL, low density lipoprotein cholesterol; HDL, high density lipoprotein cholesterol; and TAG, triacylglycerol listed as either mg/dl or mmol/L. To convert serum cholesterol values from mg/dL to mmol/L, multiply by 0.0259. To convert serum cholesterol values from mmol/L to mg/dL, multiply by 38.6. To convert serum triacylglycerol from mg/dL to mmol/L, multiply by 0.0113. To convert mmol/L to mg/dL, multiply by 88.5.

[4]TC levels above 225 mg/dl (<5.82 mmol/l) and 240 mg/dl (>6.21 mmol/l) for women and men, respectively, LDL levels above 150 mg/dl (>3.88 mmol/L) and 160 mg/dL (>4.14 mmol/l) for women and men, respectively, and TC:HDL ratios ≥5 for women and ≥5.5 for men warrant treatment according to recent recommendations. Kannel WB. Range of serum cholesterol values in the population developing coronary artery disease. *Am J Cardiol.* 1995;76:69C–77C.

ANNOTATED REFERENCES

1. Hardinge MG, Stare FJ. Nutritional studies of vegetarians. 2. Dietary and serum levels of cholesterol. *J Clin Nutr.* 1954;2:83–88.

2. Chen J-S. The effect of long-term vegetable diet on serum lipid and lipoprotein levels in man. *J Formosan Med Assoc.* 1966;65:65–77. *Note:* Vegetarians consisted of nuns and monks of 49 temples and hermitages in Taiwan, but the dietary habits of the vegetarians were not described. Of the 249 vegetarians, 62 were male and 187 were female. Of the 157 nonvegetarians, 114 were male and 43 were female.

3. Ellis FR, Path MRC, Montegriffo VME. Veganism, clinical findings and investigations. *Am J Clin Nutr.* 1970;23:249–255.

4. Sacks FM, Castelli WP, Donner A, Kass EH. Plasma lipid and lipoproteins in vegetarians and controls. *N Engl J Med.* 1975;292:1148–1151. *Note:* Vegetarians conisted of macrobiotics 40% of whom consumed fish once per week or more, 28% consumed dairy products and 11% consumed eggs.

5. Simons LA, Gibson JC, Paino C, Hosking M, Bullock J, Trim J. The influence of a wide range of absorbed cholesterol on plasma cholesterol levels in man. *Am J Clin Nutr.* 1978;31:1334–1339. *Note:* There 8 male and 12 female LOV and 21 male and 17 female NV.

6. Burslem J, Schonfeld G, Hawald MA, Weidman SW, Miller JP. Plasma apoprotein and lipoprotein lipid levels in vegetarians. *Metabol.* 1978;27:711–719.

7. Dickerson JWT, Sanders TAB, Ellis FR. The effects of a vegetarian and vegan diet on plasma and erythrocyte lipids. *Pl Fds Hum Nutr.* 1979;XXIX:85–94.

8. Simons L, Gibson J, Jones A, Bain D. Health status of Seventh-day Adventists. *Med J Aust.* 1979;2:148.

9. Armstrong B, Clarke H, Martin C, Ward W, Norman N, Masarei J. Urinary sodium and blood pressure in vegetarians. *Am J Clin Nutr.* 1979;32:2472–2476.

10. Haines AP, Chakrabarti R, Fisher D, Meade TW, North WRS, Stirling Y. Haemostatic variables in vegetarians and nonvegetarians. *Thrombosis Res.* 1980;19:139–148.

11. Huijbregts AWM, Schaik AV, Van Berge-Henegouwen GP, Van Der Werf SDJ. Serum lipids, biliary lipid composition, and bile acid metabolism in vegetarians as compared to normal controls. *Eur J Clin Invest.* 1980;10:443–449.

12. Gear JS, Mann JI, Thorogood M, Carter R, Jelfs R. Biochemical and haematological variables in vegetarians. *Br Med J.* 1980;280:1415.

13. Burr ML, Bates CJ, Fehily AM, Leger AS ST. Plasma cholesterol and blood pressure in vegetarians. *J Human Nutr.* 1981;35:437–441.

14. Armstrong BK, Brown JB, Clarke HT, et al. Diet and reproductive hormones: a study of vegetarian and nonvegetarian postmenopausal women. *J Natl Cancer Inst.* 1981;67:761–767.

15. Knuiman JT, West CE. The concentration of cholesterol in serum and in various serum lipoproteins in macrobiotic, vegetarian and non-vegetarian men and boys. *Atherosclerosis.* 1982;43:71–82. *Note:* Values for TAG are for very low density lipoprotein cholesterol (VLDL).

16. Lock DR, Varhol A, Grimes S, Patsch W, Schonfeld G. Apolipoprotein E levels in vegetarians. *Metabol.* 1982;31:917–921.

17. Ko YC. Blood pressure in Buddhist vegetarians. *Nutr Rep Int.* 1983;28:1375–1383.

18. Liebman M, Bazzarre TL. Plasma lipids of vegetarian and nonvegetarian males: effects of egg consumption. *Am J Clin Nutr.* 1983;38:612–619.

19. Kritchevsky D, Tepper SA, Goodman G. Diet, nutrition intake, and metabolism in populations at high and low risk for colon cancer. *Am J Clin Nutr.* 1984;40:921–926.

20. Roshanai F, Sanders TAB. Assessment of fatty acid intakes in vegans and omnivores. *Hum Nutr Appl Nutr.* 1984;38a:345–354.

21. Fisher M, Levine PH, Weiner B, et al. The effect of Vegetarian Diets on plasma lipid and platelet levels. *Arch Intern Med.* 1986;146:1193–1197.

22. Faber M, Gouws E, Benade AJS, Labadarios D. Anthropometric measurements, dietary intake and biochemical data of South African lacto-ovovegetarians. *S Afr Med J.* 1986;89:723–738.

23. Sanders TAB, Key TJA. Blood pressure, plasma renin activity and aldosterone concentrations in vegans and omnivore controls. *Human Nutr Appl Nutr.* 1987;41A:204–211.

24. Thorogood M, Carter R, Benfield I, McPherson K, Mann J. Plasma lipids and lipoprotein cholesterol concentrations in people with different diets in Britain. *Br Med J.* 1987;295:351–353. *Note:* Among the LOV, VEG, and NV, there were 501, 45, and 486 males, respectively, and 1049, 969, and 712 females, respectively.

25. Nieman DC, Underwood BC, Sherman KM, Arabatzis K, Barbosa JC, Johnson M, Shultz TD. Dietary status of Seventh-Day Adventist vegetarian and non-vegetarian elderly women. *J Am Diet Assoc.* 1989;89:1763–1769.

26. Kumpusalo E, Karinpää A, Jauhiainen M, Laitinen M, Lappeteläinen R, Mäenpää PH. Multivitamin supplementation of adult omnivores and lactovegetarians: circulating levels of vitamin A, D and E, lipids, apolipoproteins and selenium. *Intern J Vit Nutr Res.* 1989;60:58–66. *Note:* Values represent the average of 4 different measures taken at 4 different times during the year.

27. Thorogood M, Roe L, McPherson K, Mann J. Dietary intake and plasma lipid levels: lessons from a study of the diet of health conscious groups. *Br Med J.* 1990;300:1297–1301.

28. Phinney SD, Odin RS, Johnson SB, Holman RT. Reduced arachidonate in serum phospholipids and cholesteryl esters associated with vegetarian diets in humans. *Am J Clin Nutr.* 1990;51:385–392.

29. Slattery ML, Jacobs DR, Hilner JE Jr, Caan BJ, Van Horn L, Bragg C, Manolio TA, Kushi LH, Liu K. Meat consumption and its association with other diet and health factors in young adults: the CARDIA study. *Am J Clin Nutr.* 1991;54:930–935.

30. Pronczuk A, Kipervarg Y, Hayes KC. Vegetarians have higher plasma alpha-tocopherol relative to cholesterol than do nonvegetarians. *J Am Coll Nutr.* 1992;11:50–55.

31. Sanders TAB, Roshanai F. Platelet phospholipid fatty acid composition and function in vegans compared with age- and sex-matched omnivore controls. *Eur J Clin Nutr.* 1992;46:823–831.

32. Reddy S, Sanders TAB. Lipoprotein risk factors in vegetarian women of Indian descent are unrelated to dietary intake. *Atherosclerosis.* 1992;95:223–229.

33. Pan W-H, Chin C-J, Sheu C-T, Lee M-H. Homostatic factors and blood lipids in young Buddhist vegetarians and omnivores. *Am J Clin Nutr.* 1993;58:354–359.

34. Krajcovicová-Kudláčková M, Simoncic R, Béderová A, Ondreicka R, Klvanová J. Selected parameters of lipid metabolism in young vegetarians. *Ann Nutr Metab.* 1994;38:331–335.

35. Vuoristo M, Miettinen TA. Absorption, metabolism, and serum concentrations of cholesterol in vegetarians: effects of cholesterol feedings. *Am J Clin Nutr.* 1994;59:1325–1331. *Note:* There were 8 male and 4 female LOV.

36. Melby CL, Toohey M, Cebrick J. Blood pressure and blood lipids among vegetarian, semivegetarian, and nonvegetarian African Americans. *Am J Clin Nutr.* 1994;59:103–109. *Note:* All subjects were black Seventh-day Adventists. Of the 66 vegetarians, 16 were vegans, and 50 were lacto-ovo vegetarians, there were 46 women and 20 men. Of the nonvegetarians, 34 were women and 11 men.

APPENDIX C

Blood Pressure of Adult Vegetarians and Nonvegetarians

(REF)/year	Adjustments[1]	Group[2]/Gender (N)	Age	SDA/NSDA[3]	Systolic Blood Pressure (mm Hg)	Diastolic Blood Pressure (mm Hg)
(1) 1975	Age/Sex	LOV M/F (115)	16–62	NSDA	119	77
		NV M/F (115)	16–62	NSDA	108	63
(2) 1977	Age/Sex/BMI	LOV M (177)	30–79	SDA	126	76
		NV M (103)	30–79	NSDA	136	86
		LOV F (241)	30–79	SDA	130	76
		NV F (187)	30–79	NSDA	142	85
(3) 1978	NI	LOV M (86)	25–29	SDA	117	73
		NV M (86)	25–29	NSDA	119	77
		LOV M (86)	55–59	SDA	125	79
		NV M (86)	55–59	NSDA	137	86
		LOV F (86)	25–29	SDA	109	66
		NV F (86)	25–29	NSDA	113	71
		LOV F (86)	55–59	SDA	121	76
		NV F (86)	55–59	NSDA	138	81
(4) 1979	Age/Sex see footnotes	LOV M/F (102)	20–69	SDA	142	89
		NV M/F (102)	20–69	SDA/NSDA	148	91
(5) 1980	None	LOV/VEG M (25)	40	NSDA	128	79
		NV M (211)	50	NSDA	146	93
		LOV/VEG F (25)	44	NSDA	134	81
		NV F (71)	52	NSDA	147	92
	Age/Sex/Skin fold thickness	LOV/VEG M (25)	40	NSDA	128	79
		NV M (211)	50	NSDA	139	88
		LOV/VEG F (25)	44	NSDA	134	81
		NV F (71)	52	NSDA	139	88

(REF)/year	Adjustments[1]	Group[2]/Gender (N)	Age	SDA/NSDA[3]	Systolic Blood Pressure (mm Hg)	Diastolic Blood Pressure (mm Hg)
(6) 1981	See footnotes	LOV M (8)	40	NSDA	124	84
		NV M (50)	44	NSDA	129	83
		LOV M (21)	69	NSDA	147	87
		NV M (32)	69	NSDA	148	86
		LOV F (28)	43	NSDA	131	82
		NV F (55)	45	NSDA	129	80
		LOV F (28)	68	NSDA	156	89
		OMN F (48)	68	NSDA	148	91
(7) 1982	None	LOV M (47)	33	SDA	114	67
		NV M (59)	34	NSDA	122	73
		LOV F (51)	34	SDA	109	67
		NV F (54)	33	NSDA	117	75
	Age/BMI	LOV M (47)	33	SDA	116	69
		NV M (59)	34	NSDA	121	72
		LOV F (51)	34	SDA	109	67
		NV F (54)	33	NSDA	115	73
(8) 1983	Age/Sex/BMI	VEG M (86)	61	NSDA	128	81
		NV M (86)	61	NSDA	134	83
		VEG F (353)	60	NSDA	129	79
		NV F (353)	60	NSDA	134	82
(9) 1983	Age/Sex	OV M/F (98)	60	NSDA	126	77
		NV M/F (98)	62	NSDA	147	88
(10) 1985	None	LOV M (41)	59	SDA	119	74
		NV M (12)	51	SDA	129	77
		LOV F (93)	51	SDA	112	69
		NV F (41)	51	SDA	120	73
	Age/Sex/BMI	LOV M (41)	51	SDA	119	74
		NV M (12)	51	SDA	128	76

(REF)/year	Adjustments[1]	Group[2]/Gender (N)	Age	SDA/NSDA[3]	Systolic Blood Pressure (mm Hg)	Diastolic Blood Pressure (mm Hg)
(11) 1986	See footnotes	LOV F (93)	51	SDA	114	70
		NV F (41)	51	SDA	116	70
		LOV M/F (48)	29	NSDA	110	73
		NV M/F (41)	31	NSDA	126	80
(12) 1987	Age/Sex/BMI	VEG M (11)	32	NSDA	116	75
		NV M (11)	31	NSDA	114	66
		VEG F (11)	28	NSDA	115	70
		NV F (11)	24	NSDA	107	67
(13) 1988	Age/Sex/BMI	LOV M (14)	23	NSDA	118	59
		NV M (22)	23	NSDA	120	61
(14) 1988	None	LOV M (14)	70	SDA	129	72
		NV M (5)	70	SDA	152	82
		LOV F (34)	70	SDA	120	71
		NV F (17)	70	SDA	131	71
	Age/Sex/BMI	LOV M/F (48)	70	SDA	126	NDR
		NV M/F (22)	70	SDA	128	NDR
(15) 1988	Age/Sex/BMI	LV M/F (63)	16–65	NSDA	112	69
		VEG M/F (226)	16–65	NSDA	113	65
		NV M/F (458)	16–65	NSDA	121	76
		NV M/F (63)	16–65	NSDA	119	79
(16) 1989	Age/Sex	B-LOV M/F (55)	55	SDA	123	74
		B-NV M/F (59)	59	SDA	132	76
		W-LOV M/F (164)	52	SDA	114	66
		W-NV M/F (100)	53	SDA	116	68
	Age/Sex/BMI	B-LOV M/F (55)	55	SDA	123	74
		B-NV M/F (59)	59	SDA	130	75
		W-LOV M/F (164)	52	SDA	115	67
		W-NV M/F (100)	53	SDA	115	67

(REF)/year	Adjustments[1]	Group[2]/Gender (N)	Age	SDA/NSDA[3]	Systolic Blood Pressure (mm Hg)	Diastolic Blood Pressure (mm Hg)
(17) 1991	Age/Sex	LOV M/F (79)	18–30	NSDA	109	68
		NV M/F (4821)	18–30	NSDA	111	69
(18) 1993	None	B-LOV M (27)	69	SDA	133	76
		B-NV M (37)	65	NSDA	141	67
		W-LOV M (85)	67	SDA	121	76
		W-NV M (54)	65	NSDA	122	68
	Age/Sex/BMI	B-LOV M (27)	69	SDA	131	76
		B-NV M (37)	65	NSDA	138	75
		W-LOV M (85)	67	SDA	123	67
		W-NV M (54)	65	NSDA	123	67
(19) 1994	NI	LV/LOV M (17)	25	NI	111	72
		NV M (40)	24	NI	117	68
(20) 1994	None	LOV M/F (64)	47	SDA	117	77
		NV M/F (44)	47	SDA	120	79
	Age/sex	LOV M/F (64)	47	SDA	118	78
		NV M/F (44)	47	SDA	120	79

Notes: [1]Adjustments indicate factors controlled for when analyzing blood pressure difference.

[2]Abbreviations: LV, lactovegetarian; LOV, lacto-ovo vegetarian; VEG, vegan; OV, ovo vegetarians; NV, nonvegetarian; BMI, body mass index; NI, not indicated; SDA, Seventh-day Adventist; NSDA, non Seventh-day Adventist; and NDR, no difference reported between vegetarians and nonvegetarians although data were not provided.

[3]SDA indicates the vegetarians were specifically identified as Seventh-day Adventists whereas NSDA indicates the vegetarians were not exclusively SDAs although some SDAs may have been included in the vegetarian group. NI indicates the process by which subjects were recruited for the study was not indicated or the extent to which SDAs comprised the vegetarian groups was not possible to determine by the information provided.

ANNOTATED REFERENCES

1. Sacks FM, Castelli WP, Donner A, Kass EH. Plasma lipids and lipoproteins in vegetarians and controls. *New Engl J Med*. 1975;292:1148–1151. *Note:* Vegetarians consisted of macrobiotics 40% of whom consumed fish once per week or more, 28% consumed dairy products and 11% consumed eggs.

2. Armstrong B, Van Merwyk AJ, Coates H. Blood pressure in Seventh-Day Adventist vegetarians. *Am J Epidemiol*. 1977;105:444–449.

3. Anholm AC. The relationship of a vegetarian diet to blood pressure. *Prev Med*. 1978;7:35 (abstr a-6). *Note:* The authors indicated that more older nonvegetarians were overweight than vegetarians, but even after contolling for this difference, vegetarians still had significantly lower blood pressure.

4. Armstrong B, Clarke H, Martin C, Ward W, Norman N, Masarei J. Urinary sodium and blood pressure in vegetarians. *Am J Clin Nutr*. 1979;32:2472–2476. *Note:* Vegetarians were lighter but the authors considered this an insufficient explanation for the blood pressure differences between groups.

5. Haines AP, Chakrabarti R, Fisher D, Meade TW, North WRS, Stirling Y. Haemostatic variables in vegetarians and nonvegetarians. *Thrombosis Res*. 1980;19:139–148.

6. Burr ML, Bates CJ, Fehily AM, Leger AS ST. Plasma cholesterol and blood pressure in vegetarians. *J Human Nutr*. 1981;35:437–441. *Note:* For all age/gender groups with the exception of women under 60, the BMI of the LOV was lower than that of the NV.

7. Rouse IL, Armstrong BK, Beilin LJ. Vegetarian diet, lifestyle and blood pressure in two religious populations. *Clin Exp Pharmacol Physiol*. 1982;9:327–330. *Note:* The NV group consisted of Mormons.

8. Ko YC. Blood pressure in Buddhist vegetarians. *Nutr Rep Int*. 1983;28:1375–1383. *Note:* Vegetarian classification was based on data showing that at least 97% of calories was derived from plant products.

9. Ophir O, Peer G, Giland J, Blum M, Aviram A. Low blood pressure in vegetarians: the possible role of potassium. *Am J Clin Nutr*. 1983;37:755–762. *Note:* OV rarely used milk or milk products and consumed no more than 3 eggs per week. The OV and NV groups consisted of 48 women and 50 men each. When subjects within the OV and NV groups were compared according to weight within the range of −20% to +20% of the ideal body weight, vegetarians still had lower blood pressure.

10. Melby CL, Hyner GC, Zoog B. Blood pressure in vegetarians and non-vegetarians: a cross-sectional analysis. *Nutr Res*. 1985;5:1077–1082. *Note:* Of LOV and NV, 14% and 37%, respectively reported a history of being informed by their doctor they had high blood pressure. Of the LOV and NV, 10% and 18.5%, respectively, were taking hypertensive medications and were excluded from analysis.

11. Ernst E, Pietsch L, Matrai A, Eisenberg J. Blood rheology in vegetarians. *Br J Nutr*. 1986;56:555–560. *Note:* The LOV were equally divided between males and females, there were 29 males and 12 female NV. The LOV weighed slightly less than the NV (Broca index 0.9 vs 1.0).

12. Sanders TAB, Key TJA. Blood pressure, plasma renin activity and aldosterone concentrations in vegans and omnivore controls. *Human Nutr Appl Nutr*. 1987;41A:204–211.

13. Aalberts JS, Weegels PL, van der Heijden L, Borst MH, Burema J, Hautvast J GAT, Kouwenhoven T. Calcium supplementation: effect on blood pressure and urinary mineral excretion in normotensive male lactoovegetarians and omnivores. *Am J Clin Nutr*. 1988;48:131–138.

14. Melby CL, Lyle RM, Poehlman ET. Blood pressure and body mass index in elderly long-term vegetarians and nonvegetarians. *Nutr Rep Int.* 1988;37:47–55. *Note:* Of the LOV and NV, 32% and 62.1%, respectively, were either using hypertensive medication or exhibited medication-free blood pressure ≥240/90 mm Hg and were excluded from the analysis.

15. Sacks FM, Kass EH. Low blood pressure in vegetarians: effects of specific foods and nutrients. *Am J Clin Nutr.* 1988;48:795–800. *Note:* Vegetarians conisted of macrobiotics. See reference 1 for a description of dietary habits.

16. Melby CL, Goldflies DG, Hyner GC, Lyle RM. Relation between vegetarian/nonvegetarian diets and blood pressure in black and white adults. *Am J Public Health.* 1989;79:1283–1288.

17. Slattery ML, Jacobs DR, Hilner JE Jr. Meat consumption and its association with other diet and health factors in young adults: the CARDIA study. *Am J Clin Nutr.* 1991;54:930–935.

18. Melby CL, Goldflies DG, Toohey ML. Blood pressure differences in older black and white long-term vegetarians and nonvegetarians. *J Am Coll Nutr.* 1993;12:262–269.

19. Toth MJ, Poehlman ET. Sympathetic nervous system activity and resting metabolic rate in vegetarians. *Metabolism.* 1994;43:621–625. *Note:* Among the vegetarians, 10 were LV, and 7 were VEG.

20. Melby CL, Toohey M, Cebrick J. Blood pressure and blood lipids among vegetarian, semivegetarian, and nonvegetarian African Americans. *Am J Clin Nutr.* 1994;59:103–109. *Note:* All subjects were black; of the initial 66 vegetarians, 50 were LOV and 16 were VEG, there were 46 women and 20 men. Of the initial 45 NV, 11 were male and 44 were female.

APPENDIX D

Anthropometric Data of Female Adult Vegetarians and Nonvegetarians

(REF)/year	Group[1]/(N)	SDA/NSDA[3]	Age	Height (cm)	Weight (kg)	Body Mass Index (kg/m²)	Body fat[3]
(1) 1954	LOV (15)	SDA/NSDA	58	158.8	62.7	24.9	
	NV (15)	SDA/NSDA	57	162.6	64.5	24.4	
(2) 1975	LOV (42)	NSDA	16–40		58.0		6.0
	NV (42)	NSDA	16–40		73.0		17.0
(3) 1978	LOV (42)	SDA	57	161.3	62.6	24.1	
	NV (36)	NSDA	59	161.3	64.4	24.8	
(4) 1980	LOV/VEG (25)	NSDA	44				53.8
	NV (71)	NSDA	52				67.0
(5) 1980	LOV (13)	NSDA	26	164.6	59.8	22.1	22.4
	OMN (24)	NSDA	26	166.6	60.1	21.7	23.8
(6) 1981	LOV (28)	NSDA	43			22.4	
	NV (85)	NSDA	45			23.0	
	LOV (28)	NSDA	68			22.3	
	NV (48)	NSDA	68			24.9	
(7) 1981	LOV (46)	SDA	67	159.2	58.6	23.1	19.2
	NV (47)	SDA/NSDA	66	158.4	60.2	24.0	18.8
(8) 1982	LOV (101)	SDA/NSDA	57	161.0	61.9	23.9	27.0
	NV (107)	SDA/NSDA	62	161.5	65.3	25.0	32.1
(9) 1982	LOV (10)	NI	27	163.7	59.9	22.6	
	NV (10)	NI	26	166.8	63.8	22.7	
(10) 1983	LOV (51)	SDA	34	160.8	60.3	23.3	18.7
	NV (54)	NSDA	33	161.1	68.2	26.3	24.1
(11) 1983	LOV (14)	SDA	33	167.7	61.8	22.0	
	NV (9)	NSDA	36	164.2	63.0	23.3	

(REF)/year	Group[1]/(N)	SDA/NSDA[3]	Age	Height (cm)	Weight (kg)	Body Mass Index (kg/m²)	Body fat[3]
(12) 1985	LOV (93)	SDA	51			23.9	
	NV (41)	SDA	51			28.1	
(13) 1985	LOV (5)	NSDA	27–49			22.0	
	VEG (5)	NSDA	27–49			23.0	
	NV (5)	NSDA	27–49			22.0	
(14) 1986	VEG (10)	NSDA	18–40			21.0	
	NV (10)	NSDA	18–40			21.0	
(15) 1986	LOV (32)	NSDA	51	159.5	53.2	20.9	
	NV (60)	NSDA	52	161.9	63.8	24.3	
(16) 1986	LOV (19)	SDA/NSDA	18–40	163.5	57.7	21.5	26.6
	NV (12)	NSDA	18–40	167.8	59.7	21.1	25.4
(17) 1986	LOV (22)	NSDA	26	160.0	53.4	20.9	
	NV (18)	NSDA	22	160.0	52.9	20.7	
(18) 1987	VEG (11)	NSDA	28			20.6	13.5
	NV (11)	NSDA	24			20.6	17.3
(19) 1988	LOV (25)	NSDA	36	164.8	58.7	21.6	
	NV (21)	NSDA	38	163.3	61.5	23.1	
(20) 1988	LOV (10)	NSDA	58	160.5	57.5	22.3	
	NV (10)	NSDA	57	162.0	67.2	25.6	
(21) 1988	LOV (88)	SDA	73	159.0	62.9	31.5	39.6
	NV (278)	NSDA	79	158.3	60.1	30.1	38.4
(22) 1988	LOV (20)	NSDA	31	165.9	57.9	21.0	
	NV (16)	NSDA	29	163.6	59.8	22.1	
(23) 1988	LOV (15)	SDA/NSDA	34	164.6	61.2	22.6	
	NV (16)	SDA/NSDA	34	160.5	60.5	23.5	
(24) 1989	LOV (144)	SDA	67	161.0	64.8	25.0	NDR
	NV (146)	NSDA	66	163.0	63.6	23.9	NDR

(REF)/year	Group[1]/(N)	SDA/NSDA[3]	Age	Height (cm)	Weight (kg)	Body Mass Index (kg/m²)	Body fat[3]
(25) 1989	LV/LOV (11)	NSDA	36	167.0	59.6	21.1	
	NV (12)	NSDA	32	168.0	60.0	21.5	
(26) 1989	LOV (10)	SDA/NSDA	67	163.0	69.8	26.3	
	NV (10)	SDA/NSDA	64	163.0	67.1	25.3	
(27) 1989	LOV (23)	SDA	72	162.0	60.0	22.8	71.8
	NV (14)	SDA	71	160.0	62.5	24.2	82.8
(28) 1989	LOV (26)	NSDA	35	164.0	53.8	20.0	
	NV (36)	NSDA	49	163.0	60.5	23.3	
(29) 1989	LOV (9)	SDA	58	161.0	70.2	27.2	
	NV (10)	NI	57	161.0	58.6	22.8	
(30) 1990	LOV (12)	SDA	76	159.6	57.4	22.5	67.2
	NV (12)	SDA	72	160.4	63.9	24.7	85.0
(31) 1990	LOV (17)	NSDA	82		62.0	24.5	
	NV (216)	NSDA	72		70.0	27.3	
(32) 1990	VEG (18)	NSDA	30	161.0	59.4	22.5	
	NV (22)	NSDA	34	164.0	64.6	24.1	
(33) 1990	LOV (26)	NSDA	45			21.8	
	VEG (26)	NSDA	44			21.7	
	NV (26)	NSDA	44			22.7	
(34) 1990	LOV (8)	NSDA	27	167.0	57.0	21.1	20.6
	NV (8)	NSDA	23	164.0	60.5	21.6	21.1
(35) 1991	LOV (34)	SDA/NSDA	36	165.1	58.5	21.5	
	NV (41)	SDA/NSDA	29	164.1	59.6	22.0	
(36) 1994	LV/LOV (28)	NSDA	22	168.5	56.4	19.9	
	NV (26)	NSDA	25	167.1	60.2	21.6	
(37) 1994	LOV MF (66)	SDA	47	167.6	74.7	26.8	31.7
	NV MF (45)	SDA	47	166.6	79.4	28.6	36.3

(REF)/year	Group[1]/(N)	SDA/NSDA[3]	Age	Height (cm)	Weight (kg)	Body Mass Index (kg/m²)	Body fat[3]
(38) 1995	LV (15)	NSDA	26	166.4	58.8	21.2	24.1
	VEG (8)	NSDA	28	168.2	58.6	20.7	23.7
	NV (22)	NSDA	28	165.0	61.9	22.7	27.4
(39) 1995	LOV (22)	NSDA	20–57			21.7	
	NV (22)		20–57			21.3	

Notes: [1]Abbreviations: LV, lactovegetarian, LOV, lacto-ovo vegetarian, VEG, vegan, and NV, nonvegetarian.

[2]SDA indicates the vegetarians were specifically identified as Seventh-day Adventists whereas NSDA indicates the vegetarians were not exclusively SDAs although some SDAs may have been included in the vegetarian group. NI indicates the process by which subjects were recruited for the study was not indicated or the extent to which SDAs comprised the vegetarian groups was not possible to determine by the information provided.

[3]Reference 2, body fat calculated from subscapular thickness (mm), references 4 and 16, from sum of skinfold thickness (mm) at triceps, forearm, subscapular and suprailiac sites, references 5, 7, 10, 18 and 37 from triceps skinfold thickness (mm), references 27 and 30 from sum of triceps, suprailiac and thigh skinfolds (mm), reference 34, from hydrostatic weighing, and 38, (%) body fat based on skinfold measurements at the triceps, abdominal, suprailiac and thigh sites. Reference 21, lean body mass was calculated from the following equation 18.23 + 0.01014 × ([14.76 × weight]) + (22.07 × height) − (9.05 × age) − 1669). Reference 8 measured in mm but no details provided. Reference 22, no data provided, but no difference was reported.

ANNOTATED REFERENCES

1. Hardinge MG, Stare FJ. Nutritional studies of vegetarians. 1. Nutritional, physical, and laboratory studies. *J Clin Nutr.* 1954;2:73–82.

2. Sacks FM, Castelli WP, Donner A, Kass EH. Plasma lipids and lipoproteins in vegetarians and controls. *N Engl J Med.* 1975;292:1148–1151. *Note:* Vegetarians consisted of macrobiotics 40% of whom consumed fish once per week or more, 28% consumed dairy products and 11% consumed eggs. Values presented for females actually include 73 males in both the vegetarian and nonvegetarian groups.

3. Mason RL, Kunkel ME, Davis TA, Beauchene RE. Nutrient intakes of vegetarian and nonvegetarian women. *Tenn Farm Home Sci.* 1978;1:18–20.

4. Haines AP, Chakrabarti R, Fisher D, Meade TW, North WRS, Stirling Y. Haemostatic variables in vegetarians and non-vegetarians. *Thrombosis Res.* 1980;19:139–148.

5. Taber LAL, Cook RA. Dietary and anthropometric assessment of adult omnivores, fish-eaters, and lacto-ovo-vegetarians. *J Am Diet Assoc.* 1980;76:21–29. *Note:* Differences in BMI between LOV and NV were not statistically significant, but it was reported that 10 NV (42%) but only two LOV (15%) were considered obese.

6. Burr ML, Bates CJ, Fehily AM, Leger AS ST. Plasma cholesterol and blood pressure in vegetarians. *J Human Nutr.* 1981;35:437–441.

7. Armstrong BK, Brown JB, Clarke HT, et al. Diet and reproductive hormones: a study of vegetarian and nonvegetarian postmenopausal women. *J Natl Cancer Inst.* 1981;67:761–767.

8. Beauchene RE, Kunkel ME, Bredderman SH, Mason RL. Nutrient intake and physical measurements of aging vegetarian and nonvegetarian women. *J Am Coll Nutr.* 1982;1:131.

9. Goldin BR, Adlercreutz H, Gorbach SL, et al. Estrogen excretion patterns and plasma levels in vegetarian and omnivorous women. *N Engl J Med.* 1982;307:1542–1547.

10. Rouse IL, Armstrong BK, Beilin LJ. The relationship of blood pressure to diet and lifestyle in two religious populations. *J Hypertension.* 1983;1:65–71. *Note:* The NV consisted of Mormons.

11. Shultz TD, Leklem JE. Nutrient intake and hormonal status of premenopausal vegetarian Seventh-day Adventists and premenopausal nonvegetarians. *Nutr Cancer.* 1983;4:247–259.

12. Melby CL, Hyner GC, Zoog B. Blood pressure in vegetarians and non-vegetarians: a cross sectional analysis. *Nutr Res.* 1985;5:1077–1082. *Note:* The age of each group included data for males.

13. Carlson E, Kipps M, Lockie A, Thomson J. A comparative evaluation of vegan, vegetarian and omnivore diets. *J Plant Foods.* 1985;6:89–100.

14. Rana SK, Sanders TAB. Taurine concentrations in the diet, plasma, urine and breast milk of vegans compared with omnivores. *Br J Nutr.* 1986;56:17–27.

15. Levin N, Ratton J, Gilat T. Energy intake and body weight in ovo-lacto vegetarians. *J Clin Gastroenterol.* 1986;8:451–453.

16. Faber M, Gouws E, Benade AJS, Labadarios D. Anthropometric measurements, dietary intake and biochemical data of South African lacto-ovovegetarians. *S Afr Med J.* 1986;69:733–738.

17. Locong A. Nutritional status and dietary intake of a selected sample of young adult vegetarians. *Can Diet Assoc J.* 1986;47:101–106.

18. Sanders TAB, Key TJA. Blood pressure, plasma renin activity and aldosterone concentrations in vegans and omnivores. *Human Nutr: Appl Nutr.* 1987;41A:204–211.

19. Fentiman IS, Caleffi M, Wang DY, et al. The binding of blood-borne estrogens in normal vegetarian and omnivorous women and risk of breast cancer. *Nutr Cancer.* 1988;11:101–106.

20. Korpela JT, Adlercreutz H, Turunen MJ. Fecal free and conjugated bile acids and neutral sterols in vegetarians, omnivores, and patients with colorectal cancer. *Scand J Gastroenterol.* 1988;23:277–283.

21. Tylavsky FA, Anderson JJB. Dietary factors in bone health of elderly lactoovovegetarian and omnivorous women. *Am J Clin Nutr.* 1988;48:842–849.

22. Worthington-Roberts BS, Breskin MW, Monsen ER. Iron status of premenopausal women in a university community and its relationship to habitual dietary sources of protein. *Am J Clin Nutr.* 1988;47:275–279.

23. Kelsay JL, Frazier CW, Prather E, Canary JJ, Clark WM, Powell AS. Impact of variation in carbohydrate intake on mineral utilization by vegetarians. *Am J Clin Nutr.* 1988;48:875–879.

24. Hunt IF, Murphy NJ, Henderson C, et al. Bone mineral content in postmenopausal women: comparison of omnivores and vegetarians. *Am J Clin Nutr.* 1989;50:517–523.

25. Adlercreutz H, Fotsis T, Hockerstedt K, et al. Diet and urinary estrogen profile in premenopausal omnivorous and vegetarian women and in premenopausal women with breast cancer. *J Steroid Biochem.* 1989;34:527–530.

26. Marsh AG, Christensen DK, Sanchez TV, Mickelson O, Chaffee FL. Nutrient similarities and differences of older lacto-ovo-vegetarian and omnivorous women. *Nutr Rep Int.* 1989;39:19–24.

27. Nieman DC, Underwood BC, Sherman KM, Arabatizis K, Barbosa JC, Johnson M, Shulz TD. Dietary status of Seventh-Day Adventist vegetarian and non-vegetarian elderly womn. *J Am Diet Assoc.* 1989;89:1763–1769.

28. Millet P, Guilland JC, Fuchs F, Klepping J. Nutrient intake and vitamin status of healthy French vegetarians and nonvegetarians. *Am J Clin Nutr.* 1989;50:718–727.

29. Adlercreutz H, Hamalainen E, Gorbach SL, Goldin BR, Woods MN, Dwyer JT. Diet and plasma androgens in postmenopausal vegetarian and omnivorous women and postmenopausal women with breast cancer. *Am J Clin Nutr.* 1989;49:433–442.

30. Barbosa JC, Shultz TD, Filley SJ, Nieman DC. The relationship among adiposity, diet, and hormone concentrations in vegetarian and nonvegetarian postmenopasual women. *Am J Clin Nutr.* 1990;51:798–803. *Note:* Among the vegetarians, 6 were LV and 6 were LOV, two of whom ate fish.

31. Löwik MRH, Schrijver J, van den Berg H, Hulshof KFAM, Wedel M, Ockhuizen T. Effect of dietary fiber on the vitamin B6 status among vegetarian and nonvegetarian elderly (Dutch Nutrition Surveillance System). *J Am College Nutr.* 1990;9:241–249.

32. Reddy S, Sanders TAB. Haematological studies on premenopausal Indian and Caucasian vegetarians compared with Caucasian omnivores. *Br J Nutr.* 1990;64:331–338.

33. Thorogood M, Roe L, McPherson K, Mann J. Dietary intake and plasma lipid levels: lessons from a study of the diet of health conscious groups. *Br Med J.* 1990;300:1297–1301.

34. Oberlin P, Melby CL, Poehlman ET. Resting energy expenditures in young vegetarian and nonvegetarian women. *Nutr Res.* 1990;10:39–49.

35. Pedersen AB, Bartholomew MJ, Dolence LA, Aljadir LP, Netteburg KL, Lloyd T. Menstrual differences due to vegetarian and nonvegetarian diets. *Am J Clin Nutr.* 1991;53:879–885.

36. Krajcovicová-KudláckKovlá M, Simoncic R, Béderová A, Ondreicka R, Klvanová R. Selected parameters of lipid metabolism in young vegetarians. *Ann Nutr Metab.* 1994;38:331–335. *Note:* One-half of the vegetarians were LV, one-half were LOV.

37. Melby CL, Toohey M, Cebrick J. Blood pressure and blood lipids among vegetarian, semivegetarian, and nonvegetarian African Americans. *Am J Clin Nutr.* 1994;59:103–109. *Note:* All subjects were black Seventh-day Adventists, of the 66 vegetarians, 16 were vegans, and 50 were lactoovo vegetarians, there were 46 women and 20 men. Of the nonvegetarians, 34 were women and 11 men.

38. Janelle KC, Barr SI. Nutrient intakes and eating behavior scores of vegetarian and nonvegetarian women. *JADA.* 1995;95:180–189.

39. Kadrabova J, Madaric A, Kováciková, Ginter E. Selenium status, plasma zinc, copper, and magnesium in vegetarians. *Biological Trace Element Res.* 1995;50:13–24.

APPENDIX E

Anthropometric Data of Adult Male Vegetarians and Nonvegetarians

(REF)/year	Group[1]/(N)	SDA/NSDA[3]	Age	Height (cm)	Weight (kg)	Body Mass Index (kg/m²)	Body fat[3]
(1) 1954	LOV (15)	SDA/NSDA	55	172.7	73.6	24.7	
	NV (15)	SDA/NSDA	57	176.5	77.3	24.8	
(2) 1975	LOV (73)	NSDA	16–40		58.0		6.0
	NV (73)		16–40		73.0		17.0
(3) 1980	LOV (25)	NSDA	40				39.2
	NV (211)		50				49.3
(4) 1980	LOV (15)	NSDA	28	179.2	72.6	22.6	14.4
	NV (25)		27	179.0	78.4	24.5	17.8
(5) 1981	LOV (8)	NSDA	40			20.5	
	NV (50)		44			24.5	
	LOV (21)		69			22.7	
	NV (32)		69			24.9	
(6) 1982	LOV (52)	NSDA	35	180.0	69.0	21.4	
	NV (56)		33	178.0	77.0	24.4	
(7) 1983	LOV (47)	SDA	33	173.2	68.8	22.9	9.2
	NV (59)	NSDA	34	175.3	77.3	25.1	10.3
(8) 1984	LOV (36)	NSDA	31	179.0	74.2	23.1	24.6
	NV (18)		31	179.0	75.8	23.7	27.2
(9) 1985	LOV (41)	SDA	51			25.3	
	NV (12)		51			27.1	
(10) 1985	LOV (4)	NSDA	27–49			22.0	
	VEG (5)		27–49			23.0	
	NV (5)		27–49			24.0	

(REF)/year	Group[1]/(N)	SDA/NSDA[3]	Age	Height (cm)	Weight (kg)	Body Mass Index (kg/m²)	Body fat[3]
(11) 1985	LOV (12)	SDA	57	180.8	84.0	25.7	21.6
	NV (8)	NSDA	56	180.6	84.4	25.8	20.9
(12) 1986	LOV (14)	NSDA	28	173.0	63.7	21.3	
	NV (14)		21	175.0	66.4	21.7	
(13) 1986	LOV (60)	NSDA	55	169.0	64.9	22.7	
	NV (53)		50	172.1	75.1	25.4	
(14) 1986	VEG (8)	NSDA	18–40			21.0	
	OMN (8)		18–40			23.0	
(15) 1986	LOV (14)	SDA/NSDA	18–40	178.0	75.7	23.9	18.5
	NV (10)	NSDA	18–40	177.8	77.8	24.6	15.4
(16) 1987	VEG (11)	NSDA	32			21.1	8.8
	NV (11)		31			21.8	10.7
(17) 1988	LOV (14)	NI	23	181.0	69.7	20.9	
	NV (22)	NI	23	184.0	74.5	22.0	
(18) 1988	LOV (14)	SDA/NSDA	34	175.7	73.2	23.7	
	NV (13)	NSDA	35	174.3	76.6	25.2	
(19) 1989	LOV (11)	NSDA	37	173.0	63.4	21.2	
	NV (33)		40	175.0	76.0	24.7	
(20) 1989	LOV (15)	NSDA	29	174.0	64	20.9	
	NV (14)		27	177.0	74	23.4	
(21) 1990	LOV (20)	SDA	26	186.0	73.9	21.3	8.6
	VEG (15)	SDA	30	179.3	67.2	20.8	8.0
	NV (18)	SDA	26	178.2	75.2	23.6	14.0
(22) 1990	LOV (15)	NSDA	82		67.7	23.8	
	NV (225)		72		76.3	25.6	

(REF)/year	Group[1]/(N)	SDA/NSDA[3]	Age	Height (cm)	Weight (kg)	Body Mass Index (kg/m²)	Body fat[3]
(23) 1990	LOV (26)	NSDA	41			23.1	
	VEG (26)	NSDA	41			22.3	
	NV (26)	NSDA	41			23.1	
(24) 1994	LOV (31)	NSDA	23	180.3	71.6	22.0	
	NV (24)	NSDA	26	178.4	74.3	23.3	
(25) 1994	LVVEG (17)	NI	25	178.0	75.0	23.7	85.0
	NV (40)	NI	24	178.0	76.0	24.0	93.0
(26) 1995	LOV (22)	NSDA	20–57			22.3	
	NV (22)	NSDA	20–57			25.2	

Notes: [1]Abbreviations: LV, lactovegetarian; LOV, lacto-ovo vegetarian; VEG, vegan; NV, nonvegetarian; NI, not indicated; SDA, Seventh-day Adventist; and NSDA, non Seventh-day Adventist.

[2]SDA indicates the vegetarians were specifically identified as Seventh-day Adventists whereas NSDA indicates the vegetarians were not exclusively SDAs although some SDAs may have been included in the vegetarian group. NI indicates the process by which subjects were recruited for the study was not indicated or the extent to which SDAs comprised the vegetarian groups was not possible to determine by the information provided.

[3]Reference 2, body fat calculated from subscapular thickness (mm), references 3, 15, and 16, from sum of skinfold thickness (mm) at triceps, forearm, subscapular and suprailiac sites (data for nonvegetarians for reference 16 came from the Ten-State Nutrition Survey, 1968-1970: III Clinical, Anthropetry, Dental. DHEW Publ No. (HSM) 72:8131, 1972.), references 4 and 7, from triceps skinfold thickness (mm), reference 8 from sum of triceps and subscapular skinfolds (mm), references 11 and 21 from skinfold thickness (mm) at chest, abdomen, and thigh, and reference 24, from abdomen, axilla, biceps, calf, chest, subscapula, suprailiac, thigh and triceps skinfolds (mm).

ANNOTATED REFERENCES

1. Hardinge MG, Stare FJ. Nutritional studies of vegetarians. 1. Nutritional, physical, and laboratory studies. *J Clin Nutr*. 1954;2:73–82.

2. Sacks FM, Castelli WP, Donner A, Kass EH. Plasma lipids and lipoproteins in vegetarians and controls. *N Engl J Med*. 1975;292:1148–1151. *Note:* Vegetarians consisted of macrobiotics 40% of whom consumed fish once per week or more, 28% consumed dairy products and 11% consumed eggs. Values presented for males actually include 42 females in both the LOV and NV groups.

3. Haines AP, Chakrabarti R, Fisher D, Meade TW, North WRS, Stirling Y. Haemostatic variables in vegetarians and non-vegetarians. *Thrombosis Res*. 1980;19:139–148.

4. Taber LAL, Cook RA. Dietary and anthropometric assessment of adult omnivores, fish-eaters, and lacto-ovo-vegetarians. *J Am Diet Assoc*. 1980;76:21–29.

5. Burr ML, Bates CJ, Fehily AM, Leger AS ST. Plasma cholesterol and blood pressure in vegetarians. *J Human Nutr*. 1981;35:437–441.

6. Knuiman JT, West CE. The concentration of cholesterol in serum and in various serum lipoproteins in macrobiotic, vegetarian and non-vegetarian men and boys. *Atherosclerosis*. 1982;43:71–82.

7. Rouse IL, Armstrong BK, Beilin LJ. The relationship of blood pressure to diet and lifestyle in two religious populations. *J Hypertension*. 1983;1:65–71.

8. Latta D, Liebman M. Iron and zinc status of vegetarian and nonvegetarian males. *Nutr Rep Int*. 1984;30:141–149.

9. Melby CL, Hyner GC, Zoog B. Blood pressure in vegetarians and non-vegetarians: a cross sectional analysis. *Nutr Res*. 1985;5:1077–1082.

10. Carlson E, Kipps M, Lockie A, Thomson J. A comparative evaluation of vegan, vegetarian and omnivore diets. *J Plant Foods*. 1985;6:89–100.

11. Howie BJ, Shultz TD. Dietary and hormonal interrelationships among vegetarian Seventh-Day Adventists and nonvegetarian men. *Am J Clin Nutr*. 1985;42:127–134.

12. Locong A. Nutritional status and dietary intake of a selected sample of young adult vegetarians. *Can Diet Assoc J*. 1986;47:101–106.

13. Levin N, Ratton J, Gilat T. Energy intake and body weight in ovo-lacto vegetarians. *J Clin Gastroenterol*. 1986;8:451–453.

14. Rana SK, Sanders TAB. Taurine concentrations in the diet, plasma, urine and breast milk of vegans compared with omnivores. *Br J Nutr*. 1986;56:17–27.

15. Faber M, Gouws E, Benade AJS, Labadarios D. Anthropometric measurements, dietary intake and biochemical data of South African lacto-ovo vegetarians. *S Afr Med J*. 1986;69:733–738.

16. Sanders TAB, Key TJA. Blood pressure, plasma renin activity and aldosterone concentrations in vegans and omnivores. *Human Nutr: Appl Nutr*. 1987;41A:204–211.

17. Aalberts JS, Weegels PL, van der Hijden L, et al. Calcium supplementation: effect on blood pressure and urinary mineral excretion in normotensive male lactoovovegetarians and omnivores. *Am J Clin Nutr*. 1988;48:131–138.

18. Kelsay JL, Frazier CW, Prather E, Canary JJ, Clark WM, Powell AS. Impact of variation in carbohydrate intake on mineral utilization by vegetarians. *Am J Clin Nutr*. 1988;48:875–879.

19. Millet P, Guilland JC, Fuchs F, Klepping J. Nutrient intake and vitamin status of healthy French vegetarians and nonvegetarians. *Am J Clin Nutr*. 1989;50:718–727.

20. Bélanger A, Locong A, Noel C, Cusan L, Dupont A, Prévost J, Caron S, Sévigny J. Influence of diet on plasma steroid and sex plasma binding globulin levels in adult men. *J Steroid Biochem*. 1989;32:829–833.

21. Ross JK, Pusateri DJ, Shultz TD. Dietary and hormonal evaluation of men at different risks for prostate cancer: fiber intake, excretion, and composition, with in vitro evidence for an association between steroid hormones and specific components. *Am J Clin Nutr*. 1990;51:365–370.

22. Löwik MRH, Schrijver J, van den Berg H, Hulshof KFAM, Wedel M, Ockhuizen T. Effect of dietary fiber on the vitamin B_6 status among vegetarian and nonvegetarian elderly (Dutch Nutrition Surveillance System). *J Am College Nutr*. 1990;9:241–249.

23. Thorogood M, Roe L, McPherson K, Mann J. Dietary intake and plasma lipid levels: lessons from a study of the diet of health conscious groups. *Br Med J*. 1990;300:1297–1301.

24. Krajcovicová-KudlácKovlá M, Simoncic R, Béderová A, Ondreicka R, Klvanová R. Selected parameters of lipid metabolism in young vegetarians. *Ann Nutr Metab*. 1994;38:331–335. *Notes:* One-third of the vegetarians were LV, 2/3 were LOV.

25. Toth MJ, Poehlman ET. Sympathetic nervous system activity and resting metabolic rate in vegetarians. *Metabolism*. 1994;43:621–625. *Note:* Among the vegetarians, 10 were LV, and 7 were VEG.

26. Kadrabova J, Madaric A, Kováciková, Ginter E. Selenium status, plasma zinc, copper, and magnesium in vegetarians. *Biological Trace Element Res*. 1995;50:13–24.

Intake Ratios of N-6 to N-3 Fatty Acids on Vegetarian and Nonvegetarian Diets

Dietary Intake Ratios fo N-6 (Linolenic acid) to N-3 (α-Lenolenic acid) Fatty Acids among Vegetarians and Nonvegetarians

(Ref)/ year	Group[1]/ Gender (N)	Country	Age (years)	Linoleic acid (grams)	α-Linolenic acid (grams)	Linoleic: α-Linolenic acid acid (g:g)
(1)	LOV-F (15)	United	NI	10.5	0.2	52.5
1962	NV-F (15)	States		11.2	0.5	22.4
	LOV-M (15)			14.8	0.4	37.0
	NV-M (15)			26.3	0.7	37.6
(2)	VEG M (10)	Great	NI	31.9	1.8	17.7
1984	NV M (12)	Britain		10.7	1.0	10.7
	VEG F (10)			21.4	1.2	17.8
	NV F (12)			9.10	1.1	8.3
(3)	VEG M/F (18)	Great	5.8–12.8	16.8	0.38	44.2
1992		Britain				
(4)	LV M (23)	Taiwan	22.6	25.1	3.6	7.0
1993	NV M (20)		20.6	33.2	2.7	12.3
	LV F (32)		24.8	29.5	3.7	8.0
	NV F (39)		20.3	37.2	2.3	16.2
(5)	LOV M (16)	Great	21–40	19.2	2.1	9.1
1993	VEG M (18)	Britain	21–40	28.6	2.0	14.3
	NV M (386)		NI	14.5	2.0	7.3
	LOV F (36)		21.40	18.5	1.7	10.9
	VEG F (20)		21.40	22.4	1.5	14.9
	NV F (377)		NI	10.4	1.4	7.4

Notes: [1]Abbreviations: LV, lactovegetarian, LOV, lacto-ovo vegetarian, VEG, vegan, and NV, nonvegetarian, NI, not indicated.

ANNOTATED REFERENCES

1. Hardinge MG, Crooks H, Stare FJ. Nutritional studies of vegetarians. IV. Dietary fatty acids and serum cholesterol levels. *Am J Clin Nutr.* 1962;10:516–524.

2. Roshanai F, Sanders TAB. Assessment of fatty acid intakes in vegans and omnivores. *Human Nutr: Applied Nutr.* 1984;38A:345–354.

3. Sanders TAB, Manning J. The growth and development of vegan children. *J Human Nutr Diet.* 1992;5:11–21. *Note:* Values for linoleic and linolenic acid were converted from percentage of calories to grams per day.

4. Pan W-H, Chin C-J, Sheu C-T, Lee M-H. Hemostatic factors and blood lipids in young Buddhist vegetarians and omnivores. *Am J Clin Nutr.* 1993;58:354–359.

5. Draper A, Lewis J, Malhotra N, Wheeler E. The energy and nutrient intakes of different types of vegetarian: A case for supplements. *Br J Nutr.* 1993;69:3–19. *Note:* Values for nonvegetarians from a separate nationwide survey. Values are for polyunsaturated fat.

APPENDIX G

Protein, Calcium, Phosphorus, Sodium, and Potassium Intakes of Adult Vegetarians and Nonvegetarians

(Ref)/ year	Group¹/ Gender/(N)	Country	Kcal	Protein (grams)	Protein % Kcal	Calcium (mg)	Calcium (mg): Protein (g)	Phosphorus (mg)	Calcium: Phosphorus	Sodium (mg)	Potassium (mg)
(1) 1954	LOV M (15)	United States	3020	98.0	13.0	1700	17.3	2200	0.77		
	VEG M (14)		3260	83.0	10.2	1100	13.3	1900	0.58		
	NV M (15)		3720	125.0	13.4	1400	11.2	2200	0.64		
	LOV F (15)		2450	82.0	13.4	1600	19.5	1800	0.89		
	VEG F (11)		2400	61.0	10.2	900	14.8	1400	0.64		
	NV F (15)		2690	94.0	14.0	1000	10.6	1600	0.63		
(2) 1963	LOV F (26)	Australia	1980	52.8	10.7	813	15.4				
	NV F (25)		2115	64.6	12.2	661	10.2				
(3) 1978	LOV F (42)	United States	1600	65.0	16.3	1017	15.6	1325	0.77	2221	2817
	NV F (36)		1579	67.0	17.0	784	11.7	1114	0.70	2083	2467
(4) 1980	LOV M/F (57)	United States	2270	69.0	12.2	1200	17.4	1564	0.77	1755	3643
	LV M/F (14)		1830	56.0	12.2	856	15.3	1311	0.65	1203	4203
	VEG M/F (8)		1665	34.0	8.2	535	15.7	827	0.64	251	4127
	NV F (41)		2072	84.0	16.2	1099	13.1	1444	0.76	2289	2650
(5) 1980	LOV M (15)	United States	2624	90.0	13.7	1481	16.5	2078	0.71		
	NV M (25)		2684	112.0	16.7	1154	10.3	1889	0.61		
	LOV F (13)		2174	79.0	14.5	1386	17.5	1855	0.75		
	NV F (24)		1859	76.0	16.4	898	11.8	1240	0.72		
(6) 1981	LOV F (5)	United States	1329	51.0	15.3	723	14.2	962	0.75	1656	2356
(7) 1982	LOV F (101)	United States	1565	59.4	15.2	825	13.9	1188	0.69		
	NV F (107)		1573	68.4	17.4	782	11.4	1153	0.68		
(8) 1983	LOV M (18)	United States		79.1		1409	17.8	1536	0.92		

(Ref)/ year	Group'l/ Gender/(N)	Country	Kcal	Protein (grams)	Protein % Kcal	Calcium (mg)	Calcium (mg): Protein (g)	Phosphorus (mg)	Calcium: Phosphorus	Sodium (mg)	Potassium (mg)
(9) 1983	LOV M (20)	United States	2324	74.0	12.7	993	13.4				
	NV M (17)		2652	97.0	14.6	1244	12.8				
	LOV F (31)		1776	60.0	13.5	782	13.0				
	NV F (36)		1754	62.0	14.1	841	13.6				
(10) 1984	LOV M (25)	United States	2128	70.0	13.2	1188	17.0	1463	0.81		
	VEG M (9)		2259	66.0	11.7	762	11.5	1314	0.58		
	NV M (25)		2335	102.0	17.5	875	8.60	1406	0.62		
	LOV F (25)		1615	52.0	12.9	921	17.7	1076	0.86		
	VEG F (9)		1497	48.0	12.8	541	11.3	860	0.63		
	NV F (25)		1821	67.0	14.7	803	12.0	1117	0.72		
(11) 1985	LOV M/F (9)	Great Britain	91.8	123.7		1207				2688	4676
	VEG M/F (10)		98.0	110.2		493				2935	4855
	NV M/F (10)		100.9	134.7		937				3186	3362
(12) 1985	LOV M (17)	Great Britain	2290	66.0	11.5	1109	16.8				
	VEG M (17)		2381	61.0	10.2	577	9.50				
	NV M (17)		2313	84.0	14.5	1118	13.30				
(13) 1986	LOV M (14)	South Africa	2717	77.6	11.4	1264	16.3	1714			4092
	NV M (10)		3167	111.6	14.1	997	8.90	1756			3798
	LOV F (19)		1916	57.8	12.1	1003	17.4	1235			2911
	NV F (12)		1890	68.9	14.6	749	10.9	1152			2449
(14/15) 1986	LOV M (60)	Israel	3290	99.5	12.1	1374	13.8				
	NV M (53)		2896	121.0	16.7	1198	9.90				
	LOV F (32)		2544	74.0	11.6	1162	15.7				
	NV F (60)		2389	112.3	18.8	1142	10.2				
(16) 1986	LOV M (14)	Canada	2401	71.0	11.8	1207	17.0			3023	3656
	NV M (14)		2809	99.0	14.1	1320	13.3			3116	3588

(Ref)/ year	Group[1]/ Gender/(N)	Country	Kcal	Protein (grams)	Protein % Kcal	Calcium (mg)	Calcium (mg): Protein (g)	Phosphorus (mg)	Calcium: Phosphorus	Sodium (mg)	Potassium (mg)
	LOV F (22)	Great Britain	1760	64.0	14.5	1179	18.4			1999	3182
	NV F (18)		2097	80.0	15.3	956	12.0			2747	2691
(17) 1987	VEG M (11)		2643	73.0	11.0	671	9.2			2806	5382
	NV M (11)		2381	92.0	15.4	1089	11.8			3197	4056
	VEG F (11)		1881	55.0	11.6	437	7.9			1817	3666
	NV F (11)		1833	69.0	15.1	976	14.1			2461	3276
(18) 1988	LOV M (47)	Australia	2610	91.7	14.1					3726	4368
	NV M (59)		2767	103.6	15.0					3565	3588
	LOV F (51)		2036	72.1	14.2					3013	3432
	NV F (54)		2008	79.4	15.8					2507	2964
(19) 1988	LOV F (88)	United States	1533	54.6	14.2	823	15.1	1112	0.74	1923	2622
	NV F (278)		1633	69.9	17.1	902	12.9	1233	0.73	1897	2554
(20) 1988	LOV M (14)	United States	2444	78.2	12.8	1294	16.5				
	NV M (13)		2329	81.1	13.9	879	10.8				
	LOV F (15)		1742	53.9	12.4	860	16.0				
	NV F (16)		1656	59.2	14.3	641	10.8				
(21) 1989	LOV F (144)	United States	1474	51.8	14.1	748	14.4	1050	0.71		
	NV F (146)		1563	63.2	16.2	772	12.2	1147	0.67		
(22) 1989	LOV F (10)	United States	1612	56.0	13.9	898	16.0	1109			
	NV F (10)		1641	68.0	16.6	712	10.5	1079			
(23) 1989	LOV-B M/F (51)	United States	2406	66.8	11.1	820	12.3	1219	0.67	2385	3721
	NV-B M/F (49)		2504	97.1	15.5	960	9.9	1534	0.63	2833	3938
	LOV-W M/F (163)		2340	79.9	13.7	1113	13.9	1646	0.68	2815	4553
	NV-W M/F (89)		2225	80.8	14.5	1103	13.7	1526	0.72	2841	3945
(24) 1989	LOV F (23)	United States	1452	46.8	12.9	628	13.4	889	0.70	1930	2628
	NV F (14)		1363	55.0	16.1	633	11.5	892	0.71	1936	2342

(Ref)/year	Group[1]/Gender(N)	Country	Kcal	Protein (grams)	Protein % Kcal	Calcium (mg)	Calcium (mg): Protein (g)	Phosphorus (mg)	Calcium: Phosphorus	Sodium (mg)	Potassium (mg)
(25) 1990	LOV M (18)	Netherlands	1960	59.8	12.2	1219	20.4				
	NV M		2412	82.2	13.6	1128	13.7				
	LOV F (26)		1667	54.4	13.1	1141	21.0				
	NV F		1879	70.1	14.9	1013	14.5				
(26) 1991	LOV F (23)	United States	1939	62.0	12.8	973	15.7	1318	0.74	2462	3221
	NV F (36)		1835	76.0	16.6	770	10.1	1219	0.63	2815	2747
(27) 1991	LOV F (34)	United States	1819	63.0	13.9	931	14.8	1159	0.80	2304	2803
	NV F (41)		1700	75.0	17.6	873	11.6	1138	0.77	2649	2664
(28) 1991	LOV M/F (79)	United States	2800	95.9	13.7	1521	15.9				
	NV M/F (4821)		2980	111.0	14.9	1310	11.8				
(29) 1992	LOV F (28)	United States	1652	62.6	15.2	821	13.1	1155	0.71	2202	3012
	NV F (28)		1657	76.5	18.5	863	11.3	1250	0.69	2285	2687
(30) 1993	LOV M (16)	Great Britain	2238	66.0	11.8	995	15.1				
	VEG M (18)		2190	65.0	11.9	582	9.0				
	NV M (387)		2452	87.0	14.2	1006	11.6				
	LOV F (36)		1826	56.0	12.3	891	15.9				
	VEG F (20)		1750	47.0	10.7	497	10.6				
	NV F (377)		1733	66.0	15.2	790	12.0				
(31) 1993	LOV M/F (14)	Finland	2029					1339			
	LV M/F (6)		1913					1235			
	VEG M/F (10)		1927					1207			
	NV F (12)		1778					1351			
(32) 1994	LOV M/F (50)	New Zealand	2272	69.7	12.3	906	13.0			2800	
	VEG F (5)		1842	55.2	12.0	507	9.2			2400	
	NV M/F (50)		2608	83.2	12.8	954	11.5			3600	
(33) 1994	LV/VEG M (17)	United States	3005	100.0	13.3					3359	
	NV M (40)		2906	106.0	14.6					3575	

(Ref)/ year	Group[1]/ Gender/(N)	Country	Kcal	Protein (grams)	Protein % Kcal	Calcium (mg)	Calcium (mg): Protein (g)	Phosphorus (mg)	Calcium: Phosphorus	Sodium (mg)	Potassium (mg)
(34)	LOV M/F (64)	United	2272	72.7	12.8	720	9.9			2841	3661
1994	NV M/F (44)	States	2603	95.6	14.7	879	9.2			2833	3903
(35)	LV F (15)	Canada	2024	57.1	11.3	875	15.3	1125	0.78	2175	2884
1995	VEG F (8)		1923	51.9	10.8	578	11.1	1217	0.47	2275	3587
	NV F (22)		2086	77.1	14.8	950	12.3	1409	0.67	2789	3042

Note: [1]Abbreviations: LV, lactovegetarian, LOV, lacto-ovo vegetarian, VEG, vegan, and NV, nonvegetarian; B, Black and W, White.

ANNOTATED REFERENCES

1. Hardinge MG, Stare FJ. Nutritional studies of vegetarians. *Am J Clin Nutr.* 1954;2:73–82.

2. Hitchcock NE, English RM. A comparison of food consumption in lacto-ovo-vegetarians and non-vegetarians. *Food Nutr Notes Rev.* 1963;20:141–146.

3. Mason RL, Kunkel ME, Davis TA, Beauchene RE. Nutrient intakes of vegetarian and nonvegetarian women. *Tenn Farm Home Sci.* 1978;1:18–20.

4. Freeland-Graves JH, Bodzy PW, Eppright MA. Zinc status of vegetarians. *J Am Diet Assoc.* 1980;77:655–661. *Notes:* Of the 79 total vegetarians, 44 were reportedly male, but data for the individual vegetarians groups were not provided.

5. Taber LAL, Cook RA. Dietary and anthropometric assessment of adult omnivores, fish-eaters, and lacto-ovo-vegetarians. *J Am Diet Assoc.* 1980;76:21–29.

6. King JC, Stein T, Doyle M. Effect of vegetarianism on the zinc status of pregnant women. *Am J Clin Nutr.* 1981;34:1049–1055.

7. Beauchene RE, Kunkel ME, Bredderman SH, Mason RL. Nutrient intake and physical measurements of aging vegetarian and nonvegetarian women. *J Am Coll Nutr.* 1982;1:131.

8. Read MH, Thomas DC. Nutrient and food supplement practices of lacto-ovo vegetarians. *J Am Diet Assoc.* 1983;82:401–404.

9. Shultz TD, Leklem JE. Dietary status of Seventh-day Adventists and nonvegetarians. *J Am Diet Assoc.* 1983;83:27–33.

10. Calkins BM, Whittaker DJ, Nair PP, Rider AA, Turjman N. Diet, nutrition intake, and metabolism in populations at high and low risk for colon cancer. *Am J Clin Nutr.* 1984;40:896–905.

11. Carlson E, Kipps M, Lockie A, Thomson J. A comparative evaluation of vegan, vegetarian and omnivore diets. *J Plant Foods.* 1985;6:89–100. *Note:* The LOV, VEG, and NV groups contained 4, 5, and 5 males, respectively. Values for protein and calories are expressed as a percentage of the recommended intake for Great Britain. Calcium intake is based on the percentage of the recommended intake value of 500 mg indicated in the text. Sodium and phosphorus intakes are taken directly from the text.

12. Davies GJ, Crowder M, Dickerson JWT. Dietary fibre intakes of individuals with different eating patterns. *Human Nutr: Appl Nutr.* 1985;39A:139–148.

13. Faber M, Gouws E, Benadé AJS, Labadarios D. Anthropometric measurements, dietary intake and biochemical data of South African lacto-ovovegetarians. *S Afr Med J.* 1986;69:733–738.

14. Levin N, Rattan J, Gilat T. Mineral intake and blood levels in vegetarians. *Isr J Med Sci.* 1986;22:105–108.

15. Levin N, Rattan J, Gilat T. Energy intake and body weight in ovo-lacto vegetarians. *J Clin Gastroenterol.* 1986;8:451–453.

16. Locong A. Nutritional status and dietary intake of a selected sample of young adult vegetarians. *Can Med Assoc J.* 1986;47:101–106.

17. Sanders TAB, Key TJA. Blood pressure, plasma renin activity and aldosterone concentrations in vegans and omnivore controls. *Human Nutr: Appl Nutr.* 1987;41A:204–211.

18. Rouse IL, Armstrong BK, Beilin LJ. The relationship of blood pressure to diet and lifestyle in two religious populations. *J Hypertension.* 1983;1:65–71.

19. Tylavsky FA, Anderson JJB. Dietary factors in bone health of elderly lactoovegetarian and omnivorous women. *Am J Clin Nutr.* 1988;48:842–849.

20. Kelsay JL, Frazier CW, Prather E, Canary JJ, Clark WM, Powell AS. Impact of variation in carbohydrate intake on mineral utilization by vegetarians. *Am J Clin Nutr.* 1988;48:875–879.

21. Hunt IF, Murphy NJ, Henderson C, et al. Bone mineral content in postmenopausal women: comparison of omnivores and vegetarians. *Am J Clin Nutr.* 1989;50:517–523.

22. Marsh AG, Christensen DK, Sanchez TV, Mickelsen O, Chaffee FL. Nutrient similarities and differences of older lacto-ovo-vegetarian and omnivorous women. *Nutr Rep Int.* 1989;39:19–24.

23. Melby CL, Goldflies DG, Hyner GC, Lyle RM. Relation between vegetarian/nonvegetarian diets and blood pressure in black and white adults. *Am J Public Health.* 1989;79:1283–1288. *Note:* Of the initial 114 black subjects, 89 were females and 25 were males. Of the intial 264 white subjects, 222 were female and 42 were male.

24. Nieman DC, Underwood BC, Sherman KM, et al. Dietary status of Seventh-Day Adventist vegetarian and non-vegetarian elderly women. *J Am Diet Assoc.* 1989;89:1763–1769.

25. Brants HAM, Löwik MRH, Westenbrink S, Hulshof KFAM, Kistemaker C. Adequacy of a vegetarian diet at old age (Dutch Nutrition Surveillance System). *J Am Coll Nutr.* 1990;9:292–302.

26. Lloyd T, Schaeffer JM, Walker MA, Demers LM. Urinary hormonal concentrations and spinal bone densities of premenopausal vegetarian and nonvegetarian women. *Am J Clin Nutr.* 1991;54:1005–1010.

27. Pedersen AB, Bartholomew MJ, Dolence LA, Aljadir LP, Netteburg KL, Lloyd T. Menstrual differences due to vegetarian and nonvegetarian diets. *Am J Clin Nutr.* 1991;53:879–885.

28. Slattery ML, Jacobs DR, Hilner JE Jr, Caan BJ, Van Horn L, Bragg C, Manolio TA, Kushi LH, Liu K. Meat consumption and its association with other diet and health factors in young adults: the CARDIA study. *Am J Clin Nutr.* 1991;54:930–935. *Note:* Of the 79 vegetarians, 57 (72%) were females and of the 4,821 nonvegetarians, 2,577 (53%) were females.

29. Tesar R, Notelovitz M, Shim E, Kauwell G, Brown J. Axial and peripheral bone density and nutrient intakes of postmenopausal vegetarian and omnivorous women. *Am J Clin Nutr.* 1992;56:699–704.

30. Draper A, Lewis J, Malhotra N, Wheeler E. The energy and nutrient intakes of different types of vegetarian: a case for supplements? *Br J Nutr.* 1993;69:3–19. *Note:* Data for nonvegetarians was taken from a separate nationwide survey.

31. Lamberg-Allardt C, Kärkkäinen M, Seppänen R, Biström H. Low serum 25-hydroxyvitamin D concentrations and secondary hyperparathyroidism in middle-aged white strict vegetarians. *Am J Clin Nutr.* 1993;58:684–689. *Note:* The LOV, LV, and VEG groups each contained 8, 3, and 10 females. Calcium intake estimate from figure in references.

32. Alexander D, Ball MJ, Mann J. Nutrient intake and haematological status of vegetarians and age-sex matched omnivores. *Eur J Clin Nutr.* 1994;48:538–546. *Note:* Data for the LOV group includes data for the VEG group, which are also listed separately. There were 36 females each in the LOV and NV groups.

33. Toth MJ, Poehlman ET. Sympathetic nervous system activity and resting metabolic rate in vegetarians. *Metabolism.* 1994;43:621–625. *Note:* Of the 17 vegetarians, 10 were LV and 7 were VEG.

34. Melby CL, Toohey M, Cebrick J. Blood pressure and blood lipids among vegetarian, semivegetarian, and nonvegetarian African Americans. *Am J Clin Nutr.* 1994;59:103–109. *Note:* All subjects were black Seventh-day Adventists. Of the 66 vegetarians, 16 were vegans, and 50 were lacto-ovo vegetarians, there were 46 women and 20 men. Of the nonvegetarians, 34 were women and 11 men.

35. Janelle KC, Barr SI. Nutrient intakes and eating behavior scores of vegetarian and nonvegetarian women. *J Am Diet Assoc.* 1995;95:180–185. *Note:* Of the 15 LV, 11 ate eggs.

APPENDIX H

Iron Intake and Status of Vegetarians and Nonvegetarians

(Ref)/ year	Group/ Gender(N)	Country	Age	Iron Intake (mg)	Serum Ferritin (ng/ml)[2]	Total Iron Binding Capacity[3]	Hemoglobin (g/dl)[4]	Hematocrit (%)	Plasma or Serum Iron[5]
(1) 1974	LOV M (187)	Australia	50				14.5	46.0	
	NV M (879)		49				14.6	46.4	
	LOV F (244)		51				13.1	41.9	
	NV F (1339)		49				13.2	42.4	
(2) 1981	LOV F (39)[6]	Canada	53	12.5		312.0	13.2		107.0
	LOV F (10)[6]		53			346.0	12.9		135.0
(3) 1984	LOV M (36)	United States	31	17.0		393.0		46.0	116.0
	NV M (18)		31	18.0		373.0		45.0	104.0
(4) 1986	LOV M (24)	Germany	29		537.0		14.9		89.3
	LOV F (24)		29		537.0		12.9		89.3
(5) 1986	LOV M (14)	South Africa	29	17.9	60.7				
	NV M (10)		29	17.9	146.8				
	NV F (19)		27	11.5	16.1				
	NV F (12)		27	11.7	47.3				
(6) 1986	LOV M (60)	Israel	55	37.0		351.6			103.9
	NV M (53)		50	25.8		393.3			93.8
	LOV F (32)		51	29.7		361.8			90.6
	NV F (60)		52	21.7		409.1			96.7
(7) 1986	LOV M (14)	Canada	28	16.5	88.0				
	NV M (14)		21	16.9	107.0				
	LOV F (22)		26	14.1	33.0				
	NV (18)		22	14.9	45.0				
(8) 1987	LOV MF (93)	Australia	29		45.0				
	NV MF (37)		31		70.0				

(Ref)/year	Group[1]/Gender/(N)	Country	Age	Iron Intake (mg)	Serum Ferritin (ng/ml)[2]	Total Iron Binding Capacity[3]	Hemoglobin (g/dl)[4]	Hematocrit (%)	Plasma or Serum Iron[5]
(9) 1988	LOV F (20)	United	29	11.8	21.0	360.0	13.3	39.0	
	NV F (16)	States	31	12.7	30.0	345.0	13.9	41.5	
(10) 1989	LV/VEG M/F (13)	Sweden	47–74		52.5		13.5		15.2
	NV M/F (6)		45–69		85.7		14.5		16.8
(11) 1989	LOV M (39)	Germany	45		56.2		14.3	42.6	76.9
	NV M (52)		38		93.0		14.2	42.5	83.6
	LOV F (11)		47		19.0		13.6	41.0	102.4
	NV F (8)		49		67.4		13.7	40.8	96.0
(12) 1990	LOV F (18)	Great		13.8	10.4				
	NV F (20)	Britain		12.1	18.0				
(13) 1990	LOV M (17)	Netherlands	65–97	13.7	18%		35%		12%
	NV M (54)		65+	13.1	2%		4%		9%
	LOV F (23)		65–97	12.2	9%		4%		13%
	NV F (54)		65+	11.4	11%		1%		0%
(14) 1992	LV M (64)	Thailand	36				16.4		
	NV M (20)		33				16.6		
	LV F (68)		33				13.7		
	NV F (270)		32				14.3		
(15) 1994	LOV M (14)	New	26–30	18.7	36.6				
	NV M (14)	Zealand	26–30	15.5	105.4				
	LOV F (36)		26–30	14.4	13.6				
	NV F (36)		26–30	13.7	33.6				
(16) 1995	LOV M (23)	Taiwan	23	18.4	47.0	69.0	9.2		23
	NV M (20)		21	16.1	91.0	64.0	9.4		16
	LOV F (32)		25	15.6	12.0	72.0	7.6		17
	NV F (39)		20	11.7	27.0	69.0	7.9		17

(Ref)/ year	Group[1]/ Gender/(N)	Country	Age	Iron Intake (mg)	Serum Ferritin (ng/ml)[2]	Total Iron Binding Capacity[3]	Hemoglobin (g/dl)[4]	Hematocrit (%)	Plasma or Serum Iron[5]
(17)	LOV-F (79)	Canada	18	11.2	18.2	77.0	13.8	41.0	13.5
1995	NV-F (29)		18	11.3	20.0	78.5	13.8	41.0	14.1

Notes: [1]Abbreviations: LV, lactovegetarian; LOV, lacto ovo-vegetarian; VEG, vegan; and NV, nonvegetarian.

[2]Values for reference 13 represent the percentage of each group considered deficient.

[3]Total iron binding capacity, references 2, 3, 6, 9 (µg/dL); references 16 and 17 (umol/L).

[4]Values for reference 13 represent the percentage of each group considered deficient and for reference 16, hemoglobin is expressed as umol/L.

[5]Plasma or serum iron; references 2, 3, 4, 6 and 11 (µg/dL); references 10, 16, and 17 (umol/L) and reference 13, the percentage of of each group considered deficient.

[6]The first group of LOV are individuals who did not take iron supplements, the second group consists of supplement users.

ANNOTATED REFERENCES

1. Armstrong BK, Davis RE, Nicol DJ, van Merwyk AJ, Larwood CJ. Hematological, vitamin B12, and folate studies on Seventh-day Adventist vegetarians. *Am J Clin Nutr.* 1974;27:712–718. *Note:* Data for nonvegetarians from a separate survey.

2. Anderson BM, Gibson RS, Sabry JH. The iron and zinc status of long-term vegetarian women. *Am J Clin Nutr.* 1981;34:1042–1048.

3. Latta D, Liebman M. Iron and zinc status of vegetarian and nonvegetarian males. *Nutr Rep Int.* 1984;30:141–149.

4. Ernst E, Pietsch L, Matrai A, Eisenberg J. Blood rheology in vegetarians. *Br J Nutr.* 1986;56:555–560. *Note:* There were equal numbers of men and women, values for serum ferritin, and plasma iron were reported for the entire group, not according to gender. The normal range for ferritin was indicated to be 300–3,000 µg/l; for hemoglobin (g/l), 140–180 (men) and 120–160 (women) and for plasma iron, 800–1,800 µg/l. Thus, although all values were within the normal range for ferritin and plasma iron, they were at the very low end of the range.

5. Faber M, Gouws E, Benadé AJS, Labadarios D. Anthropometric measurements, dietary intake and biochemical data of South African lacto-ovovegetarians. *S Afr Med J.* 1986;69:733–738.

6. Levin N, Rattan J, Gilat T. Mineral intake and blood levels in vegetarians. *Israel J Med Sci.* 1986;22:105–108.

7. Locong A. Nutritional status and dietary intake of a selected sample of young adult vegetarians. *Can Med Assoc J.* 1986:101–108.

8. Helman AD, Darnton-Hill I. Vitamin and iron status in new vegetarians. *Am J Clin Nutr.* 1987;45:785–789. *Note:* There were intially a total of 120 LOV equally divided between men and women but ferritin values were reported for only 93 LOV, the proportion of men and women was not reported specifically for this subset. The nonvegetarian group initially conisted of 53 subjects, 40 women and 13 men but ferritin values were reported for only 37 nonvegetarians, the proportion of men and women was not reported specifically for this subset. Given that ferritin values are generally lower in women, and the LOV group likely contained a greater proportion of women, differences between LOV and NV are actually underestimated.

9. Worthington-Roberts BS, Breskin MW, Monsen ER. Iron status of premenopausal women in a university community and its relationship to habitual dietary sources of protein. *Am J Clin Nutr.* 1988;47:275–279. *Note:* Values were estimated from figures in reference. Approximately 43% and 30% of the LOV and NV, respectively, had serum ferritin levels (15 µg/L) considered deficient by laboratory standards.

10. Brune M, Rossander L, Hallberg L. Iron absorption: no intestinal adaptation to a high-phytate diet. *Am J Clin Nutr.* 1989;49:542–545. *Note:* Among the 13 vegetarians, there were four VEGs and 9 LVs, there were 4 male vegetarians, one of which was vegan. Among the NV, there were 3 males and 3 females, 3 of the 6 nonvegetarians were blood donors.

11. Seiler D, Nagel D, Franz H, et al. Effects of long-distance running on iron metabolism and hematological parameters. *Int J Sports Med.* 1989;10:357–362. *Note:* All subjects were long-distance runners.

12. Reddy S, Sanders TAB. Haematological studies on premenopausal Indian and Caucasian vegetarians compared with Caucasian omnivores. *Br J Nutr.* 1990;64:331–338.

13. Brants HAM, Löwik MRH, Westenbrink S, Hulshof KFAM, Kistemaker C. Adequacy of a vegetarian diet at old age (Dutch Nutrition Surveillance System). *J Am College Nutr.* 1990;9:292–302. *Note:* Values refer to the percentage of individuals in each group that were below the cutoff points considered to be within the normal range; for serum ferritin, hemoglobin, and serum iron, cutoff points were 12 µg/L, 8.1 mmol/L, and 9.0 umol/l, respectively.

14. Tungtrongchitr R, Pongpaew P, Prayurahong B, et al. Vitamin B12, folic acid, and haematological status of 132 Thai vegetarians. *Inter J Vit Nutr Res.* 1993;63:201–207.

15. Alexander D, Ball MJ, Mann J. Nutrient intake and haematological status of vegetarians and age-sex matched omnivores. *Eur J Clin Nutr.* 1994;48:538–546. *Note:* Data for female LOV included 5 VEG.

16. Shaw N-S, Chin C-J, Pan W-H. A vegetarian diet rich in soybean products compromises iron status in young students. *J Nutr.* 1995;125:212–219. *Note:* The extent to which eggs and dairy were consumed by vegetarians could not be determined from the text.

17. Donovan UM, Gibson RS. Iron and zinc status of young women aged 14 to 19 years consuming vegetarian and omnivorous diets. *J Am Coll Nutr.* 1995;14:463–472. *Note:* Twenty-nine percent of the LOV and 17.2% of the NV had ferritin levels below the cutoff point (12 µg/L) considered to be deficient.

APPENDIX I

Mineral Intake of Adult Vegetarians and Nonvegetarians

(Ref)/year	Group/Gender (N)	Country	Age	Kcal	Iron (mg)	Zinc (mg)	Magnesium (mg)	Copper (mg)	Manganese (mg)	Selenium (ug)
(1) 1954	LOV M (15)	United States	55	3020	22.0					
	VEG M (14)		51	3260	30.0					
	NV M (15)		57	3720	22.0					
	LOV F (15)		58	2450	16.0					
	VEG F (11)		49	2400	25.0					
	NV F (15)		57	2690	17.0					
(2) 1963	LOV F (26)	Australia	18–40	1980	10.1					
	NV F (25)		18–40	2115	10.5					
(3) 1978	LOV F (42)	United States	57	1600	11.2					
	NV F (36)		59	1579	10.8					
(4) 1980	LOV M/F (57)	United States	18–40	2270	17.2	11.2		3.9		
	LV M/F (14)		18–40	1830	18.1	11.3		3.4		
	VEG M/F (8)		18–40	1665	17.1	7.9		3.7		
	NV F (41)		18–40	2072	12.7	12.7		3.4		
	LOV M (32)	United States	18–40			13.3				
	LV M (8)		18–40			13.5				
	VEG M (4)		18–40			14.1				
	NV M (1)		18–40			16.8				
	LOV F (25)	United States	18–40			8.5				
	LV F (6)		18–40			8.2				
	VEG F (4)		18–40			1.5				
	NV F (40)		18–40			10.1				
(5) 1980	LOV M (15)	United States	28	2624	21.0					
	NV M (25)		27	2684	16.0					

(Ref)/year	Group/Gender (N)	Country	Age	Kcal	Iron (mg)	Zinc (mg)	Magnesium (mg)	Copper (mg)	Manganese (mg)	Selenium (ug)
(6) 1980	LOV F (13)		26	2174	18.0					
	NV F (24)		26	1859	11.0					
	LOV	India	(NI)							92.7
	NV		(NI)							84.8
(7) 1981	LOV (49)	Canada	52	1630	12.5	9.2				
(8) 1981	LOV (5)	United States	22	1329	9.2	6.4	262	1.3		
(9) 1983	LOV M (20)	United STates	36	2324	16.0					
	NV M (17)		44	2652	16.0					
	LOV F (31)		31	1776	12.0					
	NV F (36)		36	1754	11.0					
(10) 1983	LOV F (36)	Canada	69	1615				2.1	4.4	113.0
	NV F (30)		60	1727				1.6	2.6	109.0
(11) 1984	LOV M (25)	United States	39–65	2128	21.3					
	VEG M (9)		39–65	2259	22.6					
	NV M (25)		39–65	2335	15.9					
	LOV F (25)		39–65	1615	21.5					
	VEG F (9)		39–65	1497	14.9					
	NV F (25)		39–65	1821	16.3					
(12) 1984	LOV M (36)	United States	31	2532	17.0					
	NV M (18)		31	2836	18.0					
(13) 1985	LOV M/F (17)	Great Britain	34	2290	14.8	9.2				
	VEG M/F (17)		31	2381	18.5	8.8				
	NV M/F (17)		35	2313	15.9	11.4				
(14) 1986	LOV M (14)	Canada	28	2401	16.5					
	NV M (14)		21	2809	16.9					

(Ref)/year	Group/Gender (N)	Country	Age	Kcal	Iron (mg)	Zinc (mg)	Magnesium (mg)	Copper (mg)	Manganese (mg)	Selenium (ug)
	LOV F (22)		26	1760	14.1					
	NV F (18)		22	2097	14.9					
(15) 1986	LOV M (14)	South Africa	18–40	2717	17.9	11.1	467	2.4		
	NV M (10)		18–40	3167	17.9	16.2	376	2.1		
	LOV F (19)		18–40	1916	11.5	7.4	282	1.5		
	NV F (12)		18–40	1890	11.7	9.7	244	1.4		
(16) 1986	LOV M (60)	Israel	55	3290	37.0	15.2	690			
	NV M (53)		50	2896	25.8	14.7	443			
	LOV F (32)		51	2544	29.7	11.9	533			
	NV F (60)		52	2389	21.7	12.5	358			
(17) 1987	VEG M (11)	Great Britain	32	2643	25.0		571			
	NV M (11)		31	2381	16.0		424			
	VEG F (11)		28	1881	16.0		462			
	NV F (11)		24	1833	14.0		371			
(18) 1988	LOV F (88)	United States	73	1533	10.7					
	NV F (278)		79	1633	10.2					
(19) 1988	LOV M (47)	Australia	33	2619			527			
	OMN M (59)		34	2777			366			
	LOV F (51)		34	2040			396			
	OMN F (54)		33	2010			289			
(20) 1988	LOV F (20)	United States	29	1814	11.8					
	NV F (16)		31	1788	12.7					
(21) 1988	LOV M (14)	United States	34	2444	17.9	12.7	382	1.8	5.1	
	NV M (13)		35	2329	14.8	11.6	309	1.3	3.3	
	LOV F (15)		34	1742	13.9	8.8	316	1.4	4.1	
	NV F (16)		34	1656	11.0	9.0	231	1.1	2.6	
(22) 1989	LOV F (23)	United States	72	1452	12.3	6.3	283	1.4	2.2	
	NV F (14)		71	1363	11.4	6.3	226	1.0	1.3	

(Ref)/year	Group[1]/Gender (N)	Country	Age	Kcal	Iron (mg)	Zinc (mg)	Magnesium (mg)	Copper (mg)	Manganese (mg)	Selenium (ug)
(23) 1989	LOV F (10)	United	67	1612	12.3					
	NV F (10)	States	64	1641	13.3					
(24) 1989	LOV F (144)	United	67	1474		7.2	312	1.4		
	NV F (146)	States	66	1563		8.8	294	1.4		
(25) 1989	BLOV M/F (51)	United	55				368			
	BNV M/F (49)	States	56				379			
	WLOV M/F (163)		52				468			
	W-NV (89)		53				364			
(26) 1989	LOV F (26)[3]	United	29							101.0
	NV F (12)[3]	States	29							106.0
(27) 1990	LOV M (18)	Netherlands	65-97	1960	13.7	8.5[4]				
	NV M		65+		13.1	10.3[4]				
	LOV F (26)		65-97	1667	12.2	7.6[4]				
	NV F		65+		11.4	9.3[4]				
(28) 1990	LOV F (22)	Great	30	1826	13.8			1.5		
	NV F (18)	Britain	34	1779	12.1			1.4		
(29) 1991	LOV F (23)	United	35	1939	17.5	8.2	370		2.6	
	NV F (36)	States	36	1835	13.4	11.3	267		1.4	
(30) 1991	LOV F (34)	United	36	1819	20.0	13.0	323			
	NV F (41)	States	29	1700	22.0	10.0	250			
(31) 1992	LOV F (28)	United	63	1652	13.0	7.2	318	1.4		16.9
	NV F (28)	States	63	1657	15.5	7.9	266	1.0		17.4
(32) 1993	LOV M (16)[5]	Great	21-40	2238	15.4	9.4	412	1.8		
	VEG M (18)[5]	Britain	21-40	2190	18.9	10.1	939	3.4		
	NV M (386)[5]		21-40	2452	15.0	11.8	342	1.7		
	LOV F (36)[5]		21-40	1826	15.0	8.8	423	2.1		
	VEG F (20)[5]		21-40	1750	14.8	7.0	538	2.4		
	NV F (377)[5]		21-40	1733	12.9	9.0	261	1.4		

(Ref)/ year	Group[1]/ Gender (N)	Country	Age	Kcal	Iron (mg)	Zinc (mg)	Magnesium (mg)	Copper (mg)	Manganese (mg)	Selenium (ug)
(33) 1994	LOV M/F (50)	New Zealand	27	2272	16.6	11.1				39.1
	VEG F (5)		27	1842	18.7	9.3				47.8
	NV M/F (50)		27	2608	14.6	11.9				35.5
	LOV M (14)				20.2					
	NV M (14)				17.4					
	LOV F (36)				15.5					
	VEG F (5)				18.7					
	NV F (36)				13.5					
(34) 1995	LV F (15)	Canada	26	2024	13.7	8.2	337	1.6		
	VEG F (8)		28	1923	17.7	8.5	396	2.2		
	NV F (22)		28	2086	15.3	11.1	303	1.4		

Notes: [1]Abbreviations: LV, lactovegetarian; LOV, lacto ovo-vegetarian; VEG, vegan; NV, nonvegetarian; and NI, not indicated.
[2]All subjects were lactating women.
[3]Data for NV from a separate nationwide survey, data for zinc not calculated at the individual levels, but based on the average consumption of food products.
[4]Data include nutrient supplements. Data for NV from a separate nationwide survey.

ANNOTATED REFERENCES

1. Hardinge MG, Stare FJ. Nutritional studies of vegetarians. *Am J Clin Nutr.* 1954;2:73–82.

2. Hitchcock NE, English RM. A comparison of food consumption in lacto-ovo-vegetarians and non-vegetarians. *Food Nutr Notes Rev.* 1963;20:141–146.

3. Mason RL, Kunkel ME, Ann Davis T, Beauchene RE. Nutrient intakes of vegetarian and nonvegetarian women. *Tenn Farm Home Science.* 1978;1:18–20.

4. Freeland-Graves JH, Bodzy PW, Eppright MA. Zinc status of vegetarians. *J Am Diet Assoc.* 1980;77:655–661. *Note:* Zinc values for the individual male and female groups are subsets of the combined male/female groups.

5. Taber LAL, Cook RA. Dietary and anthropometric assessment of adult omnivores, fish-eaters, and lacto-ovo-vegetarians. *J Am Diet Assoc.* 1980;76:21–29.

6. Ganapathy SN, Dhanda R. Selenium content of omnivorous and vegetarian diets. *Ind J Nutr Dietet.* 1980;17:53–59.

7. Anderson BM, Gibson RS, Sabry JH. The iron and zinc status of long-term vegetarian women. *Am J Clin Nutr.* 1981;34:1042–1048.

8. King JC, Stein JC, Doyle M. Effect of vegetarianism on the zinc status of pregnant women. *Am J Clin Nutr.* 1981;34:1049–1055.

9. Shultz TD, Leklem JE. Dietary status of Seventh-Day Adventists and nonvegetarians. *J Am Diet Assoc.* 1983;00:27–33.

10. Gibson RS, Anderson BM, Sabry JH. The trace metal status of a group of post-menopausal vegetarians. *J Am Diet Assoc.* 1983;82:246–250.

11. Calkins BM, Whittaker DJ, Nair PP, Rider AA, Turjman N. Diet, nutrition intake, and metabolism in populations at high and low risk for colon cancer. *Am J Clin Nutr.* 1984;40:896–905.

12. Latta D, Liebman M. Iron and zinc status of vegetarian and nonvegetarian males. *Nutr Rep Int.* 1984;30:141–149.

13. Davies GJ, Crowder M, Dickerson JWT. Dietary fibre intakes of individuals with different eating patterns. *Human Nutr: Appl Nutr.* 1985;39A:139–148.

14. Locong A. Nutritional status and dietary intake of a selected sample of young adult vegetarians. *Can Diet Assoc J.* 1986;47:101–106.

15. Faber M, Gouws E, Benadé AJS, Labadarios D. Anthropometric measurements, dietary intake and biochemical data of South African lacto-ovovegetarians. *S Afr Med J.* 1986;69:733–738.

16. Levin N, Rattan J, Gilat T. Mineral intake and blood levels in vegetarians. *Israel J Med Sci.* 1986;22:105–108.

17. Sanders TAB, Key TJA. Blood pressure, plasma renin activity and aldosterone concentrations in vegans and omnivores. *Human Nutr: Appl Nutr.* 1987;41A:204–211.

18. Tylavsky FA, Anderson JJB. Dietary factors in bone health of elderly lactoovovegetarian and omnivorous women. *Am J Clin Nutr.* 1988;48:842–849.

19. Rouse IL, Armstrong BK, Beilin LJ. The relationship of blood pressure to diet and lifestyle in two religious populations. *J Hypertension.* 1983;65–71.

20. Worthington-Roberts BS, Breskin MW, Monsen ER. Iron status of premenopausal women in a university community and its relationship to habitual dietary sources of protein. *Am J Clin Nutr.* 1988;47:275–279.

21. Kelsay JL, Frazier CW, Prather E, Canary JJ, Clark WM, Powell AS. Impact of variation in carbohydrate intake on mineral utilization by vegetarians. *Am J Clin Nutr.* 1988;48:875–879.

22. Nieman DC, Underwood BC, Sherman KM, Arabatzis K, Barbosa JC, Johnson M, Shultz TD. Dietary status of Seventh-day Adventist vegetarian and nonvegetarian elderly women. *J Am Diet Assoc.* 1989;89:1763–1769.

23. Marsh AG, Christensen DK, Sanchez TV, Mickelsen O, Chaffee FL. Nutrient similarities and differences of older lacto-ovo-vegetarian and omnivorous women. *Nutr Rep Int.* 1989;39:19–24.

24. Hunt I-F, Murphy NJ, Henderson C, Clark VA, Jacobs RM, Johnston PK, Coulson AH. Bone mineral content in postmenopausal women: Comparison of omnivores and vegetarians. *Am J Clin Nutr.* 1989;50:517–523.

25. Melby CL, Goldflies DG, Hyner GC, Lyle RM. Relation between vegetarian/nonvegetarian diets and blood pressure in black and white adults. *Am J Public Health.* 1989;79:1283–1288.

26. Debski B, Finley DA, Picciano MF, Lönnerdal B, Milner J. Selenium content and glutathione peroxidase activity of milk from vegetarian and nonvegetarian women. *J Nutr.* 1989;119:215–220.

27. Brants HAM, Löwik MRH, Westenbrink S, Hulshof KFAM, Kistemaker C. Adequacy of a vegetarian diet at old age (Dutch Nutrition Surveillance System). *J Am College Nutr.* 1990;9:292–302.

28. Reddy S, Sanders TAB. Haematological studies on premenopausal Indian and Caucasian vegetarians compared with Caucasian omnivores. *Br J Nutr.* 1990;64:331–338.

29. Lloyd T, Schaeffer JM, Walker MA, Demers L. Urinary hormonal concentrations and spinal bone densities of premenopausal vegetarian and nonvegetarian women. *Am J Clin Nutr.* 1991;54:1005–1010.

30. Pedersen AB, Bartholomew MJ, Dolence LA, Aljadir LP, Netteburg KL, Lloyd T. Menstrual differences due to vegetarian and nonvegetarian diets. *Am J Clin Nutr.* 1991;53:879–885.

31. Tesar R, Notelovitz M, Shim E, Kauwell G, Brown J. Axial and peripheral bone density and nutrient intakes of postmenopausal vegetarian and omnivorous women. *Am J Clin Nutr.* 1992;56:699–704.

32. Draper A, Lewis J, Malhotra N, Wheeler E. The energy and nutrient intakes of different types of vegetarian: A case for supplements. *Br J Nutr.* 1993;69:3–19.

33. Alexander D, Ball MJ, Mann J. Nutrient intake and haematological status of vegetarians and age-sex matched omnivores. *Eur J Clin Nutr.* 1994;48:538–546. *Note:* Iron values for the individual male and female groups are subsets of the combined male/female groups.

34. Janelle KC, Barr SI. Nutrient intakes and eating behavior scores of vegetarian and nonvegetarian women. *JADA.* 1995;95:180–189.

APPENDIX J

Water Soluble Vitamin Intake of Vegetarians and Nonvegetarians

(Ref)/ year	Group/ Gender (N)	Country	Age	Kcal	Vit. C (mg)	Thiamin (mg)	Riboflavin (mg)	Niacin (mg)	Vit. B_6 (mg)	Folate (µg)	Pantothenic acid (mg)	Vit. B_{12} (µg)
(1) 1954	LOV M (15)	United States	55	3020	250	2.3	2.8	19.0				
	VEG M (14)		51	3260	355	2.7	1.8	26.0				
	NV M (15)		57	3720	185	2.0	2.8	23.0				
	LOV F (15)		58	2450	220	1.7	2.6	13.0				
	VEG F (11)		49	2400	280	2.1	1.5	16.0				
	NV F (15)		57	2690	185	1.5	2.1	18.0				
(2) 1963	LOV F (26)	Australia	18–40	1980	107	1.0	1.3	11.0				
	NV F (25)		18–40	2115	72	0.8	1.6	11.4				
(3) 1978	LOV F (42)	United States	57	1600	141	1.2	1.7					
	NV F (36)		59	1579	119	0.9	1.6					
(4) 1980	LOV M/F (57)	United States	18–40	2270	196	3.7	3.9	15.9				
	LV M/F (14)		18–40	1830	226	5.2	4.6	13.1				
	VEG M/F (8)		18–40	1665	584	1.8	1.5	13.9				
	NV F (41)		18–40	2072	151	2.3	2.9	15.8				
(5) 1980	LOV M (15)	United States	28	2624	217	2.7	2.3	22.0				
	NV M (25)		27	2684	121	1.4	2.2	24.0				
	LOV F (13)		26	2174	194	2.3	2.0	17.0				
	NV F (24)		26	1859	110	1.0	1.5	19.0				
(6) 1981	LOV M (11)	Great Britain	28–80	2015	94							
	NV M (18)		28–80	2300	77							
	LOV F (14)		28–80	1737	76							
	NV F (28)		28–80	1656	69							
(7) 1981	LOV F (5)	United States	22	1329	135	0.9	1.2	8.6	1.8	247		2.6

(Ref)/year	Group[1]/Gender (N)	Country	Age	Kcal	Vit. C (mg)	Thiamin (mg)	Riboflavin (mg)	Niacin (mg)	Vit. B6 (mg)	Folate (µg)	Pantothenic acid (mg)	Vit. B12 (µg)
(8) 1983	LOV M (20)	United States	36	2324	182	2.0	2.0	17.6	2.0			
	NV M (17)		44	2652	141	1.6	2.4	23.9	2.0			
	LOV F (31)		31	1776	183	1.8	1.8	14.8	1.8			
	NV F (36)		36	1754	158	1.2	1.7	17.9	1.6			
(9) 1984	LOV M (25)	United States	39–65	2128	193	2.2	2.0	21.8				
	VEG M (9)		39–65	2259	313	2.4	2.0	22.4				
	NV M (25)		39–65	2335	196	3.6	3.8	33.1				
	LOV F (25)		39–65	1615	194	2.4	1.6	14.8				
	VEG F (9)		39–65	1497	131	1.2	5.1	15.0				
	NV F (25)		39–65	1821	137	1.2	1.5	18.1				
(10) 1985	LOV M/F (17)	Great Britain	34	2290	112							2.7
	VEG M/F (17)		31	2381	156							3.0[2]
	NV M/F (17)		35	2313	117							9.2
(11) 1986	LOV M (14)	Canada	28	2401	171	2.0	2.0	27.9[3]		327		
	NV M (14)		21	2809	158	1.9	2.9	38.4[3]		252		
	LOV F (22)		26	1760	166	1.7	2.0	25.3[3]		273		
	NV F (18)		22	2097	143	1.9	2.6	30.7[3]		215		
(12) 1986	LOV M (14)	South Africa	18–40	2717	212	1.8	2.0	20.3	1.6	342		2.2
	NV M (10)		18–40	3167	115	1.5	1.9	35.4	1.9	251		7.0
	LOV F (19)		18–40	1916	178	1.2	1.4	12.1	1.1	214		1.7
	NV F (12)		18–40	1890	85	1.0	1.4	15.5	1.2	177		3.4
(13) 1987	VEG M (11)	Great Britain	32	2643	161	2.1	2.1	28.0		304		1.2
	NV M (11)		31	2381	168	1.5	2.3	26.0		233		6.5
	VEG F (11)		28	1881	115	1.6	1.7	21.0		288		1.1
	NV F (11)		24	1833	139	1.3	1.5	18.0		201		2.5
(14) 1988	LOV F (88)	Untied States	73	1533	184	1.0	1.3	11.3				
	NV F (278)		79	1633	157	0.9	1.5	13.8				

(Ref)/ year	Group/ Gender (N)	Country	Age	Kcal	Vit. C (mg)	Thiamin (mg)	Riboflavin (mg)	Niacin (mg)	Vit. B6 (mg)	Folate (μg)	Pantothenic acid (mg)	Vit. B12 (μg)
(15) 1988	LOV F (20)	United States	29	1814	169							
	NV F (16)		31	1788	144							
(16) 1989	LOV M (11)	France	37	2100	133	2.7	2.0		1.5			
	NV M (33)		40	2600	89	1.3	1.7		1.4			
	LOV F (26)		26	1700	142	2.5	1.8		1.3			
	NV F (36)		36	1800	91	1.2	1.6		1.1			
(17) 1989	LOV F (23)	United States	72	1452	155	1.4	1.5	14.3	1.6	273	3.6	2.3
	NV F (14)		71	1363	114	1.1	1.4	14.2	1.3	215	2.8	2.6
(18) 1990	LOV M (18)	Netherlands	65–97	1960	136	1.3	1.9		1.3			
	NV M[4]		65+	2412	94	1.1	1.7		1.4			
	LOV F (26)		65–97	1667	149	1.1	1.7		1.1			
	NV F[4]		65+	1879	101	0.9	1.5		1.2			
(19) 1990	LOV F (22)	Great Britain	30	1826	114					262		1.5
	NV F (18)		34	1779	69					170		5.5
(20) 1991	LOV F (23)	United States	35	1939	200	1.7		17.9	1.7	355	3.6	2.1
	NV F (36)		36	1835	134	1.4		20.1	1.5	235	3.5	4.9
(21) 1991	LOV F (34)	United States	36	1819	316				2.0	374		
	NV F (41)		29	1700	184				2.0	385		
(22) 1991	LOV MF (79)	United States	18–30	2800	264							
	NV MF (4821)		18–30	2980	197							
(23) 1992	LOV F (28)	United States	63	1652	143	1.4	1.7	14.4	1.8	255	3.6	2.5
	NV F (28)		63	1657	118	1.4	1.9	20.0	1.6	249	3.5	4.2
(24) 1992	VEG M (10)	Great Britain	32	2548	13 6							
	NV M (10)		33	2524	84							
	VEG F (10)		32	2214	151							
	NV F (10)		32	1976	82							

(Ref)/ year	Group/ Gender (N)	Country	Age	Kcal	Vit. C (mg)	Thiamin (mg)	Riboflavin (mg)	Niacin (mg)	Vit. B6 (mg)	Folate (µg)	Pantothenic acid (mg)	Vit. B12 (µg)
(25) 1993	LOV M (16)[5]	Great Britain	21–40	2238	119	1.9	2.1	33.0	2.2	366		2.7
	VEG M (18)[5]	Britain	21–40	2190	172	2.1	1.4	33.2	3.2	448		0.7
	NV M (386)[4]		21–40	2452	97	2.5	2.7	43.0	3.0	321		7.4
	LOV F (36)[5]		21–40	1826	131	1.6	1.7	27.7	2.3	354		1.8
	VEG F (20)[5]		21–40	1750	124	1.6	1.0	24.5	3.3	298		0.6
	NV F (377)[4]		21–40	1733	96	1.6	2.0	33.0	3.3	235		6.0
(26) 1994	LOV MF (50)	New Zealand	27	2272	145					455		1.9
	VEG F (5)		27	1842	155					471		0.5
	NV MF (50)		27	2608	149					343		4.2
(27) 1995	LV F (15)	Canada	26	2024	141	1.3	1.5	12.0	1.4	310	3.9	1.5
	VEG F (8)		28	1923	186	1.8	1.3	15.9	1.9	416	5.3	0.5
	NV F (22)		28	2086	116	1.6	1.7	18.7	1.6	269	5.0	3.8

Notes: [1]Abbreviations: LV, lactovegetarian; LOV, lacto-ovo vegetarian; VEG, vegan; and NV, nonvegetarian.
[2]Vegan vitamin B_{12} intake was due to the consumption of vitamin B_{12} fortified foods.
[3]Niacin as Niacin Equivalents (NE). The convention is to consider 60 mg of tryptophan as equivalent to 1 mg of niacin.
[4]Data for NV from a separate nationwide survey.
[5]Data include nutrient supplements.

REFERENCES

1. Hardinge MG, Stare FJ. Nutritional studies of vegetarians. *Am J Clin Nutr.* 1954;2:73–82.

2. Hitchcock NE, English RM. A comparison of food consumption in lacto-ovo-vegetarians and non-vegetarians. *Food Nutr Notes Rev.* 1963;20:141–146.

3. Mason RL, Kunkel ME, Ann Davis T, Beauchene RE. Nutrient intakes of vegetarian and nonvegetarian women. *Tenn Farm Home Science.* 1978;1:18–20.

4. Freeland-Graves JH, Bodzy PW, Eppright MA. Zinc status of vegetarians. *J Am Diet Assoc.* 1980;77:655–661.

5. Taber LAL, Cook RA. Dietary and anthropometric assessment of adult omnivores, fish-eaters, and lacto-ovo-vegetarians. *J Am Diet Assoc.* 1980;76:21–29.

6. Burr ML, Bates CJ, Fehily AM, Leger AS ST. Plasma cholesterol and blood pressure in vegetarians. *J Human Nutr.* 1981;35:437–441.

7. King JC, Stein JC, Doyle M. Effect of vegetarianism on the zinc status of pregnant women. *Am J Clin Nutr.* 1981;34:1049–1055.

8. Shultz TD, Leklem JE. Dietary status of Seventh-day Adventists and nonvegetarians. *J Am Diet Assoc.* 1983;27–33.

9. Calkins BM, Whittaker DJ, Nair PP, Rider AA, Turjman N. Diet, nutrition intake, and metabolism in populations at high and low risk for colon cancer. *Am J Clin Nutr.* 1984;40:896–905.

10. Davies GJ, Crowder M, Dickerson JWT. Dietary fibre intakes of individuals with different eating patterns. *Human Nutr: Appl Nutr.* 1985;39A:139–148.

11. Locong A. Nutritional status and dietary intake of a selected sample of young adult vegetarians. *Can Diet Assoc J.* 1986;47:101–106.

12. Faber M, Gouws E, Benadé AJS, Labadarios D. Anthropometric measurements, dietary intake and biochemical data of South African lacto-ovovegetarians. *S Afr Med J.* 1986;69:733–738.

13. Sanders TAB, Key TJA. Blood pressure, plasma renin activity and aldosterone concentrations in vegans and omnivores. *Human Nutr: Appl Nutr.* 1987;41A:204–211.

14. Tylavsky FA, Anderson JJB. Dietary factors in bone health of elderly lactoovovegetarian and omnivorous women. *Am J Clin Nutr.* 1988;48:842–849.

15. Worthington-Roberts BS, Breskin MW, Monsen ER. Iron status of premenopausal women in a university community and its relationship to habitual dietary sources of protein. *Am J Clin Nutr.* 1988;47:275–279.

16. Millet P, Guilland JC, Fuchs F, Klepping J. Nutrient intake and vitamin status of healthy French vegetarians and nonvegetarians. *Am J Clin Nutr.* 1989;50:718–722.

17. Nieman DC, Underwood BC, Sherman KM, et al. Dietary status of Seventh-day Adventist vegetarian and nonvegetarian elderly women. *J Am Diet Assoc.* 1989;89:1763–1769.

18. Brants HAM, Löwik MRH, Westenbrink S, Hulshof KFAM, Kistemaker C. Adequacy of a vegetarian diet at old age (Dutch Nutrition Surveillance System). *J Am College Nutr.* 1990;9:292–302.

19. Reddy S, Sanders TAB. Haematological studies on premenopausal Indian and Caucasian vegetarians compared with Caucasion omnivores. *Br J Nutr.* 1990;64:331–338.

20. Lloyd T, Schaeffer JM, Walker MA, Demers L. Urinary hormonal concentrations and spinal bone densities of premenopausal vegetarian and nonvegetarian women. *Am J Clin Nutr.* 1991;54:1005–1010.

21. Pedersen AB, Bartholomew MJ, Dolence LA, Aljadir LP, Netteburg KL, Lloyd T. Menstrual differences due to vegetarian and nonvegetarian diets. *Am J Clin Nutr.* 1991;53:879–885.

22. Slattery ML, Jacobs Jr DR, Hilner JE, et al. Meat consumption and its association with other diet and health factors in young adults: the CARDIA study. *Am J Clin Nutr.* 1991;54:930–935.

23. Tesar R, Notelovitz M, Shim E, Kauwell G, Brown J. Axial and peripheral bone density and nutrient intakes of postmenopausal vegetarian and omnivorous women. *Am J Clin Nutr.* 1992;56:699–704.

24. Sanders TAB, Roshanai F. Platelet phospholipid fatty acid composition and function in vegans compared with age- and sex-matched omnivorous controls. *Eur J Clin Nutr.* 1992;46:823–831.

25. Draper A, Lewis J, Malhotra N, Wheeler E. The energy and nutrient intake of different types of vegetarian: a case for supplements. *Br J Nutr.* 1993;69:3–19.

26. Alexander D, Ball MJ, Mann J. Nutrient intake and haematological status of vegetarians and age-sex matched omnivores. *Eur J Clin Nutr.* 1994;48:538–546.

27. Janelle KC, Barr SI. Nutrient intakes and eating behavior scores of vegetarian and nonvegetarian women. *JADA.* 1995;95:180–189.

APPENDIX K

Fat Soluble Vitamin Intake of Adult Vegetarians and Nonvegetarians

(Ref)/ year	Group[1]/ Gender (N)	Country	Age	Kcal	Vitamin A[2]	Carotene[3]	Vitamin D[4]	Vitamin E[5]	Vitamin K (µg)
(1) 1954	LOV M (15)	Untied States	55	3020	15400				
	VEG M (14)		51	3260	25570				
	NV M (15)		57	3720	14420				
	LOV F (15)		58	2450	13470				
	VEG F (11)		49	2400	19510				
	NV F (15)		57	2690	13730				
(2) 1963	LOV F (26)	Australia	18–40	1980	6800				
	NV F (25)		18–40	2115	9530				
(3) 1978	LOV F (42)	United States	57	1600	7601				
	NV F (36)		59	1579	6528				
(4) 1980	LOV M/F (57)	United States	18–40	2270	14678				
	LV M/F (14)		18–40	1830	33378				
	VEG M/F (8)		18–40	1665	19246				
	NV F (41)		18–40	2072	8069				
(5) 1980	LOV M (15)	United States	28	2624	13802				
	NV M (25)		27	2684	8189				
	LOV F (13)		26	2174	11516				
	NV F (24)		26	1859	5937				
(6) 1981	LOV F (5)	United States	22	1329	12930		92	7.4	
(7) 1983	LOV M (20)	United States	36	2324	1794				
	NV M (17)		44	2652	1806				
	LOV F (31)		31	1776	1646				
	NV F (36)		36	1754	1824				

(Ref)/ year	Group[1]/ Gender (N)	Country	Age	Kcal	Vitamin A[2]	Carotene[3]	Vitamin D[4]	Vitamin E[5]	Vitamin K (µg)
(8) 1984	LOV M (25)	United	39–65	2128	7249				
	VEG M (9)	States	39–65	2259	18115				
	NV M (25)		39–65	2335	6683				
	LOV F (25)		39–65	1615	6212				
	VEG F (9)		39–65	1497	7332				
	NV F (25)		39–65	1821	4937				
(9) 1986	LOV M (14)	Canada	28	2401	1606				
	NV M (14)		21	2809	1147				
	LOV F (22)		26	1760	994				
	NV F (18)		22	2097	1197				
(10) 1986	LOV M (14)	South	18–40	2717	10554				
	NV M (10)	Africa	18–40	3167	8009				
	NV F (19)		18–40	1916	9114				
	NV F (12)		18–40	1890	6667				
(11) 1987	VEG M (11)	Great	32	2643	204	2446		11.3	
	NV M (11)	Britain	31	2381	470	1439		6.9	
	VEG F (11)		28	1881	225	4725		12.0	
	NV F (11)		24	1833	354	3801		6.3	
(12) 1988	LOV F (88)	United	73	1533	922				
	NV F (278)	States	79	1633	875				
(13) 1989	LOV M (11)	France	37	2100	1900	8.0	1.1	14	
	NV M (33)		40	2600	1400	3.6	2.6	13	
	LOV F (26)		26	1700	1500	6.8	0.9	15	
	NV F (36)		36	1800	1400	3.9	1.8	10	
(14) 1989	LOV F (23)	United	72	1452	11081		89	6.5	
	NV F (14)	States	71	1363	7915		106	4.3	

(Ref/ year)	Group[1]/ Gender (N)	Country	Age	Kcal	Vitamin A[2]	Carotene[3]	Vitamin D[4]	Vitamin E[5]	Vitamin K (µg)
(15) 1990	LOV M (18)	Netherlands	65–97	1960	1270				
	NV M		65+	2412	1070				
	LOV F (26)		65–97	1667	1270				
	NV F		65+	1879	950				
(16) 1991	LOV F (23)	United States	35	1939	3838		104	9.0	275
	NV F (36)		36	1835	1306		127	4.1	205
(17) 1991	LOV F (34)	United States	36	1819	3760		5.3		
	NV F (41)		29	1700	2980		5.6		
(18) 1991	LOV MF (79)	United States	18–30	2800	24674				
	NV MF (4821)		18–30	2980	10549				
(19) 1992	LOV F (28)	United States	63	1652	2842				
	NV F (28)		63	1657	3015				
(20) 1992	VEG M (10)	Great Britain	32	2548				14.0	
	NV M (10)		33	2524				6.0	
	VEG F (10)		32	2214				11.0	
	NV F (10)		32	1976				5.0	
(21) 1993	LOV M (16)[6]	Great Britain	21–40	2238	538	6010	3.0	15.8	
	VEG M (18)[6]		21–40	2190	181	6710	1.9	23.1	
	NV M (386)[7]		21–40	2452	1735	2730	4.2	12.4	
	LOV F (36)[6]		21–40	1826	374	5420	2.2	16.1	
	VEG F (20)[6]		21–40	1750	172	4280	1.6	16.5	
	NV F (377)[7]		21–40	1733	1722	2530	3.3	8.7	
(22) 1993	LV MF (14)	Finland	44	2029			2.2[8]		
	VEG MF (10)		42	1927			0.3[8]		
	NV MF (12)		33	1778			4.5[8]		

(Ref)/year	Group[1]/Gender (N)	Country	Age	Kcal	Vitamin A[2]	Carotene[3]	Vitamin D[4]	Vitamin E[5]	Vitamin K (µg)
(23) 1994	LOV M/F (50)[9]	New Zealand	27	2272	5.4	5400	2.2		
	VEG F (5)		27	1842	5.2	5200	1.9		
	NV M/F (50)		27	2608	4.7	4700	3.4		

Notes: [1]Abbreviations: LV, lactovegetarian; LOV, lacto-ovo vegetarian; VEG, vegan; NV, nonvegetarian.

[2]Vitamin A as IU for references 1–6, 10, and 14. Vitamin A as RE for references 7, 9, 12, 13, 15, 16, and 19. Vitamin A as µg for references 11, 17, and 21. No information was provided for reference 18.

[3]Carotene as ug carotene for references 11, 21, and 23, and as ug β-carotene for reference 18.

[4]Vitamin D as µg for references 13, 16, 17, 21, 22, and as IU for references 6 and 13.

[5]Vitamin E as mg for references 6, 11, 16, and 20 as mg RRR-α-tocopherol (represented as the sum of the weight of RRR-α-tocopherol plus the weights of other tocopherols or tocotrienols after their equivalency as RRR-α-tocopherol), reference 14 as mg of RRR-α-tocopherol.

[6]Data includes use of supplements.

[7]Values for NV were from a separate nationwide survey.

[8]Vitamin D values were estimated from figure in reference.

[9]Values of LOV include data for the VEG that were also listed separately.

REFERENCES

1. Hardinge MG, Stare FJ. Nutritional studies of vegetarians. *Am J Clin Nutr.* 1954;2:73–82.

2. Hitchcock NE, English RM. A comparison of food consumption in lacto-ovo-vegetarians and non-vegetarians. *Food Nutr Notes Rev.* 1963;20:141–146.

3. Mason RL, Kunkel ME, Ann Davis T, Beauchene RE. Nutrient intakes of vegetarians and nonvegetarian women. *Tenn Farm Home Science.* 1978;1:18–20.

4. Freeland-Graves JH, Bodzy PW, Eppright MA. Zinc status of vegetarians. *J Am Diet Assoc.* 1980;77:655–661.

5. Taber LAL, Cook RA. Dietary and anthropometric assessment of adult omnivores, fish-eaters, and lacto-ovo-vegetarians. *J Am Diet Assoc.* 1980;76:21–29.

6. King JC, Stein T, Doyle M. Effect of vegetarianism on the zinc status of pregnant women. *Am J Clin Nutr.* 1981;34:1049–1055.

7. Shultz TD, Leklem JE. Dietary status of Seventh-Day Adventists and nonvegetarians. *J Am Diet Assoc.* 1983;27–33.

8. Calkins BM, Whittaker DJ, Nair PP, Rider AA, Turjman N. Diet, nutrition intake, and metabolism in populations at high and low risk for colon cancer. *Am J Clin Nutr.* 1984;40:896–905.

9. Locong A. Nutritional status and dietary intake of a selected sample of young adult vegetarians. *Can Diet Assoc J.* 1987;47:101–106.

10. Faber M, Gouws E, Benadé AJS, Labadarios D. Anthropometric measurements, dietary intake and biochemical data of South African lacto-ovovegetarians. *S Afr Med J.* 1986;69:733–738.

11. Sanders TAB, Key TJA. Blood pressure, plasma renin activity and aldosterone concentrations in vegans and omnivores. *Human Nutr: Appl Nutr.* 1987;41A:204–211.

12. Tylavsky FA, Anderson JJB. Dietary factors in bone health of elderly lactoovovegetarian and omnivorous women. *Am J Clin Nutr.* 1988;48:842–849.

13. Millet P, Guilland JC, Fuchs F, Klepping J. Nutrient intake and vitamin status of healthy French vegetarians and nonvegetarians. *Am J Clin Nutr.* 1989;50:718–722.

14. Nieman DC, Underwood BC, Sherman KM, et al. Dietary status of Seventh-Day Adventist vegetarian and nonvegetarian elderly women. *J Am Diet Assoc.* 1989;89:1763–1769.

15. Brants HAM, Löwik MRH, Westenbrink S, Hulshof KFAM, Kistemaker C. Adequacy of a vegetarian diet at old age (Dutch Nutrition Surveillance System). *J Am College Nutr.* 1990;9:292–302.

16. Lloyd T, Schaeffer JM, Walker MA, Demers L. Urinary hormonal concentrations and spinal bone densities of premenopausal vegetarian and nonvegetarian women. *Am J Clin Nutr.* 1991;54:1005–1010.

17. Pedersen AB, Bartholomew MJ, Dolence LA, Aljadir LP, Netteburg KL, Lloyd T. Menstrual differences due to vegetarian and nonvegetarian diets. *Am J Clin Nutr.* 1991;53:879–885.

18. Slattery ML, Jacobs Jr DR, Hilner JE, Caan BJ, Van Horn L, Bragg C, Manolio TA, Kushi LH, Liu K. Meat consumption and its association with other diet and health factors in young adults: The CARDIA study. *Am J Clin Nutr.* 1991;54:930–935.

19. Tesar R, Notelovitz M, Shim E, Kauwell G, Brown J. Axial and peripheral bone density and nutrient intakes of postmenopausal vegetarian and omnivorous women. *Am J Clin Nutr.* 1992;56:699–704.

20. Sanders TAB, Roshanai F. Platelet phospholipid fatty acid composition and function in vegans compared with age- and sex-matched omnivorous controls. *Eur J Clin Nutr.* 1992;46:823–831.

21. Draper A, Lewis J, Malhotra N, Wheeler E. The energy and nutrient intakes of different types of vegetarian: a case for supplements. *Br J Nutr.* 1993;69:3–19.

22. Lamberg-Allardt C, Kärkkäinen M, Seppänen R, Biström H. Low serum 25-hydroxyvitamin D concentrations and secondary hyperparathyroidism in middle-aged white strict vegetarians. *Am J Clin Nutr.* 1993;58:684–689.

23. Alexander D, Ball MJ, Mann J. Nutrient intake and haematological status of vegetarians and age-sex matched omnivores. *Eur J Clin Nutr.* 1994;48:538–546.

APPENDIX L

Fiber, Cholesterol, and Macronutrient Intakes of Vegetarian and Nonvegetarian School-Aged Children and Teenagers

(Ref)/ year	Group[1]/ Gender (N)	Country	Age (years)	SDA/ NSDA[2]	Kcal[3]	Protein[3] % Kcal	Fat[3] % Kcal	CHO[3] % Kcal	SF (g)	PUFA or LA (g)	PUFA: SF[4]	Cholesterol (mg)	Fiber[5]
(1) 1954	LOV-F (15)	United States	14.0	NSDA	3030	13.2			39.3	13.6	0.35	408	12.9
	NV-F (15)		14.0		4100	14.7			75.4	18.5	0.25	829	10.6
	LOV-M (15)		15.5		4450	12.7			56.4	19.0	0.34	599	17.8
	NV-M (15)		15.5		5350	13.4			95.4	25.0	0.26	1046	12.2
(2) 1982	LOV M/F (15)[6]	Great Britain	10–16	NSDA	1900								31.1
	NV M/F (12)[6]		10–16		1898								16.2
(3) 1984	LOV-M/F (34)	United States	15–17	SDA	1947	15.4	35.7	48.9	21.1	18.3	0.87	192	5.1
	NV M/F[7]		13–15	NSDA	2302	13.9	37.9	45.7	41.0	14.0	0.34	295	
(4) 1989	LOV-F (9)	United States	11.4	SDA	1650	13.7	31.5	57.6				183	4.5
	NV-F (10)		11.1	NSDA	2106	14.8	38.5	48.6				273	4.0
	LOV-M (8)		11.8	SDA	2316	11.6	27.6	63.4				188	5.0
	NV-M (12)		11.3	NSDA	2074	16.0	35.6	49.8				278	4.0
(5) 1992	LOV-F (32)	United States	16.2	SDA	1895	12.5	33.3				0.65	302	3.2
	NV-F (35)		16.7	NSDA	1742	14.9	39.3				0.43	204	2.2
(6) 1992	VEG M/F (18)	Great Britain	9.5	NSDA	1,720	12.4	31.5	59.2	9.2	16.8	1.83		37.5
	NV M/F (194)[8]		7–12	NSDA	1,700	12.3	37.0	54.0					15.6
(7) 1995	LOV-F (78)	Canada	18	NSDA	1663	12.3							14.0
	NV-F (29)		18	NSDA	1688	14.5							10.0

Notes: [1]Abbreviations: LOV, lacto-ovo vegetarian; VEG, vegan; and NV, nonvegetarian; SDA, Seventh-day Adventist; NSDA, non Seventh-day Adventist; CHO, carbohydrate; SF, saturated fat; PUFA, polyunsaturated fat; and LA, linoleic acid.

[2]SDA indicates the vegetarians were specifically identified as Seventh-day Adventists whereas NSDA indicates the vegetarians were not exclusively SDAs although some SDAs may have been included in the vegetarian group.

[3]When energy intake was listed as kilojoules, a factor of 4.2 was used to convert kilojoules into kilocalories. Values for protein, fat, and carbohydrate are the percentage of calories contributed by each nutrient. The percentage of calories contributed by protein, fat, and carbohydrate was determined by multiplying the

number of grams consumed per day, by 4, 9, and 4 calories per gram, respectively, and then dividing the calories provided by each macronutrient by the total number of calories listed in the reference. In some cases, this led to differences between the calculated percentage of calories contributed by each nutrient and the percentage listed in the reference and often resulted in the total percent not equalling 100. In cases where only the percentage of calories for each nutrient was listed and not grams, those percentages were used.

[4]PUFA (polyunsaturated fat):Sat fat ratios represent values as listed in the reference, or were determined by dividing the number of grams of PUFA or LA (linoleic acid) by the number of grams of saturated fat.

[5]Values for fiber are listed as either grams of dietary fiber (reference 2 and 6), crude fiber (references 1, 3-5) or nonstarch polysaccharide (reference 7). Typically, one gram of crude fiber represents between 3 and 4 grams of dietary fiber.

[6] The entire study initially consisted of 12 males and 22 females. Each nonvegetarian was matched for age, sex, race, and socioeconomic to a vegetarian.

[7]Data for nonvegetarians are from a separate study of adolescents residing in Cincinnati, Ohio.

[8]Data for nonvegetarians are from a separate survey of British children presented in the reference.

REFERENCES

1. Hardinge MG, Stare FJ. Nutritional studies of vegetarians. 1. Nutritional, physical, and laboratory studies. *J Clin Nutr*. 1954;2:73–82.

2. Treuherz J. Possible inter-relationship between zinc and dietary fibre in a group of lacto-ovo vegetarian adolescents. *J Plant Foods*. 1982;4:89–95.

3. Cooper R, Allen A, Goldberg R, et al. Seventh-day Adventist adolescents - life-style patterns and cardiovascular risk factors. *West J Med*. 1984;140:471–477.

4. Tayter M, Stanek KL. Anthropometric and dietary assessment of omnivore and lacto-ovo-vegetarian children. *J Am Diet Assoc*. 1989;89:1861–1863.

5. Persky VW, Chatterton RT, Van Horn LV, Grant MD, Langenberg P, Marvin J. Hormone levels in vegetarian and nonvegetarian teenage girls: potential implications for breast cancer risk. *Cancer Res*. 1992;50:578–583.

6. Sanders TAB, Manning J. The growth and development of vegan children. *J Human Nutr Diet*. 1992;5:11–21.

7. Donovan UM, Gibson RS. Iron and zinc status of young women aged 14 to 19 years consuming vegetarian and omnivorous diets. *J Am Coll Nutr*. 1995;14:463–472.

APPENDIX M

Water Soluble Vitamin Intake of Vegetarian and Nonvegetarian School-Aged Children and Teenagers

(Ref)/ year	Group[1]/ Gender (N)	Country	Age	Kcal[2]	Vit. C (mg)	Thiamin (mg)	Riboflavin (mg)	Niacin (mg)	Vit. B6 (mg)	Folate (µg)	Biotin (µg)	Vit. B12 (µg)
(1) 1954	LOV-F (15)	United States	14.0	3030	185	1.7	2.6	13.0				
	NV-F (15)		14.0	4100	210	1.5	2.1	18.0				
	LOV-M (15)		15.5	4450	210	2.3	2.8	19.0				
	NV-M (15)		15.5	5350	185	2.0	2.8	23.0				
(2) 1984	LOV-M/F (34)	United States	15–17	1947	126	1.4	2.1	19.0				
(3) 1989	LOV-F (9)	United States	11.4	1650	76	1.1	1.7	9.2				
	NV-F (10)		11.1	2106	55	1.3	1.8	17.5				
	LOV-M (8)		11.8	2316	125	1.5	3.1	13.2				
	NV-M (12)		11.3	2074	92	1.5	2.7	18.8				
(4) 1992	LOV-F (32)	United States	16.2	1895	132	1.6	2.1	13.8				
	NV-F (35)		16.7	1742	105	1.2	1.6	15.9				
(5) 1992	VEG-M/F (18)	Great Britain	9.5	1720	93	1.7	1.7	24.1	1.4	251	18.7	2.2
	NV M/F (194)[3]		7–12	1700	65	1.1	1.4	24.0	1.1	131	13.4	2.8
(6) 1995	LOV-F (78)	Canada	18	1663	119							
	NV-F (29)		18	1688	85							

Notes: [1]Abbreviations: LOV, lacto-ovo vegetarian; VEG, vegan; and NV, nonvegetarian.
[2]When energy intake was listed as kilojoules, a factor of 4.2 was used to convert kilojoules into kilocalories.
[3]Values for NV are from a separate survey of British children presented in the reference (niacin N.E.).

REFERENCES

1. Hardinge MG, Stare FJ. Nutritional studies of vegetarians. 1. Nutritional, physical, and laboratory studies. *J Clin Nutr*. 1954;2:73–82.

2. Cooper R, Allen A, Goldberg R, Trevisan M, Van Horn L, Liu K, Steinhauer M, Rubenstein A, Stamler J. Seventh-day Adventist adolescents - life-style patterns and cardiovascular risk factors. *West J Med*. 1984;140:471–477.

3. Tayter M, Stanek KL. Anthropometric and dietary assessment of omnivore and lacto-ovo-vegetarian children. *J Am Diet Assoc*. 1989;89:1861–1863.

4. Persky VW, Chatterton RT, Van Horn LV, Grant MD, Langenberg P, Marvin J. Hormone levels in vegetarian and nonvegetarian teenage girls: potential implications for breast cancer risk. *Cancer Res*. 1992;50:578–583.

5. Sanders TAB, Manning J. The growth and development of vegan children. *J Human Nutr Diet*. 1992;5:11–21.

6. Donovan UM, Gibson RS. Iron and zinc status of young women aged 14 to 19 years consuming vegetarian and omnivorous diets. *J Am Coll Nutr*. 1995;14:463–472.

APPENDIX N

Fat Soluble Vitamin Intake of Vegetarian and Nonvegetarian School-Aged Children and Teenagers

(Ref)/year	Group[1]/Gender (N)	Country	Age	Kcal	Vitamin A[2]	Vitamin D (µg)	Vitamin E[7] (mg)
(1) 1954	LOV-F (15)	United States	14.0	3030	16380		
	NV-F (15)		14.0	4100	16820		
	LOV-M (15)		15.5	4450	17920		
	NV-M (15)		15.5	5350	17230		
(2) 1984	LOV-M/F (34)	United States	15–17	1947	1421		
(3) 1989	LOV-F (9)	United States	11.4	1650	3724		
	NV-F (10)		11.1	2106	7082		
	LOV-M (8)		11.8	2316	8078		
	NV-M (12)		11.3	2074	5544		
(4) 1992	LOV-F (32)	United States	16.2	1895	4394		
	NV-F (35)		16.7	1742	3922		
(5) 1992	VEG-M/F (18)	Great Britain	9.5	1720	939	1.9	7.6
	NV M/F (194)		7–12	1700	629	1.5	4.3

Notes: [1]Abbreviations: LOV, lacto ovo-vegetarian, VEG, vegan, and NV, nonvegetarian.
[2]Vitamin A as IU (includes carotene) for reference 1, vitamin A as mg R.E. for references 2 and 5, and for references 3 and 4, vitamin A as IU.

REFERENCES

1. Hardinge MG, Stare FJ. Nutritional studies of vegetarians. 1. Nutritional, physical, and laboratory studies. *J Clin Nutr*. 1954;2:73–82.

2. Cooper R, Allen A, Goldberg R, Trevisan M, Van Horn L, Liu K, Steinhauer M, Rubenstein A, Stamler J. Seventh-day Adventist adolescents - life-style patterns and cardiovascular risk factors. *West J Med*. 1984;140:471–477.

3. Tayter M, Stanek KL. Anthropometric and dietary assessment of omnivore and lacto-ovo-vegetarian children. *J Am Diet Assoc*. 1989;89:1861–1863.

4. Persky VW, Chatterton RT, Van Horn LV, Grant MD, Langenberg P, Marvin J. Hormone levels in vegetarian and nonvegetarian teenage girls: potential implications for breast cancer risk. *Cancer Res*. 1992;50:578–583.

5. Sanders TAB, Manning J. The growth and development of vegan children. *J Human Nutr Diet*. 1992;5:11–21.

APPENDIX O

Mineral Intake of Vegetarians and Nonvegetarian School-Aged Children and Teenagers

(Ref)/year	Group[1]/Gender (N)	Country	Age	Kcal	Calcium (mg)	Iron (mg)	Zinc (mg)	Copper (mg)	Phosphorus (mg)	Sodium (mg)	Potassium (mg)
(1) 1954	LOV-F (15)	United States	14.0	3030	1700	18.0			2000		
	NV-F (15)		14.0	4100	2200	23.0			2800		
	LOV-M (15)		15.5	4450	2600	25.0			3100		
	NV-M (15)		15.5	5350	2400	28.0			3300		
(2) 1982	LOV M/F (15)[2]	Great Britain	10–15	1900			9.3				
	NV M/F (12)		10–16	1898			7.6				
(3) 1984	LOV-MF (34)	United States	15–17	1947	998	12.4			1263	2400	2800
(4) 1989	LOV-F (9)	United States	11.4	1650	1041	10.7					
	NV-F (10)		11.1	2106	1028	13.0					
	LOV-M (8)		11.8	2316	1399	17.0					
	NV-M (12)		11.3	2074	1163	13.0					
(5) 1992	LOV-F (32)	United States	16.2	1895	881	11.4					
	NV-F (35)		16.7	1742	700	9.5					
(6) 1992	VEG-MF (18)	Great Britain	9.5	1720	464	21.7	7.4	1.7			
	NV MF (194)[3]		7–12	1700	680	9.7	6.6	1.6			
(7) 1995	LOV-F (78)	Canada	17.7	1663	707	11.2	6.6				
	NV-F (29)		18.2	1688	771	11.3	7.9				

Notes: [1]Abbreviations: LOV, lacto-ovo vegetarian, VEG, vegan and NV, nonvegetarian.
[2]Initially, study consisted of 12 males and 22 females. LOV were matched for age, sex, race and socioeconomic status to NV.
[3]Data for NV are from a separate survey of British children presented in the reference.

REFERENCES

1. Hardinge MG, Stare FJ. Nutritional studies of vegetarians. 1. Nutritional, physical, and laboratory studies. *J Clin Nutr.* 1954;2:73–82.

2. Treuherz J. Possible inter-relationship between zinc and dietary fibre in a group of lacto-ovo vegetarian adolescents. *J Plant Foods.* 1982;4:89–93.

3. Cooper R, Allen A, Goldberg R, Trevisan M, Van Horn L, Liu K, Steinhauer M, Rubenstein A, Stamler J. Seventh-day Adventist adolescents - life-style patterns and cardiovascular risk factors. *West J Med.* 1984;140:471–477.

4. Tayter M, Stanek KL. Anthropometric and dietary assessment of omnivore and lacto-ovo-vegetarian children. *J Am Diet Assoc.* 1989;89:1861–1863.

5. Persky VW, Chatterton RT, Van Horn LV, Grant MD, Langenberg P, Marvin J. Hormone levels in vegetarian and nonvegetarian teenage girls: potential implications for breast cancer risk. *Cancer Res.* 1992;50:578–583.

6. Sanders TAB, Manning J. The growth and development of vegan children. *J Human Nutr Diet.* 1992;5:11–21.

7. Donovan UM, Gibson RS. Iron and zinc status of young women aged 14 to 19 years consuming vegetarian and omnivorous diets. *J Am Coll Nutr.* 1995;14:463–472.

APPENDIX P

Fiber, Cholesterol, and Macronutrient Intakes of Elderly Vegetarians and Nonvegetarians

(Ref)/ year	Group[1]/ Gender (N)	Country	Age (years)	SDA/ NSDA[2]	Kcal[3]	Protein[4] % Kcal	Fat[4] % Kcal	CHO[4] % Kcal	SF (g)	PUFA or LA (g)	PUFA: SF[5]	Cholesterol (mg)	Fiber[6]
(1) 1983	LOV F (36)	Canada	69	SDA	1615	14.5							33.2
	NV F (30)		60	NSDA	1727	15.6							20.2
(2) 1988	LOV F (88)	United States	73	SDA	1533	14.2	32.9	56.4				167	5.6
	NV F (278)		79	NSDA	1633	17.1	48.5	46.1				305	4.2
(3) 1989	LOV F (144)	United States	67	SDA	1474	14.1	30.8	58.6	15.0			155	20.0
	NV F (146)		66	NSDA	1563	16.2	34.9	49.1	20.6			243	16.0
(4) 1989	LOV F (10)	United States	67	NI	1612	13.9	36.0				0.75	194	5.2
	NV F (10)		65		1641	16.6	42.0				0.48	294	4.7
(5) 1990	LOV F (23)	United States	72	SDA	1452	12.9	31.7	60.0	12.2	9.2	0.85	89	21.5
	NV F (14)		71	SDA	1363	16.2	35.9	50.2	14.9	7.9	0.51	183	13.0
(6) 1990	LOV F (12)	United States	76	SDA	1425	13.2	31.6	60.6	10.0	7.0		72	24.0
	NV F (12)		72	SDA	1334	16.2	36.4	49.8	17.0	7.0		181	13.0
(7) 1990	LOV M (18)	Netherlands	83	NSDA	1960	12.2	37.2	50.8	15.0	8.5	0.57	200	33.7
	NV M[7]		Elderly		2412	13.6	40.8	41.8	17.3	6.8	0.39	356	27.4
	LOV F (26)		81		1667	13.1	37.3	49.8	15.8	8.3	0.53	216	28.7
	NV F[7]		Elderly		1879	14.9	40.1	43.2	17.2	6.5	0.38	294	23.7
(8) 1990	LOV M (15)	Netherlands	82	NSDA	2014	11.7	39.3	49.5					33.0
	NV M (225)		72		2414	13.6	41.0	41.6					27.0
	LOV F (17)		82		1681	12.8	39.1	48.1					28.0
	NV F (216)		72		1874	14.9	40.3	42.7					23.0
(9) 1992	LOV F (28)	United States	63	SDA/NSDA	1652	15.2	30.5	58.7	16.5	10.1		98	10.3
	NV F (28)		63	SDA/NSDA	1657	18.5	33.6	48.1	19.1	10.9		214	7.6

(Ref)/ year	Group[1]/ Gender (N)	Country	Age (years)	SDA/ NSDA[2]	Kcal[3]	Protein[4] % Kcal	Fat[4] % Kcal	CHO[4] % Kcal	SF (g)	PUFA or LA (g)	PUFA: SF[5]	Cholesterol (mg)	Fiber[6]
(10) 1993	B-LOV M (23)	United States	69	SDA	1900	14.0	30.8	59.8	13.5	15.0		84	
	B-NV M (29)		65	SDA	2487	14.5	37.1	52.3	25.5	24.7		303	
	W-LOV M (83)		67	SDA	2336	13.6	30.8	61.1	17.8	19.4		137	
	W-NV M (43)		65	SDA	2078	14.1	33.8	56.8	20.1	18.3		183	

Notes: [1]Abbreviations: LV, lactovegetarian; LOV, lacto-ovo vegetarian; VEG, vegan; and NV, nonvegetarian; SDA, Seventh-day Adventist; NSDA, non Seventh-day Adventist; NI, not indicated; CHO, carbohydrate; SF, saturated fat; PUFA, polyunsaturated fat; LA, linoleic acid; B, Black; and W, white.

[2]SDA indicates the vegetarians were specifically identified as Seventh-day Adventists whereas NSDA indicates the vegetarians were not exclusively SDAs although some SDAs may have been included in the vegetarian group. NI indicates the process by which subjects were recruited for the study was not indicated or the extent to which SDAs comprised the vegetarian groups was not possible to determine by the information provided.

[3]When energy intake was listed as kilojoules, a factor of 4.2 was used to convert kilojoules into kilocalories.

[4]Values for protein, fat and carbohydrate are the percentage of calories contributed by each nutrient. The percentage of calories contributed by protein, fat, and carbohydrate was determined by multiplying the number of grams consumed per day, by 4, 9, and 4 calories per gram, respectively, and then dividing the calories provided by each macronutrient by the total number of calories listed in the reference. In some cases, this led to differences between the calculated percentage of calories contributed by each nutrient and the percentage listed in the reference and often resulted in the total percent not equalling 100. In cases where only the percentage of calories for each nutrient was listed and not grams, those percentages were used.

[5]PUFA:Sat fat ratios represent values as listed in the reference, or were determined by dividing the number of grams of PUFA or linoleic acid by the number of grams of saturated fat.

[6]Values for fiber are listed as either dietary fiber (g) or crude fiber (g) (references 2 and 4). Typically, one gram of crude fiber represents between 3 and 4 grams of dietary fiber.

[7]Data for NV from a separate nationwide survey of elderly individuals.

REFERENCES

1. Gibson RS, Anderson BM, Sabry JH. The trace metal status of a group of post-menopausal vegetarians. *J Am Diet Assoc.* 1983;82:246–250.

2. Tylavsky FA, Anderson JJB. Dietary factors in bone health of elderly lactoovovegetarian and omnivorous women. *Am J Clin Nutr.* 1988;48:842–849.

3. Hunt I-F, Murphy NJ, Henderson C, Clark VA, Jacobs RM, Johnston PK, Coulson AH. Bone mineral content in postmenopausal women: comparison of omnivores and vegetarians. *Am J Clin Nutr.* 1989;50:517–523.

4. Marsh AG, Christensen DK, Sanchez TV, Mickelsen O, Chaffee FL. Nutrient similarities and differences of older lacto-ovo-vegetarian and omnivorous women. *Nutr Rep Int.* 1989;39:19–24.

5. Nieman DC, Underwood BC, Sherman KM, Arabatzis K, Barbosa JC, Johnson M, Shultz TD. Dietary status of Seventh-Day Adventist vegetarian and nonvegetarian elderly women. *J Am Diet Assoc.* 1989;89:1763–1769.

6. Barbosa JC, Shultz TD, Filley SJ, Nieman DC. The relationship among adiposity, diet and hormone concentrations in vegetarian and nonvegetarian postmenopausal women. *Am J Clin Nutr.* 1990;51:798–803.

7. Brants HAM, Löwik MRH, Westenbrink S, Hulshof KFAM, Kistemaker C. Adequacy of a vegetarian diet at old age (Dutch Nutrition Surveillance System). *J Am College Nutr.* 1990;9:292–302.

8. Löwik MRH, Schrijver J, van den Berg H, Hulshof KFAM, Wedel M, Ockhuizen T. Effect of dietary fiber on the vitamin B6 status among vegetarian and nonvegetarian elderly (Dutch Nutrition Surveillance System). *J Am College Nutr.* 1990;9:241–249.

9. Tesar R, Notelovitz M, Shim E, Kauwell G, Brown J. Axial and peripheral bone density and nutrient intakes of postmenopausal vegetarian and omnivorous women. *Am J Clin Nutr.* 1992;56:699–704.

10. Melby CL, Goldflies DG, Toohey ML. Blood pressure differences in older black and white long-term vegetarians and nonvegetarians. *J Am Coll Nutr.* 1993;12:262–269.

APPENDIX Q

Water Soluble Vitamin Intake of Elderly Vegetarians and Nonvegetarians

(Ref)/ year	Group[1]/ Gender (N)	Country	Age	Kcal	Vit. C (mg)	Thiamin (mg)	Riboflavin (mg)	Niacin (mg)	Vit. B6 (mg)	Folate (μg)	Pantothenic acid (mg)	Vit. B12 (μg)
(1) 1988	LOV F (88)	United States	73	1533	184	1.0	1.3	11.3				
	NV F (278)		79	1633	157	0.9	1.5	13.8				
(2) 1989	LOV F (23)	United States	72	1452	155	1.4	1.5	14.3	1.6	273	3.6	2.3
	NV F (14)		71	1363	114	1.1	1.4	14.2	1.3	215	2.8	2.6
(3) 1990	LOV F (18)	Netherlands	83	1960	136	1.3	1.9		1.3			
	NV M[2]		Elderly	2412	94	1.1	1.7		1.4			
	LOV F (26)		81	1667	149	1.1	1.7		1.1			
	NV F[2]		Elderly	1879	101	0.9	1.5		1.2			
(4) 1992	LOV F (28)	United States	63	1652	143	1.4	1.7	14.4	1.8	255	3.6	2.5
	NV F (28)		63	1657	118	1.4	1.9	20.0	1.6	249	3.5	4.2

Notes: [1]Abbreviations: LOV, lacto-ovo vegetarian and NV, nonvegetarian.
[2]Data for NV from a separate nationwide survey of elderly individuals.

REFERENCES

1. Tylavsky FA, Anderson JJB. Dietary factors in bone health of elderly lactoovovegetarian and omnivorous women. *Am J Clin Nutr.* 1988;48:842–849.

2. Nieman DC, Underwood BC, Sherman KM, et al. Dietary status of Seventh-day Adventist vegetarian and nonvegetarian elderly women. *J Am Diet Assoc.* 1989;89:1763–1769.

3. Brants HAM, Löwik MRH, Westenbrink S, Hulshof KFAM, Kistemaker C. Adequacy of a vegetarian diet at old age (Dutch Nutrition Surveillance System). *J Am College Nutr.* 1990;9:292–302.

4. Tesar R, Notelovitz M, Shim E, Kauwell G, Brown J. Axial and peripheral bone density and nutrient intakes of postmenopausal vegetarian and omnivorous women. *Am J Clin Nutr.* 1992;56:699–704.

APPENDIX R

Mineral Intake of Elderly Vegetarians and Nonvegetarians

(Ref)/ year	Group[1]/ Gender (N)	Age	Kcal	Ca (mg)	Fe (mg)	Zn (mg)	Mg (mg)	Cu (mg)	Mn (mg)	Se (µg)	Na (mg)	K (mg)	P (mg)
(1) 1983	LOV F (36)	69	1615					2.1	4.4	113			
	NV F (30)	60	1727					1.6	2.6	109			
(2) 1988	LOV F (88)	73	1533	823	10.7								
	NV F (278)	79	1633	902	10.2								
(3) 1989	LOV F (23)	72	1452	628	12.3	6.3	283	1.4	2.2		1930	2628	889
	NV F (14)	71	1363	633	11.4	6.3	226	1.0	1.3		1936	2342	892
(4) 1989	LOV F (10)	67	1612	898	12.3								1109
	NV F (10)	64	1641	712	13.3								1079
(5) 1989	LOV F (144)	67	1474	748		7.2	312	1.4					1050
	NV F (146)	66	1563	772		8.8	294	1.4					1147
(6) 1990	LOV M (18)	65–97	1960	1219	13.7	8.5							
	NV M	65+		1128	13.1	10.3							
	LOV F (26)	65–97	1667	1141	12.2	7.6							
	NV F	65+		1013	11.4	9.3							
(7) 1992	LOV F (28)	63	1652	821	13.0	7.2	318	1.4		16.9	2202	3012	1155
	NV F (28)	63	1657	863	15.5	7.9	266	1.0		17.4	2285	2687	1250

Note: [1]Abbreviations: LOV, lacto-ovo vegetarian; NV, nonvegetarian.

REFERENCES

1. Gibson RS, Anderson BM, Sabry JH. The trace metal status of a group of post-menopausal vegetarians. *J Am Diet Assoc.* 1983;82:246–250.

2. Tylavsky FA, Anderson JJB. Dietary factors in bone health of elderly lactoovovegetarian and omnivorous women. *Am J Clin Nutr.* 1988;48:842–849.

3. Nieman DC, Underwood BC, Sherman KM, Arabatzis K, Barbosa JC, Johnson M, Shultz TD. Dietary status of Seventh-Day Adventist vegetarian and nonvegetarian elderly women. *J Am Diet Assoc.* 1989;89:1763–1769.

4. Marsh AG, Christensen DK, Sanchez TV, Mickelsen O, Chaffee FL. Nutrient similarities and differences of older lacto-ovo-vegetarian and omnivorous women. *Nutr Rep Int.* 1989;39:19–24.

5. Hunt I-F, Murphy NJ, Henderson C, Clark VA, Jacobs RM, Johnston PK, Coulson AH. Bone mineral content in postmenopausal women: comparison of omnivores and vegetarians. *Am J Clin Nutr.* 1989;50:517–523.

6. Brants HAM, Löwik MRH, Westenbrink S, Hulshof KFAM, Kistemaker C. Adequacy of a vegetarian diet at old age (Dutch Nutrition Surveillance System). *J Am College Nutr.* 1990;9:292–302.

7. Tesar R, Notelovitz M, Shim E, Kauwell G, Brown J. Axial and peripheral bone density and nutrient intakes of postmenopausal vegetarian and omnivorous women. *Am J Clin Nutr.* 1992;56:699–704.

Index